Expert Praise for the PDR® Family Guide Series of Personal Health Handbooks

"Comprehensive, easy-to-understand . . . Sorts out fact from fantasy in a lucid, interesting style."
—STEPHEN BRUNTON, MD
Clinical Professor
Department of Family Medicine
University of California Irvine

"Superbly written and understandable by those we wish to help—our patients and our families."
—EDWIN C. CADMAN, MD
Ensign Professor and Chairman
Department of Internal Medicine
Yale University School of Medicine

"A must for every household where there are concerns about safe use of medications . . . An ideal way to clarify and supplement the information provided by your health care provider."
—JACK M. ROSENBERG, PharmD, PhD
Professor of Clinical Pharmacy and Pharmacology
Director, Division of Pharmacy Practice
Arnold & Marie Schwartz College of Pharmacy and Health Sciences
Long Island University

Please turn the page for more reviews. . . .

"As individuals increasingly empower themselves in a variety of areas in our society, so too are they requiring more information and input into their own medical care decisions. . . . A great resource for the patient in his or her dialogue with the physician."

—JOSEPH R. CRUSE, MD
Founding Medical Director
The Betty Ford Center

"An excellent supplement to the education that should occur during every health visit . . . Allows people to find answers when and where they need them—any time of day or night in their own home."
—BARBARA P. YAWN, MD, MS
Associate Professor of Clinical Family Medicine
and Community Health, University of
Minnesota

Published by Ballantine Books:

THE PDR® FAMILY GUIDE TO OVER-THE-COUNTER DRUGS™
THE PDR® FAMILY GUIDE ENCYCLOPEDIA OF MEDICAL CARE™
THE PDR® FAMILY GUIDE TO COMMON AILMENTS™
THE PDR® FAMILY GUIDE TO NATURAL MEDICINES AND HEALING THERAPIES™

THE PDR®
FAMILY GUIDE

TO NATURAL MEDICINES
AND HEALING THERAPIES™

BALLANTINE BOOKS • NEW YORK

A Ballantine Book
Published by the Ballantine Publishing Group
Copyright © 1999 by Medical Economics Company, Inc.

www.randomhouse.com/BB/

Library of Congress Catalog Card Number: 00-190380

ISBN 0-345-43377-7

This edition published by arrangement with Three Rivers Press, a division of Random House, Inc.

Manufactured in the United States of America

First Ballantine Edition: May 2000

10 9 8 7 6 5 4 3 2 1

Publisher's Note

may not be marketed for the diagnosis, treatment, cure, or prevention of any disease. The profiles in this book do not discuss claims made for any proprietary herbal preparation. They merely report general findings on generic botanicals and nutritional supplements.

PHYSICIANS' DESK REFERENCE®, PDR®, PDR For Ophthalmology®, Pocket PDR®, and The PDR® Family Guide to Prescription Drugs® are registered trademarks used herein under license. PDR For Nonprescription Drugs and Dietary Supplements™, PDR Companion Guide™, PDR® Medical Dictionary™, PDR® Nurse's Handbook™, PDR® Nurse's Dictionary™, The PDR® Family Guide Encyclopedia of Medical Care™, The PDR® Family Guide to Over-the-Counter Drugs™, The PDR® Family Guide to Natural Medicines and Healing Therapies™, PDR® Electronic Library™, and PDR® Drug Interactions, Side Effects, Indications, Contraindications Diskettes™ are trademarks used herein under license.

Contents

The PDR® Family Guide to Natural Medicines and Healing Therapies™

Contributors and Consultants

Editor-in-Chief: David W. Sifton
Director of New Business Development and Professional Services: Mukesh Mehta, R Ph
Design Director: Robert Hartman

Scientific Editors: Joerg Gruenwald, PhD; Thomas Brendler, BA; Christof Jaenicke, MD
Writers: Nancy K. Bannon; Brenda L. Becker; Lynn H. Buechler; Paul L. Cerrato; Steve Frandzel; Gregory A. Freeman; Kris Hallam; Ami Havens; Randi Henderson; Jayne Jacobson; Judith K. Ludwig, PhD; Barbara Klink; Lisa A. Maher; Eileen McCaffrey; Leah E. Perry; Kathleen Rodgers, R Ph; Heidi Rosvold-Brenholtz; Ronni Sandroff; David K. Silver; Theresa Waldron
Assistant Editors: Paula Benus; Gwynned L. Kelly, Ann Marevis
Editorial Production: *Director of Production:* Carrie Williams; *Manager of Production:* Kimberly H. Vivas; *Senior Production Coordinator:* Amy B. Brooks; *Senior Digital Imaging Coordinator:* Shawn W. Cahill; *Digital Imaging Coordinator:* Frank J. McElroy, III; *Electronic Publishing Designer:* Robert K. Grossman

Medical Economics Company
Senior Vice President, Directory Services: Paul Walsh
Director of Product Management: Mark A. Friedman
Associate Product Manager: Bill Shaughnessy
Director of Sales: Dikran N. Barsamian
National Sales Manager, Medical Economics Trade Sales: Bill Gaffney

Board of Medical Consultants
Chairpersons:

Richard Galbraith, MD, PhD
Director, Office of Patient Oriented
Research
College of Medicine
University of Vermont
Burlington, VT

Naomi K. Fukagawa, MD, PhD
Associate Professor of Medicine
College of Medicine
University of Vermont
Burlington, VT

How to Use This Book

The world of natural and alternative medicine is ripe with promise—and fraught with a certain amount of danger. For every genuine remedy described in this book, there's another that's completely bogus. If you make the wrong choice, you risk, at a minimum, wasting valuable time and money, and possibly damaging your health.

How can you tell a real remedy from a hyped-up fraud? It's a difficult dilemma, made no easier by the fact that doctors themselves frequently disagree. The power of suggestion alone is typically enough to provide relief, so medical scientists hold all forms of therapy—both mainstream and alternative—to extremely rigorous standards of proof. Often, there's debate over what constitutes sufficient evidence.

Many of the healing therapies in this book have yet to pass scientific tests. Some never will, and are dismissed by virtually all knowledgeable observers. Others appear to work, but remain the object of contention. Hardly any go completely unchallenged.

To cut through the controversy, this book endeavors to clearly label those claims for which there's a generally favorable consensus, and those for which there's no support. Unfortunately, very little in medicine—mainstream or otherwise—works for everyone 100 percent of the time, so there's no assurance that even an "accepted" treatment will work for you, just as some "questionable" therapies may seem to do the trick. Although we believe that the information offered here will improve your odds of success, there are no guarantees.

The book is divided into five parts.

- **Part One** provides an overview of the major types of unconventional and supportive therapy available in the United States today.
- **Part Two** offers specifics on each individual approach.
- **Part Three** does the same for

over 300 herbal and other natural medicines.

- **Part Four** provides essential information on some 50 vitamins, minerals, and other dietary elements.
- **Part Five**, the Treatment Finder, indexes the most plausible therapeutic options by the ailments they address.

Here's a closer look at what you'll find in each section.

Part One, Alternate Routes to Better Health

The four chapters in this section sketch out your options, tell where you're most likely to find them, and offer strategies for locating a qualified practitioner while avoiding charlatans and frauds.

Alternative medicine has been credited with some advantages (gentle, natural, non-toxic) that it does not invariably offer. Likewise, conventional medicine has been the focus of charges (harsh, technical, impersonal) that are often equally unjustified. The first chapter attempts to put both approaches into perspective, summarize their relative pros and cons, and abolish a few misconceptions.

Chapter 2 provides you with a closer look at the major forms of therapy available to you outside the medical mainstream. Your options range from dietary modification, physical manipulation, and the use of natural medicines to cleansing therapies, mind/body medicine, and the manipulation of various energies.

In Chapter 3, the focus shifts to the practitioners themselves. It summarizes the types of treatment that each group typically offers, the credentials you should expect a practitioner to possess, the questions you should ask, and the organizations that can give you referrals. Also included: a checklist of warning signs that you're dealing with a fraud.

Finally, Chapter 4 summarizes a few precautions that are in order no matter what course of therapy you choose to pursue:

- Get a professional diagnosis before you begin.
- Choose the approach—mainstream or complementary—that best fits the situation.
- Be quick to drop a treatment that doesn't work.
- Use even natural remedies with caution.

Part Two, Guide to Alternative and Complementary Therapies

Part Two contains profiles of over 50 forms of unconventional therapy ranging from acupressure to yoga, organized alphabetically for easy reference. Each profile includes the following standard sections:

Consider This Therapy For— This section begins with an overview of the specific ailments for which the treatment is considered most effective. If the treatment has not undergone clinical testing—as is the case with many types of bodywork—its intended benefits are given instead. To help you avoid worthless efforts and wasted time, the section ends with a brief summary of common claims that have been disproven or remain unsubstantiated.

How the Treatments Are Done—Here you'll find a description of what to expect during a typical therapy session—where the therapy is performed, how you'll be dressed, what equipment is needed, and the individual steps that you or the practitioner will be required to take. Included is the usual amount of time the treatment will last, and how frequently the treatments must be given.

What Treatment Hopes to Accomplish—This section gives the rationale for the therapy, summarizing the ways in which it is believed to confer benefit. Rationales are drawn from a wide variety of ancient and modern disciplines, ranging from oriental philosophy to current pharmaceutical research. Acupuncture, for instance, is thought to work by promoting the flow of vital energy through invisible channels throughout the body, while chelation therapy is said to cure heart disease through a chemical reaction with arterial plaque.

The section also provides you with a brief summary of each theory's scientific status. In some cases, you'll discover that a treatment has been found effective despite any evidence supporting its underlying rationale. In other instances, the opposite holds true: the

mechanism of action seems valid, but the treatment doesn't work.

Who Should Avoid This Therapy?—No matter how gentle and benign a treatment may seem, it will probably prove dangerous under certain conditions. If you have asthma, for example, aromatherapy could trigger an attack. If you have osteoporosis (brittle-bone disease), bodywork could prove risky. In this section, you'll find all such considerations spelled out.

What Side Effects May Occur?—Just as prescription drugs sometimes produce unwanted reactions, so too can many forms of alternative therapy. Although such reactions are usually mild and typically rare, you'll find whatever possibilities exist enumerated here.

How to Choose a Therapist—Many alternative therapies are offered by a variety of practitioners in settings ranging from the hospital to the YMCA. This section tells where you're most likely to find a qualified therapist, organizations that give referrals, what credentials to look for, and key questions to ask before committing to a course of therapy.

When Should Treatment Stop?—A few unscrupulous practitioners promote their treatments as "preventive medicine" or general health care tonics, and stand ready to administer them indefinitely. Unless you enjoy subsidizing an enhanced lifestyle for your therapist, you should set a measurable treatment goal and establish a deadline for reaching it.

Obviously, this isn't possible for such genuine fitness regimes as orthomolecular medicine, vegetarianism, meditation, and yoga. For other, more focused forms of treatment, however, this section provides you with model targets and deadlines. It also spells out any adverse reactions that should signal an immediate end to the treatments.

See a Conventional Doctor If ...—
Many unconventional treatments, from biofeedback to therapeutic touch, can be used in conjunction with regular medical therapy. Others, including chiro-practic and hypnotherapy, serve as replacements for standard remedies. A few, such as light therapy for seasonal affective disorder, are the only available cure. This section tells which category the treatment falls into, and lists the developments that the therapist can't be expected to handle—problems that require a return to orthodox care.

Part Three, Guide to Natural Medicines
This part of the book provides you with detailed information on over 300 natural remedies available from the garden or marketed in drugstores, health food outlets, and supermarkets as "dietary supplements." The majority are herbs and herbal extracts. A few, such as chondroitin and glucosamine, are biological agents occurring naturally in the body. The profiles are organized alphabetically by the preparation's generally accepted common name. If you know only the scientific name of the product, you can locate it through the Latin name index in Part Five of the book.

Each profile begins with the common name, Latin name, and a list of any other names by which the herb is known. The text that follows is divided into nine standard sections:

A Remedy For—First off, you'll find an itemized list of any medical problems for which the agent is generally considered effective. For approximately 150 of the herbs, this information is based on approval by the German Health Authority's "Commission E," currently the most authoritative regulatory body in the field of botanical medicines. (The U.S. Food and Drug Administration does not regulate herbal products, and proof of safety and efficacy is not required in the United States.)

For herbs that have not been considered by Commission E, itemized uses are based on positive reports in the medical literature, as documented by the respected PhytoPharm Consulting, Institute for Phytopharmaceuticals and other credible sources. Also included, as a warning, are certain common herbs that have been *disapproved* in Germany due to their toxic effects.

Following the itemized list of accepted uses, you'll usually find a summary of other, unverified applications. Included are past and present folk uses, applications in oriental medicine, and usage in homeopathy. Ailments in these categories are mentioned only as a matter of interest. There's no reason to believe that the herb will really relieve them.

What It Is; Why It Works— This section offers you a brief description of the plant and its place in history, together with an explanation of its therapeutic action.

Avoid If . . .—Like any other medication with demonstrable physical effects, herbs can be damaging or dangerous under certain medical conditions. For example, it would be unwise for someone with a weak heart to take an herb that speeds up the heartbeat. This section lists all such considerations that preclude the use of the herb.

Special Cautions—Despite their "gentle" image, herbs do have side effects. Potential problems are listed here, along with any other precautions that may be necessary while using the herb.

Possible Drug Interactions— Most herbs are mercifully free of interactions with other herbs and prescription drugs, but for a few that's not the case. The common laxative Aloe, for instance, can aggravate the side effects of water pills and increase the effect of the heart drug digitalis. If any such interactions are possible, you'll find them listed here.

Special Information If You Are Pregnant or Breastfeeding— Few herbs have been tested for safety during pregnancy, so the best policy is to avoid their use if at all possible. Some herbs are known to be dangerous during pregnancy (indeed, some have been used to provoke abortion). In such instances, you'll find a warning posted here.

How to Prepare—For many of the herbs you can pick from the garden, this section provides recipes for making tea or preparing pastes or solutions for use on the skin. Commercially available preparations are also summarized here.

Typical Dosage—This section provides you with general guidelines for use of the natural herb and whatever prepared forms may be available, such as liquid extracts, alcohol solutions, powders, and pills. Small doses are usually expressed in milligrams, larger doses in grams or milliliters. Often, larger doses are also given in teaspoonfuls, tablespoonfuls, or cups. When a special conversion factor is available, it has been used in calculating these equivalents. When no special factor is given, the following standard conversions have been employed:

5 grams = 1 teaspoonful
15 grams = 1 tablespoonful
237 milliliters = 1 cup

All amounts are approximate and apply only to general dosage forms.

Recommended doses of specific commercial preparations are likely to vary. Unless you are using the herb in its natural form, always follow the manufacturer's directions.

Overdosage—Don't forget that some of our most toxic drugs and lethal poisons are derived from plants. It's a fact that many medicinal herbs can make you sick if taken in excess—and a few can be fatal. This section gives you the symptoms of overdose, if any are known. If you suspect an overdose, don't waste any time; seek emergency treatment immediately.

Part Four, Guide to Nutritional Therapy

This part of the book offers complete how-to-use information on some 50 vitamins, minerals, and other major nutrients. The profiles are organized alphabetically by the nutrients' most familiar names, and cross-referenced by their other common names. (Thiamin, for instance, is cross-referenced under its alternate name, vitamin B_1.) Here's the information you'll find on each of the nutrients:

What It Is—This section gives you a brief overview of the nutrient's primary role in the diet, and the sources from which it is typically obtained.

What It Does—Here you'll find a description of the substance's major functions within the body.

Why You Need It—Some nutrients are used medicinally to re-lieve certain specific ailments. Others are taken as preventive measures to stave off chronic conditions such as the brittle-bone disease, osteoporosis, or deficiency diseases such as scurvy (lack of vitamin C). In this section you'll find a summary of the substance's specific effects on your health.

Can You Take Too Much?—It's definitely not true that if a little of a nutrient is good, a lot will automatically be better. Some of the most beneficial vitamins and minerals can be harmful if taken in excess. This section tells whether overdosage is a concern, and if so, what your maximum intake should be. Here you'll also learn the effects of consistent overdosage, and what the warning symptoms will be.

Recommended Daily Allowance—The optimum intake of many nutrients varies by age and gender. Experts believe, for example, that older women need more calcium than their juniors, and that all women below age 65 need more calcium than men. (Past 65, the requirement is the same for both.) This section spells out the specific recommendations, and gives the amounts supplied by various supplements—if, in fact, any supplements are really needed.

Best Dietary Sources—Most nutrition experts insist that it's usually better, if possible, to obtain all your requirements from your regular diet, rather than synthetic supplements. This section guides you to some of the foods richest in each of the nutrients.

Part Five, Treatment Finder

The first two indices in this section are designed to help you quickly identify the unconventional remedies available for a particular medical problem. The other indices assist you in locating natural remedies by name. There are five indices in all:

Alternative Therapies Indexed by Illness—This index presents you with the leading alternatives for a host of specific medical problems. Only treatments that have been scientifically verified—or show promise—have been included. Unsubstantiated and disproven treatments do not appear.

Natural Medicines Indexed by Illness—Shown here are the herbal remedies deemed useful for a long list of ailments. The majority have been pronounced effective by the German Health Authority's herbal "Commission E." Those that have not been reviewed by the commission are included on the strength of especially promising research.

Natural Medicines Indexed by Common Name—This index lists all profiles found in Part Three of the book.

Natural Medicines Indexed by Latin Name—If you know an herb only by its scientific name, this index will steer you to the appropriate profile. For each Latin title, it supplies the corresponding common name, plus the page number of the profile.

Nutritional Supplements Index—Use this index to locate entries on the vitamins, minerals, and other nutritional elements profiled in Part Four of this book. Substances are listed by both their most common and alternate names.

The Evolving World of Natural Medicine

We've tried, in this book, to provide you with a summary of what's currently known about the most common types of natural, holistic, and experimental therapy in use today. Because many of these treatments have never been subjected to formal tests, and many others are a source of bitter controversy, all statements regarding their effects must be considered provisional. As science learns more, some treatments will almost surely be validated, while others will just as surely be completely repudiated. What you'll find here is merely a snapshot of the *current* consensus as best we can determine it.

For the facts on herbal medicines, we've relied heavily on the work of PhytoPharm Consulting, Institute for Phytopharmaceuticals, an organization that has compiled one of the most extensive herbal databases available in the world today. Edited by Joerg Gruenwald, PhD, with the assistance of Thomas Brendler, BA and Christof Jaenicke, MD, the PhytoPharm database serves as the primary source for some 250 of the herbal profiles in this book. Information in the remainder of the profiles has been drawn from a variety of sources, in particular *Herbs of Choice,* by Varro E. Tyler, PhD, one of the country's leading authorities on medicinal botanicals, and *The Natural Pharmacy,* edited by Skye Lininger, DC.

Although you're unlikely to find any miracle cures in these pages, many of the natural medicines and healing therapies outlined here have worked for millions, and can improve your life too. Review the possibilities, and discuss the most promising candidates with your doctor. If this book alerts you to even one fruitful new way to deal with a stubborn ailment, it will have served its purpose.

PART ONE

Alternate Routes to Better Health

CHAPTER 1

Finding a Better Alternative

Suddenly, it seems, everybody's looking for an alternative to Establishment-style medicine. A recent national survey suggests that as many as half of all adults have already made at least some use of unconventional therapy, up from one-third in 1992. An increasing number of HMOs and medical insurance companies are beginning to cover at least a few types of nontraditional care. And—incredibly—all this is happening while mainstream medicine chalks up new scientific breakthroughs at an unprecedented pace.

To win so many converts from the world's most advanced medical system, you'd expect today's more popular alternatives to be delivering at least some of the benefits they promise. And, indeed, many of them are. Yet many others remain unproven, and some of the most avidly promoted deliver nothing at all. This book is designed to spell out exactly what you can reasonably expect, and

where results fall short of claims. Treatment by treatment, it tells what each approach aims to accomplish—and, when there's a basis for judgment, how well it succeeds.

Something for Everyone

The scores of alternative treatments available today have only two things in common: They all avoid surgery; and none use prescription drugs. Aside from that, they are as diverse as the diseases they seek to remedy. Some are centuries old; others brand new. Some are natural, others extremely high-tech. Many are harmless; a few can be dangerous. Some are scientifically proven, others have been thoroughly debunked.

Although all boast unique features enthusiastically promoted by their advocates, the majority share seven common themes:

Better Health Through Proper Diet: Although most nutritional discoveries have now been adopted by mainstream medicine, a few dietary programs are still regarded as a little beyond the pale. Among them are macrobiotic dieting, megadose supplementation, and juice therapy. While they are generally considered harmless—and sometimes even helpful—conventional physicians question their necessity.

Natural Pharmacy: Beneficiaries of the back-to-nature movement, today's burgeoning array of "green" over-the-counter remedies includes herbs, homeopathic medicines, bee products, and therapeutic enzymes. Also available in offices and clinics are oxygen therapy, cell therapy, reconstructive therapy, and neural therapy. This vast assortment of natural pharmaceuticals has to be judged on a product-by-product basis. Many herbs have proven value, many of the other remedies don't.

Cleansing Away Poor Health: As the medical representatives of the environmental movement, practitioners of these therapies blame most of our ills on the products (and by-products) of industrial society. Methods include fasting, detoxification therapies, colonic irrigation, biological dentistry, and chelation therapy, all frequently packaged together under the label "environmental medicine." Orthodox physicians regard these treatments as among the most disreputable in the entire field of health care.

Manipulating the Body's Energy: This unique area includes some of the oldest and most effective of alternative treatments, along with some of the newest and least effective. Included are acupuncture, acupressure, reflexology, therapeutic touch, magnetic field therapy, and energy medicine. Experts say that the treatments are harmless, but for some, the quackery quotient is high.

Physical Remedies: For certain specific physical problems, including tension, stress, and back pain, treatments such as chiropractic, osteopathic manipulation, and bodywork provide many with relief. Exercise programs such as tai chi and yoga serve to build and maintain good health. And tactics such as hydrotherapy and hyperthermia help to relieve minor infections, aches, and pains. Be wary, however, of applied kinesiology and craniosacral therapy. Conventional physicians warn that they're probably worthless.

Mind Over Matter: The mind really does affect the body, so the many forms of mind/body medicine have produced some astonishing results. Approaches such as hypnotherapy, biofeedback, meditation, guided imagery, neurolinguistic programming, and qigong can be relied on to relieve a variety of troubling symptoms (though they won't cure serious underlying disease). Even an oddity such as the so-called flower remedies can improve your mood—if nothing else.

A Boost from the Senses: Sensory medicine doesn't pretend to heal physical disorders, but it can improve overall health and well-being. Aromatherapy, sound therapy, and light therapy all have their uses.

For a sort of medical supermarket of these alternatives, you can visit a naturopathic physician. And for the more philosophically inclined, there's Ayurvedic medicine, a potpourri of ancient health care techniques imported from India (where they've been at least partially superseded by Western care).

You'll find a brief introduction to each of these treatments in Chapter 2, and extended discussions of their pros and cons in Part Two, Guide to Alternative and Complementary Therapies. For complete information on individual herbal products and dietary supplements, turn to Parts Three and Four.

A Kinder, Gentler Approach?

There are many reasons for seeking out alternative therapy, some justified, others misguided. As you contemplate your options, you'll need to guard against the many misconceptions that currently abound, focusing instead on proven results. Remember, no matter how appealing a procedure may sound, it's worthless unless it does the job.

Although most people use alternative therapy as a supplement to their regular medical care, some regard it as a more civil substitute for the harsh, impersonal routines of conventional medicine. Certainly, there is ample room for improvement. Medical encounters rarely unfold with the compassion exhibited on the hit television show *E.R.,* and people often complain that their doctors spent too little time with them. (Seven-minute visits are standard in managed care; and a 1994 study published in the *Journal of Family Practice* found that one group of allergy specialists spent an average of just 9½ minutes with each patient.) In a *Consumer Reports* survey of 70,000 consumers, 20 percent said their doctors didn't encourage them to ask questions; 22 percent had never had a thorough medical history taken; and 29 percent said that their doctors didn't ask their opinions about their medical condition.

Many people are also put off by the cold, abstract manner in which many doctors approach an illness. Too often, physicians seem focused on a technical malfunction within one of the body's physiological systems, while ignoring the problem's impact on the patient. This is an almost inevitable result of the microspecialization that's now required to keep pace with medicine's ever more detailed understanding of the body, but it doesn't make for optimum well-being or a happy patient.

WHY SO MUCH CONTROVERSY?

Does a treatment work or not? It seems like an easy enough question to answer. If you had a pain before the treatment, and no pain afterwards, it seems clear that the treatment worked.

Medical scientists, however, say that's not enough. Over the years, they have discovered that virtually *anything* has a chance of providing symptomatic relief as long as the patient believes in it. For example, when researchers give fake treatments called "placebos" to their patients, a certain number always report relief. For this reason, modern medicine holds its treatments to a higher standard. To be considered worthwhile, they must outdo the often impressive effects of a fake.

The so-called "placebo effect" is responsible for a tremendous amount of confusion in health care. In clinical trials, an ordinary sugar pill will produce beneficial results about a third of the time. Other bogus treatments can do even better. Acupuncture needles inserted in all the wrong spots alleviate pain roughly half the time. An impressive-looking machine connected with dummy leads to a painful area is capable of providing relief *over* half the time.

It is results such as these that lead doctors to dismiss case studies and patients' testimonials as virtually meaningless. If half of all patients gain relief simply from being told they'll get better, how much importance can you attach to any one person's experience?

The Scientific Solution

Thanks to this dilemma, the goal of medical research is to find treatments that not only work, but work *better* than a placebo. And to make the comparison valid, researchers are forced to employ some very elaborate strategies during the test.

At the outset, they must assemble a large enough group of patients to eliminate the possibility that a coincidence or mistake will alter the results. If only 10 or 20 patients are tested, one mistaken report could tip the balance for or against the treatment. Prescription drugs are typically tested on thousands of people before they are deemed effective.

Next, to avoid unconsciously favoring any particular type of patient, the researchers must assign the genuine treatment at random, leaving the remaining patients with a fake. The patients, of course, cannot be told who's getting the real thing. But there's also a very real possibility that the people administering the treatments will unconsciously communicate their expectations to the patients if they know they're giving a placebo. For this reason, the caregivers, too, must be kept in the dark. This arrangement is called a "double-blind." Adding it all up, the ideal test is referred to as a "randomized, double-blind, placebo-controlled clinical trial."

With thousands of people to be watched for months at a time, such tests are obviously very expensive. They are conducted only if a treatment shows great promise, or has significant profit potential. If herbs were required to pass such tests, all but the most potent would disappear from the market—their potential benefits simply wouldn't justify the expense of the trials. Likewise, many of the less promising alternative therapies have never been submitted to this sort of testing, and probably never will be.

Playing the Odds

If a treatment hasn't been subjected to placebo-controlled trials, there's no way to be sure it will work any better than a dose of "positive thinking," no matter how many enthusiastic testimonials it has received. It could still provide you with significant relief (for whatever the reason), but you have no way of knowing the odds of success.

One fact, however, is certain. The placebo effect has its limits. It can work actual physical changes in your body (such as lowering your blood pressure) but it can't cure a serious disease such as cancer, appendicitis, or overwhelming infection. If a treatment hasn't passed the placebo test, its chances of curing a serious, physical affliction must therefore be considered minimal. For relief of stubborn symptoms, an unverified or controversial remedy might be worth a try. But to cure life-threatening disease, your wisest course is to insist on the most thoroughly tested treatment you can find.

In response to these shortcomings, many alternative practitioners make a point of offering the warmth and concern that orthodox medicine so frequently lacks. They approach each patient as an integrated whole, ever mindful of the complex interplay between mind and body, and of the role that the body's own healing mechanisms can play. They take extra time to understand the full dimensions of a disorder, and try to address contributing and aggravating factors, as well as the immediate problem itself.

This "holistic" approach to health care can be deeply satisfying, and often yields valuable dividends through prevention of ill health and improvement in fitness and well-being. However, it's a mistake to assume that it can always provide the remedy you need. Advanced or acute physical illness (cancer, heart disease, stroke, infection) typically responds better to high-tech treatment—no matter how callously delivered—than to any holistic alternative, however reassuringly it's administered. In general, it's best to turn to holistic alternatives to maintain good health, and seek orthodox care when a breakdown occurs.

Healthy Skepticism

Despite modern medicine's amazing strides, many people still question the competence of mainstream practice. They cite the many diseases for which there's still no definitive cure: high blood pressure, diabetes, arthritis, Parkinson's disease, Alzheimer's, colitis, and more. They also point out the rapidly shifting fashions in medicine—clear evidence that conventional wisdom is often proved wrong.

Thirty years ago, for example, heart attack patients were prescribed six weeks of complete bed rest, while today we're told that they should be up and about in days. In the 1970s, the medical establishment ridiculed Nathan Pritikin for his theory that a high-fiber, low-fat diet and plenty of exercise could prevent heart disease. Now his former detractors practice exactly what he preached.

Previously, tonsillectomies, hysterectomies, and Cesarean sections were all the rage. That's no longer the case. And although we now know that most duodenal ulcers are caused by *H. pylori* bacteria, only a few years ago physicians blamed them exclusively on rich food and stress. Small wonder, then, that people no longer regard their doctors as infallible.

However, even if orthodox medicine is sometimes wrong—and always slow to change—that still doesn't mean that alternative practitioners are necessarily right. In fact, many alternative therapies are at least as wrongheaded as mainstream medicine at its worst.

Craniosacral therapists, for example, maintain that they can manipulate the plates of the skull, even though the bones fuse solid at an early age. Likewise, homeopathic physicians hold that preparations containing one molecule of medicine per billion can effect a cure. True, there may be a remote chance that such assertions are correct, but the odds make conventional medicine seem a sure bet in comparison.

In the end, there is no "medical Mafia" suppressing miracle cures for its own economic benefit. There are only cautious, conservative doctors demanding clear evidence of efficacy before they'll risk adopting a treatment. Because physicians are always in search of definitive proof, some valuable alternatives have been slow to reach general acceptance. But never forget that these promising treatments are mixed in with bogus nostrums. "Alternative" does not automatically equal "effective." You have to judge each possibility by its track record in clinical trials. (See the "Why So Much Controversy?" box nearby.)

Natural Attraction

Modern science has made some pretty horrendous mistakes—asbestos, DDT, and thalidomide, to name a few—so it's easy to see why many people are afraid to try its latest concoctions. No matter how well they're tested, potent synthetic drugs still occasionally pose unexpected threats. In just the past couple of years, two popular new pharmaceuticals—the diet drug Redux and the heart medication Posicor—had to be pulled from the market when rare, but life-threatening, side effects surfaced after their release.

It's also true that high-powered prescription drugs sometimes cause new problems even as they remedy an old one. Certain blood pressure medications, for instance, can also cause impotence. And too often, the medical response is to simply add yet another drug to the mix, risking further side effects and raising the possibility of drug interactions.

Isn't it safer, herbalists ask, to rely on mild, natural remedies that have passed the test of time? It's an attractive idea. Still, the answer is "not necessarily."

Some of the most potent poisons on earth (strychnine, for ex-ample) come from plants, and many medicinal herbs can prove fatal as well, if taken in excess. (Ephedra is a leading example. Tansy, Pennyroyal, and Rue are just a few of the others.) Fundamentally, herbs are no different than any other type of medication. They are foreign substances ingested to alter reactions within the body. The mere fact that a preparation is herbal provides no assurance of its safety.

It's worth remembering that the "natural" label is no guarantee of effectiveness either. The German Federal Health Agency, which takes a special interest in these matters, has pronounced over 150 herbal remedies genuinely effective, but has deemed an even larger number unproven. In clinical tests, many long-established folk remedies have failed to show any actual effect, while recently discovered medications such as Ginkgo Biloba have passed with flying colors.

Remember, too, that herbal products are especially unpredictable here in the United States, where there is no system for regulating their purity and quality. When analyzed, some herbal preparations have been found to contain little, if any, active ingredient. Using whole, "natural" herbs won't necessarily solve this problem either, since the active ingredients must often be extracted and refined before they'll have a measurable effect.

There's no question that many popular natural remedies—from St. John's Wort to Saw Palmetto—offer genuine relief. But to garner

HERBS IN THE MEDICAL MAINSTREAM

When a plant shows medicinal powers, scientists descend on it to find out why. The active ingredients found in this way—extracted, refined, or synthesized—now take up a significant portion of the medicine cabinet. From aspirin (white willow) to laxatives (senna) many of our favorite remedies are simply herbs in modern guise. Here are just a few examples of the herbal contribution to contemporary mainstream therapy.

- The Madagascar periwinkle, *Catharanthus roseus,* was originally believed to cure diabetes. Investigators found that, while it had little effect on blood sugar, it did inhibit the production of white blood cells in laboratory animals. Further studies led to the isolation of vinblastine and vincristine, alkaloids currently used in the treatment of Hodgkin's disease and childhood leukemia, respectively.

- In the 1930s, cortisone and other steroids were first isolated in tiny amounts from cattle glands. While their usefulness was immediately apparent, the cost of producing them was prohibitive, so a worldwide search for plant substitutes was undertaken. The result was the discovery of a type of yam, Dioscorea, which now provides a foundation for the production of several steroids and other hormones.

- Curare, the active ingredient in the toxic plants used in South America to poison arrow tips, is currently used as a muscle relaxant for surgical patients.

- Compounds obtained from the fungus Ergot are used to stop bleeding in childbirth and relieve migraine headaches.

- Foxglove, a common garden plant, initially described in the 1st century AD by Greek surgeon Dioscorides, became popular in the 18th century for the treatment of dropsy (swelling due to water retention). Today, its active ingredient, digitalis, is used to treat patients with congestive heart failure or other forms of heart disease.

- The opium poppy, praised by the Babylonians for its medicinal value, produces the pain reliever morphine.

- The snakeroot, *Rauwolfia serpentina,* has been used in India for centuries to treat mental disorders and insomnia. In 1949, researchers verified its value for treating high blood pressure. Rauwolfia's active ingredient, an alkaloid called reserpine, has been found to have a relaxing, tranquilizing effect, while lowering blood pressure and slowing the pulse.

the benefits of herbal medicine, you need to be a very discriminating shopper. In Part Three of this book, the Guide to Natural Medicines, you'll find summaries of what the experts currently know about over 300 herbs—what they've been shown to relieve, what they've traditionally been used for, and any potential dangers they pose. Turn to the Guide whenever another herbal "sensation" makes the evening news. It will give you a quick overview of the substance's past history and current status.

The Best of Both Worlds

Should you stick with conventional therapy, or try an alternative? The answer is simple: Use both. See a physician for an accurate diagnosis (alternative practitioners are little help in this area), then pursue all the treatments that offer a reasonable chance of results. For many serious problems, there are simply no better remedies than those available from mainstream medicine. (Serious infections, for example, flatly demand antibiotics.) But for many other conditions, from high blood pressure to chronic pain, promising alternatives abound. They can be used to supplement conventional treatments, or—if they work well enough—even to replace them.

How can you determine that a proposed treatment falls short? Maintain an independent outlook, and question anything—conventional or otherwise—that seems unduly extreme. You'll probably want to exhaust all other options, for instance, before allowing a conventional surgeon to replace an arthritic joint, or remove your stomach to control your weight. By the same token, if an alternative therapist suggests that you need a protracted series of enemas simply to maintain good health, or proposes to zap your troubles away with a patented energy device, you have every right to question his motives.

Indeed, it's wise to avoid investing 100 percent trust in *any* health care practitioner with whom you don't have a long-standing relationship. A managed care doctor could be steering you *away* from optimum treatment. A specialist could be steering you *toward* an unnecessary procedure. And a disreputable alternative practitioner could be selling you a worthless bill of goods. The vast majority of health care professionals—both in and out of the mainstream—are honest and well-meaning, but both worlds also have their share of quacks. It's sad to say, but in medicine as in commerce, the best rule to follow is "buyer beware."

CHAPTER 2

Sorting Out Your Options

Alternative medicine presents us with an amazing—if not downright confusing—array of choices. The treatments collected under this label range from the mundane to the mystical, the promising to the preposterous. All have been ignored by orthodox medicine, but otherwise have virtually nothing in common. This poses a severe problem: how to sift out the genuinely helpful from the well-meant but worthless.

Some forms of alternative medicine fall well within the bounds of modern science, and seem destined for the mainstream. These include the use of nutrition and diet to maximize health and stave off a variety of diseases; a host of measures for reducing stress, anxiety, and other debilitating mental states; and an assortment of techniques for improving movement and relieving various types of pain.

Other members of the alternative category are totally foreign to the Western worldview, relying on exotic theories of health and disease, mysterious diagnostic techniques, and implausible—yet often effective—forms of treatment. Especially prominent in this group are the many therapies borrowed from traditional Chinese medicine, including acupuncture, acupressure, qigong, and tai chi.

It is impossible to predict, simply from their nature, which alternatives will work best and which will fail. Some of the most unlikely candidates deliver the best results. Acupuncture, for example, claims to enhance the flow of an esoteric and undetectable life force named qi. Nevertheless, it has proved to be astonishingly effective in scientific trials.

Other treatments that sound perfectly plausible ultimately fail to deliver. The rationale for chelation therapy, for instance, seems quite "scientific." By binding with the calcium in blocked blood vessels, it's supposed to cure heart disease and poor circulation. In clinical tests, however, it works no better than a fake.

DIETING YOUR WAY TO HEALTH

Ignored for decades, nutrition is now one of the hottest fields in medicine. As scientists learn more about the protective ingredients in food, you can take advantage of their discoveries through self-help diets and supplements. Check into these popular leading options.

- Juice Therapy
- Macrobiotic Diet
- Orthomolecular Medicine
- Vegetarianism

The profiles in this book are designed to give you a closer look at the pros and cons of over 50 of these strange and unpredictable therapies, from naturopathy to neurolinguistic programming, and homeopathy to hypnosis. Although all have distinctive attributes of their own, the majority fall into a few major categories. Here's an overview of the major groupings, and a quick look at how the various treatments rate.

Dietary Remedies

Until recently, the medical profession was notorious for ignoring nutrition's role in preventing and curing disease. In the 1970s, when Nathan Pritikin theorized that a low-fat, low-cholesterol diet could reduce the risk of heart disease, he was ridiculed by most doctors. Yet today a low-fat diet is recommended by virtually all mainstream medical practitioners.

Still, it's unwise to assume that all nutritional claims are equally valid. Some programs have proven themselves; others have not. For instance, **Vegetarianism**, once a fringe movement in the U.S., is now considered a healthful and viable choice. Research has shown that vegetarians tend to have low cholesterol levels and decreased risk of heart disease, diabetes, high blood pressure, obesity, and colon cancer.

The **Macrobiotic Diet**, on the other hand, is still regarded as questionable. A modern, limited vegetarian food plan based on ancient Chinese precepts of balancing the universal opposites dubbed *yin* and *yang*, this diet offers the same benefits as ordinary vegetarianism. However, unless supplemented by fish and milk products, it can prove inadequate, even dangerous, for children and pregnant or breastfeeding women.

If food really can improve health, why not take nutrients—in capsule form—as medicine? Advocates of **Orthomolecular Medicine**, a term coined by Nobelprize-winning scientist Linus Pauling, believe that massive doses of selected nutrients can help prevent disease and aging, and even cure certain disorders. Dozens, or even hundreds, of pills a day are sometimes prescribed for patients.

· In general, standard medical authorities advise *against* such megadoses. They maintain that the preventive health effects of a diet rich in fruits, vegetables, and fiber cannot be duplicated in pill form. Natural foods, they point out, contain a whole medley of nutrients that no supplement can hope to replace. Worse yet, in large doses, some vitamins can be toxic or interfere with the body's absorption of other essential nutrients.

Some of the claims made for nutritional supplements have, in fact, failed to hold up under scientific examination. For example, Linus Pauling's conviction that massive doses of vitamin C could cure cancer was disproved in three clinical trials conducted at the Mayo Clinic. Clinical trials have also thrown doubt on the usefulness of high doses of antioxidant vitamins.

Nevertheless, studies are emerging that do confirm *some* of the benefits proposed by supplement advocates. For example, some recent studies have found that megadoses of vitamin E (400 or 800 milligrams daily) may reduce the risk of a new heart attack. Likewise, liberal intake of calcium, magnesium, and potassium can reduce high blood pressure. And some nutritional elements do

seem to have a therapeutic effect. For example, a recent Cleveland Clinic study found that taking a zinc lozenge within 24 hours of the start of a cold reduced symptoms and cut the average length of the illness from 7½ to 4½ days.

To maintain a natural mixture of nutrients while boosting your intake of beneficial vitamins and minerals, some nutritionists advocate **Juice Therapy** as a healthy alternative to artificial supplements. Take care, however. Juices lack the fat, fiber, and protein needed to maintain good health. When used as a substitute for a regular diet—as in a fasting or detoxification program—juice therapy can sap your energy, compromise the immune system, and lead to serious chemical imbalances.

Natural Medicines

Herbs were the first medicines used by man. Even today, more than one-fourth of our conventional pharmaceuticals are based on substances first found in plants. These drugs were developed by testing the various chemicals in medicinal herbs until their active ingredients had been isolated. They are still used in ways that echo the folk remedies from which they derive—a fact that has led the National Cancer Institute to test thousands of primitive remedies recommended by native shamans.

Herbal remedies have become popular for a variety of reasons. Available without a prescription, they hold the promise of relief without an expensive and frustrating encounter with the established medical system. And because they're natural, people tend to view them as safe and benign.

Unfortunately, the mere fact of being natural provides no guarantees. Just like their synthetic cousins, many herbs can be downright dangerous if overused. Others may be as safe as people imagine, but much less effective than their prescription counterparts. Since herbal products are not regulated by the Food and Drug Administration, potency and even ingredients may vary. Some dried or powdered products may even contain harmful contaminants. And because most herbs have been tested much less thoroughly than a typical prescription drug, information about side effects and possible dangers is often skimpy or completely lacking.

Nonetheless, there's mounting evidence that certain herbs are effective remedies for ailments ranging from simple fatigue to dangerous heart problems. Even the more conservative medical authorities feel that, provided you choose a reliable source, herbs can be safely used for the same sort of problems you'd treat with an over-the-counter drug.

While many alternative practitioners prescribe herbs based on experience and understanding of the active chemical ingredients, the approach known as **Homeopathy** relies on a very different rationale. Developed by late 18th century German physician

Samuel Hahnemann, the first principle of homeopathy is that "like cures like." Hahnemann used tiny doses of substances that produced unpleasant symptoms in volunteers to treat patients with similar symptoms. He theorized that this replaced the disease with a similar but weaker illness that the body's "vital force" could more easily overcome—a sort of "vaccination" for everything from headache to heart failure.

This may sound reasonable, but there are a couple of difficulties. First, although the substances Hahnemann chose could mimic the symptoms of a disease, they bore no relation to the underlying cause. Second, Hahnemann also believed that the more he diluted a remedy, the more potent it would become. As a result, many homeopathic preparations contain scarcely a molecule of the original active ingredient.

If a remedy doesn't affect the cause of a disease—and isn't in the preparation anyway—how can it possibly work? Conventional doctors say the answer is simple: It can't. Homeopaths insist that it can, explaining that even the most diluted solution retains a "trace memory" of the original substance, imprinted in the form of its electromagnetic frequency. This "imprint" has never been detected, but many people continue to say that the remedies seem to help.

Other natural medicines are less mysterious—or at least are prescribed in quantities that could

NATURE'S HELPING HANDS

These natural remedies present an appealing alternative to potent synthetic drugs. But check them out carefully. Nature plays some nasty tricks, and some natural remedies fail to fulfill their promise.

- Apitherapy
- Cell Therapy
- Enzyme Therapy
- Herbal Remedies
- Homeopathy
- Neural Therapy
- Oxygen Therapy
- Reconstructive Therapy

clearly have an effect. For instance, the venom in bee stings—an ancient cure for arthritis and joint problems—still has strong proponents today. Bee venom does contain several active ingredients, including two anti-inflammatory agents and an abundance of neurotransmitters. Among its strongest proponents are practitioners who treat multiple sclerosis. Critics believe that many of the claimed multiple sclerosis "cures" are actually due to the fact that the disease often goes into long periods of remission on its own. Nevertheless, bee therapy (also known as **Apitherapy**) is currently being tested under a research grant from The Multiple Sclerosis Society.

Bee products such as bee venom and royal jelly can produce violent allergic reactions, and have never been proven beneficial in scientifically organized clinical trials. If you want to try apitherapy anyway, be sure to get an allergy test before you begin. The treatments can be especially dangerous for people with heart trouble, diabetes, tuberculosis, and women in the midst of their menstrual periods.

Some natural medicines are accepted for one type of problem in mainstream medicine, but advocated for others by alternative practitioners. For example, conventional medicine uses enzymes (protein molecules that play a major role in digestion) to treat people with pancreatic disease, cystic fibrosis, and lactose intolerance. In the world of alternative medicine, however, **Enzyme Therapy** is touted as a remedy for cancer, AIDS, arthritis, multiple sclerosis, athletic injuries, and more. Although the need for enzymes may sound plausible, there's no evidence that they can cure anything but deficiency diseases. Indeed, since most plant enzymes are deactivated by acid the moment they arrive in the stomach, scientists say there's no chance that they can work.

Similarly, **Oxygen Therapy** is standard practice for people with breathing problems and is used in hyperbaric (high pressure) oxygen chambers to assist healing of burns and wounds. However, "enhanced" forms of oxygen such as ozone and hydrogen peroxide are still in the realm of experimental medicine. Proponents say these compounds can cure a variety of infections, and a clinical study of ozone therapy for HIV and hepatitis is now underway. As yet, however, there's no definitive proof that either compound is effective, while there's ample evidence of potentially dangerous side effects. If you opt for oxygen therapy, use it with caution.

Some natural medicines "sound" scientific, but have no accepted medical uses. For example, **Cell Therapy** promises to boost the immune system and rejuvenate the body with injections of healthy cells from various organs in animals. Although these expensive treatments have enjoyed popularity abroad, their effectiveness has never been verified. (Don't confuse these injections with the human and animal fetal cell transplants being studied for treatment of Parkinson's disease and other neurological conditions.)

Another type of injection, given to promote repair of ligaments, tendons, and cartilage (**Reconstructive Therapy**) shows more promise. The shot delivers an irritant and an anesthetic such as lidocaine to a diseased joint. This is thought to spark the body's own repair mechanisms, and some clinical trials seem to confirm that this does in fact happen.

Be skeptical, however, of another type of anesthetic injection, called **Neural Therapy**. Especially popular in Germany, this form of treatment is supposed to remove blockages in the body's electrical energy flow, thereby curing a huge assortment of ailments. Although it appears to provide some relief from chronic pain, no other effects have been proven.

Cleansing Therapies

Except in cases of outright poisoning, conventional physicians pay little attention to the toxic effects of pollution, pesticides, food additives, and the residue from pharmaceutical and recreational drugs. They argue that the body's own cleansing powers neutralize and eliminate the low-level toxins we encounter daily. Nevertheless, some alternative practitioners charge that these chemicals are overloading our immune system and interfering with elimination, circulation, and other crucial functions.

To fend off such purported dangers, these practitioners have devised a number of **Detoxification Therapies**. To cleanse the body of dietary toxins, for example, they may recommend **Fasting**, either with water-only fasts or with fruit and vegetable juice diets. (Fasting is also prescribed

---

BANISHING TOXIC BUILD-UP

Flushing toxins from the body sounds like a great idea, but most medical experts say there's no evidence of poisoning and no reason for treatment. Since some of these procedures can be expensive, painful, and dangerous, weigh them carefully before you proceed.

- Biological Dentistry
- Chelation Therapy
- Colonic Irrigation
- Detoxification Therapy
- Environmental Medicine
- Fasting

---

as the first step in an elimination diet to relieve stubborn problems such as arthritis.)

The more extreme proponents of detoxification also employ **Colonic Irrigation** (including high colonics and coffee enemas) to clear the large intestine of suspected toxic build-up. Mainstream doctors contend that the colon is self-cleansing and that no such build-up exists. Nevertheless, advocates insist that their treatments clear toxins from both the digestive system and the blood, promoting mental clarity and physical and spiritual health. Whatever the truth of the matter, if you decide to try such treatments, make sure the therapist is experienced. Colonic irrigation can cause perforation of the colon and may lead to serious infections if equipment isn't clean.

Proponents of **Biological Dentistry** find dangers elsewhere, in the mercury amalgam that dentists use to fill cavities. (Some practitioners also believe the teeth are linked to other organs in the body, and treat illness with oral acupuncture or neural therapy.) Advocates of this theory blame toxic metals in the amalgam for a variety of vague, unexplained ailments, including chronic fatigue syndrome, lack of energy, inflammatory disease, weakened immunity, and certain neurological illnesses. The remedy, they say, is to replace the fillings. Before you run up a major dental bill, however, you should know that the American Dental Association says amalgam poses absolutely no risk.

Unlike biological dentistry, **Chelation Therapy** is standard practice in conventional medicine, which uses it as a remedy for lead and heavy metal poisoning. The treatments rely on an amino acid called EDTA to bind with positively charged metals such as lead, iron, and copper and remove them from the body. Noting that

EDTA is also used by plumbers to clear calcium deposits from pipes, a number of alternative practitioners have suggested that EDTA can remove calcium-laden plaque from the veins and arteries, relieving angina and preventing strokes and heart attacks. This is a highly controversial proposition. Proponents say that treatments have worked on over half a million patients, but no mainstream medical group has ever seen fit to endorse them.

Chelation is one of the many therapies employed in **Environmental Medicine**, a self-styled specialty that blames a variety of chronic maladies on subtle allergies to environmental toxins. Advocates of this form of medicine say that detoxification with EDTA, enzymes, heat treatments, and other off-beat remedies can cure ailments ranging from headache, hay fever, and fatigue to asthma, colitis, and arthritis. Since treatment may also involve extensive and burdensome changes in lifestyle, diet, and environment, you can take comfort in the fact that mainstream critics say there's no evidence linking specific environmental factors with problems like arthritis.

Manipulating the Body's Energy

Some of the most exotic treatments in the alternative medicine repertory seek to work cures by enhancing the flow of hypothetical energies and "vital forces" within the body. Several of these approaches yield surprisingly good results.

Perhaps the best known is **Acupuncture**, a traditional Chinese therapy based on the supposition that a vital force called *qi* flows along established channels, or *meridians,* and that insertion of a needle at one point on a meridian can clear a blockage farther along the channel. There is no scientific reason why this should work, yet the experts agree that—for certain problems— it usually does. The November 1997 consensus conference of the National Institutes of Health concluded that there is clear evidence that acupuncture is effective for reducing nausea from surgery and chemotherapy, and probably nausea due to pregnancy. It can also relieve many types of pain, including postoperative dental discomfort, menstrual cramps, tennis elbow, and fibromyalgia. And since the therapy is free of drugs, the risk of side effects is slight.

Acupressure—a version of acupuncture without the needles— uses manual pressure at points along the meridians to remedy various ailments. It provides effective relief from a wide variety of muscle and joint pains, as well as tension and headache. Pressure on a particular acupoint on the inside of the wrist has been clinically proven to reduce motion sickness and postsurgical nausea. A similar form of therapy, dubbed **Reflexology**, relies on pressure at various points in the foot to remedy problems in remote parts of the body. Advocated for conditions ranging from arthritis to irritable bowel syn-

HARNESSING NATURAL ENERGY

In a field that's ripe for quackery and fraud, some exotic treatments nevertheless deliver exactly as promised. But beware of "black boxes" and extravagant claims.

- Acupressure
- Acupuncture
- Energy Medicine
- Magnetic Field Therapy
- Reflexology
- Therapeutic Touch

drome, it seems most effective for relieving headaches and improving bladder control.

Therapeutic Touch, a relatively recent healing practice akin to the ancient laying on of hands, is considered more controversial and less reliable than the traditional Chinese methods. Although it is taught in many U.S. nursing schools and used in a number of hospitals, its effectiveness in clinical trials has been spotty. The treatments rarely involve actual contact between therapist and patient. Instead, the practitioner moves her hands a few inches above the patient's body, "sensing" and correcting blockages in the patient's energy fields. This is said to reduce pain, fever, and anxiety. Some Lamaze course instructors teach the practice to reduce anxiety and discomfort during labor.

A different, more measurable sort of energy is the focus of **Magnetic Field Therapy**. The instruments used in these treatments are thought to interact beneficially with the weak magnetic field that exists throughout the body's tissues. The large magnetic devices designed to speed the healing of fractured limbs have proven their worth. However, the small magnets often used to reduce or eliminate pain remain much more controversial. For each study that finds them effective, there's another that fails to.

Ironically, manipulation of the most familiar form of energy—electricity—has produced some of the least impressive results. Although one type of treatment dubbed "transcutaneous electrical nerve stimulation" appears to be an effective remedy for pain, other electrical treatments have failed to pan out. Collectively labeled **Energy Medicine**, they include a host of dubious "black box" devices and quasi-electrical procedures that either remain untested or have already been debunked.

Physical Manipulation

Although the theories underpinning osteopathic and chiropractic medicine are rejected by the majority of mainstream physicians, both disciplines enjoy widespread favor among patients. **Osteopathy** originally focused on manipulation of the spine and joints to clear away supposed obstructions in the nervous and circulatory systems. Although a few osteopaths still offer such manipulations, the majority have joined the mainstream, performing the same diagnostic and therapeutic procedures as regular MDs. They prescribe drugs, have hospital privileges, and are licensed to practice in all 50 states.

Chiropractors, on the other hand, still do much of their work through adjustment of the joints, primarily in the spine. When chiropractic was first developed at the end of the 19th century, it was intended to cure all manner of diseases. Now it's used primarily for pain relief—especially in the lower back. Studies have shown that chiropractic treatment of low back pain (which usually goes away within a month without treatment) is at least as effective as mainstream medical approaches and may lead to greater patient satisfaction. Its value for any problem other than pain has yet to be conclusively demonstrated.

Although chiropractors receive ample training in the biological and clinical sciences, mainstream medical doctors remain concerned that they may not recognize some underlying causes of back pain, such as a tumor or collapsed vertebrae. They are also alarmed by a tendency among chiropractors to expand their practices with other forms of alternative therapy, some of dubious value. For better or worse, however, chiropractic is probably the most popular form of alternative therapy in the U.S. today. One in three back-pain patients now go to a chiropractor.

Less popular is the offshoot of chiropractic called **Applied Kinesiology**. Concocted during the 1960s, this approach combines chiropractic concepts with beliefs drawn from acupuncture. Asserting that individual muscles are somehow associated with organs elsewhere in the body, practitioners diagnose illness by searching for weak spots in muscle tissue. Cures are then effected through massage, joint adjustments, and diet. It's best to approach this therapy with skepticism. Even practitioners advise that it's a supplement to—not a replacement for—orthodox medical care, and mainstream doctors dismiss it completely.

Equally dubious is **Craniosacral Therapy**, whose practitioners insist that they can adjust segments of the skull that are known to fuse into a single bone during infancy. Craniosacral therapists say that they can nevertheless clear obstructions in the flow of the cerebrospinal fluid that bathes the brain and spine, relieving the maladies that such "obstructions" are thought to cause. The therapy is said to be effective for tension headaches, a variety of neurological problems, and even learning disabilities. Although proponents cite numerous case studies to back up their claims, the treatments have never been validated by scientific clinical trials.

For a less exotic, but perhaps more reliable, approach to stress, tension, and pain, you can turn to the array of techniques generally classified under the umbrella term "bodywork." A medley of massage, physical manipulation, and exercises, these therapies promise significant, drug-free relief from a variety of neuromuscular problems. Some, such as traditional **Massage**, **Myotherapy**, and

Trager Integration, concentrate on relief of muscular tightness and pain. Others, such as **Rolfing** and **Hellerwork**, seek to release emotional and physical tension through a more intense, deep massage. Approaches such as the **Alexander Technique**, **Aston-Patterning**, and the **Feldenkrais Method** place greater emphasis on movement training and exercise to improve posture, increase flexibility, and relieve strain.

Other forms of therapeutic exercise have their roots in traditional Chinese and Indian medicine. Although they rely on esoteric beliefs, they are nonethe-

---

"HANDS-ON" HEALING

Consider these noninvasive physical treatments for back, joint, and muscle pain. Many also enhance movement and flexibility, relieve stress, and improve your general sense of well-being. But be wary of practitioners who claim to cure serious, life-threatening illness.

- Alexander Technique
- Applied Kinesiology
- Aston-Patterning
- Chiropractic Adjustment
- Craniosacral Therapy
- Feldenkrais Method
- Hellerwork
- Hydrotherapy
- Hyperthermia
- Massage
- Myotherapy
- Osteopathic Manipulation
- Rolfing
- Tai Chi
- Trager Integration
- Yoga

less quite effective. For instance, **Tai Chi**, like acupuncture, is intended to balance and strengthen the flow of the vital force, *qi*. Whether or not it actually does this, however, it still provides proven health benefits, including reduced blood pressure and heart rate, increased flexibility, and better balance.

Likewise, the ancient Indian practice of **Yoga** seeks to prepare the body for union with the divine. Yet even stripped of its religious basis, it yields important physical dividends. Through breathing exercises, meditation, and movement routines, it aims to improve circulation, stimulate abdominal organs, stretch the muscles, and achieve normal body alignment. There's scientific evidence that regular practice can reduce blood pressure and heart rate, relieve tension, and improve concentration.

Also found under the heading of physical manipulation is **Hydrotherapy**, a set of treatments that includes an array of hot and cold compresses, hot tubs, mineral springs, and whirlpool, steam, and sitz. baths. These therapies offer simple, effective relief from a wide variety of aches and pains.

Another type of treatment, dubbed **Hyperthermia**, employs a few of the same tactics, but for entirely different ends. Based on the human body's natural response to infection (a fever), it seeks to eradicate foreign invaders with judicious applications of heat. High-tech medical research is investigating hyper-thermia as a weapon against cancer and AIDS. But low-tech natural healers also employ it in an effort to remedy infection and inflammation. Low-tech forms of the treatment include hot baths, hot blankets, hot tubs, saunas, and steam rooms.

Mind/Body Medicine

The power of mind over matter is an accepted medical fact. Although you can't wish away infections, cancer, or dangerous arterial plaque, the mind can influence a variety of supposedly involuntary bodily functions, and in the process can provide significant relief from many troubling, even debilitating symptoms.

Hypnotherapy, for instance, can focus the mind in positive ways that serve to mitigate a wide range of health problems. It has been shown effective in helping some people give up addictions to drugs, alcohol, and tobacco. Studies have also verified its value for relief of pain from chronic migraines, labor and delivery, cancer, and surgery. It can alleviate the nausea that follows chemotherapy, and can even, amazingly, cure warts.

For conscious control of unhealthy physiological responses, many physicians now recommend **Biofeedback**. This is a high-tech Western version of the Eastern arts that enable people to control "involuntary" changes in skin temperature, blood pressure, pulse, brain-wave activity, and more. Machines that signal these changes with shifting visual patterns or audible tones help to ease

POSITIVE THINKING

These safe natural therapies won't cure cancer, but they can successfully lower blood pressure, relieve pain, reduce stress, and even combat addictions. All require your active participation, but many experts say that's the best kind of medicine.

- Biofeedback
- Flower Remedies
- Guided Imagery
- Hypnotherapy
- Meditation
- Neurolinguistic Programming
- Qigong

the learning process. Clinical trials have shown that such training can help people get rid of headaches, regain urinary control, retrain muscles after an accident or surgery, and remedy circulatory problems such as Raynaud's disease.

At the low-tech end of the spectrum is **Meditation**, an age-old technique for calming and focusing the mind, usually with a combination of controlled breathing and repetition of a word or phrase, known as a mantra. The "relaxation response" that this practice evokes has been shown, in scientific studies, to reduce levels of the stress hormone, cortisol. The resulting benefits included reduced levels of tension and anxiety, as well as lower blood pressure. The technique is a scientifically verified means of reducing chronic pain. Many people also find it helpful for headaches and respiratory problems.

The beneficial physiological effects of the relaxation response can also be gained from **Guided Imagery**, a focused form of positive thinking, and from **Neurolinguistic Programming**, a form of psychotherapy that aims to solve emotional and physical problems by breaking negative habits of response. However, don't expect more from these treatments than you could reasonably expect from any other form of relaxation. Although enthusiasts have made extravagant claims, none have been verified in scientific tests.

Another excellent stress reduction technique is **Qigong**, a set of Chinese exercises originally designed to control and direct the flow of the vital energy *qi*. Although there is no evidence that qigong can cure disease, it's excellent for improving overall physical fitness, balance, and flexibility. By alleviating tension, it may also combat insomnia and certain forms of headaches.

To further quell the negative effects of stress, you can also turn to **Flower Remedies**, harmless floral essences designed to improve your mood. These remedies were developed in the early 1900s by British homeopathic physician Edward Bach, who believed that the successful treatment of negative emotions could heal physical disorders. They come with a self-diagnostic questionnaire.

Sensory Medicine

The essences used in flower therapy have no fragrance, and their mechanism of action is totally unexplained. **Aromatherapy**, on the other hand, taps into our most acute sense—smell. At least 40 oils derived from the distillation of plants can be used to influence general well-being. Lavender oil in the air, for example, has been scientifically shown to help insomnia and reduce stress. When put in the bath, it can reduce postpartum discomfort. Aromas have also been shown to affect heart rate, blood pressure, breathing, and possibly the immune system. There's no evidence, however, that they can cure any specific disease.

Sound Therapy—particularly music therapy—offers similar results. It can produce measurable, though temporary, improvements in blood pressure and heart rate, as well as boosting the mood and relieving tension and anxiety. **Light Therapy**, on the other hand, is targeted at one very specific problem: seasonal affective disorder (SAD)—the depression that strikes some people during the darker, winter months. (While light therapy is an accepted medical treatment for SAD and certain skin disorders, it is NOT recommended for other problems. Be highly skeptical of colored-light therapies and flashing, pulsing machines. Such devices have no proven effect.)

Alternative Professions

With the goal of enlisting the body's own self-healing properties, **Naturopathic Medicine** offers a whole laundry list of low-tech, noninvasive alternatives to orthodox modern therapy. Although a naturopathic physician may include standard x-rays, lab tests, and physical exams in his repertoire, he usually recommends prescription drugs or surgery only as a last resort. Instead, you'll encounter a variety of alternative treatments, including botanical medicines, nutritional supplements, homeopathic remedies, acupuncture, physical manipulation, and detoxification therapies. Some of these approaches, such as good nutrition, are now standard practice in conventional medicine. Others, such as homeopathy and detoxification, are highly suspect. When using naturopathy, you should be careful to pick and choose.

Another beneficiary of the current quest for gentle, natural treatments, **Ayurvedic Medicine** incorporates millennia-old philosophical concepts first codified in India. With the general goal of restoring the body's metabolic balance, it employs such techniques as breathing exercises,

INDULGING THE SENSES

These simple, enjoyable measures can lift your spirits and relieve tension. Most have no healing powers of their own, but they're often used to enhance the power of other therapies.

- Aromatherapy
- Light Therapy
- Sound Therapy

physical activity, herbal tonics, purification and elimination therapies, massage and meditation. Although some of its disciplines, including meditation, yoga, and massage, offer proven health benefits, others, such as purification and purging, are more likely to harm than help. As with all forms of alternative therapy, it's wise to approach Ayurvedic medicine with a critical eye, taking advantage of its benefits, while rejecting its more outmoded and questionable practices.

CHAPTER 3

Choosing the Right Practitioner

To the vast majority of Americans, nontraditional therapies are just another route to relief when conventional treatment falls short. In one recent study, people who said they used alternative therapies were found to be no more dissatisfied or distrustful of mainstream medicine than were nonusers. Fully 40 percent of the respondents said they'd employed some type of alternative medicine in the past year, yet only 5 percent said it was their primary source of care. Their main reason for using an alternative was philosophical agreement with the holistic approach that acknowledges the importance of the mind in defeating illness.

Unfortunately, not all physicians take the same attitude. A few have an almost visceral hatred of anything outside the mainstream. Many others fear (often with ample justification) that their patients will fall victim to charlatans and quacks. They are quick to dismiss any approach that hasn't been subjected to a battery of scientific tests, and slow to adopt newly discovered treatments. A growing number of doctors are experimenting with the better researched alternative therapies, but the majority remain aloof. Today's reality, therefore, is that many of us are left to our own devices when it comes to finding reputable alternative practitioners.

To make matters more confusing, the world of alternative therapy is a maze of specialists and generalists. You'll need to find a specialist, for example, if you want hypnotherapy, massage, or one of various forms of bodywork such as Rolfing, Hellerwork, Myotherapy, and the like. On the other hand, you'll never find a specialist in such treatments as orthomolecular medicine, colonic irrigation, and light therapy. Instead, you need to look for someone with a general alternative practice, such as a naturopathic physician or a chiropractor. For the best place to turn for each form of therapy, check

WHERE TO FIND IT

Alternative medicine spans a broad spectrum of disciplines. Depending on the treatment you're seeking, potential sources range from maverick MDs to health food clerks. The table below shows some of the more common providers of each type of therapy. Don't be surprised, though, if you find some of them being offered in other venues.

	Acupuncturist	Chiropractor	Naturopath	Osteopath	Chinese medicine	Ayurveda	Other
Acupressure	yes	some		some	yes		some MDs
Acupuncture	yes	some		some			some MDs
Apitherapy							specialty practitioners
Applied kinesiology							specialty practitioners
Aromatherapy		some					massage therapists
Ayurveda			yes			yes	
Biofeedback							specialty practitioners
Biological dentistry							specialty practitioners
Bodywork							trained instructors
Cell therapy							European clinics
Chelation			yes				
Chinese medicine	some		yes		yes		massage therapists
Chiropractic adjustment		yes					
Colon therapy			yes			yes	
Craniosacral therapy		some					specialty practitioners
Detoxification therapy			yes			yes	
Energy medicine					yes	yes	
Environmental medicine			yes				
Enzyme therapy			yes				
Fasting			yes			yes	

	Acupuncturist	Chiropractor	Naturopath	Osteopath	Chinese medicine	Ayurveda	Other
Flower remedies			yes				specialty practitioners
Guided imagery							hypnotherapists
Herbs	some		yes		yes	yes	
Homeopathy	some	some	yes	some			some MDs
Hydrotherapy			yes	yes			
Hyperthermia			yes				
Hypnotherapy							some therapists
Light therapy							some MDs
Macrobiotics				yes			
Magnetic field therapy		yes					
Meditation					yes	yes	
Neural therapy							popular in Germany
Neurolinguistic programming							specialty practitioners
Orthomolecular	some		yes				
Osteopathic manipulation				yes			
Oxygen therapy							popular in Germany
Qigong	yes				yes		
Reconstructive therapy				some			some MDs
Sound therapy							specialty practitioners
Therapeutic touch							specialty practitioners
Vegetarianism			yes		yes		
Yoga						yes	trained instructors

Adapted from: Eisenberg, DM. *Annals of Internal Medicine*. July 1, 1997, 127:61-68.

the nearby "Where To Find It" table and the profiles in the "Alternative and Complementary Therapies" section of this book.

While some generalists claim to take care of all or most of their patients' health needs, keep in mind that many alternative practitioners—even those with medical licenses—do not have hospital privileges. This means that if you require hospital care, you'll be taken care of by another—unfamiliar—physician. For this reason, as well as a desire for "the best of both worlds," the overwhelming majority of people who use an alternative therapist also retain the services of a mainstream MD.

Negotiating the Mainstream and Alternative Worlds

Given the contempt with which many doctors greet the subject of alternative medicine, dare you tell your physician you're getting nontraditional therapy? Despite any qualms you may have, the answer is an unqualified yes. Attitudes *are* changing and many of today's MDs are quite open to a discussion of alternatives. But even if your doctor is not among the openminded, it's still important that he know about all the treatments you're receiving (including over-the-counter nutrients and herbs) because some can interact with mainstream therapy. For example, certain herbs counteract or increase the effect of prescription medicines for heart problems and bleeding disorders. Likewise, if you're taking a prescription medication that reduces liver or kidney function, it could increase the effects of certain herbs and supplements.

Your doctor can also warn you if a product or procedure can be dangerous or toxic. For example, the popular herb Ephedra (also known as ma huang) can be deadly, and in fact has caused recent fatalities. Overdoses of Pennyroyal, Tansy, Coltsfoot, and Colchicum may also prove lethal. And alternative therapies such as colonic irrigation, cell therapy, and apitherapy also pose dangers when administered carelessly or given to the wrong people.

Warning Signs of Hype and Fraud

Because "natural," "gentle," and "holistic" methods have won a positive image for alternative medicine, it's easy to be too trusting. Remember that only a few alternative treatments have been thoroughly tested, and that even the most reliable are good for only certain specific problems. In the largely unregulated world of "natural" medicine, it's all too easy for frauds and hustlers to hang out a shingle and start raking in the fees.

Unfortunately, there's no simple way to distinguish between sincere practitioners and those out to fleece the sick and desperate. In a world where even a medical license is no guarantee, you always face the risk of stumbling into a quack. Nevertheless, you can improve your odds of satisfaction by checking the background of each potential therapist and, if a license is required in your state, making certain he has it. (See the nearby box for state requirements.) Then remain alert for high-pressure sales tactics that almost always signal fraud:

- Grandiose promises to cure conditions that mainstream medicine believes are still incurable (Alzheimer's, Parkinson's, certain cancers).
- Claims that a treatment can reverse a condition that's currently regarded as irreversible (aging, for example).

- Pressure to use an alternative therapy for serious disease *instead* of the mainstream treatments you're already taking.
- Expressions of hostility or derision toward mainstream medicine.
- Charges that a medical "conspiracy" is keeping a treatment from the public.
- Claims that "natural" remedies are automatically better than prescription drugs. ("Natural" does not equal "safe." Snake venom is natural. So is poison ivy.)
- Insistence on a continuous, frequent, and expensive treatment regimen without setting a target date for success.

How Unscrupulous Practitioners String You Along

The quacks that infest the world of alternative medicine sell their treatments by appealing to our fears, beliefs, and vulnerabilities. They offer cures for every imaginable disease . . . including some that don't even exist . . . and promise to keep us free of vague conditions that can't really be confirmed. Favorite ploys to keep patients in the fold include:

- Promises to "detoxify" the body of various poisonous accumulations (few of which have been shown to exist).
- Pitching a treatment as a "tonic" to prevent a wide range of ailments (when they fail to appear, it's said to be proof that the treatment is working).
- Puffing up trivial problems into

warning signs of a fundamental "imbalance" or "deep-seated" trauma (vague causes that are difficult to demonstrate or disprove).
- Offering "painless," "nontoxic" substitutes for reliable, but frightening treatments.

Unscrupulous practitioners are quick to attach themselves to the disease *du jour* (such as chronic fatigue syndrome, environmental illness, hypoglycemia, or mercury-amalgam toxicity); quote or misquote scientific references; and back up their assertions with testimonials from purportedly satisfied patients.

If a diagnosis seems unfocused or offbeat, take it as a signal to be wary. And when faced with a sales pitch for a universal, "one-size-fits-all" style of therapy, remember that enthusiasm (and even sincere conviction) isn't proof of efficacy and safety. Unless you're suffering from a deficiency disease, no single diet, nutritional supplement, or herb can cure a chronic illness. Likewise, no single product or diet is known to work against all forms of cancer, heart disease, chronic fatigue, or any other health-compromising condition.

Questions to Ask a Prospective Practitioner

As often as not, people choose an alternative practitioner on the basis of a friend's enthusiastic referral. "It worked for me" is a compelling recommendation. Beware, however, of the honeymoon effect. Positive expectations often produce instant cures that later fade away. Be sure to ask your friend how long the therapy has been working, and whether he or she finds it burdensome in terms of costs, daily requirements, or time spent on appointments.

Once you've reached the practitioner, there are several issues to explore before you decide to proceed. Try to get a clear answer to each of the following questions:

- Is the practitioner's belief in the effectiveness of the therapy based on clinical experience with similar patients? If so, is it possible to speak to one of the patients?
- What does the therapy involve and how frequently is it administered?
- How soon will we know whether the therapy is working?
- What is the cost of the initial work up and each subsequent visit? Does the cost include medications? What is the expected total cost for the full course of therapy? Is insurance reimbursement available?
- What are the potential side effects of the treatments?
- Are you willing to share diagnostic findings, therapeutic plans, and follow-up with my regular physician? Are there any limitations on this communication?

A Quick Guide to Alternative Practitioners

Acupuncture. There are about 3,000 U.S. medical doctors and doctors of osteopathy (DOs) who have attended courses in acupuncture and incorporate the therapy in their practice. In addition, there are about 6,500 other acupuncture practitioners. Licensing requirements and regulations vary from state to state. To find an accredited acupuncturist, contact the National Commission for the Certification of Acupuncturists, Washington, DC (202-232-1404) or the American Association for Acupuncture and Oriental Medicine, Catasauqua, Pennsylvania (610-266-1433).

Ayurvedic Medicine. There is no licensing program for Ayurvedic medicine in the U.S. Physicians, chiropractors, nutritionists, and other healers practice it, and the best and most responsible of these encourage patients with serious illness to also see mainstream physicians. Meditation is the most popular of the many Ayurvedic techniques. It has been marketed as Transcendental Meditation and popularized in the work of Deepak Chopra. Training for practitioners and referrals are available from The Ayurvedic Institute, Albuquerque, New Mexico (505-291-9698) and the College of Maharishi AyurVeda Health Center, Fairfield, Iowa (515-472-5866).

Traditional Chinese Medicine. This complete system of health care has been in use for over 3,000 years. In contemporary China, however, it is now used in conjunction with modern Western-style medicine. Practices include acupuncture, acupressure,

TOP ALTERNATIVE TREATMENTS IN THE U.S.

Chiropractic	16%
Lifestyle, diet	8
Exercise/movement	7
Relaxation	7

Source: Astin, JA, *Journal of the American Medical Association*, May 20, 1998, V279, No19: pgs. 1548–1553.

qigong, tai chi, and herbal medication. Most practitioners specialize in either acupuncture or massage. Many states regulate acupuncture but not other aspects of Chinese medicine. For the names of local practitioners contact the American Association of Acupuncture and Oriental Medicine, Raleigh, North Carolina (919-787-5181).

Homeopathy. Homeopathic practitioners are licensed in only four states, and homeopathic remedies are not regulated by the Food and Drug Administration. Medical doctors who offer homeo-

pathic remedies may advertise as such in telephone book listings. Practitioner referrals are available from The National Center for Homeopathy, Alexandria, Virginia (703-548-7790) and The International Foundation for Homeopathy, Seattle, Washington (206-324-8230).

Naturopathy. There are over 1,000 licensed naturopathic doctors (NDs) and two accredited naturopathic medical colleges in the U.S. today. Although a majority of states have no licensing requirements for naturopaths, about 100 insurance companies

MOST FREQUENTLY CITED HEALTH PROBLEMS

Chronic pain	37%
Anxiety	31
Chronic fatigue	31
Sprains/muscle strain	26
Addictive problems	25
Arthritis	25

Source: Astin, JA, *Journal of the American Medical Association*, May 20, 1998, V279, No19: pgs. 1548–1553.

LICENSE REQUIRED

If your state licenses the type of practitioner you're planning to use, make sure that anyone you consider has one. Chiropractors, osteopaths, and of course MDs are licensed in all 50 states.

	Naturopathy	Acupuncture	Massage	Homeopathy
Alabama				
Alaska	•			•
Arizona	•		•	•
Arkansas		•		
California	•			
Colorado	•			
Connecticut	•	•	•	•
Delaware		•		
District of Columbia	•	•		•
Florida	•	•		•
Georgia				
Hawaii	•			•
Idaho				
Illinois	•			
Indiana				
Iowa	•	•		
Kansas				•
Kentucky				
Louisiana	•	•		
Maine	•	•		•
Maryland	•	•		
Massachusetts	•	•		
Michigan				
Minnesota	•			

in the U.S. and Canada now cover naturopathic care. Some health care programs use naturopaths as primary care doctors, requiring them to refer patients to mainstream medical specialists as necessary. Referrals are available from the National Association of Naturopathic Physicians, Seattle, Washington (206-323-7610) and the National College of Naturo-pathic Medicine, Portland, Oregon (503-255-4860).

Chiropractic. This is said to be the most commonly used alternative therapy in the U.S. today. All 50 states require a license, and practitioners must usually attend four years at an accredited institution to be eligible for licensure. Some chiropractors believe im-

	Naturopathy	Acupuncture	Massage	Homeopathy
Mississippi				
Missouri				
Montana	•			•
Nebraska		•		
Nevada	•		•	
New Hampshire	•	•		•
New Jersey	•			
New Mexico	•	•		
New York	•	•		
North Carolina	•			
North Dakota		•		
Ohio		•		
Oklahoma				
Oregon	•	•		•
Pennsylvania	•			
Rhode Island	•	•		
South Carolina	•	•		
South Dakota				
Tennessee	•	•		
Texas	•	•		
Utah	•	•		•
Vermont	•			
Virginia	•	•		
Washington	•	•	•	•
West Virginia	•			
Wisconsin	•			
Wyoming				

proper spinal alignment is the cause of all illnesses; others (the majority today) are mixed types who grant that there are other causes of disease. Many also offer nutritional and wellness advice (although this is not within the scope of their training). For referrals for mixed-type practitioners, contact the American Chiropractic Association, Arlington, Virginia (703-276-8800). For practitioners who rely on spinal manipulation for virtually all ailments, contact the International Chiropractors Association, Arlington, Virginia (703-528-5000).

Osteopathy. Although osteopathy is rooted in manipulation of the spine and joints, in much the same way as chiropractic, it now includes a complete range of mainstream medical techniques. Today, osteopathic physicians are licensed to practice and prescribe in all 50 states, and are covered by health insurance in the same way as medical doctors. Doctors of osteopathy (DOs) complete four years of medical training, followed by one-year internships. Many also complete two-to-six-year residencies in one of 120 medical specialties. For information on "full-service" osteopathy, contact the American Osteopathic Association, Chicago, Illinois (800-621-1773). For information on DOs who specialize in osteopathic manipulative treatments, call the American Academy of Osteopathy, Indianapolis, Indiana (317-879-1881).

Bodywork. Hands-on therapy, often accompanied by movement training, is now available in over 100 different varieties. Some, such as Rolfing and Hellerwork involve deep, forceful massage aimed at releasing ingrained tension. Others, such as the Alexander Technique, the Feldenkrais Method, and Aston-Patterning, focus on movement and posture. Most of these specialized disciplines have their own societies and accreditation schemes. Regular massage is licensed in 25 states.

For more information, contact the following:

Alexander Technique: National Society of Teachers of the Alexander Technique, Minneapolis, Minnesota (800-473-0620).

Aston-Patterning: The Aston Training Center, Inclined Village, Nevada (702-831-8228).

Feldenkrais Method: The Feldenkrais Guild, Albany, Oregon (800-775-2118).

Hellerwork: Hellerwork International, Mount Shasta, California (800-392-3900).

Massage: American Massage Therapy Association, Evanston, Illinois (847-864-0123); National Certification Board for Therapeutic Massage and Bodywork, McLean, Virginia (703-610-9015).

Rolfing: The Rolf Institute, Boulder, Colorado (800-530-8875; 215-545-8079).

Trager Integration: The Trager Institute, Mill Valley, California (415-388-2688).

CHAPTER 4

Necessary Precautions

In the not-too-distant past, the one in three consumers who sought alternative treatments were regarded as ignorant, gullible, or "end-stage neurotic" by the medical establishment. In fact, they tended to be better educated, more affluent, and more health conscious than the average adult.

The idea that aficionados of alternative medicine are a small band of hard-core fanatics is also a myth. In fact, only a small percentage of the patients who make use of alternative medicine have abandoned conventional care. It's much more common to see alternative medicine used in conjunction with mainstream therapies. People employ the safer, gentler forms of alternative medicine to boost their fitness and control troublesome symptoms, while relying on conventional therapy to eradicate underlying disease.

This is as it ought to be. Ideally, traditional and alternative medicine *should* work together, because no single approach can address every aspect of an illness.

Indeed, the best medicine is complementary medicine. In this scenario, traditional medicine identifies the nature of a disorder, and a team of practitioners—both orthodox and alternative—remedy the cause of the problem and its various effects.

It's relatively easy (and safe) to pursue this scenario, provided you take some basic precautions. To get the best of both worlds without falling into the hands of an incompetent or a quack, follow these four simple steps.

Step 1: Make Sure You Know What's Wrong.

The typical alternative practitioner—whether a chiropractor, acupuncturist, or bodywork specialist—is not equipped with the diagnostic skills of the average MD. So when a problem develops, your first stop should always be a mainstream office or clinic. If the ailment lends itself to alternative treatments, you're always free to move on. But at least when you do so, you'll have the assurance that

CONDITIONS THAT THREATEN IRREVERSIBLE DAMAGE

If you suspect you have any of the disorders listed below, be sure to see a conventional physician—even if you're already under the care of an alternative practitioner. These damaging and potentially life-threatening problems must be attacked with everything that modern medicine can offer.

Anemia
Arthritis
Asthma
Cancer
Circulation problems
Coronary artery disease
Depression
Diabetes
Eye disorders
Fractures or dislocations
High blood pressure
Infections
Irregular heartbeat
Poisoning
Stroke

a debilitating or life-threatening disorder isn't waiting undiscovered in the wings.

Diagnosis is one of conventional medicine's greatest strengths, and even a routine check-up can sometimes be a lifesaver. An x-ray, Pap smear, CAT scan, EEG, EKG, mammogram, colonoscopy, or blood test can reveal the presence of disease long before the symptoms become obvious to the patient. While it's true that no test is infallible, Western medical doctors are unquestionably the best at diagnosing disease. And the optimum treatment requires the most accurate diagnosis.

Step 2: Match the Approach to the Problem.

Generally speaking, conventional medicine works best on the source of a problem, while alternative therapy works best on the symptoms. For example, orthodox chemotherapy can eradicate many cancers, while acupuncture can relieve the resulting nausea. Likewise, surgery is mandatory for a burst appendix, while hypnotherapy or transcutaneous electrical nerve stimulation can play an important role in relieving the accompanying pain.

There are, of course, plenty of exceptions. Chiropractic adjustment often proves better for low back pain than conventional drugs or surgery. Likewise, for some arthritis victims, reconstructive therapy (shots in the joints) may prove more effective than the usual prescription drugs.

Nevertheless, as a rule of thumb, it's wise to seek immediate conventional treatment for any sudden, severe problem or life-threatening disorder. You need the very best of high-tech medicine when faced with cancer, stroke, heart attack, respiratory difficulties, severe infection, or serious injury.

Where Alternatives Can Shine

Prevention of serious disorders is an entirely different matter. In this area, alternative strategies often produce results that are as good as—or better than—those of traditional medicine. For example, many experts believe that changes in diet can reduce the risk of cancer. Careful diet plus chromium supplements may alleviate diabetes. Relaxation techniques, a low-fat diet, and vitamins E and B_6 can reduce the risk of heart attack, and may even reverse heart disease. Mineral supplements, meditation, biofeedback, and yoga can all relieve mild high blood pressure as effectively as prescription drugs. Yoga (as well as tai chi and movement training) can also minimize the frequency of injuries among women being treated for osteoporosis.

Alternative medicine holds special promise for the many chronic conditions that still defy conventional treatment. While no one would dispute the importance of discoveries such as anesthesia, antibiotics, the polio vaccine, or open heart surgery, it's clear that traditional Western medicine has yet to fully solve such problems as diabetes, asthma, arthritis, and Alzheimer's disease. For these ailments, certain unconventional treatments offer the possibility of another route to recovery.

Poorly understood conditions characterized by general unwellness or malaise, such as fibromyalgia, chronic fatigue syndrome, environmental illness, food allergies, and some recurrent infections are other potential targets for alternative therapy. Likewise, strains, sprains, and muscle pain often benefit more from bodywork than from any of the treatments that mainstream medicine can offer.

Indeed, chronic and recurring pain are ideal candidates for unconventional therapy. Prescription drugs offer effective relief, but impose significant side effects, and can't be used indefinitely. Bodywork, acupuncture and acupressure, biofeedback, hypnotherapy, and meditation, on the other hand, all hold the promise of genuine pain relief—without danger and without drugs. Many have been found effective for pain ranging from migraines to menstrual cramps. Provided you've ruled out a dangerous underlying cause of the pain, any or all of them are well worth a try.

Other problems deemed susceptible to alternative therapy include the so-called "self-limiting" conditions that usually clear up

DANGER: THESE THERAPIES POSE RISKS

Even the most benign alternative therapy represents a health risk if it's used as a substitute for, rather than as an adjunct to, proven medical treatment for life-threatening or potentially disabling disorders. However, many therapies pose other, more specific dangers for selected individuals. The most significant concerns are listed below. Check the individual therapy profiles for additional cautions.

- *Apitherapy* . . . dangerous for individuals who are allergic to bee venom; pregnant women; and people with heart problems, diabetes, tuberculosis, and other infections.
- *Aromatherapy* . . . risky for pregnant women and individuals with asthma or skin allergies.
- *Biofeedback* . . . a hazard for individuals with a pacemaker or a serious heart condition.
- *Chiropractic* . . . best avoided if you have a fracture, rheumatoid arthritis, or any kind of bone disease.
- *Heat therapy* . . . dangerous for pregnant women and individuals with diabetes, circulation problems, a heart condition, high blood pressure, or decreased sensitivity to hot and cold.
- *Light therapy* . . . not for people with cataracts, glaucoma, or other eye problems.
- *Macrobiotic diet* . . . not recommended for infants, children, or pregnant women without careful medical supervision and nutritional supplementation.
- *Massage* . . . risky for people with a skin disease, circulation disorder, a bone fracture, a dislocation, or cancer.
- *Prolonged fasting* . . . dangerous for children, women who are pregnant or nursing, people on medication, and individuals who have problems with their heart, lungs, or kidneys.
- *Yoga* . . . a hazard after surgery or a recent back injury, and best approached with caution by individuals with heart disease. Some of the more advanced positions can be dangerous for people with high blood pressure and for pregnant women.

on their own, but often take their time doing it. Digestive problems, skin conditions, insomnia, and mild recurrent infections are a few examples. While conventional medicine has excellent remedies for individual outbreaks of such ailments, it has a bit more trouble preventing recurrences. Although there's little definitive evidence in their favor, many forms of alternative therapy do promise a more lasting sort of relief.

Whatever the condition, the best time for alternative treatments and preventive measures is early, before the problem gets out of hand. By the time you're in the hospital undergoing your third angioplasty, it's too late for orthomolecular medicine and yoga to make much difference.

Step 3: Be Quick to Move On When a Treatment Doesn't Work.

There's good reason to be skeptical, impatient, and demanding whenever you undertake an unconventional form of therapy. The majority of these treatments are backed only by testimonials from satisfied recipients, while all the failures go unpublicized. Except for a few of the most widely used alternatives, such as acupuncture, hypnotherapy, biofeedback, yoga, meditation, and nutrition, none of the alternative therapies in use today have been verified by the kind of scientific trials that every new medication is routinely forced to pass.

That doesn't mean a particular alternative won't work for you. After all, most mainstream therapies have never been validated either. A 1978 report from the Congressional Office of Technology Assessment found that no more than 10 to 20 percent of all medical procedures then in use had been proven with randomized, double-blind, placebo-controlled trials (tests in which

neither the patient nor the doctor knows whether the treatment is genuine or fake). And in 1985, the National Academy of Sciences noted that there was still no systematic evaluation of new medical procedures before they came into use.

Still, the lack of critical standards is especially prevalent in the alternative world, and it makes treatment failure a very real possibility. Keep this in mind as you weigh your various alternatives. If you have a progressive or potentially life-threatening condition, you can't afford to waste time on an experimental, unreliable, or phony treatment. You may not get a second chance.

The "Opportunity Cost" of Useless Therapy

Even a harmless alternative treatment can be dangerous to your health if it is used as a substitute for more reliable mainstream care. For instance, guided imagery, acupuncture, herbal remedies, and other alternative treatments can improve your well-being while you're undergoing conventional cancer treatment, but they cannot be used as a substitute for it.

Your mother was right: a stitch in time does, indeed, save nine. The sooner a life-threatening or disabling disease is diagnosed and mainstream treatment begun, the better your chances of survival. An experimental treatment such as hyperthermia may someday be proven useful as a weapon in the fight against cancer, for

WATCHDOG GROUPS

These organizations keep an eye peeled for health care fraud. If you're suspicious of a proposed product or procedure, they may be able to allay your fears—or confirm them.

American Council on Science and Health
1995 Broadway
New York, NY 10023
Phone: 212-362-7044

American Medical Association
Library Answer Center
515 North State St.
Chicago, IL 60610
Phone: 312-464-4818

Consumer Health Information Research Institute
Medical Information Retrieval Center
3521 Broadway
Kansas City, MO 64111
Phone: 816-753-8850

National Council Against Health Fraud
P.O. Box 1276
Loma Linda, CA 92354
Phone: 800-821-6671, 909-824-4690

example, but until then, surgery, radiation, and chemotherapy remain your best bet.

To avoid a potentially dangerous waste of irreplaceable time, look carefully into every treatment suggested to you, regardless of its source, especially if there's any risk involved. Determine how long the treatment has been around and how commonly it's currently being used. Find out how long the treatment should take. Inquire about expected outcomes, or success rates. Be aware of any potential side effects. Ask whether there are better or more proven treatments to accomplish the same goals. If you have any doubts, check on the legitimacy of the treatment with one of the organizations listed in the nearby box.

Step 4. Self-Medicate with Caution.

The resurgence in the popularity of medicinal herbs is at least partly a result of the widespread belief that "natural" remedies are somehow better than conventional drugs. It's an assumption that fails to stand up to careful examination.

For starters, many of today's most popular pharmaceuticals are simply refined herbal extracts, basically every bit as "natural" as their unprocessed cousins. Among them are such old standbys as digitalis, quinine, and aspirin, along with such newly discovered drugs as taxol, an ovarian cancer treatment that's extracted from a species of yew tree. They differ from unprocessed herbal preparations primarily in their potency and purity, both of which are superior.

Many people also have a tendency to think of herbs as safer than conventional drugs; and this too can be false. Most prescription pharmaceuticals are actually extremely safe: although some do indeed have unpleasant, debilitating or dangerous side effects, the majority rarely cause problems. Conversely, while many herbs are in fact as mild and harmless as people suppose, a few can be dangerous . . . or even deadly.

For example, Coltsfoot and Comfrey contain alkaloids proven to cause cancer. Arnica, an herb recommended for bruises and sprains, can cause contact dermatitis. Angelica, Rue, and the wildly popular St. John's Wort can cause an allergic reaction to light. Large quantities of Ginseng can cause sleeplessness, tight muscles, and water retention. Ephedra, source of the popular decongestant drug ephedrine, stimulates the heart and can be extremely dangerous for those with a heart condition. As little as a teaspoonful of the oil in Pennyroyal (a remedy for indigestion) can prove fatal.

Check Potency and Purity

The FDA does not regulate herbal remedies, so strength and quality vary widely from brand to brand, even batch to batch. Some herbal products may contain little if any of the active ingredients you seek. Others may occasionally contain more than you expect, posing the risk of side effects. For instance, herbal constipation remedies—such as Aloe, Buckthorn berries, and Senna—are risky to use, since it's difficult to measure dosages or predict results.

To improve your chances of getting a genuine remedy, ask your doctor and pharmacist about each herb you plan to take, and where to find a reliable source. Try to stick with manufacturers you recognize, and select brands labeled with "standardized" amounts. Don't assume that whole herbs are better than extracts: a purified extract is usually more effective than the unprocessed plant, and a whole herb may contain toxins along with its active ingredient. Don't bother paying extra for "organic" herbs either. The Environmental Protection Agency guards against unacceptable pesticide residues in all plant products.

Be Alert for Interactions

Learn as much as you can about any herb you're taking, not just

THESE HERBS CAN DO HARM

Many people believe that because herbs are "natural," they must be safe. This is not always the case. Ephedra, for example, a plant used in China to treat upper-respiratory ailments for two thousand years (and now taken in the U.S. to boost energy and promote weight loss) has recently caused an estimated 15 deaths. Here's a selection of herbs that the U.S. Food and Drug Administration recommends not be taken orally, as drugs, foods, or beverages.

Common Name	Botanical Name
Arnica, Wolf's Bane, Leopard's Bane, Mountain Tobacco	Arnica montana
Belladonna, Deadly Nightshade	Atropa belladonna
Bittersweet, Dulcamara, Woody Nightshade	Solanum dulcamara
Bloodroot, Red Root	Sanguinaria canadensis
Broomtops, Irish Broom	Cytisus scoparius
Buckeyes, Horse Chestnut	Aesculus hippocastanum
Calamus, Sweet Root, Sweet Cane, Cinnamon Sedge	Acorus calamus
Hemlock, Spotted Hemlock, Spotted Parsley, Spotted Crowbane	Conium maculatum
Henbane, Devil's Eye, Poison Tobacco	Hyoscyamus niger
Jimson Weed, Apple Peru, Jamestown Thornapple	Datura stramonium
Lily-of-the-Valley, May Lily	Convallaria majalis
Lobelia, Indian Tobacco, Wild Tobacco, Asthma Weed, Emetic Weed	Lobelia inflata
Mandrake, Mandragora	Mandragora vernalis
Mandrake, Podophyllum, May Apple, Wild Lemon	Podophyllum peltatum
Mistletoe	Viscum album
Periwinkle, Greater and Lesser Periwinkle	Vinca major and minor
Tonka Bean, Tonquin Bean	Dipteryx odorata
Wahoo Root Bark, Burning Bush, Spindle Tree	Euonymus atropurpureus
Wormwood, Absinthe	Artemisia absinthium

the claims about its effectiveness, but also its potential toxicity and possible drug interactions. Most herbs won't interfere with regular prescription medications, but there are a few exceptions. Be especially cautious if you are taking heart medications, antidepressant drugs, steroid medications, and certain high blood pressure drugs; some herbs can increase their effects.

As with conventional medications, it's best to avoid herbal remedies during pregnancy and while nursing. Virtually none have been tested for safety, and some are known to induce miscarriage. Check with your doctor before taking *any* over-the-counter remedy, herbal or otherwise.

Your Safest Course

To cherry-pick the best that conventional and alternative medicine can offer without compromising your own safety, try to find an up-to-date primary care physician who remains open to innovative therapeutic approaches without advocating any single "complementary" technique. The ideal candidate would be a board-certified family practitioner or an internist affiliated with a teaching hospital who is willing to coordinate a holistic approach to your health, steering you toward appropriate high-quality alternative therapies and away from fraud and quackery.

If you can't find such an ideal mentor, at least choose a doctor you can talk with frankly, a qualified MD who is willing to listen to your concerns, react to your plans, and warn you when an alternative treatment could threaten your health. Likewise, when you seek out an alternative practitioner, select someone who proposes realistic options, targeting specific problems with tested techniques. Avoid miracle-workers who promise to improve every aspect of your health with a single medical "discovery."

If you feel any practitioner— conventional or alternative—isn't doing enough to help, or you want to overcome a condition diagnosed as incurable, discuss the issue openly. If you're not satisfied, consult another professional, preferably one who is regarded as an authority in the field. Trust your instincts, and above all, never be driven by fear or desperation. You have a right to be treated as an intelligent, involved, and critical member of the health care team.

PART TWO

Guide to Alternative and Complementary Therapies

Acupressure

Consider This Therapy For

Clinical studies of this traditional Chinese therapy have yielded encouraging—though not conclusive—results in the treatment of postsurgical nausea and vomiting, including nausea after Cesarean section. The technique also shows promise for relief of nausea and vomiting during pregnancy ("morning sickness") and for prevention of motion sickness. Pressure at a special point on the inside of the wrist, from either the fingers or a small elastic band, has been shown to relieve nausea better than "sham" acupressure delivered elsewhere. Some doctors also regard acupressure as a reasonably effective remedy for headache pain, using points on the hands and feet as well as the neck. And there is general agreement that the technique can relieve muscle and joint aches and pains, promote deep relaxation and relief of tension, and improve general vitality.

On the other hand, although both acupressure and acupuncture have been proposed as weight-loss aids, neither has been found effective during clinical trials. Likewise, the contention that acupressure strengthens disease resistance has not been confirmed by any scientific evidence of improved immune function. Reports that the technique can ease breathing for patients with chronic obstructive lung disease also seem premature.

How the Treatments Are Done

Often called "acupuncture without needles," acupressure seeks to remedy illness through the application of deep finger pressure at points located along an invisible system of energy channels called meridians. Shiatsu is the Japanese version of acupressure. Tuina is a Chinese variation that involves more massage-like kneading motions.

Acupressure may be performed on a floor mat or massage table, and the person receiving the treatment usually wears light, loose clothing. Practitioners may administer pressure to various points using elbows and feet as well as thumbs and fingertips.

Treatment Time: A typical session lasts 30 minutes to 1 hour.

Treatment Frequency: Although Westerners typically seek out acupressure for a particular complaint, such as a stiff neck or aching back, traditional Oriental medicine views this therapy as a way to maintain health and keep vital energy in balance. For this purpose, acupressure may be administered on a regular basis; and pressure on many points can be self-administered as often as desired for relief of minor daily problems such as headache, tired eyes, and nervous tension.

What Treatment Hopes to Accomplish

According to the principals of traditional Oriental medicine, the body's vital energy (called *ch'i* or *qi* in Chinese and *ki* in Japanese) flows along 14 meridians that connect vital organs throughout the body. Over the several thousand years that this system has been in use, Oriental physicians have mapped hundreds of sensitive "acupoints" along these meridians. A blockage in the flow of *ch'i* at one point on a meridian can, it's believed, cause disease and discomfort in an organ or tissue further down the line. Hence, an acupressurist may seek to relieve a problem in the head by using deep massage to break up a blockage of *ch'i* in the foot.

Western medical science has found no evidence that meridians exist, although some acupoints have been shown to coincide with nerve trigger points. However, as with any massage, acupressure can definitely be relaxing (although it may cause some transient discomfort in sensitive or tense areas). Some researchers also theorize that acupressure, like acupuncture, may work by prompting the body to release natural pain-killing compounds such as endorphins.

Who Should Avoid This Therapy?

Although treatments are administered in a slow, steady manner, they can involve very forceful pressure, and thus may not be a prudent choice for a person with brittle bones (osteoporosis) or a history of spinal or other orthopedic injury or easy bruising. They should also be avoided if you have a bleeding disorder, take anticoagulant drugs, or are undergoing long-term steroid therapy, which can make the tissues fragile.

Acupressure is traditionally recommended to ease discomforts of pregnancy and childbirth. However, as with any treatment during pregnancy, it's best to consult a doctor first, and to avoid any pressure near the abdominal area.

Acupressure in the legs and feet could prove damaging if you have circulation problems resulting from diabetes or varicose veins. It could also aggravate carpal tunnel syndrome, which is, at the outset, a result of pressure on a nerve. Caution should also be used near fragile or irritated skin, sores, and wounds.

What Side Effects May Occur?

After an acupressure session, some people report feeling light-headed or slightly groggy for a while. Lasting soreness is also a possibility. Usually attributed to "released energy" or "released toxins," it is more often the result of trauma to soft tissue or tendons that may already be inflamed. If treatments are painful, or result in extended discomfort, be sure to let the therapist know.

How to Choose a Therapist

Acupressure is administered by a wide variety of practitioners under many styles and guises. Elements of the technique are found in many types of bodywork and massage therapy. Some practitioners hew to a traditional Oriental style of practice, sometimes combined with other components of traditional Oriental medicine such as herbology. Other, more Westernized practitioners dismiss the philosophical angle and regard the meridians as a system of neurological trigger points.

There is currently no widely accepted, standard credentialing agency for acupressure. The National Commission for the Certification of Acupuncturists and Oriental Medicine has recently begun a certification program for practitioners of "Oriental body-work therapy," including acupressure and Shiatsu, but fewer than 100 practitioners have applied for and received certification thus far.

When Should Treatment Stop?

If you regard acupressure as a way of toning the body and tuning up your general health and well-being, then "treatment" is more like preventive maintenance, and may be continued indefinitely. For acute problems, several weeks of therapy is a reasonable time in which to expect some relief.

See a Conventional Doctor If . . .

Acupressure alone is not considered an effective form of therapy for any major or life-threatening ailments, although it can certainly be used to complement conventional Western medical regimens as a means of relieving tension and stress. If you have any symptoms that could signal an acute medical problem (such as chest pain) or symptoms that become worse (such as a headache that is unusually severe or won't go away), consult a physician.

Resources

ORGANIZATIONS

Acupressure Institute
1533 Shattuck Ave.
Berkeley, CA 94709
Phone: 510-845-1059
This organization, which provides training in various styles of

acupressure, also offers the public general information and a mail-order catalog of publications.

National Commission for the Certification of Acupuncturists and Oriental Medicine (NCCAOM)
1424 16th St., NW, Suite 501
Washington, DC 20036
Phone: 202-232-1404
Web: www.nccaom.org

FURTHER READING

The Complete Illustrated Guide to Shiatsu: The Japanese Healing Art of Touch for Health. Elaine Liechti. Rockport, MA: Element Books Inc., 1998.

Acupuncture

Consider This Therapy For

Acupuncture is promoted as a treatment for pain—and there is absolutely no question that it does in fact provide short-term benefit for many of the people who try it. By some estimates, between 50 and 70 percent of patients with chronic pain receive at least temporary relief when treated with acupuncture, and some experience long-term relief as well.

However, doctors are still debating whether this type of therapy has any effect beyond that of a placebo (a fake treatment with no real activity). It's a difficult question to resolve because most placebos are actually quite potent. Dummy pills typically achieve a relief rate of 30 to 35 percent, and a sham procedure, accompanied by suitably impressive instruments and rituals, can be effective more than 50 percent of the time. Indeed, in tests comparing genuine acupuncture with an imitation, patients receiving the fake treatment usually enjoy just about as much relief (50 percent) as those given the real thing.

Of course, if your only concern is pain relief (as opposed to a cure of the underlying problem), it doesn't really matter whether acupuncture's effects are physical or merely psychological, as long as you feel better. And there is, in any event, mounting proof of acupuncture's genuine value. According to an expert consensus panel convened by the National Institutes of Health (NIH) in 1997, well-performed scientific studies have provided evidence of acupuncture's efficacy in relieving pain after dental surgery and in reducing the nausea and vomiting associated with pregnancy ("morning sickness"), chemotherapy, and anesthesia. Other research suggests that acupuncture may be useful—along with other, more conventional therapies—for asthma, osteoarthritis, low back pain, headache (both tension and migraine), menstrual cramps, carpal tunnel syndrome, fibromyalgia, and other conditions that cause chronic pain.

Two other intriguing areas are currently under research. One is the use of acupuncture in easing withdrawal from addiction to hard drugs and alcohol; acupuncture, especially of the outer ear, is in use at many detoxification clinics in the United States. (Similar results have not been observed for tobacco addiction, however.) Another possibility is that acupuncture therapy may speed rehabilitation and limit damage after a paralyzing stroke.

How the Treatments Are Done

The "puncture" in acupuncture refers to insertion of tiny needles at certain very specific points on the surface of the body. The treatments vary widely, depending on the individual practitioner and the style of acupuncture. There are several "schools," including Chinese, Korean, Japanese, and a westernized version (based on neurology, not Oriental medical philosophy) called trigger-point therapy. Most practitioners of Oriental-style acupuncture perform at least a partial physical examination at the first visit (including extensive pulse-taking and, possibly, examination of the tongue and palpation of the abdomen). They also tend to take a very detailed medical history, including nutritional habits and other environmental factors.

The actual insertion of the hair-thin, disposable needles has been described as feeling like a mosquito bite. After insertion, the needles may be stimulated by twirling them or connecting them to a mild electrical current (there is no risk of electrical shock). This stimulation may cause a mild tingling or aching sensation referred to as "de qi." The nee-

dles may be inserted from a fraction of an inch up to about one inch deep. They can either be withdrawn a few seconds after insertion or kept in place for up to 30 minutes.

Treatment Time: Typically, you should allow 20 minutes to 1 hour per session. The initial visit may take longer.

Treatment Frequency: This varies according to the problem. You may start out with several treatments per week, then taper to weekly or less often. Duration of therapy may range from a few treatments for acute, temporary problems to regularly scheduled treatments over several months for chronic conditions.

What Treatment Hopes to Accomplish

Acupuncture has been practiced in China for several thousand years, although this traditional healing art didn't catch Americans' interest until the early 1970s, when a Western reporter in Beijing received acupuncture for postoperative pain (after undergoing an appendectomy under conventional general anesthesia).

How acupuncture works remains a mystery. According to ancient Chinese medical theory, the life force (called *qi* or *ch'i* and pronounced "chee") flows through the body via 14 invisible channels (called meridians), regulating all physical and mental processes. Opposing forces within the body, called yin and yang, must be balanced to keep *ch'i* flowing properly. The meridians supposedly run deep within the body's tissues and organs, surfacing at some 360 places identified as acupuncture points, sometimes called acupoints. Certain meridians are identified with organs such as the bladder or liver, and the points all along such meridians—even in the hands or feet—are believed capable of affecting the associated internal organ. Stimulating these points is said to balance and restore the flow of *ch'i*.

An explanation proposed by Western scientists is that acupuncture may trigger the release of natural pain-killing substances within the body called endorphins, thus blunting the perception of pain. It may also alter the body's output of neurotransmitters such as serotonin and norepinephrine, and of inflammation-causing substances such as prostaglandins. Like the manipulation of *ch'i*, however, this explanation has yet to be conclusively documented.

Whatever the cause may be, the pain-relieving effects of acupuncture seem to have a delayed onset; they increase slowly, even after removal of the needles, and may become more evident after several treatments. The effects may diminish after acupuncture treatments are ended.

Who Should Avoid This Therapy?

In general, there are no medical conditions that rule out the use of acupuncture except, perhaps, a morbid fear of needles. People at risk of easy bruising or excessive bleeding (for example, patients with clotting disorders and those taking a blood-thinning medication) would be prudent to avoid acupuncture, since there is a slight risk of damage to blood vessels. Pregnant women should avoid needle insertion on or near the abdomen.

What Side Effects May Occur?

Acupuncture has no inherent side effects. However, careless application of the technique can present certain hazards. There have been documented cases of hepatitis B transmission and serious bacterial infection due to improperly sterilized needles, a problem that has been controlled by the widespread use of disposable needles. Improperly performed acupuncture can also cause bleeding (if a blood vessel is punctured) or injury to organs, nerves, or tissue, making it important to find a skilled and reputable practitioner.

How to Choose a Therapist

At least 35 states require some form of licensure or certification for the practice of acupuncture. In unregulated states, acupuncture is technically illegal unless performed by a physician, although this ban is rarely enforced.

Educational requirements for licensure vary by state, and this regulatory patchwork makes it difficult to judge an acupuncturist's credentials. Even the titles vary; an acupuncturist may be "licensed," "certified," or "registered," and in a few states may even have the title of "doctor" of acupuncture or Oriental Medicine. Just to make matters more confusing, these titles bear no consistent relationship to educational requirements, which range from 1,300 to 2,600 hours of training (usually in an accredited school or college of acupuncture). Surprisingly, the least qualified practitioners may be physicians, who are permitted to practice acupuncture with no training at all (although most have attended at least a few courses).

There are about 10,000 licensed, registered, or certified acupuncturists in the U.S., and an additional 3,000 medical doctors (MDs) or doctors of osteopathy (DOs) who practice the technique. To learn more about qualification standards and practitioners in your state, contact the groups listed under "Resources." Two of them may prove particularly helpful. The Accreditation Commission for Acupuncture and Oriental Medicine sets standards for acupuncture schools throughout the United States, and can send you a list of accredited schools. The National Certification Commission for Acupuncture and Oriental Medicine (NCCAOM) administers a standardized examination testing theoretical and practical knowledge of acupuncture. Those passing this test must meet continuing education requirements every two years in order to retain certification. There are currently 5,000 practitioners who have achieved certification, and an increasing number of states are using the examination as part of the requirements for acupuncture licensure. When choosing a therapist, you should check to see whether he graduated from an accredited school and whether he has received NCCAOM certification.

Unfortunately, no degree or license can reveal the most important variable: skill and talent. Before undergoing treatment, you may also wish to learn more about the practitioner's approach and philosophy. Some practitioners combine acupuncture with other aspects of traditional Chinese medicine, such as the use of traditional herbal remedies and the technique called moxibustion (applying a smoldering cone of herbal material to the skin at an acupuncture point). If your experience with one acupuncturist is negative, remember that it's possible for a different practitioner to produce better results.

When Should Treatment Stop?

According to the NIH panel, if you haven't obtained relief after 10 sessions of acupuncture, the therapy isn't working and should be stopped. In general, chronic pain relief should be perceptible after about six sessions if it's going to happen at all; relief of conditions such as asthma tends to take longer, sometimes months. A responsible acupuncturist will acknowledge when treatment seems to be ineffective and won't pressure you to continue.

See a Conventional Doctor If . . .

Check with a doctor if you develop any symptoms that might signal a serious illness. Even if traditional Chinese medical theory holds true, and acupuncture has overall health-giving benefits, there are better treatments available for many specific illnesses. Pain, whether chronic or acute, is a red flag for countless medical conditions—some minor, some life-threatening. Any new, persistent, or worsening pain should be evaluated by a medical doctor before you seek relief through acupuncture.

Resources

ORGANIZATIONS

National Commission for the Certification of Acupuncturists and Oriental Medicine (NCCAOM)

1424 16th St., NW, Suite 501
Washington, DC 20036
Phone: 202-232-1404
Web: www.nccaom.org
This group provides certification for practitioners of acupuncture, Chinese herbology, and Oriental bodywork therapy such as Shiatsu.

Accreditation Commission for Acupuncture and Oriental Medicine (ACAOM)

Phone: 301-608-9680
This group sets standards for acupuncture schools and can provide a list of accredited institutions.

American Academy of Medical Acupuncture (AAMA)

Phone: 800-521-2262
This is a telephone referral service for acupuncturists who are also medical doctors.

American Association of Acupuncture and Oriental Medicine (AAAOM)

Phone: 610-266-1433
This group can provide nationwide referrals for licensed or registered practitioners.

National Acupuncture and Oriental Medicine Alliance (NAOMA)

Phone: 253-851-6896
Web: www.acuall.org
This group provides general information on acupuncture and referrals by mail for state licensed or nationally certified acupuncturists.

FURTHER READING

Between Heaven and Earth: A Guide to Chinese Medicine. Harriet Beinfield and Efrem Korngold. New York: Ballantine Books, 1991.

Acupuncture: How It Works, How It Cures. Peter Firebrace and Sandra Hill. New Canaan, CT: Keats Publishing Inc., 1994.

The Web That Has No Weaver. Ted Kaptchuk. New York: Congdon & Weed, 1983.

The Layman's Guide to Acupuncture. Yoshio Manaka. Weatherhill, 1972.

Alexander Technique

Consider This Therapy For

The goal of this discipline is to bring the body's muscles into natural harmony. Hence it can aid in the treatment of a wide variety of neurological and musculoskeletal conditions, including disorders of the neck, back, and hip; traumatic and repetitive strain injuries; chronic pain; arthritis; breathing and coordination disorders; stress related disorders; and even migraine.

People with sciatica, scoliosis, osteoporosis, osteoarthritis, rheumatoid arthritis, and neck and low back syndrome may find the Alexander Technique useful in improving overall strength and mobility. Others with Lyme disease, chronic fatigue syndrome, lupus, or fibromyalgia may use it for pain management. It is also used to improve functioning in people with multiple sclerosis, stroke, or Parkinson's disease.

Because the technique requires active participation by the patient, it's impossible to test its effectiveness with customary scientific procedures, such as "placebo controls," in which some patients are given a fake remedy, and "double-blind trials," in which neither the patients nor the therapists know who's receiving genuine treatment. Nevertheless, many people who've undertaken this therapy, including the likes of John Dewey and Aldous Huxley, vouch for its benefits.

How the Treatments Are Done

Alexander Technique sessions are most often conducted one-on-one with a teacher, but group classes may be available as well. Students wear comfortable clothing, and perform everyday actions, such as walking, bending, standing, or sitting, while the teacher encourages the students to shed ingrained—and inappropriate—muscular reactions and allow healthy natural reflexes to take over. To encourage the release of natural reactions, the teacher will lead a student through various movements, occasionally touching the neck, back, or shoulder to help trigger the proper reflexes. Some sessions may have the student lying down most of the time, while others involve mostly sitting and standing. If there is a specific movement the student wishes to improve, such as working at a computer keyboard, holding a telephone, or driving a car, the teacher may work with the student on those as well. Teachers stress that the Alexander Technique is not a passive experience, such as a massage. However, the sessions are not strenuous or physically taxing. No machinery is used.

Treatment Time: The length of each session varies from teacher to teacher, but usually ranges from 30 to 45 minutes.

Treatment Frequency: Sessions may be weekly or more often, depending on the teacher and your needs. The recommended series is a set of 30 lessons.

What Treatment Hopes to Accomplish

With advancing age, most people seem to fall into a variety of common, but unnatural, habits of movement and posture. Depending on the amount of energy and tension these habits commandeer, the results can range from subtle changes in mood to outright pain. The Alexander Technique attempts to remedy these problems by discouraging habitual, counterproductive muscular reactions and allowing efficient natural reflexes to take over.

When you begin training in the Alexander Technique, the goal is to inhibit your habitual muscular responses by deliberately and consciously "doing nothing" so that your body can revert to its inherent natural movements. This is not an exercise in relaxation, per se, but rather a way of reclaiming an efficiency and ease of movement lost through years of poor postures and unnatural muscular response. As you "unlearn" inappropriate habits in the formal sessions, you'll be encouraged to practice your new freedom of movement as you go about your normal activities.

Unlike other bodywork disciplines, such as the Feldenkrais Method, the Alexander Technique focuses on the relationship of head, neck, and torso, which teachers call "primary control." Alexander Technique teachers believe that when these three are properly aligned, the head will lift upward and release the neck and spine, improving overall muscular function and allowing you to move your whole body in a harmonious way. Central to the technique are the four "Concepts of Good Use," which focus on freeing the muscles from unneeded tension:

Allow your neck to release so your head can balance forward and up;

Allow your torso to release into length and width;

Allow your legs to release away from your pelvis;

Allow your shoulders to release out to the sides.

The Alexander Technique was developed in the early 1900s by Australian actor F.M. Alexander, who felt that his own bad posture had caused his voice-loss problems. He began working on a system to teach simple, efficient movements that would help improve balance, posture, and coordination while relieving pain. The resulting technique became popular in the U.S. after the first World War, especially among artists, performers, and intellectuals, and has been practiced successfully ever since. Today, the Alexander Technique is used not only by those seeking pain relief, but also by many actors, dancers, athletes, and other performers who use their bodies intensively.

Who Should Avoid This Therapy?

The Alexander Technique is generally considered safe for everyone. However, if you have any chronic health problems, it's wise to check with your doctor before undertaking any form of alternative therapy.

What Side Effects May Occur?

With its emphasis on efficient release of natural muscular reflexes, the Alexander Technique has no known side effects.

How to Choose a Therapist

Make sure your teacher is certified by the North American Society of Teachers of the Alexander Technique. This professional organization has well-established programs and requires members to take at least 1,600 hours of training over a three-year period, observe minimum teacher-to-student ratios, and follow set guidelines for conducting their classes. While no special background is required to become a teacher, many practitioners are dancers or other performers who have found the technique useful in their own lives.

When Should Treatment Stop?

You may continue the Alexander Technique classes as long as you wish.

See a Conventional Doctor If . . .

Because the scope of the Alexander Technique is limited to problems with movement and posture, you'll need to continue regular medical treatment for any non-muscular disorders such as infection or inflammation. Check with your doctor, too, if you experience any new symptoms while participating in Alexander Technique sessions.

Resources

ORGANIZATIONS

American Center for the Alexander Technique (ACAT)
129 West 67th St.
New York, NY 10023
Phone: 212-799-0468

North American Society of Teachers of the Alexander Technique (NASTAT)
3010 Hennepin Ave. South
Minneapolis, MN 55408
Phone: 800-473-0620

FURTHER READING

The Alexander Technique: How to Use Your Body Without Stress. Wilfred Barlow, MD. Healing Arts Press, 1991.
Back Trouble. Deborah Caplan. Triad Publishing, 1987.
Body Learning. Michael J. Gelb. Henry Holt, 1996.
Your Guide to the Alexander Technique. John Gray. St. Martin's Press, 1991.

Apitherapy

Consider This Therapy For

The exotic substances produced by bees have been invested with assorted medicinal powers since the dawn of history. The venom from bee stings, for instance, has been recommended as a remedy for arthritis since the time of the ancient Egyptians. And modern advocates of apitherapy still hold great faith in the powers of so-called royal jelly, which they say can boost energy and ease the symptoms of premenstrual syndrome. Apitherapy has, in fact, been promoted for everything from chronic pain, back pain, and migraines to such disorders as hair loss, poor vision, gout, asthma, certain skin conditions, loss of memory, and poor bladder control.

Despite all these claims, modern clinical testing has failed to reveal any medicinal value in the various by-products of bees. Indeed, the only currently accepted application of apitherapy is in desensitization treatments for people with a potentially life-threatening allergy to bee stings. For such individuals, controlled exposure to tiny amounts of bee venom can help build a protective tolerance.

Lately there has also been much speculation about a potential role for bee venom in the treatment of multiple sclerosis. The Multiple Sclerosis Society has provided a research grant to study the possibility, and The International Apiary Society reportedly is tracking 4,500 people with multiple sclerosis for the same purpose. However, the jury remains out on the treatment's real value, and few doctors recommend it—at least for now.

What Treatment Hopes to Accomplish

Five bee-generated substances fall under the rubric of apitherapy. Each is credited with various health benefits, though none has been conclusively shown to deliver them.

BEE VENOM

Advocates contend that bee venom, when injected directly into the joints, provides an effective remedy for rheumatoid arthritis. They believe that the highly inflammatory venom triggers such an outpouring of anti-inflammatory hormones that there are plenty left over to ease the pain and swelling of the disease. However, while some arthritis victims have indeed reported relief, the effectiveness of such therapy has never been confirmed by scientific tests.

ROYAL JELLY

This substance has a major impact—on bees. When fed to an ordinary female bee, it extends her life twenty-fold and enables her to produce twice her weight in eggs. Perhaps it's this life-giving effect on the queen bee that suggested the possibility of an energizing property in humans. Unfortunately, there's no scientific evidence that any such property exists.

BEE POLLEN

Promoted as an energy boosting nutritional supplement, the pollen collected by bees does in fact contain vitamins, minerals, sugar, protein, and fat. However, so does ordinary food, and the purported advantages of bee pollen over other sources of nutrition are debatable at best. Don't, for instance, rely on bee pollen as a good source of protein. Ounce for ounce, you'll get more from a sirloin steak.

Some athletes claim that bee pollen supplements improve their athletic performance. However, scientific tests have so far failed to reveal any difference. Other advocates believe that bee pollen helps fight infection. In this case, quite the opposite seems to hold true: not only does bee pollen fail to kill infection, it actually helps feed the invading germs. Another enduring myth holds that bee pollen slows the aging process. However, this claim is based on the longevity of a particular group of people who, when ultimately studied, didn't appear to consume any bee pollen whatsoever.

RAW HONEY

Advocates tout raw honey as a quick source of energy and a natural supply of several minerals and B-complex vitamins. To the extent that it contains glucose, the form of sugar most readily converted to energy, these claims are no doubt true. However, the amount of difference this makes in actual practice is subject to debate.

PROPOLIS

Bees manufacture this waxy substance from a tar-like material they collect from trees. Advocates say it has antioxidant properties that can protect the body's cells from damage by free radicals. Its beneficial effects have yet to be scientifically verified, however.

Who Should Avoid This Therapy?

Before undertaking any type of apitherapy, be sure to get tested for an allergy to bee venom. Life-threatening allergic reactions have occurred after a single exposure to the venom—or to a single dose of royal jelly. Even if you've been stung in the past without apparent harm, you may still have developed an allergy since then. Allergies usually don't surface with the first sting, but once you've been sensitized, a second sting can send you into shock.

For some people, even the slightest risk of a reaction simply can't be justified. If you have a heart condition, for instance, you should avoid all forms of apitherapy. Those with diabetes, tuberculosis, or other types of infections should also be wary. It's wise, too, to avoid apitherapy during pregnancy.

What Side Effects May Occur?

People receiving bee venom treatments are likely to experience pain, inflammation, stiffness, soreness, and itching . . . as anyone who has ever had a bee sting knows. Of more concern is the possibility of a severe and potentially life-threatening reaction in someone unaware that he's allergic. Due to the danger of such a reaction, many practitioners believe treatments should be administered only in the presence of a physician.

How to Choose a Therapist

According to the American Apitherapy Society, which has 1,600 members, there are some 10,000 people who perform apitherapy. For more information, or for a referral, contact the society at 800-823-3460. Check with your physician as well. Doctors who believe in apitherapy can often make referrals.

When Should Treatment Stop?

It is probably wise to discontinue treatment if the discomfort becomes intolerable or the therapy isn't helping.

See a Conventional Doctor If . . .

If your symptoms fail to improve, or any new symptoms appear, your best course is to discuss the situation with your doctor. For most problems, other, more effective remedies are available.

Resources

ORGANIZATIONS

American Apitherapy Society, Inc. (AAS)
P.O. Box 54
Hartland Four Corners,
VT 05049
Phone: 800-823-3460

Applied Kinesiology

Consider This Therapy For

A melange of concepts derived from chiropractic, acupuncture, and nutrition, applied kinesiology claims to be both a diagnostic technique and an approach to therapy. It holds that various muscles are associated with specific organs and glands, and that weakness in a muscle can signal a problem elsewhere in the body (for instance, a weak deltoid muscle may reflect a problem in the lungs or a nutritional deficiency affecting the respiratory system). Likewise, correcting a muscular problem can relieve a disorder in associated organs (for instance, strengthening certain leg muscles can stimulate the adrenal glands).

There is no evidence that such relationships exist, and even practitioners of applied kinesiology say the technique should be used in conjunction with "other standard diagnostic methods." They recommend it for a variety of muscle problems, for treatment of temporomandibular joint (jaw) disorders, and for diagnosis of various nutritional deficiencies and food allergies. Mainstream physicians dismiss it completely, saying it plays "no role in scientific health care."

How the Treatments Are Done

Each applied kinesiologist has his own style, but most practitioners are likely to begin with an analysis of your posture, gait, and range of joint motion. The session is likely to include tests to see whether various muscles can hold a given position against manual pressure from the practitioner. A muscle that can do so is considered "fixed," "strong," or "locked." A muscle that gives way immediately is considered "weak" or "unlocked."

The practitioner may also ask you to touch certain areas of your body while he repeats the muscle test. This is believed to help isolate the source of your trouble. To evaluate nutritional deficiencies, he may assess muscle strength while touching various points along the acupuncture meridians (the pathways along which, according to traditional Chinese medicine, the life force is believed to flow). Some practitioners also test nutrients by placing them on the tongue for 10 to 20 seconds at a time. (If a taste of the substance strengthens a weak muscle, you are said to have a deficiency.) Alternatively, you might be told to hold a box containing capsules of the nutrient against your abdomen.

Treatments vary according to the diagnosis, but may include deep massage, joint manipulation and realignment, cranial therapy (supposed adjustment of the bones that, fused together, make up the skull), meridian therapy, nutritional therapy, and diet management.

What Treatment Hopes to Accomplish

Applied kinesiology is a relatively recent outgrowth of chiropractic. It was devised in the 1960s by George J. Goodheart, Jr., a chiropractor who focused on muscular dysfunction rather than joint abnormalities. Its goals, as set forth by the International College of Applied Kinesiology, are to:

- Provide a non-equipment-intensive assessment of the patient's functional health status,
- Restore postural balance, correct impaired gait, improve range of motion,
- Restore normal neuromuscular function,
- Achieve balance of endocrine, immune, digestive, and other internal functions, and
- Permit early intervention in degenerative diseases.

Although weakness in a specific muscle is said to be a clue to possible problems in its associated organ or gland, practitioners do not claim that the results are diagnostically definitive. They say that improper performance in a manual muscle test may be due to nerve dysfunction, nutritional inadequacy, toxic chemicals, abnormal circulation of the cerebrospinal fluid that bathes the brain and spinal cord, tension in the membranes surrounding the brain and spinal cord, poor circulation of blood or lymph fluid, or "meridian system imbalance."

Likewise, the International College of Applied Kinesiology warns that muscle testing alone is not sufficient for determining a person's nutritional needs. Indeed, there is no known physiological mechanism that explains how evaluation of muscles could reveal nutritional status, or how a brief exposure to a nutrient could correct a deficiency severe enough to cause muscle weakness. (Some practitioners have theorized that nutrient deficiencies disrupt the flow of energy within the body, and that the energy emanating from nutrients held in the mouth or against the abdomen can re-establish the flow and restore muscle function.)

Attempts to verify the effectiveness of applied kinesiology through scientific testing have met with scant success. One recent review in a chiropractic journal found little favorable clinical research in support of the technique. Another critique of 20 reports published by the International College of Applied Kinesiology found that none excluded the possibility that the results were simply due to chance.

Comparisons between applied kinesiology and other diagnostic techniques have also fared poorly. A study that evaluated the thyroid function of 65 people using standard methods and applied kinesiology techniques concluded that a doctor using clinical and laboratory observations has the greatest assurance of a correct diagnosis, and that applied kinesiology enhanced but did not replace standard diagnosis of thyroid function. In another study, diagnosis of nutritional deficiencies by three applied kinesiologists proved no more accurate than random guessing. The practitioners agreed with each other in only 12 of 44 instances.

Who Should Avoid This Therapy?

There are no medical conditions that preclude the use of applied kinesiology. Remember, however, that it should be used only as an adjunct to conventional diagnosis and treatment, and that the practitioner should have substantial medical training.

What Side Effects May Occur?

No major side effects are likely.

How to Choose a Therapist

The discipline's professional society, the International College of Applied Kinesiology, suggests using only a health care professional licensed to diagnose medical problems, such as an MD, DO, or chiropractor. It warns that others who use applied kinesiology techniques lack the expertise to properly perform examinations and interpret findings.

To be considered a bona fide applied kinesiologist, a doctor or chiropractor must complete 100 hours of training from a teacher certified by the College and must pass the College's exam. Certified teachers, in turn, must log at least 300 hours of study under another certified teacher, complete 5,000 hours of practical experience, write two research papers per year, and pass written and practical examinations.

To locate a practitioner meeting these standards, check with the International College (see "Resources," on page 65).

When Should Treatment Stop?

Because the effectiveness of this technique is considered doubtful by the majority of medical experts, don't hesitate to seek an different form of therapy if immediate improvement fails to appear.

See a Conventional Doctor If . . .

There is a very real possibility of misdiagnosis if you rely solely on applied kinesiology. Your wisest course is to get a second opinion from a standard physician, no matter what your applied kinesiology practitioner may recommend.

Resources

ORGANIZATIONS

International College of Applied Kinesiology
6405 Metcalf Ave., Suite 503
Shawnee Mission, KS 66202
Phone: 913-384-5336
Fax: 913-384-5512
Web: www.icakusa.com

FURTHER READING

Alternative Medicine: The Definitive Guide. The Burton Goldberg Group. Puyallup, WA: Future Medicine Publishing, Inc., 1994.

Applied Kinesiology: Muscle-Testing for "Allergies" and "Nutrient Deficiencies." S. Barrett. Quackwatch, May 1998 (www.quackwatch.com).

Applied Kinesiology Status Statement. International College of Applied Kinesiology-USA, June 16, 1992 (www.icakusa.com).

Reader's Guide to Alternative Health Methods. J.F. Zwicky, et al. Chicago, IL: American Medical Association, 1993.

Aromatherapy

Consider This Therapy For

Aromatherapy is one of those rare forms of treatment that can improve your quality of life whether or not it has any other benefits. That's just as well, because few doctors believe it has any significant effects on health. Whatever relief it confers, they speculate, stems from emotional response to aromatherapy's pleasing scents, rather than any physiological effects.

Used as a comforting ritual to reduce stress, enhance relaxation, and relieve anxiety, aromatherapy may indeed improve your well-being, relieve psychosomatic symptoms, and alleviate some emotionally-related disorders. For some people, it has provided a respite from insomnia. Others have found it an effective remedy for impotence. A few people even report that it eases the pain of arthritis and relieves postpartum discomfort. However, medical science can find no physical reason for these effects.

How the Treatments Are Done

Although many gift boutiques have taken to marketing scented candles, pomanders, and potpourri as "aromatherapy," genuine treatments rely on the use of highly concentrated essential oils extracted from various healing herbs. In most cases, these oils are produced by steam distillation or cold pressing from a plant's flowers, leaves, branches, bark, rind, or roots. The volatile, flammable oils are then mixed with a "carrier"—usually a vegetable oil such as soy, evening primrose, or almond—or diluted in alcohol before being applied to the skin, sprayed in the air, or inhaled.

Although you can pursue treatments under the supervision of a certified aromatherapist, many people simply use the oils as a form of home remedy. There is a notable lack of agreement on such issues as the amount of oil necessary to achieve a desired effect, the most effective method of administration, and the length of time necessary to continue treatment.

However, some of the more typical approaches are as follows:

Inhalation: For problems with respiration, try adding 6 to 12 drops of essential oil to a bowl of steaming water. Place a towel over your head, and deeply breathe the scented vapors.

Diffusion: Aromatherapists often suggest spraying oil-containing compounds into the air. This technique is said to calm the nerves, enhance a feeling of well-being, and even to improve respiratory conditions. In any case, it freshens the air. Commercially available spray units can be used. Add 10 drops of an essence to 7 tablespoonfuls of water. If you will not be using the entire amount at one time, add 1 tablespoonful of vodka or pure alcohol as a preservative. Shake the mixture and fill the sprayer.

Massage: Rubbing aromatic oil into the skin may be either calming or stimulating, depending on the type of oil used. Some people use it as a remedy for muscle sprains and soreness. Most preparations contain 5 drops of essential oil blended with a light base oil. A higher concentration could irritate the skin.

Bathing: Use no more than 8 drops in a bath. Add the oil to a tubful of water. You can also add 10 to 15 drops to a Jacuzzi or hot tub, 4 to 5 drops to a foot bath, or 3 to 4 drops to a hand bath (for chapped skin). If you shower, after washing yourself, dip a wet sponge or cloth in an oil-water mixture and apply to your skin while you are under the spray. Do not use this technique if you have any skin allergies.

Hot and cold compresses: For muscle aches or pains, bruises, or headaches add 5 to 10 drops of oil to approximately 4 ounces of water. Soak a cloth in the solution and apply to the sore area.

Other aromatherapy techniques include placing 2 or 3 drops of essential oil on a pillow or shoe rack, heating the essential oil in a ring burner, or sprinkling the oil over the logs in a fireplace.

Warning: Never take aromatherapy oils internally. They are extremely potent and many can be poisonous.

What Treatment Hopes to Accomplish

Fragrant oils have been used for thousands of years to lubricate the skin, purify infectious air, and repel insects. However, aromatherapy as we know it today dates from the late 1930s, when René-Maurice Gattefosse, a French chemist, dunked his badly burned hand into a container of pure lavender oil. Amazingly, the pain and redness disappeared and the burn healed within hours. In later experiments he found that other oils also alleviated skin problems. Other French scientists who were impressed with his research, developed techniques that are still in use today.

Aromatherapy first appeared on this side of the Atlantic in the early 1980s, when there was an upsurge in the popularity of "natural," nontoxic healing methods that cost less than conventional medications and produced fewer side effects. Practitioners in California used essential oils to treat everything from viral and bacterial infections to depression, anxiety, and sexually transmitted diseases. They insisted aromas could heal wounds, stimulate the immune system, cure skin disorders, improve circulation, relieve pain, reduce swelling, and even improve memory. According to these enthusiastic therapists, fragrant oils had the power to heal malfunctioning ovaries, kidneys, veins, adrenal glands, and many other organs. However, none of these claims has ever been scientifically substantiated.

Indeed, relatively few attempts to verify aromatherapy's purported benefits have ever been made at all, and of those, only a few have delivered promising results. In one trial for arthritis pain, some of the participants were able to reduce the dosage of their potent anti-inflammatory drugs. In another study, the scent of lavender successfully put insomniacs to sleep. Other research has documented improvement in cases of erectile dysfunction, and a reduction in pain following childbirth. However, attempts to prove that aromatherapy can cure shingles have failed (although fragrant creams can reduce some of the pain). And a 1958 paper extolling the ability of essential oils to fight and conquer infections could cite no positive human or animal tests.

Advocates of aromatherapy propose a variety of mechanisms for its reported effects. The most widely accepted theory suggests that fragrances do their work via the brain. When aromatic molecules enter the nasal cavity and stimulate the odor-sensing nerves, the resulting impulses are sent to the limbic system—the part of the brain that's believed to be the seat of memory and emotion. Depending on the scent, emotional responses then kick in to exert a calming or energizing effect on the body.

Alternatively, some proponents suggest that certain aromas may work by stimulating the glands, prompting the adrenal glands, for example, to produce steroid-like hormones that fight pain and inflammation. Others believe that the essential oils, whether inhaled or rubbed into the skin, react with hormones and enzymes in the bloodstream to produce positive results.

Whatever the truth of the matter, aromatherapists assign specific properties to each essence. Here are typical claims for some of the more common essential oils.

Lavender: Heals burns and cuts; destroys bacteria; relieves depression, inflammation, spasms, headaches, respiratory allergies, muscle aches, nausea, menstrual cramps; soothes bug bites; lowers blood pressure.

Peppermint: Alleviates digestive problems; cleans wounds; decongests the chest; relieves headache, neuralgia, and muscle pain; useful for motion sickness.

Eucalyptus: Lowers fever; clears sinuses; has antibacterial and antiviral properties; relieves coughs; useful for boils and pimples.

Tea Tree: Fights fungal, yeast, and bacterial infections; useful for skin conditions such as acne, insect bites, and burns; helps clear vaginitis, bladder infections, and thrush.

Rosemary: Relieves pain; increases circulation; decongests the chest; relieves pain, indigestion, gas, and liver problems; lessens swelling; fights infection; helps alleviate depression.

Chamomile: Reduces swelling; treats allergic symptoms; relieves stress, insomnia, and depression; useful in treating digestive problems.

Thyme: Lessens laryngitis and coughs; fights bladder and skin infections; relieves digestive problems and pain in the joints.

Tarragon: Stimulates digestion; calms neural and digestive tracts; relieves menstrual symptoms and stress.

Everlasting: Heals scars; reduces swelling after injuries; relieves sunburn; fights infections such as bronchitis and flu; treats pain from arthritis, muscle injuries, sprains and strains, tendonitis.

Who Should Avoid This Therapy?

Many essential oils can trigger bronchial spasms. If you have asthma, do not use any form of aromatherapy without first consulting your doctor.

If you have any skin allergies, do not use essential oils in your bath. To check whether you are allergic to an oil, place one drop on the inside of your elbow and wait 24 hours to see if it produces a reaction.

As with any medication, it's best to avoid aromatherapy during pregnancy. Be especially wary of sage, rosemary, and juniper oils. These herbs have been known to cause uterine contractions when taken in excessive amounts.

Infants and young children are especially sensitive to potent essential oils. Keep the oils away from their faces. Do not use peppermint oil on children under the age of 30 months.

What Side Effects May Occur?
Because essential oils are highly concentrated, taking them internally can easily lead to a toxic overdose. Do not ingest even the tiniest amount without your doctor's approval.

Except for lavender, do not use any highly concentrated, undiluted oils on your skin. Be careful to keep the oils away from your eyes. Close your eyes while inhaling aromatic vapors.

Many essential oils will cause skin irritation if used too frequently. They can also increase your sensitivity to sunlight, making it easier to burn. Excessive inhalation of fragrant vapors can cause headache and fatigue. Remember, too, that certain oils, such as peppermint, can *cause* insomnia rather than relieve it.

How to Choose a Therapist
If you choose to pursue aromatherapy under the guidance of an expert (which is not a bad idea), start by checking for availability of a certified aromatherapist in your neighborhood. Several of the organizations listed under "Resources" conduct certification programs and can provide referrals.

There is no formal licensing procedure for aromatherapists in the United States, so you will find that it is offered by a wide range of practitioners with licenses in other fields, including chiropractors, psychologists, and massage therapists.

When Should Treatment Stop?
If the treatments seem to help, they generally can be continued as long as needed. However, if you develop an allergy to any of the products you are using, stop treatment immediately and seek another form of therapy.

See a Conventional Doctor If . . .
Continued symptoms, or the development of new ones, are a signal to check with your doctor. Many seemingly minor symptoms can be evidence of a serious underlying problem. You owe it to yourself to get a professional diagnosis whenever your condition changes for the worse.

Resources
ORGANIZATIONS

American Alliance of Aromatherapy
P.O. Box 750428
Petaluma, CA 94975-0428
Phone: 707-778-6762

American Aromatherapy Association
P.O. Box 3679
South Pasadena, CA 91031
Phone: 818-457-1742

Aromatherapy Seminars
3379 South Robertson Blvd.
Los Angeles, CA 90034
Phone: 800-677-2368

National Association for Holistic Aromatherapy
P.O. Box 17622

Boulder, CO 80308-0622
Phone: 303-258-3791

The Pacific Institute of Aromatherapy
P.O. Box 6842
San Rafael, CA 94903
Phone: 415-479-9121

FURTHER READING

The Complete Aromatherapy Handbook: Essential Oils for Radiant Health. Suzanne Fisher-Rizzi. New York: Sterling Press, 1991.

Aromatherapy Workbook. Marcel Lavabre. Rochester, VT: Healing Arts Press, 1990.

Aromatherapy for Common Ailments. Shirley Price. New York: Simon & Schuster, 1991.

The Aromatherapy Book: Applications & Inhalations. Jeanne Rose. Berkeley, CA: North Atlantic Books, 1992.

Aromatherapy to Heal and Tend the Body. Robert Tisserand. Santa Fe, NM: Lotus Light Press, 1988.

The Practice of Aromatherapy. Jean Valnet. Rochester, VT: Inner Traditions, 1990.

Aston-Patterning®

Consider This Therapy For

This specialized program of physical training and massage is designed to relieve muscle tension and pain, speed recovery from injuries, and aid in general relaxation and stress-reduction. It's particularly well-suited for such problems as back and neck pain, headache, and repetitive stress injuries like tennis elbow.

Like most forms of bodywork and movement training, Aston-Patterning does not lend itself to controlled clinical trials, and its effectiveness has therefore not been scientifically verified. Remember, too, that it requires a significant commitment on your part; it is much more than a program of passive massage.

How the Treatments Are Done

Aston-Patterning sessions are conducted one-on-one with a trained practitioner. They include massage, movement training, fitness exercises, and advice on changes in the home and work environments. When you begin the program, the practitioner will conduct an extensive evaluation of your general fitness, including your history, physical measurements, and movement habits. Movements tested range from simple acts of sitting and standing to "arcing," an Aston-Patterning flexion/extension movement of the whole body

The massage segment of the treatment employs a special "spiraling" technique that relaxes tense muscles and loosens stiff joints without causing pain. The goal is to release tightness and tension, thus permitting the body to revert to a healthier posture.

Movement training during the sessions is designed to reinforce the results of massage, bringing your routine habits of motion into harmony with the unique configuration of your body. This may require intensive drilling in certain movements that the practitioner selects to correct your posture and the way you bear your weight. These repetitive drills are likely to continue until relaxed, efficient movement becomes second nature to you.

Employed as an adjunct to movement training, the fitness exercises typically encountered in Aston-Patterning concentrate on improving muscle tone, joint resiliency, and lightness of movement. These exercises are backed up by counseling on ways to achieve healthier movement and posture in your daily routine. Recommended environmental adjustments can range from simply changing the height of a chair to employing a variety of cushions, knee supports, and side body supports to keep the spine and other areas of the body in proper alignment and prevent postural compression. (A patented line of Aston devices is available.)

Treatment Time: Sessions generally last 1 to 2 hours.
Treatment Frequency: Governed by the severity of the problem.

What Treatment Hopes to Accomplish

Aston-Patterning practitioners, along with the advocates of many other types of bodywork, believe that relaxed, efficient movement and a balanced, effortless posture can relieve unconscious stress, thus improving emotional and physical well-being.

The Aston-Patterning techniques were developed by dancer Judith Aston during her recovery from a pair of automobile accidents. It is an extension of Rolfing, a form of deep massage therapy aimed at improving the body's alignment (see the profile on Rolfing). After her successful rehabilitation through Rolfing, Aston devised a program of movement training and exercise aimed at maintaining the benefits of massage.

Who Should Avoid This Therapy?

The Aston-Patterning drills and exercises can be extremely demanding. If you have a heart condition or respiratory problems, check with your doctor before undertaking this form of therapy, and if you proceed, make sure the practitioner is aware of your disorder. The program can be adjusted to meet the needs of older adults, those in poor health, and patients with special rehabilitation requirements.

The deep massage employed in Aston-Patterning could prove dangerous if you have brittle bone disease (osteoporosis) or a tendency to bruise easily. Also avoid this therapy if you have a bleeding disorder, take anticoagulant drugs, or are undergoing long-term steroid therapy, which can make the tissues fragile.

If you have circulation problems such as those resulting from diabetes or varicose veins, be wary of massage in the legs and feet. Remember, too, that excessive pressure can aggravate carpal tunnel syndrome, which is itself a result of pressure on a nerve that passes through the wrist.

What Side Effects May Occur?

For people in good physical condition, most complications are the result of overly intensive training. Exhaustion and pain are the principal dangers. Be sure to give the practitioner plenty of feedback during the sessions. An experienced practitioner will know how hard to push and when it's best to stop.

How to Choose a Therapist

Although Aston-Patterning incorporates elements of both massage and movement training, it is not available from standard bodywork practitioners or physical therapists. For authentic treatment, you'll need to see a certified graduate of the Aston Training Center in Nevada. These practitioners—who are typically physical or occupational therapists or nurse practitioners— must complete several 2-week training sessions over a 3-year period in order to qualify. You can contact the Aston Training Center for referrals.

Because you'll be working closely with the practitioner for an extended period of time, it's important to interview the prospects before making a commitment. If you feel that you cannot place complete trust in the individual, seek another therapist.

When Should Treatment Stop?

At the outset, set specific goals with your therapist. When you've achieved them, treatment can stop. In cases of severe injury or rigid emotional resistance, this could take years. Usually, however, only a few weeks or months are required.

See a Conventional Doctor If . . .

If the Aston-Patterning techniques don't relieve your pain (or make it worse) see your doctor for further diagnostic work. Pain sometimes signals a serious disorder in a seemingly unrelated part of the body. It's important to establish its cause—*especially* if healing therapies such as Aston-Patterning fail to make a difference.

Resources

ORGANIZATIONS

The Aston Training Center
P.O. Box 3568
Inclined Village, NV 89450
Phone: 702-831-8228

FURTHER READING

Bodywork. C. Thomas. William Morrow & Co., 1995.

Conservative Care of Low Back Pain. B. Miller. Williams & Wilkins, 1992.

Alternative Medicine: The Definitive Guide. The Burton Goldberg Group. Puyallup, WA: Future Medicine Publishing, Inc., 1993.

Mind Body Medicine. D. Goldman and J. Gurin. Yonkers, NY: Consumer Reports Books, 1993.

The Alternative Medicine Handbook. B.R. Cassileth. New York: W.W. Norton & Co., 1998.

Take Care of Yourself. D. Vickery and J. Fries. Addison-Wesley Publishing Co., 1988.

Alternative Medicine or Magical Healing. G.A. Ulett. St. Louis, MO: Warren H. Green Inc., 1996.

Ayurvedic Medicine

Consider This Therapy for

Strictly speaking, Ayurvedic medicine is not a treatment. Rather, it is an entire medical system whose goal is the prevention of disease through the proper balance of three "irreducible principles" at work in the body.

Derived from philosophical theories propounded in India over 2,000 years ago, the principles of Ayurvedic medicine have never been substantiated by contemporary medical science—and no medical conditions have been proven to respond to Ayurvedic treatments. Certain Ayurvedic exercises, such as the meditation and gentle stretching exercises of yoga, afford people relief from tension and stress. However, any impact these exercises have on chronic conditions such as high blood pressure appears to be momentary, and can't be considered a lasting remedy.

How the Treatments Are Done

Ayurvedic medicine encompasses a wide range of treatments and lifestyle measures, including dietary recommendations, massage, medicinal herbs, and the meditation and breathing techniques of yoga. Some practitioners also recommend intestinal "cleansing" through the use of laxatives or enemas. Depending on your specific ailments and condition, you could be prescribed any or all of these various modes of therapy.

Ayurvedic practitioners generally begin by taking a comprehensive personal and medical history to determine your physical and spiritual "type," and then prescribe and treat accordingly. Expect detailed questions about your emotional temperament, skin type, food preferences, and other quirks. The practitioner is also likely to examine your tongue and spend a significant amount of time taking your pulse. (In the Ayurvedic view of medicine, the pulse is a critical diagnostic tool, revealing imbalances in the three basic principles at work in the body.)

Much like traditional Oriental medicine, the Ayurvedic system aims not just to treat diseases, but to maintain and balance the energy and health of both mind and body. It emphasizes avoidance of stress and a moderate, balanced lifestyle. The version of Ayurvedic medicine commercialized in the United States is a relatively recent "reconstruction" of ancient Indian medical practices, refined and tailored to meet

Western expectations and tastes. In India itself, Western-style medicine is replacing many of the older practices.

The frequency and duration of Ayurvedic treatments vary widely. Many aspects of Ayurvedic practice, such as dietary choices and yoga, can be self-administered on a regular basis or as needed. Typical measures may include massage with warm sesame oil; avoidance of certain types of foods (based on flavor, not nutritional content) and emphasis on others; breathing exercises, such as breathing alternately through one nostril and then the other; and herbal saunas or enemas to "detoxify" the body. A comprehensive program of treatments, called *panchakarma*, aims at overall "purification" and rejuvenation, and may be offered at some Ayurvedic clinics, centers, or spas.

What Treatment Hopes to Accomplish

The complex Indian system of healing called Ayurveda (from the Sanskrit words for "knowledge of life") has been around for millennia, but was first popularized in the United States by the Maharishi Mahesh Yogi, founder of the Transcendental Meditation movement. Later, the physician-author Deepak Chopra, MD seized the baton, promoting the system in a string of books and lectures during the 1980s and 90s.

According to Ayurveda, there are three doshas, or basic metabolic types: kapha, pitta, and vata. Each dosha is rooted in specific organs of the body and asso-ciated with two of Ayurveda's elements (earth, water, fire, air, and space, or "ether"). Combinations of these doshas in various proportions are said to yield a total of 10 body types which determine each individual's physical and emotional make-up.

The Ayurvedic practitioner's job is to identify the individual's "tridosha," a unique combination of the three doshas, and prescribe dietary patterns, exercises, lifestyle changes, and therapies designed to bring the tridosha into balance. People described as predominantly "vata" are thought to be thin, quick, and energetic; "pitta" types are considered competitive and hot-tempered; "kapha" types are regarded as calm and stolid. Each type is considered prone to characteristic ailments (for example, "pitta" types are thought to be more vulnerable to ulcers, inflammation, or rashes).

Identification of one's tridosha determines an array of recommendations, ranging from dietary choices to the best types of exercise. Ayurvedic dietary advice is based on a food's flavor rather than its nutritional content as defined by Western science. Increasing your intake of sweet, sour, and salty foods, for instance, is said to balance "vata." Herbal prescriptions are drawn from a vast selection of traditional Indian remedies, most of them unfamiliar to Westerners. (Don't make assumptions. Even familiar herbs may be used for different purposes than those documented by Western medical research.) Attempts to "purify" the body through excretion are also stressed, including herbal enemas and steam treatments. (Induced vomiting, a purgative technique used in Indian Ayurvedic practice, has—not surprisingly—been avoided by American practitioners.)

Who Should Avoid This Therapy?

Because none of the treatments endorsed by Ayurvedic medicine have been tested and found effective in regular clinical trials, Western physicians rarely recommend them for anyone. At best, Ayurvedic techniques are seen as means of attaining balance and harmony in your physical and emotional life—certainly not as a cure for a specific disease.

In any event, it's wise to be especially wary of the purgative treatments sometimes recommended by Ayurvedic practitioners. Overuse of laxatives and enemas can lead to serious chemical imbalances within the body. Laxatives, in particular, should never be taken in the presence of abdominal pain, nausea, or vomiting without first consulting a regular doctor.

Likewise, if you must follow dietary restrictions in order to manage a serious disorder such as diabetes or heart disease, it's advisable to consult a physician or registered dietitian before adopting an Ayurvedic diet plan. Because Ayurvedic recommendations are based mainly on the flavor of food, they may be at odds with the body's requirements as understood by contemporary medical science.

What Side Effects May Occur?

Meditation and the gentle stretching and breathing exercises of yoga are unlikely to have any adverse effects on most individuals. Likewise, gentle massage with warm oil, another mainstay of Ayurveda, is generally harmless. Ayurvedic herbal medicines, however, are a different matter. There's little published information on them, and many herbs have potent—and not necessarily desirable—effects when overused. If you develop any unforeseen symptoms while taking an Ayurvedic remedy, regard them as a signal to check with a mainstream doctor or pharmacist.

How to Choose a Therapist

Ayurveda is not recognized as a medical discipline in the United States, and there is no licensure system in place for its practitioners. A few medical doctors and osteopaths combine Ayurvedic philosophy and practice with contemporary medicine and other types of alternative health care. For practitioners trained by the followers of the Maharishi Mahesh Yogi, contact the Ayur-Veda Health Center listed on the next page.

When Should Treatment Stop?

If you are using Ayurvedic techniques such as meditation and yoga to combat stress and improve your general well-being, you can probably continue indefinitely. However, if a specific complaint fails to respond to Ayurvedic herbs or dietary adjustments within a matter of weeks, the wisest course is to discontinue the treatment and seek alternative therapy.

See a Conventional Doctor If . . .

Even if you find an Ayurvedic program to be a helpful tonic, it's best to regard it as an adjunct to other forms of medicine. If you develop any serious or alarming symptoms, seek diagnosis and treatment from a mainstream physician. Remember, even in India most health care professionals now use at least some modern medical techniques.

Resources

ORGANIZATIONS

The Raj, Maharishi Ayur-Veda Health Center
1734 Jasmine Ave.
Fairfield, IA 52556
Phone: 800-248-9050
This spa-like Ayurvedic health center is affiliated with a university founded by Maharishi Mahesh Yogi, the Indian spiritual leader who devised Transcendental Meditation. The center provides general information on Ayurveda and referrals to graduates of their Ayurvedic training program.

FURTHER READING

Ayurvedic Secrets to Longevity and Total Health. Peter An-

selmo with James S. Brooks, MD. Paramus, NJ: Prentice Hall, 1996.

Ayurveda: The A-Z Guide to Healing Techniques from Ancient India. Nancy Bruning and Helen Thomas. New York: Dell, 1997.

Maharishi Ayur-Ved: TM Goes Health Food. Stephen Barrett, MD, and Victor Herbert, MD, JD, in *The Vitamin Pushers.* Amherst, NY: Prometheus, 1994.

Perfect Health: The Complete Mind-Body Guide. Deepak Chopra, MD. New York: Harmony Books, 1991.

The Complete Book of Ayurvedic Home Remedies. Vasant Lad. New York: Harmony Books, 1998.

The Book of Ayurveda. Judith H. Morrison. New York: Fireside, 1995.

Yoga and Ayurveda. J. Raso in *"Alternative" Healthcare: A Comprehensive Guide.* Amherst, NY: Prometheus, 1994.

Biofeedback

Consider This Therapy For

This specialized type of training allows people to gain control over physiological reactions that are ordinarily unconscious and automatic. Malfunctions in these automatic responses contribute to a wide variety of medical problems. In study after study, biofeedback has shown the ability to help bring such counterproductive reactions back into line, providing significant relief for many of the people who try it.

Although it's not a sure cure, biofeedback helps many people with chronic pain, including the pain of arthritis, muscle spasms, and headache (both migraine and tension headache). It can reduce tension and anxiety, combat chronic insomnia and fatigue, alleviate depression, reduce hyperactivity and attention deficit disorder, and even help overcome alcoholism and drug addiction. Some people have found it helpful for controlling high blood pressure or an abnormal heart rate. It's also useful for retraining, reconditioning, and strengthening muscles after an accident or surgery, restoring control lost due to pain or nerve damage, and overcoming urinary (or bowel) incontinence.

For asthmatics, biofeedback offers the possibility of controlling bronchial spasms and reducing the severity of attacks. Many victims of Raynaud's disease (periodic loss of circulation in the fingers) have been able to rectify the problem through biofeedback. The technique has helped others deal with digestive disorders such as ulcers, irritable bowel syndrome, acidity, dysfunction of the esophagus, and difficulty swallowing.

Biofeedback is under study as a potential aid in the treatment of a number of other ailments as well, although results are more mixed. It may help relax the muscles in temporomandibular joint syndrome (TMJ). It appears to reduce the severity and frequency of seizures in some (though not all) epileptics. It can help ease the symptoms of chronic fatigue syndrome. It has even been tried as a remedy for chronic constipation, motion sickness, and the uncontrollable tics and compulsions of Tourette's syndrome.

How the Treatments Are Done

Biofeedback is not a passive treatment. It requires your intensive participation as you learn to control such normally involuntary ("autonomic") functions as heart rate, blood pressure, brain waves, skin temperature, muscle tension, breathing, and digestion.

At your first session, you'll be asked a few questions about your own health and that of family members. The biofeedback therapist will then apply sensors to various points on your body. The location depends on the problem that needs treatment. If you have migraines, sleep problems, and mood disorders, for example, the electrodes are often attached to your scalp; to treat heart problems and muscle tension, they will be placed on your skin. Other possible sites include the hands, feet, or fingers.

The sensors are connected to a computer, a polygraph, or another piece of monitoring equipment that provides instant feedback to you on the function you're trying to control, such as the tension in a particular set of involuntary muscles or circulation to a specific part of the body. Some biofeedback machines signal changes graphically on a computer display, others beep, buzz, or blink to indicate the strength or level of the function you're targeting.

The therapist will teach you mental or physical exercises that can help you affect the function that's causing a problem. You can easily gauge your success by noting any changes in the intensity, volume, or speed of the signals from the machine. Gradually, you'll learn to associate successful thoughts and actions with the desired change in your involuntary responses.

Once you've thoroughly learned an effective pattern of actions, you'll be able to assert control without the aid of the feedback device.

Among the feedback instruments you're most likely to encounter are the following:

Electromyographs (EMGs) measure muscle tension. Therapists use them to relieve muscle stiffness, treat incontinence, and recondition injured muscles.

Skin Temperature Gauges show changes in the amount of heat given off by the skin, a measurement that indicates any change in blood flow. These gauges are used in the treatment of Raynaud's disease, high blood pressure, anxiety, and migraines.

Galvanic Skin Response Sensors (GSRs) use the amount of sweat you produce under stress to measure the conductivity of your skin. They are often used to reduce anxiety.

Electroencephalographs (EEGs) measure brain-wave activity. Conditions that may benefit from training on these machines include attention deficit/hyperactivity disorder, tooth grinding, head injuries, and depression (including bipolar depression and seasonal affective disorder).

Electrocardiographs (ECGs) monitor the heart rate and may be useful in relieving an overly rapid heartbeat and controlling high blood pressure.

Respiration feedback devices concentrate on the rate, rhythm, and type of breathing to help lessen symptoms of asthma, anxiety, and hyperventilation and promote relaxation.

Along with biofeedback training, the therapist may also give you instruction in deep breathing, meditation, visualization, and muscle relaxation—all of which may aid in relieving stress-related symptoms.

Treatment Time: Sessions usually last between 30 minutes and 1 hour.

Treatment Frequency: In most cases, people can learn to raise or lower their heart rate, relax specific muscles, lower blood pressure, and control other functions in 8 to 10 sessions. Some problems, such as attention deficit/hyperactivity disorder, take longer—sometimes up to 40 sessions.

Depending on the severity of the problem and the technique used, therapists suggest you attend 1 to 5 sessions per week.

What the Treatment Hopes to Accomplish

Biofeedback is a "mind over matter" form of therapy that has only recently begun to filter into mainstream medicine. Although ancient Greek, Chinese, and Indian healers were convinced that the mind could influence the body, either causing illness or curing disease, the concept fell into disrepute as Western medicine began to discover the infectious agents and chemical malfunctions that lie at the root of so many familiar ailments. It was only when modern instrumentation made it possible to measure subtle changes in unconscious physical reactions that medicine once more turned its attention to the mind-body connection.

Although biofeedback promises to remedy certain ailments through disciplined mental effort, it has nothing in common with other forms of mind-body therapy such as meditation and yoga. It does not rely on maintenance of some sort of theoretical balance or harmony in order to achieve its effects. Instead, it seeks control over specific, measurable physiological reactions that have somehow gone awry. As such, it can prove especially useful for any disorder caused or aggravated by involuntary muscular tension or tightening. Like other forms of mind-body therapy, it's entirely useless for fighting infections, curing cancer, relieving allergies, or healing injuries.

Who Should Avoid This Therapy?

If you use a pacemaker or have a severe heart disorder, check with your doctor before using a biofeedback device that measures your perspiration output. These machines use a small amount of electricity to produce readings, and, even though no problems have been reported to date, there is a chance that they may affect your pacemaker or damage your heart.

What Side Effects May Occur?

Like other mind-body forms of therapy, biofeedback is notably free of side effects. Indeed, it's often turned to by people seeking a respite from the side effects of conventional medicines.

How to Choose a Therapist

Select a biofeedback therapist with training in psychology and, ideally, physiology. He or she should be certified by the Biofeedback Certification Institute of America. Directories of biofeedback practitioners are available from the Institute.

You may also check with a biofeedback association in a major city near you, ask your physician for a recommendation, or (as a last resort) find a therapist in the Yellow Pages.

When Should Treatment Stop?

If you see no improvement in 10 to 20 sessions, or if your problem worsens, you're probably one of the people for whom biofeedback doesn't work. You should discontinue the training and ask your doctor about other alternatives.

See a Conventional Doctor If . . .

Although biofeedback is harmless—and can often be helpful—it is not a substitute for regular visits to the doctor if you have a serious chronic condition such as diabetes, epilepsy, heart disease, or high blood pressure. For such problems, failure to continue conventional care can be more dangerous than any alternative you care to try.

Likewise, if you try biofeedback to help ease depression, do not suddenly drop other forms of treatment. Continue to see your doctor. Eventually, he may be able to reduce the dosage of your antidepressant medication as you continue your training.

Remember, too, that if your biofeedback techniques suddenly fail to work, you may be facing a new medical problem for which biofeedback is ineffective. At such times, it's wise to see your doctor for a thorough diagnosis.

Resources

ORGANIZATIONS

Association for Applied Psychotherapy and Biofeedback (AAPB)
10200 West 44th Ave.
Suite 304
Wheatridge, CO 80033
Phone: 303-422-8436

Biofeedback Certification Institute of America (BCIA)
10200 West 44th Ave.
Suite 304
Wheatridge, CO 80033
Phone: 303-420-2902

Center for Applied Psychophysiology
Menninger Clinic
P.O. Box 829
Topeka, KS 66601-0829
Phone: 913-273-7500 (ext)5375

Mind-Body Medical Institute
Division of Behavioral Medicine
New England Deaconess Hospital
183 Pilgrim Rd.
Boston, MA 02213
Phone: 617-732-9330

Society for the Study of Neuronal Regulation (SSNR)
4600 Post Oak Pl.
Suite 301
Houston, TX 77027
Phone: 713-552-0091

FURTHER READING

Biofeedback: An Introduction and Guide. David G. Danskin and Mark Crow. Palo Alto, CA: Mayfield Publishing Co., 1981.

The Future of the Body: Explorations into the Further Evolution of the Human Species. Michael Murphy. Los Angeles: Jeremy P. Tarcher, Inc., 1992.

Third Line Medicine. Melvyn R. Werback. New York: Third Line Press, 1988.

Biological Dentistry

Consider This Therapy For

The various therapies encompassed by biological dentistry all share a single basic premise: They are founded on the idea that the teeth can affect the general health of the body, and vice versa.

For example, the theory for which biological dentistry is best known asserts that the mercury in amalgam fillings can make you sick, leading to recurrent health problems, such as neurologic disorders, chronic fatigue, and arthritis. To remedy these ailments, proponents say, you need only have all your amalgam fillings removed and replaced with less toxic alternatives, such as nonmetallic quartz-based fillings or porcelain inlays.

Many dentists and oral surgeons can and often do remove amalgam fillings at their patients' request. However, before you embark on what could become a very expensive and uncomfortable series of dental procedures, you should consider the fact that both the American Dental Association and the National Institutes of Health have specifically rejected the amalgam theory. There is no scientific evidence, they say, of any detrimental effects from amalgam.

Of course, the so-called amalgam problem is not the only reason that people seek out biological dentists. The various unconventional treatments outlined below seek to cure a broad spectrum of ailments—ranging from headache to heart disease—through operations on the teeth and mouth. Some people adopt these therapies as "natural" or "nontoxic" alternatives to mainstream treatment. However, none of them have been proven effective in scientific tests.

How the Treatments Are Done

Many biological dentists work in conjunction with other alternative health care providers, such as homeopathic practitioners and holistic medical doctors. The dental procedures most commonly offered in the United States include neural therapy, oral acupuncture, cold laser therapy, and mouth balancing. To enhance the effectiveness of these therapies, the practitioner may prescribe homeopathic remedies and make recommendations concerning diet and nutrition.

NEURAL THERAPY

According to practitioners of neural therapy, biological energy flows throughout the human body and enters each cell at a specified frequency range. If the energy flow stays within the appropriate range, it's believed that the individual will stay healthy. However, a breakdown of this flow can theoretically cause a disruption of cell function, eventually leading to a number of chronic disorders.

According to this theory, injury, inflammation, or infection in the mouth signals a blockage in the energy flow elsewhere in the body. Hence, it's thought that a problem in a distant organ can be remedied by restoring the normal flow of energy at the site of the dental problem. To accomplish this, biological dentists inject a local anesthetic, such as procaine, around the offending tooth.

Treatment Time: 2 to 3 seconds for the injection.

Treatment Frequency: Varies according to the body's response to the injection. If it's not clear which tooth is involved, the practitioner may experiment with 4 to 5 treatments over a period of 2 to 4 weeks to identify the location of the energy blockage.

ORAL ACUPUNCTURE

Acupuncture seeks to balance the flow energy along 14 channels, or meridians, throughout the body. It's thought that the flow can be adjusted through application of needles at specific "acupoints" along the meridians. Oral acupuncture uses injections of saline water, weak local anesthetics, or homeopathic solutions at acupoints within the mouth. When the energy flow has been properly balanced at these points, practitioners believe, problems elsewhere on the meridian will be rectified. Hence, this form of therapy is used for problems ranging from sinusitis and allergies to digestive problems and neuralgia.

Treatment Time: 1 to 2 seconds for the injection.

Treatment Frequency: Varies de-

pending upon the body's response to the injection. Patients typically undergo no more than 3 treatments over a period of 2 to 3 weeks.

COLD LASER THERAPY

Cold laser therapy is an alternative form of oral acupuncture available to patients who dislike needles. The low-power beam used in this procedure is incapable of causing any thermal damage to the body's tissues; hence the name "cold." The beam is typically aimed either directly at the teeth to prepare them for treatment or at an acupoint within the mouth. The therapy is usually recommended to reduce swelling and hasten healing.

Treatment Time: When used directly on the teeth, 30 seconds to 1 minute; when used on acupoints, 1 to 5 minutes.

Treatment Frequency: Depending upon the body's response, 2 to 3 applications may be recommended.

HOMEOPATHY

Homeopathic remedies are extremely weak herbal solutions given to stimulate the body's healing powers. Advocates regard them as a nontoxic alternative to drugs, although they have never been proven effective in standard clinical trials. Biological dental practitioners use them to temporarily alleviate pain or discomfort during dental emergencies. They are also used to aid the body in eliminating supposed mercury toxicity after the removal of amalgam fillings. Other dentists prefer to use them to enhance "detoxification" during the actual amalgam removal process.

Treatment Frequency: May be used every 15 minutes in dental emergencies. For amalgam detoxification, treatments range from 2 to 3 months up to 2 to 3 years or longer.

MOUTH BALANCING

Often recommended as a remedy for painful temporomandibular joint syndrome (TMJ), headaches, and eye problems, this form of therapy aims to bring the facial muscles, ligaments, and jaws into the proper relationship so that the muscles do not endure too much stress. The alignment of the teeth, jaws, and muscles undergo an initial evaluation, typically with the aid of a computer, as the practitioner looks for muscle dysfunction and jaw vibrations. If any deformities are identified, custom orthopedic braces are produced to be worn in the mouth and realign the jaw, thus eliminating associated pain. Note that although this procedure sounds similar to standard orthodontics, its claims are considerably more expansive.

Treatment Time: Depends upon the severity of the deformity, but can last up to 12 months, perhaps longer in severe cases.

Treatment Frequency: Appliance adjustments must be made on a regular basis. Between 5 and 20 appointments are typically required.

DIET

Most biological dentists recommend that you supplement their treatments with certain vitamins and foods. For example, patients who have undergone the removal of amalgam are told to include magnesium, selenium, vitamin C, vitamin E, and folic acid in their diets to promote the excretion of mercury from their system. (These ingredients can be found in a variety of popular multivitamin supplements.) Patients are also given a long list of things to avoid, often including sugar, alcohol, caffeine, chocolate, soft drinks, refined carbohydrates, milk, cheese, margarine, and fish. (Note, however, that none of these products, eaten in moderation, has been shown to have any adverse effect upon health.)

What Treatment Hopes to Accomplish

Two schools of thought run through biological dentistry. One asserts that the materials used in mainstream dentistry are toxic and can promote serious disorders elsewhere in the body. By weakening the immune system or attacking the nervous system, these materials are said to cause ailments ranging from Alzheimer's disease, chronic fatigue syndrome, and arthritis to kidney problems and heart disease. Removing the offending materials is therefore supposed to effect a cure. Although various case studies are advanced to demonstrate the validity of this theory, there is no scientific evidence to support it.

The second school of thought holds that the teeth and surrounding tissues are linked to other organs in the body through a network of energy channels. Although these channels—such as the meridians of acupuncture—have never been verified by modern science, clinical trials have shown that acupuncture-type techniques can in fact relieve certain types of pain. Claims for oral acupuncture include relief of toothaches, tooth sensitivities, jaw pain, gingivitis, neuralgia, sinusitis, and pain in distant parts of the body. In addition, the oral acupuncture points behind the last upper and lower molars have been used to treat shoulder and elbow pain, neck pain, restricted neck movement, low back pain, and TMJ. Although the jury is still out on the true value of acupuncture, it's possible that it could provide some relief.

Who Should Avoid This Therapy?

Mainstream dentists regard amalgam removal and detoxification as an expensive scam, and the American Dental Association has declared it unethical.

Other forms of biological dentistry, such as oral acupuncture, are generally considered safe for anyone, although you may want to avoid the use of needles if you tend to bleed easily.

What Side Effects May Occur?

Proponents of biological dentistry point with pride to its lack of side effects. Occasionally a patient may experience nausea from the detoxification process during and after amalgam removal. However, biological dentists say that patients are more likely to experience tooth sensitivity and allergic reactions in traditional dentistry than in the biological variety.

How to Choose a Therapist

There is no certification criteria for biological dentists. In fact, the treatments can be offered by any licensed dentist or oral surgeon. To locate a practitioner in your area, you can contact one of the several holistic, biological dental organizations that provide lists of biological dentists free of charge.

Before choosing a dentist, try to schedule a consultation visit with the leading contenders. Find out which ones offer the type of procedure you desire. Ask what other services they provide. Check on the safety precautions taken in the dental chair. If you are seeking amalgam removal, ask what measures the dentist uses to eliminate mercury from the body's tissues and what materials he uses in replacement fillings. Finally, ask for some patient references and see what they say.

When Should Treatment Stop?

Many biological dentists promote the technique as a process, not a definitive treatment. They point out that, like any sort of treatment, holistic therapies may not necessarily cure all problems completely—indeed, some can last a lifetime and may require constant monitoring. Many biological dental patients, for example, continue to see their dentists on a weekly, monthly, or annual basis for bite adjustments.

If you agree with this philosophy, the treatments—and your payments—can last indefinitely. To make sure continued therapy remains worthwhile, try skipping a treatment once in a while. If your problem remains in check, you may be able to cut back or eliminate the therapy entirely.

See a Conventional Doctor If . . .

In many cases, people turn to biological dentistry after mainstream treatments have failed. Nevertheless, if any serious new symptoms arise, the only safe course is to return to your doctor for a professional medical diagnosis. Unfamiliar symptoms could signal new and unrelated problems that require a whole new course of treatment.

Resources

ORGANIZATIONS

American Academy of Biological Dentistry
P.O. Box 856
Carmel Valley, CA 93924
Phone: 408-659-5385

International Academy of Oral Medicine and Toxicology
P.O. Box 608531

Orlando, FL 32860-8531
Phone: 407-298-2450

Environmental Dental Association
9974 Scripps Ranch Blvd.,
Suite 36
San Diego, CA 92131
Phone: 800-388-8124;
619-586-7626

FURTHER READING

Are Your Dental Fillings Poisoning You? Guy S. Fasciana, DMD. Keats Publishing Inc., 1986.

The Complete Guide to Mercury Toxicity from Dental Fillings. Joyal Taylor, DDS. Scripps Publishing Co., 1988.

Dentistry Without Mercury. Sam Ziff and Michael Ziff. Bio-Probe Inc., 1993.

It's All in Your Head. Hal Huggins, DDS. Life Science Press, 1986.

Mercury Poisoning from Dental Amalgam—A Hazard to the Human Brain. Patrick Stortebecker, MD, PhD. Bio-Probe, 1986.

Cell Therapy

Consider This Therapy For

Cell therapy seeks to reverse the ravages of degenerative disease by injecting healthy animal cells (or cell extracts) into the patient's bloodstream. A variety of claims have been made for the treatments, which achieved considerable popularity among the rich and famous during the mid-20th century. The injections have been promoted as a way to improve overall health, boost the immune system, enhance vitality, counteract the effects of aging, cure impotence, stimulate healing, relieve arthritis, reverse Parkinson's disease, and even fight cancer. They've also been used to treat painful menstruation, infertility, herpes, prostate problems, bronchial disorders, epilepsy, hardening of the arteries, bladder infections, skin problems, hepatitis, heart problems, circulatory disorders, and menopause.

Unfortunately, despite numerous testimonials, there are no studies verifying cell therapy's purported beneficial effects, and the treatments have been banned in the United States since 1985 due to the danger of infections and allergic reactions. (Unlike blood transfusions and bone marrow transplants, which are carefully matched to the recipient, animal-cell injections can trigger serious immune rejection reactions.) One highly publicized achievement of cell therapy— the alleviation of Down's syndrome—has been conclusively *disproven*. In clinical trials, children receiving cell therapy showed no improvement in mental ability.

How the Treatments Are Done

The cells used in this type of therapy are usually taken from unborn sheep or pigs. In its original form (pioneered by Swiss physician Paul Niehans in the 1930s), the therapy called for live cells, which were prepared for injection by finely mincing the animals' tissues or glands and mixing them with a special saline solution. The injections were typically made within one hour of the donor animal's death to ensure that the cells maintained their vitality and to avoid the breakdown of the living material into toxic substances.

Today, however, therapists are more likely to use freeze-dried cells or antibodies produced from the cells. These preparations are said to offer the same benefits as live-cell therapy with less danger of infection or immune reactions. The newer forms of treatment are also less costly.

Prior to treatment, the therapist will probably give you a physical exam and take a health history to determine whether cell therapy is appropriate. (If a specific organ or gland is the target of the treatments, it must retain enough vitality to respond to stimulation.) The therapist will then give a test injection to make sure you won't suffer an allergic reaction. If any sensitivity is detected, additional injections will be canceled and you'll be advised to seek another form of treatment.

A variety of injections are available. The preparations most commonly employed today by the leading practitioners in the field include:

A COMBINATION OF VARIOUS CELL TYPES

These injections are used primarily for revitalization purposes. The patient is injected with four types of cells—pituitary, liver, connective tissue, and male or female reproductive glands—plus a fifth type selected according to the patient's specific need. For example, if the patient has liver problems, liver cells will be included in the preparation.

WHOLE EMBRYO ULTRAFILTRATE INJECTIONS

This type of injection is intended to stimulate connective tissues and muscles, increase fluid content in the tissues, and retard aging. The preparation contains material from all areas of the embryo, and is therefore considered effective for the whole body. As with the combination injections, if a patient is experiencing problems in a particular area, such as the liver or kidney, the injections can be supplemented with cells from those organs as well.

THERAPEUTIC IMMUNOLOGY (ANTIBODY INJECTIONS)

This more sophisticated variation of the treatments relies on antibodies rather than the cells themselves. The injections are produced by administering the cells to an animal, whose immune system then manufactures antibodies in response. These antibodies are then harvested from the animal's blood, purified, and administered to the patient in much the same way that shots of gamma globulin are given to boost immunity.

Such use of antibodies is actually one of the hottest research areas in medicine today. Antibodies produced by genetic engineering are being used experimentally to treat autoimmune diseases such as lupus and rheumatoid arthritis. Several products are already under FDA review.

Cell therapists who use antibody preparations claim they have no side effects. To enhance effectiveness and prevent potential reactions, the antibodies are administered via both injection and suppository in low doses over a period of several weeks or months. Cell extracts containing ribonucleic acid, the material that transmits genetic information from the DNA, are often added to the antibodies to enhance the effectiveness of therapy.

BIO-NUTRITIONAL THERAPY

These treatments offer a potpourri of cells, cell extracts, and antibodies combined with various nutrients and adenosine triphosphate (ATP), a compound that stores and transfers energy within cells, and which is thought to promote cellular and tissue regeneration. Practitioners typically administer this preparation either under the tongue or through the nasal or rectal passage, where it is quickly absorbed.

Treatment Time: For each method discussed, patients typically receive 2 to 5 doses per session.
Treatment Frequency: Varies according to the method employed and the body's response;

some cases may require only one session, while other patients may undergo additional sessions for a period of 6 months, 1 year, or perhaps up to 2 years.

What Treatment Hopes to Accomplish

Traditional cell therapy is founded on the belief that, when injected into a human patient, certain animal fetal cells will automatically travel to the same organ from which they were procured and revitalize its activity. For example, it's thought that fetal liver cells introduced into the human body will naturally migrate to the host liver and stimulate regeneration; kidney cells will migrate to the kidney; and so forth. The newer, antibody form of therapy relies less on regeneration of specific organs and more on general stimulation of the immune system.

Depending upon how the treatment is administered and for what condition, the benefits of cell therapy are sometimes reported to appear in as little as 36 hours, as in the case of a hepatitis patient said to have experienced almost immediate rejuvenation after a liver cell injection. However, most recoveries take 4 to 6 months, and proponents say that the overall long-term healing process can take several years, as the body begins to accept the transplanted cells, resumes normal activity, slowly rebuilds stamina, and increases blood supply.

Who Should Avoid This Therapy?

Cell therapy is not recommended for those with kidney disease, liver failure, or acute infections and inflammatory diseases, such as ulcerative colitis, a chronic disease of the large intestine and rectum. (Note, however, that this may not necessarily apply to the genetically engineered antibody treatments currently under investigation in the United States. These products are being tested for use in patients who do in fact have ulcerative colitis and other inflammatory bowel diseases, particularly Crohn's disease.)

Of course, patients who show an allergic reaction to a test injection during the screening process should not receive treatments.

What Side Effects May Occur?

There are a number of potential side effects of which individuals considering this therapy should be aware. Any type of cell therapy is likely to produce fatigue, typically from the time of injection to as much as 2 weeks afterwards. Allergic reactions are also quite possible.

With live cell therapy, there is a distinct danger that the body's immune system will reject the material, as it can an organ transplant. Among the signs of rejection are high fevers.

How to Choose a Therapist

Although cell therapy is practiced in Europe, the Bahamas,

Switzerland, and Mexico, in the United States it is unapproved—and is likely to remain so until solid proof of its effectiveness can be found. Intraspecies cell transplants—human to human—are currently under study in the U.S. for treatment of Parkinson's disease and diabetes. However, these treatments are quite different from those offered by overseas cell therapists.

Before committing to a trip abroad for this serious form of alternative treatment, you should give serious consideration to the following issues:

Travel: Those who wish to pursue "classic" cell therapy are, of course, required to leave the U.S. Keep in mind that the uncertainty of treatment outcomes and absence from family, friends, and familiar surroundings may create yet another stress level. Compounding these anxieties may be language barriers and stark cultural differences.

Treatment Success: Because there is little scientific information on these treatments, it's important to quiz potential therapists about such concerns as success rates, side effects, length of treatment, and duration of beneficial effects. Ask for documented cases and testimonials, and seek to clarify response time and quality of life issues.

Also, ask for referrals to patients who have actually undergone the same treatment plan with the same physician, and consider obtaining as much information as possible via telephone and mail. A good starting point is the International Clinic of Biological Regeneration North American Information Office, which can provide general information and referrals. (See "Resources" on the next page.)

Also, once treatment has been rendered, be sure to clarify any instructions that must be followed to ensure maximum success. For example, should you follow a special diet? Is a special exercise program needed?

Finances: Don't forget that these treatments will require a major investment. They often cost several thousand dollars and are rarely covered by insurance. Establish up front, in writing, what the total cost will be and how payment is to be made.

When Should Treatment Stop?

Since many cell therapy treatment plans are undertaken to combat the ongoing aging process, it's conceivable that you could undergo treatment indefinitely, returning to the clinic every few years for the same treatment, as long as you are satisfied with the results.

However, if you are taking the treatments to correct a specific medical problem, don't be overly patient. If your symptoms fail to improve—or get worse—be quick to seek a different therapeutic alternative.

See a Conventional Doctor If . . .

For most diseases, a wide array of potential treatments are available to you—and the longer they're delayed, the more serious your condition can become. If cell therapy doesn't yield significant improvement within a matter of months, seek other forms of care. If you have cancer or some other life-threatening illness, finding a more effective type of treatment is particularly urgent.

Likewise, if the treatments cause persistent side effects such as severe fatigue or allergies, there is no compelling reason to put up with them. Check with one or more doctors for a less troublesome—and possibly more effective—treatment regime.

Resources

ORGANIZATIONS

International Clinic of Biological Regeneration North American Information Office
P.O. Box 509
Florissant, MO 63032
Phone: 800-826-5366;
314-921-3997

International Society for the Application of Organ Filtrates, Cellular Therapy and Onco-Biotherapy
Robert Bosch Strasse, 56a
D-6909 Walldorf, Germany
Phone: 0620276-3268
Fax: 062227-6330

The Stephan Clinic
27 Harley Place, Harley Street
London, England W1N 1HB

Phone: 071-636-6196
Fax: 071-255-1626

FURTHER READING

Forever Young: A Practical Guide to Youth Extension. Michael E. Molnar. Witkower Press, 1985.

Introduction to Cellular Therapy. Paul Niehans, MD. Cooper Square Publishers, Inc., 1960.

Options: The Alternative Cancer Therapy Book. Richard Walters. Avery Publishing Group, 1992.

Third Opinion. John M. Fink. Avery Publishing Group, Inc., 1992.

Chelation

Consider This Therapy For

Chelation therapy, which clears a variety of heavy metals from the body, leads a double life. In mainstream medicine, it's considered a standard treatment for poisoning with lead, iron, copper, zinc, aluminum, manganese, and other metals. Alternative medicine, however, credits it with far more sweeping medicinal powers.

Thanks to its ability to remove calcium—an ingredient in arterial plaque—it is seen as a cure for hardening of the arteries, and hence for heart disease and a variety of problems resulting from poor circulation, including leg cramps and gangrene. Advocates have also promoted it as a treatment for Alzheimer's disease, multiple sclerosis, muscular dystrophy, thyroid problems, Parkinson's disease, arthritis, psoriasis, and cancer, and often recommend it to boost energy, improve mental alertness, and prevent strokes.

Although these claims are enticing—particularly if you are facing open heart surgery or an angioplasty to clear the coronary arteries—they suffer from a fatal flaw. When submitted to the kind of "double-blind," "placebo-controlled" testing required of any new drug (trials in which neither the doctors nor the patients know who's receiving the treatment and who's receiving a fake) chelation treatments for anything other than poisoning simply haven't proved out.

How the Treatments Are Done

Chelation clears minerals from the body with a chemical called ethylenediaminetetraacetic acid (EDTA). This substance is administered through an IV needle inserted in a vein in your finger or the back of your hand. (The solution usually contains vitamins and minerals as well.) The treatments are relatively painless, and are usually given in the doctor's office or clinic. During the treatments you can lie back in a comfortable reclining chair, sleep, read, watch television, drink, eat, walk around, or even go to the restroom, if necessary.

Before starting chelation, you'll be given a thorough physical exam. When questioned about your health and that of family members, be sure to mention any allergies and list all the medications you are taking. If you are undergoing the treatments as a remedy for heart problems, you'll probably be given

a stress test, electrocardiogram, and chest x-ray. If heavy metal poisoning is suspected, the doctor will probably send a sample of your hair to a laboratory for analysis of its metal levels. You may also have other tests to determine how well your kidneys are working and how well your blood is circulating.

During and after the treatments, your doctor will continue to take your blood pressure, check your cholesterol and blood sugar levels, and test your heart and kidneys to see how well they're doing.

Treatment Time: Each treatment takes between 3 and 4 hours, although in some cases, a session may last longer.

Treatment Frequency: Advocates of this therapy usually recommend between 20 and 50 treatments. People being treated for clogged arteries may need as many as 100 infusions of EDTA solution, while those who are getting chelation merely as a preventive measure may only get 10. Treatments are typically given at a rate of 1 to 3 per week.

What the Treatment Hopes to Accomplish

The term "chelation" is derived from the Greek word *chele*, meaning "claw." Like a claw, EDTA grabs, or binds onto, the metals in the bloodstream and carries them through the system so they can be excreted in the urine.

Until the late 1940s, EDTA was more familiar to plumbers than to physicians. It was first used to remove calcium from pipes and boilers. In 1948, it was found effective for treating workers who had developed lead poisoning while working in a battery factory. The U.S. Navy began using it for sailors who had absorbed lead from the paint they used on ships and docks.

Then, in the early 1950s, Dr. Norman Clark and other physicians noticed that patients treated with EDTA for lead poisoning reported less pain from angina; improved memory; better sight, hearing, and smell; and an increase in energy. The doctors speculated that EDTA might grab onto and remove calcium-laden plaque from the arteries in the same way as it removed harmful metals from the blood. Convinced from tests with rabbits that EDTA could clear out clogged arteries, some doctors began to use chelation on humans.

Later, as the popularity of the treatments grew, advocates developed another rationale for its effects. Noting that free radicals— compounds that cause oxidation and tissue damage in the body— had been implicated in the development of heart disease, they suggested that chelation could reverse this damage by removing the excess metals that foster free radicals. With the free radicals in check, the arteries could heal, shedding their plaque and relieving the symptoms of heart disease and poor circulation.

Mainstream physicians dismiss these theories. They point out that EDTA cannot pass through the membranes of the cells in the arteries to reach calcium deposits, and that even if it could, the amount of calcium it could "bind" is negligible. In addition, they say, merely removing the calcium from plaque is not sufficient to make it disintegrate. As for free radicals, they note that the chelation of iron actually *increases* production of these damaging compounds. And to top it off, the vitamin C often added to the chelating solution can further increase the damage.

Why, then, are there so many case reports of successful chelation treatments? Perhaps, say mainstream doctors, because chelation is accompanied by an array of other therapeutic measures. The EDTA solution usually contains additional ingredients, such as vitamins and minerals. Patients are also advised to take vitamin and mineral supplements, follow a low-fat diet, stop smoking, limit alcohol and caffeine consumption, reduce stress, and exercise regularly. These nutritional and lifestyle changes, alone, can improve health.

Chelation advocates respond by citing the thousands of papers submitted to the American Academy for the Advancement of Medicine, a group of pro-chelation physicians. They say that over 500,000 patients have been successfully treated in the U.S. alone, and insist that the treatments are a safe, effective, inexpensive alternative to coronary bypass surgery or balloon angioplasty to clear the arteries. Indeed, they charge that these procedures fail to extend life, and hint darkly that the operations are extremely profitable for the surgeons who perform them.

Despite these arguments, every major institution in the medical establishment has dismissed the evidence for chelation as biased and inadequate. None of them—from the Food and Drug Administration and the National Institutes of Health to the American Medical Association, American College of Physicians, American College of Cardiology, and American Osteopathic Association—have endorsed the therapy.

Who Should Avoid This Therapy?

For anything other than metal poisoning (which is a dangerous emergency), chelation treatments are not recommended if you have kidney damage, liver disease, or a brain tumor. You should also avoid chelation if you are pregnant or are trying to conceive.

What Side Effects May Occur?

Like the effectiveness of chelation therapy, its side effects are a source of controversy. Mainstream physicians warn that EDTA can produce serious—even fatal—kidney damage. According to the American Heart Association, other reported side effects include anemia, blood clots, bone marrow damage, fever, headache, insulin shock, irregular heartbeat, joint pain, low

blood pressure, painful and difficult urination, severe inflammation of the area where the needle is inserted, and stroke.

Physicians and other professionals who favor chelation strongly dispute these findings. They argue that while some of these side effects were reported in the therapy's infancy, the picture is entirely different today. In the 1950s and early 1960s, patients received 6 grams of EDTA over a period of 30 minutes. The current dosage is 50 milligrams for every 2.2 pounds of body weight (roughly 4 grams for a 180 pound individual) given over 3 to 4 hours.

Although patients with severe kidney problems may be supersensitive to EDTA, proponents say that in the vast majority of cases, when the treatments are performed correctly, no serious side effects occur. Indeed, some advocates say that chelation is safer than aspirin—and hundreds of times safer than bypass surgery.

How to Choose a Therapist

Chelation therapy is usually performed by physicians (medical doctors or osteopaths) with specialized training and certification from a chelation-oriented organization such as The American College for Advancement in Medicine or The American Board of Chelation Therapy (see "Resources," on the next page).

Advocates recommend that you choose a doctor who has several years of experience in the therapy. If a nurse administers the solution, a qualified physician should be on-site at all times.

When Should Treatment Stop?
If you develop any serious side effects, stop chelation therapy immediately and seek traditional medical treatment.

See a Conventional Doctor If . . .
If you have a serious medical condition such as heart disease, kidney failure, cancer, or liver problems, chelation is especially risky. Be sure to discuss your treatment options with a conventional physician before deciding whether to go ahead with this form of therapy.

Resources
ORGANIZATIONS

American Board of Chelation Therapy
70 West Huron St.
Chicago, IL 60610
Phone: 312-266-7246

American College of Advancement in Medicine
P.O. Box 3427
Laguna Hills, CA 92654
Phone: 714-583-7666

Great Lakes Association of Clinical Medicine, Inc.
70 West Huron St.
Chicago, IL 60610
Phone: 312-266-7246

The Rheumatoid Disease Foundation
5106 Old Harding Rd.

Franklin, TN 37064
Phone: 615-646-1030

FURTHER READING

40-Something Forever. Harold and Arline Brecher. New York: Health Savers Press, 1992.

Bypassing Bypass. Elmer Cranton and Arline Brecher. Troutdale, VA: Hampton Roads, 1990.

The Alternative Medicine Handbook. Barrie R. Cassileth, PhD. New York: W.W. Norton & Company, 1998.

The Scientific Basis of EDTA Chelation Therapy. Bruce Halstead. Colton, CA: Golden Quill Publishers, Inc., 1979.

What Your Doctor Won't Tell You. J. Heimlich. New York: HarperCollins Publishers, 1990.

The Healing Powers of Chelation. John P. Trowbridge and Morten Walker. Stamford, CT: New Way of Life, Inc., 1992.

Chiropractic

Consider This Therapy For
The "hands-on" joint manipulation known as chiropractic is considered particularly valuable for relief of acute (temporary) pain in the lower back. This type of pain usually subsides on its own within 3 months, but chiropractic treatment can often bring it to an end immediately. (See also the entry on osteopathic medicine.)

In many cases, chiropractic can also ease pain—due to either a temporary condition or aggravation of a chronic problem—in areas such as the mid-back, neck, or joints. Additionally, it is sometimes used to relieve the pain of headaches, muscle spasms, and nerve inflammation. Its effectiveness for relief of sciatica (pain or numbness along the sciatic nerve, generally in the back, buttocks, hips, or adjacent parts) remains controversial.

After the common cold, low back pain is the most common reason for doctor visits. It's an especially frustrating problem because there's frequently no simple medical explanation for it—and therefore no easy cure. However, there's now mounting evidence that spinal manipulation can be a genuine source of relief. In 1994, the Agency for Health Care Policy and Research (AHCPR) released its Guidelines on Acute Low Back Problems in Adults. This report identified manipulation (defined as certain specific techniques used to re-align or readjust a joint) as the preferred method of treatment for relief of acute back pain. Traction, bed rest, corsets, or drug therapies were not recommended.

Similarly, a report from the RAND Corporation published in the prestigious *Annals of Internal Medicine* found manipulation effective for the relief of acute low back pain. (It was not, however, deemed as successful in the treatment of chronic or recurrent low back pain, sciatica, asthma, high blood pressure, or pain caused by neurological conditions.) Chiropractors, RAND pointed out, perform 94 percent of spinal manipulations (though not necessarily with the same techniques employed in the study).

To date, there's no scientific confirmation of chiropractic's effectiveness for anything other than low back pain. However, in a few years we should know more. In early 1998, the National Institutes of Health's Office of Alternative Medicine, and the National Institute of Arthritis and Musculoskeletal and Skin Diseases awarded a research grant to support the first federally funded Center for Chiropractic Research.

How Treatments Are Done

Although the back is the primary focus of chiropractic, the manipulations can be applied to any muscle or joint in the body. Techniques vary among practitioners. Typically, after preparation and proper positioning, the chiropractor creates tension around the offending joint, then applies pressure to return it to its proper position. A popping sound is often heard—and sometimes felt—following this maneuver. The noise is similar to the one you hear when cracking your knuckles. It results from the sudden release of built-up pressure in the joint, and is generally painless. As the joint snaps into place, pain is relieved and proper function is restored. Other techniques you may encounter include soft tissue manipulation, trigger-point manipulation, or deep tissue massage.

On your first visit to a chiropractor, you'll probably be asked to complete a questionnaire about your personal and family medical history. Be sure to discuss any illnesses that run in the family. Although chiropractors are not prepared to diagnose the full gamut of disease, they are trained to perform physical examinations in much the same way as a general medical practitioner. For example, you may be given a blood test to rule out infection and a reflex test to rule out neurological problems. Your blood pressure, pulse, and respiration will also be measured.

Once these general readings have been taken, the examination will begin to zero in on your musculoskeletal system—the muscles and bones in your body—with particular attention to your spine. The chiropractor will also analyze your posture, and will probably perform some orthopedic tests as he examines your articulations (a chiropractic term for joints). These tests usually involve moving a particular limb in search of joints that are "fixated" (not moving) or moving with impaired range.

If the chiropractor identifies a fixated joint, he will then attempt to determine whether there is any risk involved in restoring normal movement to the joint and what other parts of the musculoskeletal system have been affected by the joint's dysfunction. It is common for a "healthy" joint to overcompensate by moving excessively when another joint is not working correctly. The healthy, hyperactive joint might be near the fixated joint or in an entirely different part of the musculoskeletal system. Overcompensation can result in new, incorrect structural configurations that cause discomfort or pain.

To rule out any conditions that would preclude treatment, chiropractors usually take an x-ray of the region causing your pain before beginning the manipulations. Some chiropractors also take x-rays to locate subluxations (partial dislocations). Most chiropractors have basic x-ray equipment on-site and all chiropractors are trained to read x-ray images. If a specialized view is required, you may be referred to a center that has advanced technology, such as magnetic resonance imaging (MRI) equipment, or other equipment that provides a comprehensive image.

About 90 percent of chiropractors use x-rays. However, full-spinal x-rays in search of subluxations are considered controversial by many practitioners, and constitute less than 17 percent of all x-rays performed by chiropractors, according to the American Chiropractic Association. Many practitioners, chiropractic and otherwise, believe that full-spinal x-rays yield little if any useful information, and thus expose patients to radiation needlessly.

The chiropractor will also examine your muscles to determine if they are balanced. Just as healthy joints compensate for injuries in other structures, muscles may also exhibit "compensated distortion." When one muscle or group of muscles is contracted, for example, those on the other side may be abnormally relaxed.

Once the chiropractor has all the information he needs, treatment will proceed. Therapeutic equipment common to virtually all chiropractors is a specialized table designed to conform to a patient's body. The table has mechanized parts that can be adjusted in accordance with the patient's size and the region of the body that requires treatment. For example, the surfaces where the face, pelvis, and other body structures lie will yield independently as the chiropractor applies controlled force to these areas during treatment.

According to the American Chiropractic Association, more than 90 percent of chiropractors use techniques common to physical therapy, especially in preparation for manipulation. Your practitioner may use a broad, pad-like vibrator to relax your back muscles. He may apply hot or cold compresses to increase circulation and relax painful muscle spasms, or use traction to ease pressure. Ultrasound is often used as a "micro massage" to stimulate circulation and remove fluid from the area around a damaged joint and nearby tissues.

Some chiropractors also recommend and teach relaxation techniques as a way to prevent future strain, and prescribe rehabilitative exercises as part of an extended treatment plan. Some also prescribe and sell dietary supplements and herbs, although

such products fall outside the realm of chiropractic.

Treatment Time: The initial visit typically lasts at least 1 hour. Subsequent visits usually take between 10 and 30 minutes.

Treatment Duration: On average, a course of treatment involves 3 to 5 visits per week for 2 weeks. Several studies have noted that consumers using chiropractic care are more satisfied with treatment than patients who receive medical care. Chiropractors are perceived as spending more time face-to-face with the patient, although no studies have been done to verify this.

What Treatment Hopes to Accomplish

The primary goals of chiropractic therapy are relief of musculoskeletal pain and restoration of mobility. However, many consumers use (or misuse) chiropractors for a wide variety of unrelated ailments. In a 1993 survey of more than 5,000 chiropractors, musculoskeletal complaints did in fact dominate the list of conditions they treated, but respondents also reported "routinely" seeing patients with headaches, and "often" seeing patients with high blood pressure problems, allergies, or obesity. Seen less frequently were patients with nutritional disorders, menstrual irregularities, asthma, and diabetes.

Chiropractic has long drawn criticism from the medical world for its failure to provide valid proof of its effectiveness, and for the exaggerated claims of some practitioners, who have touted spinal adjustment as a cure for everything from chronic pain to sinus infections. Indeed, until 1980 the American Medical Association (AMA) labeled as unethical the referral of patients to chiropractors, only lifting the prohibition when challenged in a successful antitrust suit.

Lately, with growing proof of spinal manipulation's effectiveness for low back pain, chiropractic has gained newfound respectability. Collaboration between medical specialists and chiropractors is on the increase, and some managed care plans have begun covering chiropractic treatments. Still, critics say there is little evidence that chiropractic relieves anything other than acute back pain. Few reliable studies support chiropractic for the treatment of chronic musculoskeletal disorders, although some studies of chiropractic treatment for headache show promising results.

The version of chiropractic currently gaining medical favor is far different from the original discipline. Developed by Daniel David Palmer in Davenport, Iowa, in 1895, chiropractic started out as a natural healing method freighted with a variety of spiritual and metaphysical concepts. Palmer's theory suggested that an Innate Intelligence flows through the nervous system and can be obstructed by a "subluxation"—or misalignment—of one or more of the 24 joints in the vertebral column, thus interfering with the blood supply and the body's full expression of healthy functioning. Palmer believed that, because all parts of the body are connected through the nervous system, all diseases were caused by one or more subluxations. Thus, any disease could be cured by manipulating or realigning the vertebrae in order to allow the body to heal itself.

A significant misalignment of the vertebrae is rare—and, as in scoliosis, is usually quite noticeable. Conversely, many people have asymmetrical spines with slight imperfections in alignment, yet suffer no adverse effects on their health. Many contemporary chiropractors therefore have begun to discuss subluxation less in terms of misalignment and more in terms of loss of function, since even a joint in perfect alignment may fail to work properly and tend to cause pain.

Over the years, different branches of chiropractic developed that emphasized one or more principles of Palmer's original theories to greater or lesser degrees. Historically, chiropractors categorized themselves as "straights" or "mixers" to describe how closely they adhered to Palmer's philosophy. "Straights" were purists, using only manipulation and focusing exclusively on the spine; "mixers" supplemented manipulation with other forms of treatment, such as nutritional counseling and physiotherapy, and acknowledged that diseases were caused by problems other than subluxations. Chiropractic schools and professional associations developed along these lines.

Today, these distinctions are breaking down. According to a 1997 report from the Agency for Health Care Policy and Research, more than two-thirds of chiropractors use techniques other than manipulation, such as exercise, nutritional counseling, and physiotherapy, although 93 percent retain spinal adjustment as their primary approach to treatment.

Who Should Avoid This Therapy

Chiropractic is not recommended for disorders of other than musculoskeletal origin, and should be avoided for certain musculoskeletal problems as well. For instance, it is not recommended for osteoporosis, bone or joint infections, bone cancer, acute rheumatoid arthritis, and diseases of the spinal chord or bone marrow. It should also be avoided in an area that has been operated on, such as a spinal fusion, and near acute fractures and dislocations or healed fractures and dislocations with signs of ligament damage. Chiropractors do not treat fractures.

Scoliosis, a condition in which the spine curves to the side, is generally considered a target for chiropractic therapy. However, *idiopathic* scoliosis, which develops over time instead of being present at birth (congenital scoliosis), is not appropriate for treatment by a chiropractor.

What Side Effects May Occur?

Serious side effects from spinal manipulation appear to be rare. Strokes have been reported following manipulation of the neck, presumably as a result of damage to one of the arteries supplying blood to the brain. However, the incidence of adverse events from manipulation of the neck region is estimated to be 1 in 1 million procedures, according to the Agency for Health Care Policy and Research. Likewise, the Agency pegs the risk of a serious side effect from manipulation of the lower back at 1 case in 100 million manipulations.

Minor side effects of spinal manipulation have not been systematically analyzed. The adverse reactions reported by one study, such as headache, radiating discomfort, and fatigue following manipulation, were not clearly shown to be a result of the treatment.

How to Choose a Therapist

Choose a chiropractor as you would any other health care professional. Discuss your condition with him and clearly establish the type of treatment he plans to provide, its expected outcome, how long it will last, and how much it will cost. Ask about his training and treatment philosophy, bearing in mind that chiropractic is generally considered effective only for temporary back and joint pain. Find out whether the chiropractor is part of a team of health care providers, and see whether he will provide referrals if necessary. Be suspicious of a practitioner who attempts to sell you expensive nutritional supplements or devices that purport to improve your health.

There are approximately 50,000 chiropractors in the United States. They are licensed in every state and must pass an examination with the National Board of Chiropractic Examiners. Restrictions on the procedures they may perform vary from state to state. To be admitted to a managed care plan, they must often pass additional tests.

The 16 chiropractic colleges in the U.S. are accredited by the Council on Chiropractic Education, a federally recognized accrediting agency. Typical academic training and clinical internships include four years of training at an accredited institution after a minimum of two years of college; more than 2,000 study hours of biological and clinical sciences; more than 1,000 study hours of chiropractic sciences, including body mechanics, spinal analysis and adjustments, diagnostic imaging, and x-ray interpretation; internships in clinical radiology and interpretation; and at least 900 hours of clinical practice and patient care. Some chiropractors have additional postgraduate or continuing education in the fields of sports injuries, occupational health, orthopedics, or neurology.

When Should Treatment Stop?

In many cases, relief is immediate. If pain persists, allow some time for improvement to appear—

2 weeks is generally sufficient in cases of acute low-back pain. If there's still no change, or if the condition becomes worse, stop the treatments and seek alternative therapy. Many chiropractors refer patients to specialists for further evaluation when a condition persists.

See a Conventional Doctor If . . .

Despite chiropractic's original contention that all health problems stem from subluxation, your wisest course is to check with an MD if the problem isn't clearly related to the back or joints. Likewise, if a chiropractor discovers any dangerous problems that need immediate medical attention, he's likely to refer you to a medical specialist without delay. Tumors, fractures, or other suspicious findings viewed on an x-ray are common reasons for immediate referral.

Resources

ORGANIZATIONS

The American Chiropractic Association
1701 Clarendon Blvd.
Arlington, VA 22209
Phone: 703-276-8800;
800-986-4636
Web: http://www.amerchiro.org

The International Chiropractors Association
1110 North Glebe Rd.,
Suite 1000
Arlington, VA 22201
Phone: 703-528-5000
Web: http://www.chiropractic.org

FURTHER READING

The American Holistic Health Association Complete Guide to Alternative Medicine. William Collinge, MPH, PhD. New York: Warner Books, 1987.

Chiropractic: The Victim's Perspective. George Magner. Amherst, NY: Prometheus Books, 1995.

The Alternative Health & Medicine Encyclopedia. James E. Marti. Detroit: Visible Ink Press, 1995.

Quackwatch. Website at http://www.quackwatch.com

Dr. Rosenfield's' Guide to Alternative Medicine. Isadore Rosenfield, MD. New York: Random House, 1997.

The New Wellness Encyclopedia. The editors of the University of California at Berkeley Wellness Letter. New York: Houghton Mifflin Company, 1995.

Understanding Acute Low Back Problems, Consumer Version. Clinical Practice Guideline No. 14, U.S. Department of Health and Human Services, Public Health Service, Agency for Health Care Policy and Research, Publication No. 95-0644, December 1994. Write: ACHPR Publications Clearinghouse, P.O. Box 8547, Silver Spring, MD 20907; Call: 1-800-358-9295.

Colonic Irrigation

Consider This Therapy For

Before the advent of antibiotics and other modern medicines, "cleansing" the bowels was a popular therapy for everything from infections to heart disease, high blood pressure, arthritis, and depression.

Today, mainstream medicine rejects not only the therapy, but even the rationale for its use. Opponents deny its ability to cure any sort of ailment, and warn that careless administration of the treatments can spread disease and cause serious—even life-threatening—problems.

Modern advocates of this extremely passé procedure say it's an important way of maintaining general health and preventing illness. There are, however, no scientific studies to support this contention, and virtually all medical experts continue to dismiss the therapy as worthless.

How the Treatments Are Done

The goal of this procedure is to flush "built-up" toxins from the bowel. The treatments are usually given in an office, a special clinic, or a spa. Before the procedure begins, you'll need to change into a hospital-style gown with an opening in the back and may be asked to take an enema.

During the session, you'll lie on a treatment table while the therapist gently inserts a small rigid tube called a speculum about 5½ inches into your rectum. He or she will then attach the speculum to a plastic hose connected to a colon irrigation machine. This device will slowly fill the five-foot length of your colon with warm, purified water. Herbs or enzymes are sometimes added to the water in hope of increasing the benefits of the treatment.

The water causes the muscles that line the colon to contract and expand rhythmically, forcing out the fecal matter (undigested food, water, and bacteria), gas, and mucus through an evacuation tube that leads back to the machine. While the water is in the bowel, the therapist may massage portions of your abdomen to help loosen and remove as much fecal material as possible from the pockets and folds that line the walls of the colon. Some therapists also find reflexology and special breathing and relaxation techniques useful for ridding the colon of waste.

After the first infusion of water has been expelled, the procedure will be repeated until a total of 20 to 30 gallons of water have been flushed through the bowel. Although you should not have any pain, you may feel a sensation of warmth as the cleansing proceeds. The cause, say some practitioners, is the presence of toxins in the fecal matter leaving your body.

In preparation for the treatment, you'll be told to eat light meals on the day before therapy. Many practitioners suggest that you stick to small portions of fruits and vegetables for breakfast and lunch and take even less for supper. On the day of the procedure, eating will probably be forbidden until the treatment is over. Some colon therapists suggest that you take a "cleansing" drink, such as psyllium powder and bentonite, and use a mild laxative the night before treatment, while others say no special preparation is necessary.

After the session, practitioners typically advise eating easy-to-digest, nourishing foods such as vegetable soups and broths, fruit and vegetable juices, or peppermint tea. To help restore the bacterial balance in your colon, the therapist may insert acidophilus in your rectum or instruct you to drink a product containing acidophilus for the following 2 weeks.

Treatment Time: Each session lasts between 30 and 50 minutes.
Treatment Frequency: While some practitioners advise 1 or 2 sessions, and others recommend 4 to 8, a few insist that to maintain a well-functioning colon, you need treatments every 3 to 6 months.

What the Treatment Hopes to Accomplish

Like many of the alternative medical practices currently enjoying a renaissance, colon therapy has its roots in Egypt, Greece, and India, where enemas and physics have been used for many centuries to cleanse the body of disease. In early times the procedure was performed in rivers, using a hollow reed. By the 1890s, it had reached the New World. Thousands of Americans flocked to spas that promised radiant health and rejuvenation through "high colonic" enemas.

Perhaps the most famous early therapist was John Harvey Kellogg, who later founded the cereal company that still bears his name. In his sprawling Battle Creek, Michigan, sanitarium, he treated 40,000 patients with gastrointestinal disease. All but two of them, according to his accounts, avoided surgery through his ministrations.

The "high colonic" craze reached its peak in the 1920s and 1930s. Machines for flushing out the colon appeared in hundreds of physicians' offices and hospitals, and thousands of Americans seemed fixated on bowel movements. Then, as more effective treatments were discovered, colonic irrigation slowly vanished from the conventional medical scene.

Contemporary advocates still insist that "high colonics" can cure ailments ranging from asthma to cancer. They regard the colon as a fertile breeding ground for damaging toxins and insist that regular cleansing is necessary to maintain good health.

The colon, a tube-shaped organ also called the large bowel, processes undigested food passed on to it from the small intestine, absorbing water into the system and slowly propelling the solid remnant to the rectum, where it is eliminated from the body. The movement of the broken-down food is accomplished by peristalsis, the rhythmic contraction of the muscles lining the walls of the colon.

Proponents of colonic irrigation contend that thick, gluey fecal matter—mostly undigested cellulose, bacteria, viruses, fungi, and, perhaps, parasites—can accumulate in the pockets and folds that line the walls of the colon and become backed-up along the passageways of the colon. As more and more feces pack the bowel, elimination becomes increasingly difficult.

This, they say, is where all the trouble begins. They believe that, as the fecal matter builds up and stagnates, it begins to produce toxic substances. This condition not only can affect the normal function of the colon, but, because the toxic matter is absorbed into the bloodstream, can also have a negative impact on the liver, lymphatic system, lungs, kidneys, thyroid, and other vital organs. The body, they theorize, regards toxic molecules of undigested foods as foreign bodies and produces antibodies to fight them. In the process, the antibodies can also destroy healthy tissue.

The villain, according to proponents of this treatment, is the modern diet: high in fats and sugar, low in fiber. Also to blame, they say, is the tendency of most Americans to defecate infrequently. They strongly advocate having at least one movement for every meal eaten and heading to the bathroom immediately upon feeling "the urge."

Irrigation becomes necessary, according to this theory, whenever a build-up interferes with normal elimination. The cleansing treatments, they say, rid the colon of the potentially poisonous encrusted stool. Normal peristalsis is restored, bowel movements become regular, the blood is cleansed of toxins, the immune system returns to normal, and the body becomes healthy.

Mainstream medical practitioners question virtually every aspect of this theory. They point out that both Americans and Europeans are needlessly obsessed with constipation, and there is absolutely no scientific proof that people need to defecate frequently. They argue that accumulation of fecal matter is actually a rather rare event, and that a high-fiber diet with liberal fluid intake is sufficient to remedy the problem when it occurs.

Furthermore, they point out that there is no evidence that the modern American diet produces any toxins in the bowel, or that accumulated fecal matter turns poisonous. In fact, the toxins postulated by colon therapists have never been identified and have never been found in any organ or in the bloodstream. Colonic irrigation, they observe, isn't even the most effective remedy for intestinal parasites, which can be more reliably eliminated by standard drug treatments.

To all these objections, they add that the treatments pose the risk of a chemical imbalance in the body, a perforated bowel, or an infection. Worse yet, if the treatments take the place of effective therapy, disorders that could be cured may go unchecked, causing needless pain and risk.

Who Should Avoid This Therapy?

Because these treatments do pose certain risks, check with your doctor before proceeding. Avoid this therapy completely if you have Crohn's disease, diverticulitis, hemorrhoids, tumors of the large intestine or rectum, or ulcerative colitis.

What Side Effects May Occur?

Therapists often use laxatives and enemas as part of the treatment, and critics warn that overuse of these products can damage your colon. They also feel that the vast quantity of water used can stretch the bowel to such an extent that it can no longer function properly.

Other possible side effects may include general weakness and deficiencies or imbalances of enzymes that work on fat, fat-soluble vitamins, and calcium.

The most dangerous potential side effect is inadvertent perforation of the colon by a nozzle.

How to Choose a Therapist

As late as the early 1980s, sanitary conditions at some treatment centers in this country were appalling. Because facilities were not kept clean and equipment was often not sterilized adequately, clients ran the risk of developing amebic dysentery and other potentially serious—even fatal—infections.

Today, fortunately, things have

changed radically. Most treatment centers now use disposable applicators and adhere to rigorous standards of cleanliness as established by such certification organizations as the International Association of Colon Hydrotherapy. This organization, for example, requires that applicants for initial certification submit photos of every section of their facility, including treatment rooms and bathrooms, and that they complete a detailed questionnaire. Despite these generally improved standards, it's wise to inspect the cleanliness of the office before signing up for therapy. Make certain, too, that the equipment is sterilized between patients.

Most practitioners of colon therapy are naturopaths, holistic doctors, acupuncturists, hygienists, or chiropractors. If you are considering this treatment, try to find an experienced therapist. Look, too, for certification by one of the organizations listed under "Resources" below.

When Should Treatment Stop?

If you develop an infection, feel weak, or have any other serious symptoms following therapy, stop treatment and check with a doctor.

Remember that the risk of side effects increases with the frequency of treatments. Limit them to the minimum number necessary for improvement. If you see no benefit after the recommended course of therapy, discontinue the treatments and seek a better alternative.

See a Conventional Doctor If . . .

If you pursue colon therapy at all, use it as a general health maintenance measure. Medical experts stress that it will not cure any major physical or psychological problem. If you develop any new symptoms, see a physician for a professional diagnosis.

Resources

ORGANIZATIONS

American Association of Naturopathic Physicians
2366 Eastlake Ave.
Suite 322
Seattle, WA 98102
Phone: 206-323-7610

American Colon Therapy Association
17739 Washington Blvd.
Los Angeles, CA 90066
Phone: 310-572-6223

California Colon Hygienists Society
P.O. Box 588
Graton, CA 95444
Phone: 707-829-0984

International Association for Colon Hydrotherapy
P.O. Box 461285
San Antonio, TX 78246-1286
Phone: 210-366-2888

FURTHER READING

The Alternative Medicine Handbook. Barrie R. Cassileth, PhD. New York: W.W. Norton & Company, Inc., 1998.
Dr. Rosenfeld's Guide to Alternative Medicine. Isadore Rosen-

feld, MD. New York: Random House, 1996.

Alternative Medicine: The Definitive Guide. The Burton Goldberg Group. Puyallup, WA: Future Medicine Publishing, Inc., 1994.

Craniosacral Therapy

Consider This Therapy For

This controversial form of hands-on therapy seeks to cure disease by manipulating the bones of the skull. Practitioners assert that certain disorders are caused by obstructions in the normal flow of the cerebrospinal fluid that bathes the brain and spinal cord. By gently nudging the head, spine, sacrum (lower spine), rib cage, and limbs, they believe they can break up these obstructions, reestablish the natural rhythm of cerebrospinal flow, and thus relieve associated illnesses.

Among the disorders targeted by craniosacral therapy are trigeminal neuralgia (stabbing pains in the jaw), headaches, sinusitis, visual disturbances, strabismus (an imbalance in the eye muscles), transient cerebral ischemia (temporary "mini-strokes"), traumatic brain injury, vertigo, and certain cases of mental retardation. Some proponents also suggest it for asthma, sinusitis, ear-nose-throat problems, cerebral palsy, and muscle tension headache ("to the degree that biomechanical problems cause these conditions"). Others recommend it for children with learning disabilities, attention-deficit-hyperactive disorders, pervasive developmental delay, cerebral palsy, ear infections, genetic and neurological disorders, and autism. It is also proposed for certain soft tissue injuries to the head, torso, and extremities.

Advocates of craniosacral therapy (also known as cranial osteopathy) cite numerous case studies as proof of its effectiveness. Nevertheless, mainstream physicians and medical organizations refuse to recommend it. They say that manipulation of the bones of the skull is impossible, since they are all fused together. They add that, whether the bones move or not, there have been no scientifically controlled clinical trials to prove the technique's success.

How the Treatments Are Done

Unlike the chiropractic adjustments that pop a joint back into proper alignment, craniosacral therapy is done with light touches to the head, spine, sacrum, ribs, and extremities. The version of the therapy propounded by Dr. John Upledger is particularly noted for its light touch—equivalent to the weight of a nickel in the palm of the hand.

Treatment Time: Sessions typically last 30 minutes to 1 hour.
Treatment Frequency: Varies with the problem and patient.

What Treatment Hopes to Accomplish

Cranial osteopathy—the initial form of this therapy—is a neglected subspecialty of general osteopathy (treatment of disease through adjustment of the bones). Developed in the 1930s by William Garner Sutherland, DO, it attempts to diagnose medical problems by evaluating the motion of the skull and sacrum, and by feeling the "cranial rhythmic impulse" throughout the body. (This impulse is said to reflect the flow of cerebrospinal fluid, as well as the motion of the brain, spinal cord, and surrounding membranes, along with movement in the skull bones and sacrum. It's said that a trained practitioner can feel it.)

Cranial osteopaths hold that trauma to the head or body can alter or hinder the flow of fluids or change the skull's natural configuration, thereby causing illness. Birth trauma, for example, is said to lead to colic, chronic ear infections, inability to suck or swallow, and developmental delays. Manipulations that restore the normal flow of fluids are thought to relieve such problems.

While cranial osteopathy is included in the general osteopathic curriculum and appears in the osteopathic board exams, few osteopaths include it in their practice. Out of more than 40,000 DOs in the United States, only 1,000 are members of The Cranial Academy, cranial osteopathy's professional organization.

A more recent variation of this therapy, emphasizing a light, gentle touch, was developed in the 1970s by John Upledger, DO. Dr. Upledger's interest in this area was ignited when, while assisting in surgery, he observed movement of the membrane that lines the skull and covers the brain and spinal cord. His work built upon that of Dr. Sutherland. Much like cranial osteopaths, his followers hold that touching the head, feet, or other areas can reveal restrictions in the "craniosacral rhythm." The same touch that finds the rhythm is also said to relieve symptoms.

Is there really a craniosacral rhythm, and can manipulating the skull really affect it? According to most mainstream doctors, the answers are clear-cut. It's a well-known, long-established, physically evident fact, they say, that the bones of the skull fuse into a single unit around the age of two, and can't be manipulated thereafter.

Craniosacral therapists, however, simply don't accept this. They say that research reported in the Journal of the American Osteopathic Association as recently as 1996 has confirmed the existence of motion around the sutures of the skull bones. Using infrared markers attached to acupuncture needles or stuck to the skin, the researchers say they not only detected movement, but actually identified a cranial rhythmic impulse.

Dr. Upledger himself made intensive efforts to establish the existence of the craniosacral system, working with anatomists, physiologists, biophysicists, and bioengineers at Michigan State University's College of Osteopathic Medicine from 1975 to 1983. He cites many published reports in support of the existence of a craniosacral system. In the end, however, he argues that "positive patient outcomes ... should weigh greater than data from designed research protocols."

Who Should Avoid This Therapy?

According to its critics, no one should try this therapy, since it can't possibly help. And even its practitioners say its not worth trying unless the problem has a biomechanical origin (is caused by abnormal pressure or stress).

Whatever your problem, you should definitely forego craniosacral therapy if you have a known or suspected brain hemorrhage or aneurysm, or have any other condition that makes it ill-advised to alter the pressure of intracranial fluid. The treatments are also considered unwise for small children with only recently fused skull bones, although no problems have actually been reported.

What Side Effects May Occur?

Even critics of this therapy view it as physically harmless, and the chances of triggering an adverse reaction seem extremely slight. Nevertheless, problems have been reported in traumatic brain injury patients receiving craniosacral therapy as part of an outpatient rehabilitation program. The symptoms included headache, vomiting, diarrhea, cardiac palpitation, angry thoughts, paranoia, explosive behavior, and a total body spasm. Whether they were caused by the therapy or

the underlying injury remains undetermined.

How to Choose a Therapist

Two organizations can give you referrals.

The Cranial Academy, a component society of the American Academy of Osteopathy, issues certificates of competency to members who have passed written, oral, and practice competency testing, and have completed 3 years of clinical practice. The Academy certifies only fully licensed professionals such as doctors, osteopaths, and, in some states, dentists. It provides names of members, but does not vouch for their competence.

The Upledger Institute offers courses in craniosacral therapy to medical doctors, doctors of osteopathy, psychologists, occupational therapists, physical therapists, massage therapists, bodyworkers, and lay persons. However, neither the American Academy of Osteopathy nor the American Osteopathic Association grant continuing medical education credits for these courses.

When Should Treatment Stop?

If you find the treatments helpful, they can safely be continued indefinitely.

See a Conventional Doctor If . . .

Craniosacral therapy is not recommended for such life-threatening problems as heart disease, cancer, or medical emergencies. In addition, if your therapist is not an MD or DO, you should check with a doctor whenever a worrisome new symptom appears.

Resources

ORGANIZATIONS

The Cranial Academy
8202 Clearvista Parkway, #9-D
Indianapolis, IN 46256
Phone: 317-594-0411

The Upledger Institute
11211 Prosperity Farms Rd.,
D325
Palm Beach Gardens, FL 33410
Phone: 561-622-4334

FURTHER READING

CranioSacral Therapy. R. Desjarlais. In *Dermascope*, September/October, 1997, p. 96–100.
Differences Separate Cranio-Sacral Therapy from Cranial Osteopathy. J.E. Upledger. In *Massage & Bodywork*, Fall 1995, pp. 20-22.
Quackwatch. Website at http://www.quackwatch.com
Reader's Guide to Alternative Health Methods. J.F. Zwicky, A.W. Hafner, S. Barrett, W.T. Jarvis. Chicago, IL: American Medical Association, 1993.

Detoxification Therapy

Consider This Therapy For

A product of environmental concerns and nostalgia for the more natural lifestyles of the past, these treatments aim to free the body from a build-up of various artificial toxins. The poisons targeted by these therapies are not necessarily the high-profile carcinogens we've all come to fear. More often, they are unspecified pollutants and by-products thought to have a generally negative impact on health.

Although the offending substances are frequently nameless and vague, advocates of detoxification believe that, as a group, these chemicals are somehow at the root of all disease. Eliminating them, proponents believe, eases the load on the immune system and gives the body a chance to heal itself. In this way, they say, detoxification can prevent cancer, heart disease, arthritis, and diabetes; lower blood pressure; increase vitality; improve mental function; and slow down the aging process.

Since no single, specific toxin is typically identified for elimination, it's impossible to say whether the treatments have succeeded in removing it, or whether it was causing a problem in the first place. Most mainstream scientists therefore dismiss the whole approach as unproven—and unprovable. And there are, in fact, no clinical studies supporting the effectiveness of these treatments.

How the Treatments Are Done

Naturopathic practitioners and an assortment of maverick physicians have devised a number of methods to rid the body of the toxins we are presumed to build up. You'll find the more popular of these approaches summarized on pages 110–112.

In all cases, you're likely to be given a brief physical before treatment begins. The therapist will start by taking a complete history that covers both your own health and that of family members. He or she will then take your blood pressure; check your lungs, heart, joints, and reflexes; arrange for x-rays; and send a sample of your urine and blood to a laboratory for analysis. Some practitioners will also order analysis of a sample of your hair to check for the presence of heavy metals. Others may feel it helpful to analyze the contents of your sweat. You may also receive a battery of questions about your diet, your workplace, and your everyday activities.

CHELATION

This relatively painless procedure is the antidote for heavy-metal poisoning, and is also used in attempts to reverse hardening of the arteries. It usually takes place in a physician's office or clinic. You will lie back in a comfortable reclining chair while the doctor or a staff member inserts a tiny needle in a vein in your finger or the back of your hand. An intravenous solution containing ethylenediaminetetraacetic acid (EDTA) is then administered in hope of preventing health problems or clearing excess calcium from the arteries. Each session usually takes between 3 and 4 hours. In most cases, physicians recommend between 20 and 50 treatments at a rate of 1 to 3 a week.

For more information, turn to the profile on chelation.

COLONIC IRRIGATION

These treatments aim to cleanse the bowel of purportedly toxic fecal matter, which is thought to build up and leak poisons into the bloodstream. The sessions may take place in an office, a special clinic, or a spa. During the treatments, a special colon irrigation machine pumps warm, purified water into the lower bowel to loosen and remove the built-up fecal matter supposedly clinging to the walls. These instillations are repeated until a total of 20 to 30 gallons of water have been washed through the bowel. Each session takes between 30 and 50 minutes. While some practitioners say only 1 or 2 sessions are necessary, others recommend 4 to 8, and a few insist that you should be treated every 3 to 6 months. For additional details, turn to the profile on colonic irrigation.

A variation of this approach is the coffee enema, a technique devised in the 1940s by Dr. Max Gerson to treat cancer, which, he believed, was caused by artificial ingredients, environmental pollution, sugar, starch, and salt. Today, this form of colon therapy is still practiced at the Gerson Clinic in Mexico, and in other clinics near Tijuana. The caffeine in the enemas is thought to stimulate the production of detoxifying bile. The enemas are usually given on an inpatient basis, one an hour for a period of weeks or months.

FASTING

Whether you fast or follow a special detoxification diet (see below), therapists consistently recommend that during treatment—and after—you should avoid all chemicals, refined foods, food additives, sugar, tobacco, and alcoholic beverages. Many also request that you stop taking medications. (Because discontinuing certain medications can be dangerous, check with your doctor before you comply.) You will also be instructed to drink a great deal of filtered or mineral water.

There are two basic types of fasts: water fasts and juice fasts. The water fast is exactly what its name implies. For 24 to 36 hours you must drink not less than 4, nor more than 8 pints of water—and nothing else. This type of fast is usually done over a weekend. You may be allowed to take raw fruits and vegetables along with your water on Sunday. Some therapists suggest you fast this way every weekend for a few months. Others say you should start with three weekends a month and gradually reduce your fasts until your tongue no longer feels furry and you have no more headaches (see "Side Effects" on page 114).

Juice fasts include various forms of vegetable juices: carrot, celery, green bean, parsley, watercress, and zucchini are among the most popular. Some therapists also allow vegetable broths, herbal teas, miso (fermented soy paste), and powdered algae. One suggests you also drink a mixture of garlic, lemon juice, grapefruit juice, and olive oil at bedtime. (The combination is thought to detoxify the liver.) Juice fasts usually last around 10 days. Since they are fairly long and restrictive, these fasts should not be undertaken too frequently, critics say.

For more information, see the profiles on fasting and juice therapy.

SPECIAL DIETS

So-called "detoxification" diets usually emphasize organically grown, pesticide-free fresh fruits and vegetables (cooked or steamed); yogurt containing live cultures; whole grains and seeds; herbal teas such as mint, lemon, and chamomile; and plenty of water (at least 32 ounces a day). Some diets also allow beans, nuts, low-fat dairy products, fresh fish, or organically raised poultry. In any case, you will have to avoid all sugar, salt, saturated fat, coffee, alcohol, and nicotine.

Your therapist may also put you on a diet that restricts you to only one food (for example, grapes, apples, papaya), one type of food (whole grains, potatoes), or only raw foods. You will probably be told to eat slowly; chew well (some practitioners insist you must chew each morsel 30 to 60 times); finish your meals by 6:30 PM; cook only in iron, stainless steel, glass, or porcelain pots; and substitute natural remedies for synthetic drugs. To aid in detoxification, the regimen may also call for additional fiber or frequent enemas. Depending on the nature of the diet, it can end in a few weeks or go on for months or years.

HYPERTHERMIA AND OTHER HYDROTHERAPY TREATMENTS

All of these techniques assume that heat can detoxify the body. You may sit in a steam room or cabinet; take a sauna (hot, dry heat) followed by a cold shower or a dip in a cold pool; or soak in a hot solution of baking soda, sea salt, or even chlorine bleach. When undertaking these treatments, you must be careful to observe strict time limits, since excessive hyperthermia can be dangerous. Limit sessions in a Turkish bath or steam room to about 20 minutes, and remain in a steam cabinet for no more than 1 hour. If you take a sauna, you will need to take a cold shower or plunge into a cold pool every 5 to 10 minutes during treatment, and at the end of your session. You can stay in a detoxifying bath until the water cools. For more information, see the profiles on hyperthermia and hydrotherapy.

LYMPHATIC STIMULATION

Your therapist may massage your body lightly in the areas where lymph glands are present, for example, around your ribs.

NUTRITIONAL SUPPLEMENTS

Therapists often recommend massive quantities of vitamin C for people undergoing detoxification.

Other suggested supplements include vitamins A and E, the B vitamins (especially niacin), and minerals such as zinc, selenium, potassium, and magnesium. L-cysteine and methionine are also popular among detoxification practitioners, and some therapists favor herbs such as garlic, cayenne, and echinacea. They often suggest adding extra fiber to the diet, as well.

What the Treatment Hopes to Accomplish

In the "good old days," say the proponents of detoxification therapy, the air was clean, the water pure, and the foods natural. Today, they warn, we have sealed our own doom with chemicals, additives, preservatives, and other forms of environmental pollution.

Overlooked in this flattering view of the past are the industrial dust, fumes, and soot that used to fill the air, the horse droppings that dirtied the streets, and the spoiled food that threatened illness at every meal. Nevertheless, many people now fear that the many synthetic chemicals we've used to improve our world could have unexpected consequences on our health.

To detoxification advocates, this is more than a danger. They firmly believe that we are living in an age of "toxic overload," and that the herbicides, pesticides, insecticides, rancid oils, artificial colors and flavors, food additives, and preservatives we use or ingest every day eventually interfere with the normal functioning of our bodies. They find danger lurking in paints, household cleaning products, cosmetics, prescription and over-the-counter medications—even clothes made from synthetic products. The refined and processed foods in our diet pose additional threats, they say, along with our high intake of fat, caffeine, and alcohol.

Although the government has tested all these substances and certified them safe, advocates of detoxification therapy insist that these chemicals (or their by-products) can remain in the body for years, causing serious damage to essential organs such as the liver, kidneys, adrenals, and thyroid, and compromising the immune system. A healthy diet (no artificial ingredients or refined foods, and little fat) and a chemical-free home and workplace can, they say, get you started on the road back to health, but won't fully undo the damage caused by years of toxic build-up. For that you need the treatments (or fasts, or diets) that they happen to prescribe.

While it's clear that excessive intake of almost any chemical can have severe repercussions, few experts see any danger in the trace amounts we're currently exposed to. They also dismiss the idea that unidentified toxins can build up in the body and cause ill health. They charge that many of the recommended treatments are ineffective. And they warn that many can be dangerous as well.

Chelation, for instance, is deemed effective only for removing heavy metals from the bloodstream. There is no proof that it stops the production of dangerous free radicals, opens up the arteries by removing calcium from artery walls, or increases blood flow. It has not been effective for reversing heart disease and other plaque-related problems.

Colonic Irrigation, mainstream physicians point out, is based on a false assumption. Fecal matter rarely builds up on the lining of the bowel, and has never been shown to produce toxins. Furthermore, rather than curing diseases, this therapy can cause a host of health problems, including bowel dysfunction, infections, and even intestinal perforation.

Coffee Enemas, which are supposed to stimulate the flow of bile from the liver and thus carry toxins away, have never been proven effective, and could be dangerous.

Fasting, critics warn, does not clear out stored toxins and allow the body to heal itself. Indeed, they say, it can do the opposite. Fasting lowers blood sugar levels, so that the body is forced to get energy from the protein in muscle tissue. In a prolonged fast, this can raise levels of ammonia and nitrogen so high that the undernourished kidneys and liver cannot get rid of the excess. Uric acid levels may rise (leading to gout), and calcium and potassium levels may be disturbed (affecting the heart rhythm). Ultimately, the kidneys and liver could fail. The body's ability to fight infection is also compromised.

Special Diets can also be dangerous. Programs that eliminate or severely restrict nutrients such as fats or proteins can weaken the system instead of strengthening it.

Hyperthermia, doctors point out, can relieve pain and improve circulation, but it won't kill bacteria and viruses, and doesn't rid the body of poisons or cure disease.

Vitamin C is also not a miracle cure, say most physicians. Detoxification advocates claim that vitamin C combines with and destroys toxins produced by environmental and chemical pollutants. Not true, physicians reply. A host of double-blind clinical studies have failed to prove that it cures anything, including the common cold.

Who Should Avoid This Therapy?

Do not take **any type** of detoxification therapy if you are pregnant, nursing, elderly, weak, or underweight. Also avoid all forms of detoxification if you have diabetes or suffer from ulcers.

Avoid **chelation** if you have kidney or liver problems.

Avoid **colonic irrigation** if you have Crohn's disease, ulcerative colitis, or any other type of bowel inflammation. Avoid it, too, if you suffer from diverticulitis, hemorrhoids, or tumors of the large intestine or rectum.

Avoid **fasting** if you have advanced cancer, heart problems, kidney disease, liver disease, diabetes, lung problems, or tuberculosis.

Avoid **hyperthermia** if you have asthma, epilepsy, heart disease, high or low blood pressure, or multiple sclerosis. Also steer clear of this therapy if you are very young or very old, have recently had surgery, or have a history of blood clots.

What Side Effects May Occur?

Excessive use of **chelation** has been known to cause anemia, blood clots, bone marrow damage, fever, headache, insulin shock, irregular heartbeat, joint pain, low blood pressure, painful and difficult urination, inflammation of the area where the needle is inserted, and stroke.

Possible side effects from **colon therapy** include enzyme deficiencies or imbalances, general weakness, infection (if the facility is not sterile), bowel dysfunction, intestinal perforation, and alternating bouts of constipation and diarrhea.

Early side effects from **fasting** may include headache and a furry tongue. An extremely long fast can end with anemia, body aches, decreased sex drive, depression, dizziness, fainting, fatigue, gout, irregular heartbeat, irritability, kidney or liver failure, low blood pressure, low blood sugar, lowered resistance to infection, nausea, osteoporosis, and weakness.

High doses of **vitamin C** can cause diarrhea and other digestive problems and the formation of kidney stones.

How to Choose a Therapist

If you decide to undergo **chelation** therapy, select a physician (a medical doctor or osteopath) with several years of experience and specialized training and certification from a major professional organization such as The American College for Advancement in Medicine or The American Board of Chelation Therapy. (See addresses and telephone numbers below.)

When seeking **colonic irrigation**, look for a therapist certified by one of the following organizations: American Association of Naturopathic Physicians; American Colon Therapy Association; California Colon Hygienists Society; or the International Association for Colon Hydrotherapy. (See addresses and telephone numbers below.)

To find an expert on **fasting**, you might want to check with the American Association of Naturopathic Physicians. (See addresses and telephone numbers below.)

When Should Treatment Stop?

If you develop an infection, feel weak, or have any other serious symptoms, stop treatment and see your physician.

See a Conventional Doctor If . . .

Check with your doctor before undertaking any type of detoxification therapy, and be certain to ask your doctor before discontinuing any medication. While under-going therapy, seek medical advice immediately if new symptoms develop or you fail to make progress.

Do not undertake a long fast without medical supervision. Short fasts are usually safe for people in good health. If you have a heart problem, you may need frequent EKGs (electrocardiograms) to make sure the fast is not affecting your heart.

Do NOT rely on detoxification alone to cure any life-threatening disease, such as cancer or heart disease. There simply isn't enough evidence in its favor to justify the risk.

Resources

ORGANIZATIONS

Chelation:
American Board of Chelation Therapy
70 West Huron St.
Chicago, IL 60610
Phone: 312-266-7246

American College of Advancement in Medicine
P.O. Box 3427
Laguna Hills, CA 92654
Phone: 714-583-7666

Colon Therapy:
American Association of Naturopathic Physicians
2366 Eastlake Ave.
Suite 322
Seattle, WA 98102
Phone: 206-323-7610

American Colon Therapy Association
17739 Washington Blvd.

Los Angeles, CA 90066
Phone: 310-572-6223

California Colon Hygienists Society
P.O. Box 588
Graton, CA 95444
Phone: 707-829-0984

International Association for Colon Hydrotherapy
P.O. Box 461285
San Antonio, TX 78246-1286
Phone: 210-366-2888

Fasting:
American Association of Naturopathic Physicians
2366 Eastlake Ave.
Suite 322
Seattle, WA 98102
Phone: 800-206-7610

American College of Nutrition
301 E. 17th St.
New York, NY 10003
Phone: 212-777-1037

American Society for Clinical Nutrition
9650 Rockville Pike
Bethesda, MD 20814
Phone: 301-530-7110

FURTHER READING

Body/Mind Purification Program.
Leon Chaitow. New York: Simon and Schuster/Gaia, 1990.
Staying Healthy with Nutrition.
Elson Haas. Berkeley, CA: Celestial Arts, 1992.
What Your Doctor Won't Tell You.
J. Heimlich. New York: HarperCollins Publishers, 1990.

The Complete Guide to Health and Nutrition. Gary Null. New York: Delacorte Press, 1986.
Diet for a Poisoned Planet. David Steinman. New York: Ballantine Books, 1990.
The Healing Powers of Chelation. John P. Trowbridge and Morten Walker. Stamford, CT: New Way of Life, Inc., 1992.

Energy Medicine

Consider This Therapy For

Electricity plays a prominent role in modern medicine. The charged paddles used to jolt the heart back into action are a common sight in emergency rooms everywhere. Electroencephalograms (EEGs) record electrical brain waves and electrocardiograms (EKGs) read the rhythms of the heart. Electrical devices ranging from the common x-ray to the gigantic MRI (magnetic resonance imaging) machine routinely give us an accurate diagnosis.

The contraptions and procedures promoted under the rubric of "energy medicine" are, however, an entirely different matter. They are either extremely controversial or totally unproven. Some are simply electrified versions of other alternative therapies such as acupuncture. Others are the last remnants of a fascination with "black box" cures that extends from the dawn of the electrical age through the present.

Of all the electrical therapies currently available, *transcutaneous electrical nerve stimulation (TENS)* is the closest to adoption in the mainstream. It can be used for any type of localized physical pain, although it is most commonly advocated for arthritis, sciatica, neuralgia, and chronic back pain. It is sometimes used after knee, hip, or lower back surgery (usually in combination with other analgesic treatments). And it has also been used for dental pain, jaw muscle pain, cancer pain, angina pectoris, menstrual pain, migraine, carpal tunnel syndrome, repetitive strain injuries, pain from nerve damage, musculoskeletal trauma, and the pain of shingles.

All other forms of energy therapy remain either untested or unverified. Among the leading examples, *electroacupuncture* and *auricular acupuncture* (acupuncture limited to the ear) are advocated for treatment of disorders throughout the body. Similarly, a device called the *MORA* delivers electromagnetic energy to various acupuncture points, purportedly relieving headaches, migraines, muscular aches and pains, circulation disorders, and skin disease. Another variation on this theme—*electroacupuncture biofeedback*—is promoted as a diagnostic tool capable of revealing the presence of toxins, food allergies, and "imbalances."

Moving beyond acupuncture, the *Electro-Acuscope* promises to relieve pain by running current through damaged tissues. It is generally applied to such conditions as muscle spasms, migraines, jaw pain, bursitis, arthritis, surgical incisions, sprains and strains,

neuralgia, shingles, and bruises. *Microcurrent Electrical Therapy (MET)* is also promoted for pain relief in the muscles and joints, and is said to speed wound healing as well. A device called the *Light Beam Generator* is advocated for healing throughout the body.

Other unproven devices attempt to use sound and radio waves therapeutically. *Cymatic Instruments*, supposedly tuned to the "frequency" of various tissues, are said to diagnose aberrations and restore the tissues to health. Likewise, the *Sound Probe* is employed to kill viruses, bacteria, and fungi. A device called the *Diapulse* employs radio waves to reduce swelling and inflammation following surgery.

In almost all cases, there is little if any published research in reputable journals to back up the claims made for these instruments. It's conceivable that some of them may actually be effective, but the odds are not strongly in their favor.

How the Treatments Are Done

Transcutaneous Electrical Nerve Stimulation. These treatments are administered with a small electronic unit that sends pulsed currents to a set of electrodes stuck to the skin. The electrodes are usually placed near the painful area (often on either side), over a main nerve leading to the painful area, on the spine one or two segments above the spinal nerve receiving the pain, or at acupuncture points. Treatments are typically given 3 to 4 times per day for 30 to 40 minutes a session, or intermittently at the physician's and user's discretion.

Electroacupuncture. Typically, the therapist inserts 4 to 20 thin disposable needles into the patient's skin, either directly into the area of pain or into traditional acupuncture points. Once the needles are in place, they are stimulated with a low-level electrical charge. The treatment generally takes 15 to 30 minutes.

Auricular Acupuncture. Practitioners of this form of therapy believe that each area of the ear is linked to a corresponding part of the body. The therapist may apply gentle pressure to the part of the ear associated with the problem, either by hand, or with small acupuncture needles and a weak electrical current or laser or infrared light. Electrical therapy entails a very brief, 10-second burst of current at about 100 microamperes or less.

Microcurrent Electrical Therapy. For these treatments, electrodes are placed over the painful area on opposite sides of the body, so that the current will run through it. Treatment time varies with the size of the injured or diseased site. The effect of the treatments is said to be cumulative, so at least three treatments are typically needed before pain relief sets in.

What Treatment Hopes to Accomplish

Transcutaneous Electrical Nerve Stimulation. The pulsed currents delivered in TENS are believed to "drown out" pain signals in the affected nerves, thus preventing the pain message from reaching the brain. The method is based on the "gate theory" of pain, which hypothesizes that pain impulses must pass through a "gate" in the spinal cord. TENS units are also believed to stimulate the production of endorphins, the body's natural painkillers.

Although TENS has been intensively tested, its degree of efficacy is still a subject of debate. While a large 1990 study reported in *The New England Journal of Medicine* pronounced TENS ineffective, several other trials have deemed it capable of relieving pain, although it may be more helpful for mild to moderate discomfort than for severe pain. The type of tissue may also be a factor; one study suggests that TENS works on skin and connective tissue but not on muscle or the outer layers of the bones.

Electroacupuncture. Also called electro-acutherapy, this form of treatment operates on essentially the same principles as regular acupuncture, with the addition of a weak electrical current applied to the needles. As in other forms of acupuncture, the goal is to correct purported blockages in the flow of the life force *qi*, thus restoring balance and health.

Advocates of electroacupuncture say that it's better suited to surgical anesthesia than manual therapy, since it reaches a large number of acupoints simultaneously. (However, use of any sort of acupuncture as the sole painkiller during surgery is a feat that's rarely attempted.)

Auricular Acupuncture. The scientific basis of regular acupuncture has never been explained, and acupuncture limited solely to the ear is doubly mysterious. A few studies in the early 1980s—including one Italian trial with 724 patients—claimed support for auricular therapy. However, the technique was discredited by the American Medical Association in 1984 when a study of 36 pain patients failed to show a significant difference between those receiving the therapy and those receiving a fake.

Electroacupuncture Biofeedback. Employing a device called the Dermatron, advocates of this procedure attempt to diagnose illness by measuring electrical resistance at various acupuncture points that correspond to specific organs and tissues. An abnormal reading at any particular point is the signal to check the other points associated with the organ in question. Such devices have thus far been approved only on an experimental basis in the U.S.

Cymatic Instruments. According to proponents, each organ and tissue in the body emits sounds at a particular harmonic frequency, which can be recognized by the cymatic device. Furthermore, it's said that any disturbances can be remedied by bathing the site of the problem with sounds tuned to the frequency pattern found in the organ's healthy state. The existence of such frequencies has not, however, been accepted by mainstream science.

The Diapulse. This device emits radio waves that are said to produce short, intense electromagnetic pulses capable of penetrating tissue to improve blood flow, reduce pain, and improve healing. Mainstream critics charge that its value has yet to be verified in independent scientific tests.

The Electro-Acuscope. This device is said to reduce pain, not by stimulating the affected nerves as in TENS, but by promoting tissue repair. As the treatments progress, the current is adjusted to alter the resistance from the damaged tissue and thus accelerate recovery. Again, the treatments await validation by independent scientific tests.

The Light Beam Generator. According to its proponents, this instrument works by radiating light photons that assist in restoring the cells' normal energy state, thus promoting healing. Mainstream critics are dubious.

Microcurrent Electrical Therapy. Proponents of this therapy believe that electrical stimulation of a wound or injured muscle promotes healing. MET is one of the more intensively researched of the energy therapies. To date, however, there is no consensus regarding its effectiveness.

The MORA. This instrument is supposed to receive electromagnetic signals directly from the body, detect any aberrant wave patterns, and replace them with "normal" waves delivered back to the patient via the acupoints that correspond to the diseased area. As in traditional Chinese acupuncture, this is thought to correct imbalances in the flow of the life force, and thus the disorder. To grant this machine credibility, you must assume the manufacturers know which waves are "normal" and which are not, that sending "normalized" waves into the body will correct them, and that these electromagnetic maneuvers can affect the undetectable life force posited by Chinese medicine. There is no accepted scientific evidence for any of these contentions.

The Sound Probe. According to its advocates, this device emits a pulsed tone of three alternating frequencies that can destroy any foreign matter, such as viruses and bacteria, that is not in resonance with the body.

Who Should Avoid This Therapy?

In general, people with pacemakers and those who are pregnant should avoid all forms of electrotherapy unless their doctor approves.

In addition, transcutaneous electrical nerve stimulation can't be used during electrocardiography or heart monitoring, and while the patient is running a fever. The electrodes should not be applied near the heart, head, front of the neck, or eyes. Although a few studies have examined use of TENS for labor pains, the electrodes should not be placed on the abdomen, because safety in pregnancy has not been proven.

All forms of electroacupuncture should be strictly avoided during pregnancy, since there's a danger of triggering premature uterine contractions. Techniques employing needles can't be used on people with bleeding disorders. It's also best to avoid this form of therapy if you have a fever or any sort of irregular heartbeat.

What Side Effects May Occur?

Transcutaneous electrical nerve stimulation, the most thoroughly studied of these therapies, appears to have no side effects. The situation with the other forms of treatment is really unknown. Remember, however, that with most of them you are playing with electricity.

How to Choose a Therapist

Most of these devices have never undergone rigorous clinical testing, and many lack FDA approval.

Be extremely wary of therapists that propose their use. Check the practitioner's credentials carefully, and try to get a second opinion from a doctor you trust.

Transcutaneous electrical nerve stimulation, the most widely accepted of these therapies, is available from many physicians—particularly those specializing in pain management, physical medicine and rehabilitation, sports medicine, or orthopedic surgery. The other forms of treatment are typically offered by acupuncturists, physical therapists, rehabilitation therapists, chiropractors, and naturopathic physicians.

When Should Treatment Stop?

Virtually all of these therapies promise to relieve pain or correct a specific disorder. If you see no improvement, drop the treatment and move on. Pain treatments such as transcutaneous electrical nerve stimulation can be stopped as soon as the pain subsides. Microcurrent electrical therapy should be discontinued as soon as improvement seems to be leveling off. No matter how short the duration of treatment, additional therapy will provide no further benefit.

See a Conventional Doctor If . . .

If you have pain of unknown origin, it is extremely important to see a conventional physician for an initial diagnosis *before* undergoing any energy therapy. Pain is frequently the warning of a serious condition which electrotherapy such as TENS could temporarily mask.

Do not rely on electroacupuncture biofeedback, cymatic instruments, or the MORA to provide you with a firm diagnosis. Seeking a second opinion is your wisest course.

Resources

ORGANIZATIONS

American Holistic Health Association
P.O. Box 17400
Anaheim, CA 92817
Phone: 714-779-6152

The National Institute of Environmental Health Sciences
P.O. Box 1233
Research Triangle Park,
NC 27709
Phone: 919-541-3345

The Office of Alternative Medicine
National Institutes of Health
P.O. Box 8218
Silver Spring, MD 20907
Phone: 888-644-6226;
301-496-4000

FURTHER READING

The Body Electric: Electromagnetism and the Foundation of Life. Robert O. Becker and Gary Selden. New York: William Morrow and Company, 1987.

Environmental Medicine

Consider This Therapy For

Environmental medicine aims to relieve disorders that its practitioners blame on pollutants and toxins in the modern environment. If you are allergic to particular elements in your diet—or to substances in the air—some of the techniques employed by environmental practitioners could remedy the problem. (A mainstream allergist could also help.) Food allergies, hay fever, nasal congestion, sneezing, ear infections, and sinus headaches are all potential targets for environmental therapies.

Many environmental therapists believe, however, that pollution's impact on health extends far beyond allergies that can be clearly linked to a particular irritant. Indeed, they insist that virtually all chronic maladies are caused—or at least aggravated—by a host of natural and artificial environmental pollutants. This proposition is considered far more dubious than the widely documented allergies we're all familiar with. In fact, there are no scientific studies that support it.

How the Treatments Are Done

The physicians who target disorders of a presumably environmental nature use a wide array of treatments, ranging from diet to a combination of holistic, homeopathic, and pharmaceutical therapies. You may encounter some very trendy, over-the-top treatments when you visit an environmental practitioner, but the majority fall into four categories:

- *Nutritional Therapies*: the use of oral and intravenous vitamins, minerals, and other important nutrients. (For more information, see the profile on "Orthomolecular Medicine.")
- *Detoxification*: the removal of metals and chemicals from the body. (For more information, see "Detoxification Therapy.")
- *Immunotherapy*: treatments to strengthen the immune system.
- *Desensitization*: the process of retraining the immune system to eliminate allergies.

Before you begin therapy, the doctor will put you through a battery of tests to help pinpoint the nature of the problem, and will take a very comprehensive medical history. Many physicians have developed their own treatment programs. However, here's a brief look at some of the more popular approaches:

DIET MODIFICATION

Diet and nutrition are the staples of many environmental medical treatments. The goal is to identify various food allergies so that the offending items can be removed from the diet.

The doctor may begin by recommending elimination of certain foods on a trial basis. If symptoms subside in a food's absence, then return in its presence, it's probably the source of the problem. Alternatively, the doctor may administer a "provocation" or "neutralization" test. In this procedure, a small amount of a suspected allergen is either injected just beneath the skin or placed under the tongue. If the skin turns red and forms a raised wheal at the injection site, you have a positive response. (Don't jump to conclusions, however. False positives are very common in skin tests for food allergies, and additional tests may be needed.)

The most common food allergies are to milk and milk products, wheat, yeast, corn, eggs, soybeans, tomatoes, peanuts, other nuts, citrus fruits, and shellfish.

ENZYME POTENTIATED DESENSITIZATION (EPD)

This technique calls for administration of extremely small doses of an allergen in order to cure your sensitivity to it. A natural enzyme called beta glucuronidase is included to boost desensitization. The treatments are intended to "train" the immune system to tolerate the allergen. They are given intravenously, and are recommended only for those in good nutritional health.

Treatments are typically given at two-month intervals initially; then less often as the patient begins to respond. For hay fever, 1 or 2 treatments per year are sufficient. House dust and mite allergies are typically treated with 2 doses given 2 to 3 months apart.

For stubborn disorders, results can take as long as two years to appear. Most people must continue EPD for a lifetime, although many are able to skip treatments for as long as 5 or 6 years before resuming.

CHELATION THERAPY

These treatments use intravenous administration of a man-made amino acid called ethylenediaminetetraacetic acid (EDTA) to flush heavy metals from the body. EDTA binds with molecules of metals such as lead, iron, copper, calcium, magnesium, zinc, plutonium, and manganese and carries them out of the system through the intestinal tract, urinary tract, skin, or saliva. It is a standard treatment for heavy metal poisoning. Many proponents also promote it as a treatment for coronary artery disease, circulatory disorders, and stroke; but its effectiveness for anything other than poisoning has never been confirmed. For more information, see the profile on "Chelation Therapy."

HEAT DEPURATION

Like chelation therapy, these treatments seek to rid the body of chemicals such as lead, copper, iron, and other toxins. Patients are placed in a sauna heated to as high as 150 degrees Fahrenheit, a temperature that is thought to mobilize the chemicals from deep stores within the body. The treatments are often administered in conjunction with chelation therapy and other forms of detoxification. For example, patients may spend a full day undergoing heat treatments, exercise sessions, a massage, and nutritional therapy counseling.

Each treatment lasts from 15 to 40 minutes, and 3 or 4 may be given during the course of a day. Advocates say that an average of 20 eight-hour sessions are needed to completely clear the body of toxins.

OTHER TREATMENTS

Some environmental practitioners offer other, more controversial, types of therapy. They may prescribe DMSO (dimethyl sulfoxide), a solvent that is sometimes used externally to relieve pain and swelling from strains, sprains, and arthritis, and that is taken internally for certain bladder infections. You might also encounter DHEA (dehydroepiandrosterone), a hormone that some advocates say can reduce the risk of cancer, control immunity, regulate blood sugar, maintain tissue integrity, reduce blood pressure, and relieve allergies. Claims for both drugs are considered largely unproven in the mainstream medical community.

What Treatment Hopes to Accomplish

Almost any type of illness or disorder, from hay fever to heart disease, can be treated with some form of environmental medicine, according to those who practice these controversial techniques. As with most medical treatments, however, there are no guarantees, and practitioners say that, in general, their overall goal is to help individuals cope with the daily hazards of their environment and, in the process, become healthier and, in many cases, disease-free individuals.

In practice, these treatments are most commonly sought out to remedy food allergies, mold and pollen allergies, chemical sensitivities, and rheumatoid arthritis. Advocates say that once these disorders are treated, many other underlying diseases and illnesses, such as migraine headaches, asthma, and colitis may also improve.

Other conditions said to be relieved by environmental medicine include heart disease, high blood pressure, chronic pediatric disorders such as recurrent ear infections and bed wetting, premenstrual syndrome, hypoglycemia, irritable bowel syndrome, gastroenteritis, diarrhea, and various abdominal pains.

Who Should Avoid This Therapy?

Some of the treatments offered by environmental practitioners can be harmful under certain medical conditions. You should, for example, avoid chelation therapy if you have kidney or liver disease. It's also wise to avoid heat treatments if you have asthma, epilepsy, heart disease, blood pressure problems, or multiple sclerosis.

What Side Effects May Occur?

During allergy testing and desensitization, there's always a chance of an unpleasant reaction. Likewise, almost any intravenous infusion can occasionally cause a reaction, or at least minor discomfort and bruising at the site of the injection. Heat treatments and other detoxification leave some people weak, dizzy, nauseous, or shaky (a result, say therapists, of the toxins mobilized into the bloodstream).

Be particularly cautious about chelation therapy. At typical dosage levels, patients experience little more than occasional nausea, dizziness, or headache immediately following treatment. However, in higher dosages, the EDTA used in the treatments has been known to cause anemia, blood clots, bone marrow damage, insulin shock, irregular heartbeat, and more.

How to Choose a Therapist

Many of the diagnostic techniques and treatments used in environmental medicine require the oversight of an MD or DO, so it's best to stick with a licensed physician. A number of doctors offer both environmental and conventional medical services. They come from a variety of specialties, but typically have a background in internal medicine, pediatrics, allergies, gynecology, or psychiatry. To their conventional expertise, they add training in such nontraditional areas as applied toxicology, immunology, nutritional biochemistry, free radical medicine, and molecular biology.

For specialized treatments, it's best to look for a physician with specific training in the desired field. If you're contemplating chelation therapy, for instance, try to find a doctor who has completed courses from the American College of Advancement in Medicine (ACAM), chelation's professional society.

As you should when selecting any type of therapist, be sure to discuss the proposed treatment regime, its possible side effects, and the outcomes to expect. Don't be afraid to ask for the names of patients who have been treated for the same illness with the same techniques, and don't hesitate to contact them.

Most physicians practicing environmental medicine in the United States will treat you on an outpatient basis. However, if you're looking for an inpatient experience, the Occupational and Environmental Unit at Tri-Cities Hospital in Dallas, Texas can accommodate you.

When Should Treatment Stop?

Environmental practitioners stress the importance of a strong commitment to therapy and rigorous compliance with treatment guidelines. The complexity and toxicity of the modern environment, they say, often make it difficult to reach a specific diagnosis and treatment plan. They warn that persistence and patience are important, and that in some cases a complete change in lifestyle may be needed.

If you enjoy taking this much responsibility for your health, and agree that environmental toxins are making you sick, you may find yourself continuing the treatments for years. Remember, however, that other forms of therapy may offer faster relief. If your health doesn't seem to be improving at all, don't hesitate to shop around.

See a Conventional Doctor If . . .

Many of the treatments used in environmental medicine are deemed ineffective by the majority of physicians. If you have any serious chronic disease, you owe it to yourself to try all the more reliable forms of mainstream therapy before turning to these less promising substitutes.

Resources

ORGANIZATIONS

American Academy of Environmental Medicine
P.O. Box 16106
Denver, CO 80216
Phone: 303-622-9755

Environmental Health Center
8345 Walnut Hill Lane,
Suite 205
Dallas, TX 75231
Phone: 214-368-4132

Human Ecology Action League
P.O. Box 49126
Atlanta, GA 30359
Phone: 404-248-1898

Occupational and Environmental Unit Tri-Cities Hospital
7525 Scyene Rd.
Dallas, TX 75227
Phone: 214-275-1430

FURTHER READING

Alternative Healing. Mark Kastner and Hugh Burroughs. Halycon Publishing, 1993.

An Alternative Approach to Allergies. Theron G. Randolph, MD, and Ralph W. Moss. Bantam Books, 1987.

Brain Allergies: The Psychonutrient Connection. William H. Phipott, MD, and D.K. Kalita. Keats Publishing, 1987.

Detecting Your Hidden Allergies. William G. Crook, MD. Professional Books/Future Health, 1988.

Dr. Mandell's 5-Day Allergy Relief System. Marshall Mandell, MD, and L. Scanlon. Harper & Row, 1988.

Help for the Hyperactive Child. William G. Crook, MD. Professional Books, 1991.

Is This Your Child? Discovering and Treating Unrecognized Allergies. Doris Rapp, MD. William Morrow and Company, Inc., 1991.

Enzyme Therapy

Consider This Therapy For

Advocates say that enzyme supplements can cure an astonishing array of maladies. Acne, arthritis, AIDS, allergies, bronchitis, cataracts, colds, sciatica, and shingles are only a few of the problems that digestive enzymes are said to relieve. Fever, headaches, swelling, and pain can also be banished, along with myasthenia gravis, pancreatitis, lung and tooth infections, bone fractures, kidney disease, liver disorders, and general weakness. According to enthusiasts, even multiple sclerosis, cancer, and aging will succumb to regular enzyme supplementation.

Is there any truth to these claims? The good news is that the supplements can indeed be helpful—if you have one of the rare conditions that cause enzyme deficiency (cystic fibrosis, Gaucher's disease, and celiac disease are the leading culprits). Certain enzymes can also help people with specific digestive problems such as lactose intolerance, bloating, and gas. For the rest of us, however, the supplements are thought to be completely unnecessary and are said to have no scientifically validated effect.

How the Treatments Are Done

For genuine cases of enzyme deficiency, verified by blood tests and assessment of digestive status, doctors prescribe supplements such as Donnazyme, Cotazyme, Creon, Pancrease, Ultrase, and Zymase. For people with lactose intolerance, there's the over-the-counter remedy Lactaid. And for those troubled by chronic gas, there's a product called Beano.

Enzyme products promoted for other disorders are typically sold as dietary supplements, a category that's not regulated by the Food and Drug Administration. It's illegal to claim that these products can cure any specific disease, and any such claims can be considered bogus.

What Treatment Hopes to Accomplish

Enzymes are catalysts for virtually every biological and chemical reaction in the body, and digestive enzymes are crucial for the breakdown of food into nutrients the body can absorb. Without sufficient digestive enzymes, the fat, starch, and sugar that we eat can't be fully digested, and this, in turn, can disrupt absorption of minerals and fat-soluble vitamins.

Various digestive enzymes are produced at different points along the digestive tract, ranging from the salivary glands to the small intestine. Other digestive enzymes, including several of the most important, are produced in the pancreas. If the pancreas is chronically infected or damaged by a disease such as cystic fibrosis, the result is severe malabsorption, diarrhea, and malnutrition. In such cases, enzyme supplements can be a life-saver.

Likewise, if the small intestine fails to produce enough of the digestive enzyme lactase, the milk sugar called lactose will move down the intestinal tract unabsorbed, causing gas, bloating, and diarrhea. A shortage of the enzyme alpha galactosidase can also have unpleasant consequences, leading to incomplete digestion of certain carbohydrates in foods such as beans and cabbage, and thus causing gas.

"Enzyme therapy" does not, however, concern itself with these specific deficiencies. Instead, it seeks to maintain peak digestion by bolstering the body's natural enzymes with ample supplements from other sources. This is thought to reduce the body's workload, allowing the immune system to flourish and ridding the system of toxic, only partially digested nutrients.

Enzyme advocates are particularly worried about absorption of partially digested protein molecules into the bloodstream, where they can be mistaken as foreign invaders and attacked by the immune system. The resulting circulating immune complexes (CICs) can, they say, put stress on the immune system, accumulate in the tissues, and provoke inflammation, arthritis, allergies, ulcers, sciatica, and a variety of pains.

How is it that we supposedly lack sufficient enzymes to prevent these dire consequences? Many proponents of enzyme therapy blame it on our preference for cooked food. At the high temperatures used in food preparation, the destruction of enzymes, minerals, and vitamins is a well-accepted fact. Faced with a shortage of these dietary enzymes, the theory goes, the body's digestive system is forced to compensate by increasing its own enzyme production. Advocates of enzyme therapy say a shortfall remains. Mainstream scientists respond that the supply is more than sufficient.

Who Should Avoid This Therapy?

According to virtually all medical experts, unless you've been diagnosed with a clear-cut deficiency, enzyme supplements are a waste of money. Diabetics in particular should be wary of high-enzyme diets that may conflict with the carefully balanced menus they need to keep their blood-sugar levels under control.

What Side Effects May Occur?

High doses of pancreatic enzymes can interfere with kidney function. Liver disorders and digestive problems are also possibilities. Lung problems and immune disorders could be aggravated as well; and diabetics may experience wide variations in blood sugar levels.

How to Choose a Therapist

Among the ranks of enzyme therapists you'll find osteopaths, chiropractors, and physicians. When selecting a practitioner, it's wise to go for the maximum amount of medical training and experience.

When Should Treatment Stop?

If your symptoms persist, seek another form of therapy without delay.

See a Conventional Doctor If . . .

Clinical research suggests that, for most problems, your odds of success with enzyme therapy are low, while another, more tightly targeted form of treatment might quickly remedy the problem. Certainly for any sort of serious illness, substituting enzyme therapy for standard treatment could be a serious mistake. Try to exhaust all your mainstream medical options before turning to enzymes.

Be especially wary of experimental cancer treatments with pancreatic enzymes and vitamins A and C. Although these treatments are supposed to mobilize the immune system and stimulate tumor necrosis factor, there are no scientific studies supporting such claims. Be sure to get a second opinion if anyone proposes this or similar forms of therapy.

Resources

ORGANIZATIONS

Digestive Disease National Coalition (DDNC)
711 Second St. NE, Suite 200
Washington, DC 20002
Phone: 202-544-7497
Fax: 202-546-7105

National Digestive Diseases Information Clearinghouse (NDDIC)
Two Information Way
Bethesda, MD 20892-3570
Phone: 301-654-3810
Fax: 301-907-8906

American Dietetic Association (ADA)
216 W. Jackson Blvd., Suite 800
Chicago, IL 60606
Phone: 312-899-0040;
800-366-1655
Fax: 312-899-1979

FURTHER READING

The Alternative Medicine Handbook. B.R. Cassileth. New York: W.W. Norton & Company, 1998.

Alternative Medicine: The Definitive Guide. The Burton Goldberg Group. Puyallup, WA: Future Medicine Publishing, Inc., 1996.

Enzymes & Enzyme Therapy. Anthony J. Cichoke. New Canaan, CT: Keats Publishing, Inc., 1994.

Guide to Alternative Medicine. Isadore Rosenfeld, MD. New York: Random House, 1996.

Food Enzymes. Humbart Santillo. Prescott, AZ: Hohm Press, 1987.

Fasting

Consider This Therapy For
Prolonged fasting is an extremely effective—though not necessarily desirable—way to lose weight in a hurry. Much depends on the type of fast you undertake. Total fasts, which were popular in the 1960s, promote the loss not only of body fat, but of muscle tissue and other body proteins as well. The modified fasts developed more recently solve this problem by allowing intake of protein. Total fasts also tend to produce unpleasant—sometimes even dangerous—side effects, another problem that the modified, protein-sparing diet generally eliminates. Both approaches, however, have one major drawback in common: Whatever weight you shed during the fast usually returns once it ends.

While the purpose of these long-term fasts is to help one shed unwanted pounds, many advocates of naturopathic medicine recommend shorter periods of therapeutic fasting to help alleviate diseases like arthritis, irritable bowel syndrome, eczema, depression, asthma, and psoriasis, and to "detoxify" the body from environmental poisons that have built up over the years (see also the profile on "Detoxification Therapy"). The value of this sort of fasting is much more dubious, although short fasts followed by a carefully restricted vegetarian diet have shown promise for relieving arthritis.

How the Treatments Are Done
WEIGHT-LOSS FASTS

Currently, two variations of the protein-sparing modified fast are used to assist in weight loss. Both are recommended only for people who are dangerously overweight. They are not for those who've gained a few pounds over the winter and are trying to get back into shape for the beach.

Version One calls for a daily intake of 1.5 grams of protein per 2.2 pounds of your *ideal* body weight. In practical terms, that means consuming about 75 grams daily if you're a woman, or 100 if you're a man— roughly the daily amount in the typical American diet. The protein should be high-quality (meat, fish, or fowl), and should be supplemented with a multiple vitamin tablet plus extra potassium and calcium.

Version Two substitutes a premixed formula rich in milk or egg protein for the meat and vitamins used in Version One. Such formulas usually provide about 50 to 70 grams of protein daily, 40 milligrams of carbohydrate, and a little fat. Critics fault them for failing to include enough protein, the requirement for which goes up as your calorie intake goes down. They also point out that it's cheaper to buy the components separately than in premixed form. Aside from these minor differences, however, the two diets are much the same.

Typically, a modified fasting program lasts for several months, furnishing no more than 600 calories a day—an amount much lower than that needed to maintain weight. (A non-pregnant woman under age 50 usually needs between 1,600 and 2,500 calories. A man in the same age range needs 2,500 to 3,000.)

"DETOXIFICATION" FASTS

Some proponents of detoxification recommend brief, intense, water-only fasts. However, a three-day fast supplemented with vegetable and fruit juices is more typical. The procedure often begins with a "pre-fast." On the day before the fast starts, you're instructed to eat lightly, finishing the day with a meal of fresh fruits and vegetables. During the fast itself, you're expected to drink 3 to 4 eight-ounce glasses of juice, preferably fresh squeezed. Most therapists also recommend avoiding coffee and soft drinks, and getting lots of rest. Often the entire procedure is scheduled for a weekend, when you can conserve energy and take naps as needed. It's also best to avoid vigorous exercise, although short walks or stretching are considered acceptable.

You will notice that, as the fast progresses, your body temperature will fall and your blood pressure, pulse, and rate of breathing will slow down—all signs of a decline in your metabolic rate. Since the drop in body temperature may make you feel colder than those around you, be sure to wear extra clothing to keep warm. During the first day of the fast, you'll lose 3 to 5 pounds. That's a water loss that will come right back after you start eating again. To break the fast, experts suggest that you introduce solid foods slowly, in limited portions.

What Treatment Hopes to Accomplish

Although modified, protein-sparing fasts are considered a reasonably safe way for the dangerously obese to quickly bring down their weight, this approach is no longer favored by most doctors due to the abrupt rebound that almost invariably occurs when the patient resumes eating. Instead, most physicians now recommend a gradual weight-loss program accompanied by a sustained effort to modify bad eating habits.

Likewise, few doctors believe that fasting, in itself, has any lasting therapeutic effects. (Indeed, extended fasts can be quite harmful.) However, as part of a larger dietary modification program, some fasts have delivered encouraging results. During an experiment reported in the respected medical journal *Lancet,* Norwegian researchers put 27 patients with rheumatoid arthritis on a 7 to 10 day partial fast, followed by a special vegetarian diet free of refined sugar, citrus fruit, milk products, eggs, and gluten—the protein found in many grains.

The diet plan required participants in the study to slowly reintroduce foods, one by one, every second day, and to watch for the return of symptoms. If they reappeared within 48 hours, the food was eliminated permanently. At the end of 3 to 5 months, the participants were left on the resulting vegetarian diet.

Although the symptoms of arthritis often improve while a patient is fasting, they usually return as soon as eating resumes. In the *Lancet* experiment, however, the patients enjoyed lasting results. By the end of four weeks, patients on the experimental diet had significantly fewer swollen, tender joints, less pain, better grip strength, and improved lab-test results. Those volunteers who stayed off the regime didn't fare nearly as well.

Some researchers attribute these results to the elimination of foods which, they theorize, act as "arthritic allergens," causing the immune system to produce antibodies that attack the joints and produce symptoms. Others speculate that a vegetarian diet may alter the bacterial population in the large intestine, somehow relieving the disease. The truth of the matter has yet to be established; but if you suffer from arthritis, you might want to give the program a try regardless of the explanation.

Who Should Avoid This Therapy?

Prolonged, modified fasts should be avoided by all but the seriously obese, and should be undertaken only under the supervision of a physician who has plenty of experience and training in this kind of treatment. Experts also advise that even with adequate supervision, a modified fast should not extend beyond 16 weeks.

Shorter fasts are safer, of course, but for many people it's wise to avoid even a three-day fast. Pregnant mothers, for instance, risk depriving their baby of much-needed proteins, fats, and other nutrients whenever they fast. Similarly, nursing mothers compromise the quality of their breast milk. Others who should avoid any sort of fast are those with ulcers, diabetes, or diseases of the liver, heart, kidneys, and lungs, as well as anyone with advanced cancer.

Children are not very good candidates for even a one-day fast. In one study, children who fasted from dinnertime until noon the next day had poorer scores on tests that measured memory and the ability to recognize various types of visual stimuli. As you might expect, those who were already undernourished did the worst.

It's also wise to check with your doctor before attempting even a one-day fast if you are taking any prescription medications. Many drugs need to be taken with food to improve their absorption, or to minimize their harsh effects on the stomach and intestinal tract. In other instances, the biochemical changes that occur during fasting may alter the way the body handles the drug.

What Side Effects May Occur?

In the late 1970s, a popular "liquid protein" diet product was linked to a number of sudden deaths. The victims suffered fatal heart disturbances typically brought on by protein and mineral deficiencies, and it was discovered that the protein these folks were taking was actually collagen, which is useless as a source of nutritional protein.

The formulas available today are, needless to say, much safer and rarely cause any serious cardiac side effects (although they are still best reserved for those with severe weight problems and should always be taken under a doctor's supervision). There are, however, other risks that continue to accompany any stringent weight-loss regime.

Potassium deficiency, which can cause severe irregularities in the heart rhythm, remains a threat. So does protein depletion. And the rapid burning of fat that occurs when the body is deprived of carbohydrates can lead to a build-up of by-products called ketones, which, in turn, can interfere with elimination of uric acid, triggering a painful attack in those who suffer from gout.

Any rapid weight-loss program—including fasting—also poses a risk of gallstones. In addition, salt and water depletion can lead to light-headedness and dizziness when first standing up. Other potential side effects include constipation, dry skin, and menstrual irregularities.

If you are in good health and are doing a brief, 1-to-3 day fast, it's not uncommon to experience some light-headedness, fatigue, or a headache. If you've been a heavy coffee drinker, for instance, and stop for 3 days, you'll probably suffer a caffeine withdrawal headache. On the plus side of the equation, many fasters report mild euphoria or an increased sense of well-being and clearer thinking.

If you fast for only 24 hours, you may not experience the build-up of ketones that accompanies a longer fast. That's because during the first day, your body is busy burning the stored carbohydrates referred to as glycogen. After that, as the body begins to metabolize fat stores, you may notice that your breath takes on a sweet or fruity aroma. That's produced by acetone, one of the ketones produced when fat stores are burned. The symptom is harmless.

How to Choose a Therapist

If you are interested in a modified fast to help you lose weight, you'll want to find a doctor who is specially trained in weight loss, a specialty called bariatrics. One of your best approaches would be to contact the American Society of Bariatric Physicians for a referral. (See the "Resources" section for details.)

If, on the other hand, you're looking for a therapist to supervise a brief detoxifying fast, a licensed naturopathic physician might be a better choice. The American Association of Naturopathic Physicians maintains a list of qualified practitioners.

When Should Treatment Stop?

If you're under the supervision of a qualified practitioner, consult with him or her before discontinuing your fast.

See a Conventional Doctor If . . .

Although most of the side effects you'll encounter during a fast aren't a cause for concern, an irregular heartbeat requires immediate medical attention. Call your doctor or go to an emergency room at once.

Resources

ORGANIZATIONS

The American Society of Bariatric Physicians
5600 South Quebec St., Suite 109A
Englewood, CO 80111
Phone: 303-779-4833
(for patient referrals)
Fax: 303-779-4834

American Association of Naturopathic Physicians
2366 Eastlake Ave., Suite 322

Seattle, WA 98102
Phone: 206-323-7610

FURTHER READING

Krause's Food, Nutrition, and Diet Therapy. L.K. Mahan and S. Escott-Stump. Philadelphia: W.B. Saunders, 1996.

Encyclopedia of Natural Medicine. M. Murray and J. Pizzorno. Rocklin, CA: Prima Publishing, 1998.

Feldenkrais Method

Consider This Therapy For

The Feldenkrais Method is not a treatment or cure. Rather, it is a type of supportive therapy that can help in any situation where improved movement patterns (and awareness of those patterns) can help with recovery from illness or injury. Practitioners consider it useful for many types of chronic pain, including headache, temporomandibular joint disorder, other joint disorders, and neck, shoulder, and back pain. It is sometimes used as supportive therapy for people with neuromuscular disorders, such as multiple sclerosis, cerebral palsy, and stroke. It's also helpful for improving balance, coordination, and mobility; many athletes, dancers, and other performers use the Feldenkrais Method as part of their overall conditioning.

How the Treatments Are Done

The Feldenkrais Method has two components; you may use either or both of them, depending on your needs. One component, called Functional Integration, consists of hands-on sessions with a Feldenkrais practitioner, who uses touch to help you sense and improve your movement patterns. As you sit, stand, or lie comfortably, the practitioner may gently manipulate your muscles and joints. Unlike some forms of bodywork, Feldenkrais manipulations are all within the usual range of motion, without pain or "cracking" of joints.

The second component is a type of training called Awareness Through Movement, which focuses on slow, non-aerobic movement and specific motions from everyday life, such as sitting and standing. Practitioners consider the two components to be equivalent, complementary ways of achieving the same results. Loose, comfortable clothing is worn for both. Practitioners emphasize that the method does not involve traditional calisthenics.

Treatment Time: Functional Integration sessions typically last about 45 minutes. Awareness Through Movement sessions run 45 minutes to an hour.

Treatment Frequency: Both Functional Integration and Awareness Through Movement are typically offered in a series of 4 to 6 sessions, meeting once a week.

What Treatment Hopes to Accomplish

The Feldenkrais Method aims to help you relearn how to move your body, replacing old ways of movement with new, more efficient habits. It focuses on improving flexibility, coordination, and range of motion. Feldenkrais practitioners don't make any extravagant claims that the method will cure a specific ailment. They do say that it helps people become aware of how they move, and teaches them how to reduce stress on joints and muscles, and how to move more comfortably.

Feldenkrais practitioners believe that people develop habits of movement as young children, and retain those patterns for life. If the movements are adequate for daily life, the patterns remain unnoticed, even if there are more efficient, comfortable ways to move. But if the patterns are not adequate, or if the body is stressed through illness, accident, or simply age, they argue that the body will become stiff, or uncomfortable, or experience pain. For people trying to optimize their movements, such as athletes or dancers, the most efficient method of movement is of paramount concern.

The method was developed by Russian-born Israeli Moshe Feldenkrais (rhymes with "rice"), a scientist who was himself recovering from an injury. A lifelong athlete and martial artist, he began synthesizing his knowledge of anatomy, physics, and psychology when his own doctors couldn't fully restore movement to his injured knee. The method first became popular in the U.S. during the 1970s. With its emphasis on the importance of making movement a conscious act, it is similar to other mind-body therapies, including the Alexander Technique.

Who Should Avoid This Therapy?

The Feldenkrais Method is generally considered safe for everyone as a supportive form of treatment.

What Side Effects May Occur?

There are no known side effects to the Feldenkrais Method.

How to Choose a Therapist

Because the terms Feldenkrais, Functional Integration, and Awareness Through Movement, are registered service marks of the Feldenkrais Guild, only practitioners trained in an accredited program are entitled to offer Feldenkrais lessons. The technique requires 160 days of training over almost four years. There are over 30 training programs in the U.S. You can check with the Guild for referrals, or to verify a practitioner's training.

No medical background is required for people who wish to be practitioners, but the method has been adopted by many physical therapists. You may want to see what other credentials a potential therapist has obtained.

When Should Treatment Stop?

The Feldenkrais Method may be continued as long as it is comfortable and beneficial to you.

See a Conventional Doctor If . . .

Because most Feldenkrais practitioners are not schooled in medical diagnosis, you should see a doctor to rule out the possibility that a serious disorder is causing your problems. Also check with your doctor if you experience any new symptoms while participating.

Resources

ORGANIZATIONS

Feldenkrais Guild
P.O. Box 489
Albany, OR 97321
Phone: 503-926-0981;
800-775-2118

FURTHER READING

Awareness Heals: The Feldenkrais Method for Dynamic Health. Steven Sharfman. Addison-Wesley, 1997.

Awareness Through Movement: Easy Exercises to Improve Personal Growth. Moshe Feldenkrais. Harper, 1991.

Mindful Spontaneity. Ruthy Alon. North Atlantic Books, 1996.

Flower Remedies

Consider This Therapy For

The flower extracts recommended in this form of therapy are intended to relieve various unwanted, counterproductive emotional states. Advocates say that diminishing these negative emotions can, in turn, remedy any physical symptoms the emotions may have fostered.

Although many physicians would agree that emotional stress can contribute to illness, the ef-

fect of flower remedies on emotions has never undergone formal clinical trials, and there is no scientific proof that the remedies have any therapeutic value.

How the Treatments Are Done

The extracts used in this form of therapy are extremely diluted solutions produced from 38 different blooms. The so-called "mother tinctures" are made by either floating the blossoms in water for a number of hours or boiling them for half an hour. Each tincture is preserved by mixing it 50/50 with full-strength, 80-proof brandy. Drops of this mixture are diluted in additional brandy and bottled for personal use. Before ingesting, patients are advised to further dilute the remedy by putting two drops in a 30-milliliter (1-ounce) dropper bottle and filling it with mineral water. The bottle should be refrigerated.

The entire set of remedies is intended as a self-help system simple enough to use without professional advice. Manufacturers provide self-administered questionnaires to aid in the selection of the proper flowers, each of which is thought to correspond to an emotional or psychological state. Users are advised to ignore any overt illness, instead asking themselves how they feel and what emotions they are experiencing, since the remedies are intended to treat psychological states, not physical disease. Remedies can be combined, but no more than six or seven should be used at once.

The problems that the remedies purport to relieve range from fear of the unknown to intolerance. Here's a complete list.

Agrimony . . . mental torture behind a cheerful face

Aspen . . . fear of unknown things

Beech . . . intolerance

Centaury . . . the inability to say "no"

Cerato . . . lack of trust in one's own decisions

Cherry Plum . . . fear of the mind giving way

Chestnut Bud . . . failure to learn from mistakes

Chicory . . . selfish, possessive love

Clematis . . . dreaming of the future without working in the present

Crab Apple . . . the cleansing remedy, also for self-hatred

Elm . . . for those overwhelmed by responsibility

Gentian . . . discouragement after a setback

Gorse . . . hopelessness and despair

Heather . . . self-centeredness and self-concern

Holly . . . hatred, envy, and jealousy

Honeysuckle . . . living in the past

Hornbeam . . . procrastination, tiredness at the thought of doing something

Impatiens . . . impatience

Larch . . . lack of confidence

Mimulus . . . fear of known things

Mustard . . . deep gloom for no reason

Oak . . . for the plodder who keeps going past the point of exhaustion

Olive . . . exhaustion following mental or physical effort

Pine . . . guilt

Red Chestnut . . . for those overly concerned for the welfare of loved ones

Rock Rose . . . terror and fright

Rock Water . . . self-denial, rigidity, and self-repression

Scleranthus . . . inability to choose between alternatives

Star of Bethlehem . . . shock

Sweet Chestnut . . . extreme mental anguish and hopelessness

Vervain . . . overenthusiasm

Vine . . . dominance and inflexibility

Walnut . . . protection from change and unwanted influences

Water Violet . . . pride and aloofness

White Chestnut . . . unwanted thoughts and mental arguments

Wild Oat . . . uncertainty over one's direction in life

Wild Rose . . . drifting, resignation, apathy

Willow . . . self-pity and resentment

There is also a combination remedy called Rescue Remedy.

If you feel you need help with your diagnosis, you can consult a practitioner trained in selecting the remedies. He or she will question you about your emotions and attempt to intuit the emotional state underlying your condition.

However, practitioners are expected to encourage patients to choose their own flower therapies once they're sufficiently knowledgeable.

Treatment Frequency: Take 4 drops of each diluted remedy 4 times a day. Alternatively, put 2 drops of the solution from the manufacturer's bottle into a glass of water and sip from the glass at least 4 times daily.

What Treatment Hopes to Accomplish

Flower remedies were developed in the early 1900s by Dr. Edward Bach, an English homeopathic physician, who believed that negative emotional or psychological states underlie physical illnesses. The remedies are designed to treat these emotional states rather than any specific disease. For this reason, people with similar physical conditions may need different remedies, based on their psychological needs.

Dr. Bach identified the 38 wildflowers used in the remedies while searching the English countryside for blooms with healing effects. He determined which flower helped which emotional state by trying various plants on himself when he experienced a particular feeling.

Who Should Avoid This Therapy?

Although the brandy used as a preservative is taken in extremely diluted form, recovering alcoholics and those who wish to avoid alcohol for other reasons may wish to forego these preparations. Alternatively, the concentrated drops can be boiled to evaporate the alcohol without affecting the remedy's potency.

What Side Effects May Occur?

Proponents of the remedies warn that they may "(stir) up repressed feelings that need to be cleansed before complete healing can be achieved." Mainstream physicians, however, seem unconcerned. Most regard the remedies as harmless unless they're substituted for needed medical care.

Advocates cite no physical side effects. Indeed, they say that the remedies can be taken more frequently in moments of crisis without risk of overdose, addiction, or tolerance. The solutions do not affect other courses of treatment, and are unaffected by them. Some practitioners add that the remedies are a self-limiting form of treatment, asserting that the need for and effectiveness of the remedies decrease as the patient's emotional health improves.

How to Choose a Therapist

Practitioners using the original 38 remedies developed by Dr. Bach are certified by The Bach Foundation, and sign a Code of Practice that includes ethical standards. The code specifies that practitioners are not licensed to diagnose medical illness or otherwise practice medicine. (You can find the complete text of the code on the Foundation's website.) About 350 practitioners are registered with the Foundation, according to a 1997 report.

Floral essences are available from a number of sources. Some lines, however, may include plants excluded by Dr. Bach, or offer other herbal therapies prepared using the Bach method.

When Should Treatment Stop?

When you feel that the emotional problem you've addressed has been resolved, you can discontinue therapy immediately. There's no need to taper off the remedies. According to the Bach Centre and Foundation, the remedies should be used only to relieve existing emotional problems, not as a means of preventing their development.

See a Conventional Doctor If . . .

Check with your doctor if there is any suspicion of an ailment that can be treated through standard medical means. Bach flower remedies are not a substitute for medical treatment, but can be used along with conventional care.

Resources

ORGANIZATIONS

American Council on Science and Health
1995 Broadway, 2nd Floor
New York, NY 10023
Phone: 212-362-7044
Fax: 212-362-4919
Web: http://www.acsh.org

The Dr. Edward Bach Centre and Foundation
Mount Vernon, Bakers Lane
Sotwell, Oxon OX10 0PZ, UK
Phone: 011-44-1491-834678
Fax: 011-44-1491-825022
Web: http://www.bachcentre.com

FURTHER READING

Alternative Medicine: The Definitive Guide. The Burton Goldberg Group. Puyallup, WA: Future Medicine Publishing, Inc., 1994.

A Concise Guide to Alternative Medicine. K. Butler and S. Barrett, editors. Buffalo, NY: Prometheus Books, 1992.

Guided Imagery

Consider This Therapy For

Guided imagery seeks to make beneficial physical changes in the body by repeatedly visualizing them. A form of mind-body therapy, it has been advocated for a number of chronic conditions, including stress, anxiety, high blood pressure, and headaches, and for people undergoing conventional cancer therapy or surgery.

Although another mind-body technique, biofeedback, has been tested extensively and has been found effective for a variety of ailments, including certain types of chronic pain, guided imagery has no such track record. Currently there is no evidence that it can relieve any type of disease, though it does seem capable of promoting relaxation.

How the Treatments Are Done

Guided imagery is taught in small classes or one-on-one. Practitioners emphasize that it's not a passive experience; you're expected to be an active participant in each session. You will be asked to wear comfortable clothing, and will either sit comfortably in a chair or lie on a table or a floor mat. The practitioner will not touch you, and no instruments will monitor you. Some practitioners use music as a background to aid relaxation.

Sessions usually begin with general relaxation exercises, then move on to a specific visualization, described by the practitioner. You'll be asked to build a detailed image in your mind, using all five senses, and then repeat the exercise with a different image. If you have a specific medical complaint, the practitioner may ask you to picture your body free of the problem. If it's a localized disorder, you'll probably be encouraged to picture the affected organs working properly, visualizing, for instance, your heart beating regularly, your lungs breathing freely, a tumor shrinking, or your legs moving strongly. For more generalized problems, you may need to picture your entire body as healthy, strong, and calm. Athletes or performers picture themselves moving well and competing or performing perfectly.

Between sessions, you can use a book or audiotape to help you practice visualization on your own.

Treatment Time: Guided imagery sessions are typically 20 to 30 minutes long, or longer as needed.

Treatment Frequency: Sessions are usually held once or twice a week, or more frequently if needed.

What Treatment Hopes to Accomplish

Also known as creative imagery, mental imagery, or creative visualization, guided imagery aims to help you focus your mind on positive images and, in so doing, work changes in your body. It is often used along with other mind-body techniques. Unlike its cousins meditation and hypnosis, guided imagery doesn't ask you to focus your mind on a single word or image, but instead takes you on a journey through several visualizations. It's been described as a "focused daydream" by some practitioners.

Like other mind-body techniques, guided imagery is based on the assumption that the mind can indeed affect the functions of the body. Exactly how this might transpire is not completely understood, but there is certainly compelling evidence that it happens. Numerous studies have confirmed the ability of both biofeedback and meditation training to lower blood pressure and control heart rate; and there is some evidence that guided imagery can do so as well. However, claims that it relieves pain, reduces anxiety, improves the effectiveness of drugs, and has psychological benefits have yet to be verified. Further studies are under way.

How can visualizing something make it so? One theory proposes that picturing something and actually experiencing it are equivalent as far as brain activity is concerned. Brain scans have verified this effect, and proponents suggest stimulating the brain through imagery can therefore have a direct effect on both the nervous and endocrine systems, ultimately producing changes in the immune system and other body functions.

Whatever the truth of the matter, if you have cancer, you should be aware of a specialized type of guided imagery called the Simonton Method. Developed by oncologist O. Carl Simonton and his wife, Stephanie Matthew-Simonton, this technique is designed to help patients who are undergoing standard treatments for cancer. Emphasizing the use of imagery to complement (not replace) other therapies, it requires patients to visualize their immune systems fighting and destroying cancer cells. While considered a useful tool by many, it has not been proven to increase survival time.

Who Should Avoid This Therapy?

Used as a supplement to standard treatments, guided imagery is generally considered safe for everyone.

What Side Effects May Occur?

There are no known side effects of guided imagery.

How to Choose a Therapist

Guided imagery is offered by many types of practitioners, including psychologists, nurses, and social workers, as well as others with no health care background. There is no central licensing or certification required for practitioners, so it is up to you to check into the credentials of the practitioner you choose. The national organizations listed below may be helpful in locating a practitioner in your area.

If you wish, you can also try to learn guided imagery from books or audiotapes.

When Should Treatment Stop?

Practitioners say there is an incremental increase in benefit over time, so you should allow several weeks before deciding whether guided imagery is working for you. If it's not, move on to other alternatives without delay.

See a Conventional Doctor If . . .

Because guided imagery is at best a supplement to other forms of treatment, you should also get standard care for whatever problems you're seeking to remedy.

Resources

ORGANIZATIONS

Academy for Guided Imagery
P.O. Box 2070
Mill Valley, CA 94942
Phone: 800-726-2070

American Imagery Association
4016 Third Ave.
San Diego, CA 92103
Phone: 619-794-8814

American Imagery Institute
P.O. Box 13453
Milwaukee, WI 53213
Phone: 414-781-4045

International Imagery Association
P.O. Box 1046
Bronx, NY 10471
Phone: 914-423-9200

FURTHER READING

Healing Yourself: A Step-by-Step Program for Better Health Through Imagery. Martin L. Rossman, MD. New York: Pocket Books, 1994.

Healing With the Mind's Eye. Michael Samuels. New York: Random House, 1992.

Rituals of Healing: Using Imagery for Health and Wellness. Jeanne Achterberg MD, Barbara Dossey RN, and Leslie Kolkmeier. New York: Bantam Books, 1994.

Staying Well With Guided Imagery. Belleruth Naparstek. New York: Warner Books, 1995.

Hellerwork

Consider This Therapy For
A combination of deep tissue massage and "movement reeducation," Hellerwork is advocated by its practitioners for a variety of problems related to muscle tension and stress. It is said to relieve respiratory problems, sports injuries, and pain in the back, neck, and shoulders. Like most forms of bodywork, it has undergone little in the way of scientific testing; but many of those who've tried it say that it helps.

How the Treatments Are Done
Hellerwork therapy consists of a series of eleven sessions aimed at helping you get in touch with different parts of your body and the emotions that affect it. The first Hellerwork session, for instance, focuses on the chest, seeking to release unconscious tensions that interfere with easy, natural breathing. To accomplish this, the practitioner will engage you in a discussion designed to draw out any emotional attitudes that may be impeding normal movement.

Therapy then moves on to the feet and arms, followed by the "core" muscles deep in the body. At each step, the practitioner uses physical manipulation of the tissues to help release built-up tensions. In the final session, the practitioner endeavors to pull all the work together, fashioning a better understanding of the relationship between mind and body.

Treatment Time: Each session lasts approximately 90 minutes.

Treatment Frequency: The interval between each of the eleven Hellerwork sessions can vary.

What Treatment Hopes to Accomplish
An offshoot of the deep-tissue massage therapy known as Rolfing, Hellerwork was developed by Joseph Heller, a NASA aerospace engineer. Like Rolfing, Hellerwork holds that tense, stressed muscles eventually lose their flexibility, throwing the body out of vertical alignment. Once this abnormal tension is

banished, the theory goes, the body can return to its proper alignment, producing a general improvement in well-being.

Hellerwork treatment begins with an exploration of the way the body works and how emotions can help . . . or interfere. As you begin to comprehend these forces, treatment progresses to physical release of muscular tension and retraining in healthy movement and posture. Through practice in the proper ways of sitting, standing, walking, running, and lifting, you learn how to use your body more efficiently while eliminating unnecessary stress. The practitioner may take "before and after" videotapes to show you the specific aspects of your posture and movements that need to be changed and, then, to demonstrate how treatment is progressing. As your body becomes more flexible, you should begin to feel more limber and relaxed.

Who Should Avoid This Therapy?

The deep muscle massage encountered in Rolfing and Hellerwork is not advisable if you have cancer, rheumatoid arthritis, or any other inflammatory condition.

What Side Effects May Occur?

No side effects have been reported. Remember, however, that no full-fledged studies have been done.

How to Choose a Therapist

There are more than 300 practitioners trained in the Hellerwork approach. To find one in your area, contact the organization called The Body of Knowledge/Hellerwork (see "Resources" below). This group maintains a referral directory of practitioners and also has information on their training and certification.

When Should Treatment Stop?

Unlike some forms of therapy that threaten to go on without end, Hellerwork is over after eleven sessions. Even so, if you experience severe or worsening muscle pain during the course of the treatments, it may be advisable to quit before the end.

See a Conventional Doctor If . . .

Before you begin therapy, consult a doctor to make sure that there's no dangerous medical problem underlying your symptoms. If Hellerwork fails to relieve the symptoms, or makes them worse, see the doctor again.

Resources

ORGANIZATIONS

The Body of Knowledge/Hellerwork
406 Berry St.
Mount Shasta, CA 96067
Phone: 916-926-2500

FURTHER READING

Bodywise. Joseph Heller and William Henkin. Berkeley, CA: Wingbow Press, 1991.

Homeopathy

Consider This Therapy For

Homeopathic remedies are *extremely* diluted solutions (usually 1 part per million or less) of assorted herbs, animal products, and chemicals. Indeed, the vast majority are so diluted that it's impossible to detect the original active ingredient in laboratory tests.

This leads to a certain amount of confusion. Many people tend to think of homeopathic products as herbal remedies when, in fact, they contain little if any of the desired herb. According to homeopathic practitioners, the solutions do continue to hold a "trace memory" of the original substance. Mainstream scientists, however, find them completely devoid of any meaningful amount of medicine.

What, then, can homeopathic remedies do for you? As far as science can determine, the answer is Nothing. On the other hand, advocates of this therapy say that clinical research has shown certain homeopathic medicines to be more effective than a placebo (dummy pill) in the treatment of seasonal allergies, asthma, and influenza. Proponents also claim verified benefits for a variety of other conditions, from easing labor and childbirth to speeding the healing of a sprained ankle. Still, these claims have yet to be confirmed by the kind of broad-based, carefully controlled testing demanded for other types of medication.

There are literally thousands of homeopathic remedies, and their alleged benefits cover just about every disease symptom imaginable. Since they are as safe as bottled water (in fact, often *are* bottled water), there's no harm in trying them for relief of annoying conditions such as colds, flu, headache, and indigestion. It would be unwise, however, to use them as the sole remedy for any serious medical condition. Not only would you be foregoing the possibility of a speedy cure when faced with an ailment like an infection, you'd also be risking dangerous complications when suffering from progressive conditions like heart disease and cancer.

How the Treatments Are Done

Homeopathic medicines are available without a prescription, so anyone can read up on the remedies suggested for a particular symptom, buy them, and try them on their own. If you visit a homeopathic practitioner, however, you'll be introduced to a whole "through-the-looking-glass" approach to medicine unlike anything in standard health care.

A homeopathic practitioner (who may be a physician, chiropractor, or unlicensed entrepreneur) typically begins by taking a lengthy medical history, including detailed information on an individual's temperament, preferences in diet and lifestyle, and emotional state. From these findings, a "classical" homeopathic practitioner will build a "symptom picture" against which to match homeopathy's extensive array of remedies. More eclectic (or opportunistic) practitioners may also employ props such as "electrodiagnostic devices" that beep and give read-outs when a probe is pressed to the skin.

Remedies (in the form of alcohol or water solutions or sugar pills) are usually prescribed one at a time, although they may be combined. Homeopathic practitioners may rely solely on homeopathy, or may complement this approach with standard medicine or other alternative therapies such as naturopathy. For instance, a homeopathic physician might try homeopathic remedies to relieve a child's ear infection, turning to antibiotics only if the homeopathic products fail to work a cure.

What Treatment Hopes to Accomplish

Homeopathy was developed around 1800 by Samuel Hahnemann, a German physician. At the time, it was a welcome alternative to the damaging and ineffective practices of traditional medicine, which included bloodletting, application of leeches, and purging with high doses of life-threatening substances, including mercury and lead.

At the turn of the 19th century, little was known about the causes of disease, so Hahnemann focused on the symptoms instead. Noting that cinchona, a malaria remedy, produced malaria-like symptoms when taken by a healthy volunteer, Hahnemann concluded that "like cures like":

a substance that causes certain symptoms should also relieve them. He then proceeded to test a vast number of plant, animal, and mineral substances on himself and others in a procedure called "proving," observing the symptoms they produced and categorizing them as cures for disorders that cause similar troubles.

The idea that like cures like wasn't new; it had been suggested by the ancient Greek physician Hippocrates, among others. But Hahnemann added a twist called the "Law of Infinitesimals." Because large doses of many remedies were quite poisonous, he began to experiment with smaller and smaller amounts, ultimately coming to believe that minute doses were actually more effective. Hence it became a tenet of homeopathy that the more diluted a substance is, the more powerful its healing action will be.

To maximize the effect of his remedies, Hahnemann therefore invented a system for "potentizing" them. Each substance was repeatedly diluted and shaken until, at the "higher" potencies, not one molecule of the original substance remained. For example, a homeopathic remedy labeled "12X" has been diluted by a factor of ten, 12 times in a row, to produce a dilution of 1 part in a trillion.

Since it's impossible for such a solution to have any physical effect, homeopaths ascribe the therapeutic action of their remedies to an "essence," "memory," or "energy imprint" that can mobilize the body's "vital forces." Medical science, on the other hand, attributes any relief either to coincidence (when an illness runs its course) or the placebo effect (the power of suggestion).

Despite the implausibility of homeopathic theories, results of clinical research have not been entirely negative. In 1997, an international team of researchers reviewed over 100 controlled studies that had claimed positive results from homeopathy. The team deemed 26 of these experiments to have been designed and carried out according to the most rigorous standards. By themselves, none of these studies showed homeopathy to be clearly effective. However, when taken as a group, they seemed to indicate that homeopathy produced somewhat greater benefit than placebo.

Noting the lack of any scientific theory to explain the results, the team simply said they showed the need for more intensive research. Some baffled scientists commented that if placebo-controlled clinical trials could show some effectiveness for homeopathy, then the trials themselves must be subject to as-yet-unidentified bias on the part of the researchers. Others simply ascribed the results to luck, noting that if you perform enough trials, a few will deliver positive results merely by chance.

Proponents of homeopathy respond that conventional medicine still uses a variety of drugs that were shown effective by trial and error long before their mecha-

nism of action was understood. Homeopathic practitioners also point to vaccination as an example of "like curing like," and note that smaller doses of certain standard drugs (such as aspirin to prevent heart attack) are more effective than larger doses. To critics, however, these examples are irrelevant. Neither aspirin nor vaccines would have any effect if diluted to the strengths found in homeopathic products. Furthermore, say opponents, homeopathy's emphasis on matching remedies to symptoms, and not to underlying disease states, discards the vast body of discoveries made since the time when Hahnemann proposed his theory.

Who Should Avoid This Therapy?

If you choose to experiment with this therapy, you can rest assured that it's safe for virtually anyone, including children. If you need to avoid alcohol, however, you'll need to forego homeopathic remedies with an alcohol base (tinctures).

What Side Effects May Occur?

Even placebos have been known to cause side effects, so there's always a chance that you could experience an adverse reaction. For practical purposes, however, the odds are very slim.

Unlike vitamins and herbal remedies, which are sold as "dietary supplements," homeopathic remedies are marketed as over-the-counter medications—

but with a unique exemption from standard regulatory procedures. In 1938, U.S. Senator Royal Copeland of New York—a leading homeopath—included a special release for homeopathic remedies in the landmark Federal Food, Drug, and Cosmetic Act, allowing them to be sold without proof of safety. Today they continue to be marketed without the evidence of safety and efficacy required of other medications. Their labels must, however, include ingredients, directions, dilution, and at least one indication (what the medication is to be used for).

How to Choose a Therapist

Homeopathy is practiced as an acceptable medical discipline in many nations, but is minimally regulated in the United States. Homeopathic practitioners may be medical doctors, osteopaths, chiropractors, naturopathic physicians, or other licensed medical professionals. (They may also be unlicensed freelancers.) They may be self-educated in homeopathy, or may have undergone extensive training. To avoid a potentially dangerous misdiagnosis of your condition, it's best to seek a licensed MD or DO.

The vast majority of homeopathic remedies do not require a prescription, so any motivated individual may in effect become an amateur homeopath by consulting reference books and taking remedies available at health food stores, pharmacies, or by mail order. In many states, however, prescribing even non-prescription medications (including homeopathic ones) for other people without a medical license is illegal.

When Should Treatment Stop?

Some homeopathic remedies are recommended for use every few hours during an acute condition; others, for use on a daily basis to support resistance to disease or strengthen various aspects of health. You can quickly tell whether the remedy is relieving an acute condition, and move on to other treatments if it isn't. Remedies taken to improve resistance are more insidious, since there's no specific way to judge their effect.

See a Conventional Doctor If . . .

It's safe to take homeopathic remedies for temporary symptoms of minor illness, but don't rely on these products for treatment of any serious illnesses or injury. Even reputable homeopaths don't do that; nor do they claim that homeopathy can cure life-threatening conditions such as cancer or diabetes. If your symptoms persist or any new problems develop, see a licensed physician for a conventional diagnosis.

Although homeopathy is often recommended as a "safe and gentle" alternative therapy for children, always keep in mind why it's so safe. If symptoms such as diarrhea, headache, fever, or abdominal pain fail to clear up, see a doctor before the situation gets worse.

Resources

ORGANIZATIONS

The National Center for Homeopathy
801 North Fairfax St., Suite 306
Alexandria, VA 22314
Phone: 703-548-7790
Web: www.homeopathic.org
This organization offers general information and practitioner referrals, publishes a newsletter, and sponsors educational programs.

Homeopathic Educational Services
2124 Kittredge St.
Berkeley, CA 94704
Phone: 510-649-0294
Web: www.homeopathic.com
This resource center offers books, tapes, software, and medicinal products.

FURTHER READING

The Alternative Medicine Handbook. Barrie R. Cassileth, PhD. New York: W.W. Norton & Company, 1998.

The Complete Homeopathy Handbook. Miranda Castro. New York: St. Martin's Press, 1990.

Everybody's Guide to Homeopathic Medicines (third revised edition). Stephen Cummings, MD, and Dana Ullman, MPH. New York: Tarcher/Putnam, 1997.

The Family Guide to Homeopathy: Symptoms and Natural Solutions. Andrew Lockie. New York: Simon & Schuster, 1993.

Let Like Cure Like. Vinton McCabe. New York: St. Martin's Press, 1997.

The Consumer's Guide to Homeopathy. Dana Ullman. New York: Tarcher/Putnam, 1996.

Hydrotherapy

Consider This Therapy For

Although the use of water to treat illnesses is a time-honored medical technique, it has recently declined in popularity among mainstream physicians. The application of hot and cold water or water-soaked compresses to manage the pain and swelling of soft tissue injuries and burns is still standard practice, and has been proven effective in a variety of well-controlled clinical trials. Likewise, physical therapy performed in water is still a common treatment for the disabled. However, other forms of hydrotherapy are no longer routinely used in hospitals, and most medical schools no longer teach the techniques. The hydrotherapy formerly used in psychiatric clinics is now considered obsolete.

In the world of natural healing, however, hydrotherapy continues to claim devoted proponents. Techniques such as constitutional hydrotherapy and hot fomentation, both of which seek to rid the body of toxins, are advocated for a wide range of diseases. Watsu®, a sort of aquatic version of Chinese deep-tissue massage, is said to help pain, stiff joints, spasticity, and tension. Although none of these techniques have been validated through clinical trials, practitioners point to a growing file of case studies as proof of their success.

Among hydrotherapy's more conventional uses are treatment of soft-tissue injuries, musculoskeletal injuries, back pain, arthritis, premenstrual syndrome, menstrual cramps, diabetes, and other diseases that impair circulation, balance disorders, and muscle weakness.

In the alternative medicine realm, claims for procedures such as constitutional hydrotherapy and hot fomentation tend to be much more extravagant. They include treatment of ear infections, high fever, multiple sclerosis, cancer, fractures, migraine, digestive problems, prostatitis, kidney and bladder infections, depression, attention deficit disorder, and anxiety.

How the Treatments Are Done
CONSTITUTIONAL HYDROTHERAPY

Typically given in the practitioner's office, this form of therapy combines systematic application of hot and cold wet towels with administration of mild electrical stimulation to various muscle groups.

Before starting therapy, the practitioner may conduct a physical examination to diagnose your condition. The sophistication of the exam will depend on the type of practitioner you're seeing. The recommended number of sessions will be based on the therapist's assessment of your condition. Here's how a typical session progresses:

First, as you lie face-up on an examination table, the therapist will cover your torso with two hot, wet towels, wrung out so that they are moist but not dripping, and folded in half. The temperature of the towels will be about 120 degrees Fahrenheit. Once the towels are in place, the therapist will pull a wool blanket up to your shoulders, leaving it loose so that air can circulate around the body. The towels are left in place for 5 minutes.

Next, the therapist will pull the blanket down and place a new set of hot towels over the original ones, which will have cooled. He will then flip the towels so that new ones are next to your body, and remove the old ones. Next, he will place folded cold towels, described by one practitioner as at "gasping temperature," over the hot towels and flip the towels again. The cold towels remain in place on the chest for 10 minutes. Again, you'll be covered by a blanket.

During application of the cold wet towels, the therapist will place "sine wave" (electrical) pads on either side of your spine just below the shoulders. The pads will deliver a mild electrical current to the muscles. This current feels like a buzzing or tickling sensation. It isn't painful, but it should be firm. The sine wave machine will run for 10 minutes. You'll be able to control the strength of the current. (When used to encourage healing after a fracture—once the bones have been set—the sine wave pads are positioned directly over the injured bone.)

After 10 minutes, the therapist will remove the cold towels and reposition the pads, with one placed on the center of the lumbar or lower back area and the other located just under your rib cage in the solar plexus region. The sine wave machine will then run for another 10 minutes, without the benefit of new towels.

The entire process is then repeated as you lie face-down. At the end of the treatment, the therapist will rub your back down with a dry towel—sort of a "wake-up" call for the skin and body.

Treatment Time: Each session takes about 45 minutes to 1 hour.

Treatment Frequency: Depending on the condition, as many as 15 sessions may be recommended; children may require fewer treatments. For an acute condition, like the flu, for example, a practitioner may suggest constitutional hydrotherapy every day for 3 or 4 consecutive days. For a chronic condition, therapy is often recommended 2 to 3 times a week. According to practitioners of constitutional hydrotherapy, the treatments are most successful when administered close together.

HOT FOMENTATION

These treatments are like constitutional hydrotherapy minus the electrical stimulator. They are administered in the practitioner's office, where patients with serious, chronic conditions can be monitored if need be. Here's what to expect:

As you lie on your back, the therapist will place hot towels over your torso. He will then put hot packs atop the towels, place others under your back, and cover you with a wool blanket. Herbs may be added to the hot water in the towels.

This technique can also be used on specific regions of the body to relieve specific symptoms, such as menstrual cramps or PMS. Other variations include placing your feet in hot water while the hot towels are being applied to your chest, or putting a cold compress on your forehead while you're wrapped in the blankets. A rubdown over the chest with a cold towel sometimes follows the hot towel application.

Treatment Time: Each session lasts about 1 hour.

Treatment Frequency: Sessions may be repeated once a week or more frequently, depending on the illness under treatment.

OTHER HOT/COLD TREATMENTS

Some naturopathic practitioners recommend a procedure called a "wet T-shirt treatment" for use at home. To relieve symptoms of a cough, for example, the patient is told to stand in a hot shower long enough for steam to build up. He then dries off, wrings out a T-shirt that's been soaking in ice water, puts it on, covers it with a wool or flannel shirt or sweater, and goes to bed under several layers of blankets. A comparable treatment for children or infants who can't stand in a shower involves cold, moist socks covered by dry, warm socks.

Many primary care physicians recommend a variation of this procedure for colds, coughs, and congestion, especially in young children and infants. Parents are instructed to sit with the child in the bathroom while the running shower creates steam. After about 15 minutes in the steam, the parent then holds the child's face in front of the opened freezer compartment of the refrigerator, while encouraging the child to inhale the cold air. If the weather is cold enough, a brief trip outside, holding the child in a blanket, may achieve the same effect. This process should be repeated several times.

AQUATIC PHYSICAL THERAPY

This form of water-supported exercise is recognized by many insurance providers. Still known as hydrotherapy in Europe, it is recommended for patients whose medical condition causes pain during physical therapy outside of water, or whose rehabilitation will be aided by a water environment. Procedures range from immersion in a whirlpool bath to movement therapy in a swimming pool.

WATSU®

This unique form of therapy has been described as water ballet, though it is wholly passive on the patient's part. The therapist holds, floats, tosses, or stretches patients through the water in a specific sequence of movements. The effect is somewhat like aquatic yoga combined with maneuvers from shiatsu, or Chinese massage.

What Treatment Hopes to Accomplish

CONSTITUTIONAL HYDROTHERAPY

The practice of constitutional hydrotherapy originated with Otis G. Carroll in 1908. To earlier forms of water treatment, Carroll added electrical stimulation, shortening the application times for the hot and cold packs. He believed that this regimen could change the constitution of the cells in the body.

Today, advocates claim that the treatments detoxify the system and bring it back into balance. They believe that alternate applications of heat and cold can increase the body's white cell count, and hence boost its ability to fight infection and disease. They claim that, since the nerves in the skin are connected to the central nervous system, the hot/cold treatments can also help reestablish normal neurological functions. They add that the therapy can be expected to improve circulation and metabolism in the digestive organs and increase the amount of oxygen in the bloodstream. The mild electrical current administered during the treatments is believed to promote the production of digestive enzymes by stimulating the smooth muscle in the lining of the stomach and the ducts of the pancreas, gallbladder, and liver.

Despite all these purported benefits, many patients feel worse, rather than better, after a course of these treatments. Advocates of constitutional hydrotherapy (and hot fomentation) explain this reaction as a "healing crisis" said to occur when the body becomes strong enough to throw off harmful toxins. For example, if constitutional hydrotherapy is used to cure a sinus infection, the body is said to eliminate its toxins through the mucus in the sinuses, thus causing what appears to be a relapse. Patients also tend to experience a mild, flu-like feeling for a couple of days as the body restores itself. On the plus side, advocates promise that once the body has experienced a healing crisis it won't succumb to the same illness as severely in the future.

Critics of these treatments suggest that almost any activity, from taking a cold shower to getting too much sleep, can boost the body's infection-fighting T cells. They add that although many of the treatment's actions may sound plausible, there's no evidence that they actually occur.

HOT FOMENTATION

Some practitioners believe that hot fomentation aids the body in destroying cancer cells, viruses, and bacteria, all of which have a narrow tolerance to high temperatures. (The goal when treating cancer, for instance, is to raise the body temperature to 102 to 105 degrees for 30 to 45 minutes.)

Other practitioners recommend these heat treatments to *relieve* fever. The theory here is that fever-reducing medications disrupt the body's normal regulatory mechanisms, ultimately destroying its ability to bring the fever to an end. By raising body temperature to between 101 and 103 degrees, hot fomentation is said to reestablish the natural fever cycle, allowing the body to break the fever itself.

AQUATIC PHYSICAL THERAPY

The uplifting effect of immersion in water can relieve the pain of a compression injury in a joint or the spine. Hydrotherapy can also improve circulation and reduce swelling or fluid build-up in the legs. And exercising in water can help patients achieve a more efficient heart rate.

WATSU®

Watsu, created by Harold Dull, at the School of Shiatsu and Massage in Harbin Springs, California, has sparked controversy among physical therapists. Although some consider its methods helpful for some patients, others find its intimate, though nonsexual, nature uncomfortable. It is typically recommended to relieve stiffness and tension.

Who Should Avoid this Therapy?

Hot/cold treatments, including constitutional hydrotherapy and hot fomentation, are ill-advised for anyone suffering from loss of sensation in a part of the body to be exposed to the treatments. You should also avoid this type of therapy if you have asthma, kidney disease, a weak heart, a bleeding disorder, or an organ transplant. Likewise, frail people such as the elderly may not tolerate the treatments well. Constitutional hydrotherapy, in particular, is inadvisable for people with metal implants or pacemakers, due to the electrical stimulation used during treatment.

Aquatic physical therapy and techniques such as Watsu are best avoided if you have inner ear problems, a disorder of the spine, multiple sclerosis (in warm water), an acute orthopedic injury or unstable joint, or a condition that makes breathing in water difficult. Avoid Watsu, in particular, if you have a head injury or a dislike of intimate contact.

What Side Effects May Occur?

The "healing crisis" often encountered in constitutional hydrotherapy and hot fomentation is an unpleasant, but short-lived, side effect. Procedures that leave one tightly wrapped in towels and blankets sometimes trigger feelings of claustrophobia in those prone to the problem. The heat used in many of the treatments can also prove overwhelming to some patients. For the majority, however, these treatments are usually harmless.

How to Choose a Therapist

The "detoxifying" forms of hydrotherapy are especially popular among naturopathic physicians—practitioners who focus on helping the body heal itself. The noninvasive, nontoxic nature of these therapies fits in well with naturopathy's emphasis on the "healing power of nature." Indeed, naturopaths are the only alternative medicine practitioners who receive formal training in hydrotherapy techniques.

When choosing a naturopathic practitioner, check with the American Association of Naturopathic Physicians (AANP) to make sure he or she is licensed or accredited. (Only 11 states currently require a license.) Physicians recommended by the AANP must complete four years of graduate-level naturopathic medical school, receiving training in the same basic sciences covered in conventional medical schools. There are currently two such schools in the United States. Avoid graduates of correspondence courses.

If you need to consider water-based physical therapy, look for a certified professional experienced in this special type of treatment. Many physical therapists, occupational therapists, physical or athletic trainers, and massage therapists offer aquatic therapy. It was recognized as a special interest area by the American Physical Therapy Association in 1992.

If you're not sure whether aquatic therapy is right for you, consult a licensed physical therapist. He or she can provide an assessment and treatment plan for your condition, and recommend a specialist.

When Should Treatment Stop?

"Detoxification" with hydrotherapy is usually discontinued as soon as a "healing crisis" occurs. Ordinarily, several sessions are required to trigger the crisis. An additional session or two may be recommended to help you through the symptoms.

Other forms of hydrotherapy can be stopped when symptoms subside—or when the treatments no longer help.

See a Conventional Doctor If . . .

Although some practitioners advocate hydrotherapy as a treatment for cancer, there is absolutely no scientific evidence that it works. Using hydrotherapy as a substitute for conventional treatment will therefore put your life at risk. Continue to see an MD or DO if you have cancer or any other serious illness.

Likewise, if you have chest pains, a rapid pulse, and difficulty with exertion—or even suspect you have a heart condition—get mainstream medical care. Most natural healing programs don't even *attempt* to remedy acute cardiac problems (though many seek to prevent them).

Recurrent fevers, infections, or pain may be signs of a serious chronic illness. If such symptoms return or are made worse by hydrotherapy, turn to a conventional doctor for further evaluation.

Resources

ORGANIZATIONS

American Association of Naturopathic Physicians
601 Valley St., Suite 105
Seattle, WA 98109
Phone: 206-298-0126
Referral line: 206-298-0125
Web: www.naturopathic.org

American Physical Therapy Association
1111 North Fairfax St.
Alexandria, VA 22314-1488
Phone: 703-706-3248
Web: www.apta.org

FURTHER READING

Home Remedies: Hydrotherapy, Massage, Charcoal, and Other Simple Treatments. Agatha Moody Thrash, MD. New Lifestyle Books, 1981.

Lectures in Naturopathic Hydrotherapy. Wade Boyle and Andre Saine. Eclectic Medical Publications, 1998.

National Council Against Health Fraud. Website at www.ncaf.org

Quackwatch: Website at www.quackwatch.com

Hyperthermia

Consider This Therapy For

Hyperthermia—treatment of disease with heat—is gaining popularity in two diametrically opposed camps—the sophisticated world of high-tech medicine and the "kinder, gentler" field of natural healing. Cutting-edge physicians are experimenting with a variety of space-age high-temperature treatments for cancer and AIDS. At the same time, practitioners of natural healing advocate more down-to-earth heat treatments for ailments such as colds, flu, and other respiratory infections, bladder problems and urinary tract infections, and other types of infection and inflammation throughout the body. Many also regard such treatments as a means of ridding the body of stored-up toxins that presumably cause ill-health.

How the Treatments Are Done

Defined as any temperature above the body's normal level of 98.6 degrees Fahrenheit, hyperthermia can be applied to specific trouble spots in the body or administered globally to create an artificial fever.

In a procedure known as diathermy, high-tech doctors use electrical currents, ultrasonic waves, or microwave radiation to boost the temperature at selected points in the body. They may also resort to extracorporeal heating, removing blood from the body, heating it, and returning it to the body at a higher temperature—a procedure that has been used in the battle against human immunodeficiency virus (HIV). To get any of these treatments, you'll probably need to check into a medical center.

Natural healing practitioners, on the other hand, tend to favor less exotic forms of treatment that can be given on an outpatient basis in the office or clinic. The equipment required is typically nothing more than a bathtub, sauna, or steam room.

Whole-body immersion is an especially common approach. It's usually done in a deep, stainless steel tub. The water is typically heated to between 101 and 108 degrees Fahrenheit, although temperatures as high as 115 degrees are sometimes used if the patient can tolerate them. The goal is to keep the body temperature at between 102 degrees and 104 degrees Fahrenheit for about 20 minutes.

Locally applied hyperthermia may also be used, for example in the treatment of a hand or foot wound, and many practitioners use a combination of hyperthermia and cold baths or compresses to help stimulate circulation. For example, one leading hyperthermia clinic, the Uchee Pines Institute, employs the following treatments for headaches:

- Hot footbath with cold compresses to the head.
- Alternate hot/cold footbath (3 minutes hot, 30 seconds ice water) and cold compresses to the head.
- Alternate hot/cold applications to the head, starting with hot compresses at the base of the head and ice water compresses at the face, temples, ears and forehead. After 3 minutes, the areas of heat and cold are switched; the complete cycle is repeated two more times.

Although treatments often amount to little more than sitting in a very hot tub, do-it-yourself hyperthermia is not recommended due to the extremely high temperatures required.

Treatment Time: For whole-body immersion, a typical treatment requires approximately 30 minutes—10 minutes while the body temperature rises and 20 minutes while the high temperature is maintained. The time required for other forms of treatment varies widely.

Treatment Frequency: The course of treatment depends on your problem and the type of therapy. For upper and lower respiratory infections, patients typically undergo only 1 or 2 treatments. For more serious conditions, however, therapy can take much longer. Cancer patients typically begin with 15 treatments over a 3-week period followed by a 3-week rest. The cycle is then repeated 4 more times.

What Treatment Hopes to Accomplish

Whole-body hot water or steam hyperthermia is usually prescribed to combat infections. Because many germs cannot tolerate high temperatures as easily as our bodies can, these invading organisms often die from the extreme heat before any harm befalls the surrounding tissues. While hyperthermia may not kill all of the invaders, it can reduce their numbers to a point where the immune system can easily dispatch the remainder.

Other, more intensive hyperthermia treatments are used to treat viral infections. For example, much research has been done recently on the use of hyperthermia in the treatment of HIV infections. Some studies have shown that HIV is temperature-sensitive and becomes much less active at temperatures above 98.6 degrees Fahrenheit.

In the treatment of cancer, some studies have shown that hyperthermia can modify cell membranes in a manner that actually protects the healthy cells and makes the cancer cells more susceptible to chemotherapy and radiation treatments. Used as an adjunct, hyperthermia may thus permit lower doses of these potent and toxic forms of therapy.

Much research is also being conducted on hyperthermia's beneficial effect on the immune system. Researchers have found that although the white cell count appears to drop immediately following hyperthermia treatment, it rebounds strongly within a few hours. Furthermore, the cells' ability to destroy invaders appears to be enhanced.

Among many natural healing practitioners, hyperthermia is also viewed as a means of ridding the body of toxins such as pesticides, food additives, and other chemicals thought to disrupt the immune system. There is currently no evidence that it works in this manner.

Who Should Avoid This Therapy?

Although many of these treatments seem "natural" and benign, for some people hyperthermia can actually be quite dangerous. For example, it should be strictly avoided during pregnancy due to potential danger to the unborn child. People with peripheral vascular disease or loss of sensation should avoid it due to the risk of burns. Likewise, it's not for those with temperature regulation problems, especially the elderly and the very young. You should avoid it if you have a heart disorder such as an irregular heartbeat or an abnormally rapid pulse. And it's best to forego this type of therapy if you have extremely high or low blood pressure.

A number of other conditions can increase your sensitivity to extreme temperatures. If you have anemia, heart disease, diabetes, a thyroid problem, a seizure disorder, or tuberculosis, you may need to either reduce the number of treatments you take, exercise more precautions, or perhaps seek another method of treatment altogether. Before beginning the treatments, you should also give the doctor a list of all the medications you're taking. High temperatures can increase the impact of certain drugs— theophylline, for example—to the point where they become toxic.

What Side Effects May Occur?

The risk of side effects rises with the body temperature; most occur at temperatures above 106 degrees Fahrenheit. Among the most commonly reported side effects are herpes outbreaks, liver toxicity, and injuries to the

nervous system. In the very young, there's a risk of seizures. In the very old, there's a greater danger of heart failure during the treatments.

Keep in mind, also, that those seeking this type of treatment for an acute illness such as pneumonia may have a more difficult time tolerating extreme temperatures at the outset. The treatments can also cause a temporary flare-up of some chronic conditions such as herpes. However, these initial side effects may subside after a fever is initiated.

How to Choose a Therapist

There are no special certification programs in hyperthermia. Your best course is to seek out a conventional licensed physician with one year of additional training in these treatments. The physicians who offer hyperthermia services typically come from backgrounds in sports medicine or family practice.

As when choosing any physician or therapist, it's important to ask questions regarding the length of treatment, expected outcomes, and side effects. The doctor should be able to give you specific answers in all of these areas, as well as information related to your unique situation and state of health.

When Should Treatment Stop?

Typically, conditions such as lower or upper respiratory infections may require only one or two treatments before improving, usually within a few days or weeks. For more severe problems, such as cancer, treatments may continue for as long as a year.

See a Conventional Doctor If . . .

If you experience any side effects, stop the treatments immediately and seek standard care. For problems other than cancer or AIDS, you should begin to see improvement after the first few treatments. If you don't, consider other forms of therapy without further delay.

Resources

ORGANIZATIONS

Bastyr University Natural Health Clinic
1307 North 45th St., Suite 200
Seattle, WA 98103
Phone: 206-632-0354

National College of Naturopathic Medicine
11231 Southeast Market St.
Portland, OR 97216
Phone: 503-255-4860

FURTHER READING

Alternative Medicine: The Definitive Guide. The Burton Goldberg Group. Future Medicine Publishing, Inc., 1994.

Dr. Rosenfeld's Guide to Alternative Medicine. Isadore Rosenfeld, MD. Random House, 1996.

Home Remedies: Hydrotherapy, Massage, Charcoal, and Other Simple Treatments. Agatha Thrash, MD. New Lifestyle Books, 1981.

Hypnotherapy

Consider This Therapy For

With its ability to enhance the power of suggestion, hypnosis has been found effective for a variety of problems that hinge on emotions, habits, and even the body's involuntary responses. It won't cure underlying physical disorders such as cancer, heart disease, or infection, but it can relieve virtually all types of pain, no matter what the source—including the pain of surgery. It is also helpful against anxiety, tension, depression, phobias, and compulsions, and can sometimes help break an addiction to smoking, alcohol, or drugs.

Hypnosis doesn't work for everybody. For those who are susceptible, however, it has successfully alleviated an amazing range of symptoms, including those of asthma, allergy, stroke, multiple sclerosis, Parkinson's disease, cerebral palsy, and irritable bowel syndrome. It can control nausea and vomiting from cancer medications, reduce bleeding during surgery, steady the heartbeat, and bring down blood pressure. It has helped some people lose weight, controlled severe morning sickness in others, and given many relief from muscle spasms and even paralysis.

How the Treatments Are Done

During your initial visit, the first task will be to determine whether you're a good candidate for hypnosis. (Roughly 1 person in 10 can't be hypnotized.) There are several tests the therapist can use:

Stanford Hypnotic Susceptibility Scales: This test requires you to complete 12 exercises that range from closing your eyes and falling forward (or backward) to imagining your hand to be so heavy that you can't hold it up (or lift it). The last couple of exercises test your response to "posthypnotic suggestions." You might, for example, find yourself changing chairs spontaneously whenever the therapist taps his fingers after the test. Most people can perform the first few exercises; only a few can do them all. The further you get, the greater your chances of being hypnotized.

Barber Suggestibility Scale: This battery of exercises is similar to the Stanford Scales, but includes only 8 tasks. For example, you may have to imagine that you are extremely thirsty; or you may be expected to respond with a spontaneous cough every time the therapist makes a clicking sound after the test. Again, the more tasks you can complete successfully, the better a candidate you are for hypnosis.

Harvard Group Scale of Hypnotic Susceptibility: Like the Stanford Scales, this test includes 12 exercises, but is given to a group. Since the presence of other people can prove distracting, it is not considered as reliable a predictor as the other two.

Other ways of measuring your susceptibility for hypnosis include:

The Eye-roll Test: In this exercise, you'll first be asked to open your eyes wide, then roll them up. Then you'll have to lower your eyelids without rolling your eyes down. Ability to complete these tasks is not, however, a foolproof predictor of your ability to be hypnotized.

The Light Test: You may also be asked to stare at a small spot of light in a dark room. While most people are convinced the light is moving, those who see it change directions most frequently are supposedly the best subjects for hypnosis.

The Lemon Test: Some therapists ask first-time patients to imagine looking at, feeling, picking up, and slicing a lemon in half. They must then picture themselves squeezing some of the juice into a container, smelling it, and drinking a little. Those who are aware of salivating after performing the exercise once (or, in some cases, more than once) are more likely to be good candidates than those who do not salivate more than usual.

After the testing, the therapist will discuss the medical or psychological condition you wish to work on, as well as any other goals you may have in mind. This helps the therapist determine the approach to use during your upcoming sessions.

When therapy begins, you'll be asked to remove all jewelry and other accessories that may distract you and lie on a reclining chair or couch. There are several techniques the therapist can use to put you into a "hypnotic trance." The most common are:

- Asking you to watch a moving object as it swings back and forth, then suggesting in a monotonous, soothing voice that your eyes are getting so heavy you can't keep them open.
- Telling you to concentrate on the therapist's voice as he gives you instructions.
- Having you count backward slowly from 30 to 0.

As you slip into the trance, you'll feel deeply relaxed. Your conscious mind will no longer control every thought and emotion as it does when you are "awake." Your surroundings will become less important as you become increasingly aware of your inner feelings and sensations. At this point, you will be asked to stop thinking "consciously" and concentrate on something that will make you feel peaceful, such as walking through the woods or watching a sunset. With all troubles, pains, and other negative thoughts cleared from your mind, you'll find yourself able to focus intently on the instructions the therapist gives you.

Now the therapist may make suggestions. He may tell you how you can make an unwanted symptom or habit disappear. For example, if you have pain in your stomach, you may be told to visualize the pain as a small fish and then to imagine a shark snatching the fish and swimming away with it. With the fish gone, the therapist may suggest, you will be pain-free when you awake.

Analytical hypnotists use a technique called "regression." While you are in a relaxed "trance" state, the therapist will ask you to recall buried memories or emotions that may have caused your problem. (This is an accepted therapeutic technique when limited to your conscious life. Be alert, however, for mystics who promise to prod you into "remembering" events that happened in your mother's womb, or say they can regress you to a "past life" that supposedly occurred generations—or even centuries—ago. Whatever this may be, it's not therapy.)

The therapist may also implant posthypnotic suggestions while you are in the trance. You may be asked to remember or forget something or behave a certain way in response to a given signal after you awaken. For example, you may be told to feel nauseated every time you hear the sound of a cigarette lighter or see a certain type of food. Or the therapist may suggest you ignore a pain after you come out of the trance.

At the end of the session, the hypnotist will suggest how you should feel afterward and will order you to wake up. You may feel normal right away, or you may be sleepy for a few hours. Even if the hypnotist were to leave you alone, you would not remain in a trance. After slipping into a natural sleep, you would wake up by yourself.

To reinforce your treatment, the therapist will also teach you self-hypnosis. (You can learn this technique from audio and videotapes, but most professionals strongly urge that you take lessons from a qualified hypnotherapist.)

When performing self-hypnosis, sit or lie in a quiet, comfortable place, such as your favorite chair. Then try to relax completely, letting all your muscles go limp and allowing all tension to flow away.

To induce the hypnotic "trance," or focused state of mind, you can imagine yourself walking down a long path or descending a long staircase; concentrate on an object and breathe slowly and deeply; count backward from 10 to 0; tell yourself over and over that your eyes are heavy, your limbs are numb, or your face is warm or cool; or repeat a word or phrase.

Once you have achieved a hypnotic state, tell yourself how you want to feel, or listen to a tape on which you have recorded the message. To wake up, count slowly upward from 0 to 10, or reverse the image you used to put yourself under—for example, walk up the staircase. Tell yourself you will awaken feeling wonderful.

Treatment Time: Sessions with a hypnotherapist usually last from 60 to 90 minutes. Self-hypnosis sessions typically take 20 to 30 minutes.

Treatment Frequency: Most people see the therapist once a week. Proponents of self-hypnosis suggest you hypnotize yourself every day.

What Treatment Hopes to Accomplish

Modern hypnotherapy relies on induction of a "trance-like" state to reach the unconscious level of the mind—the level over which people usually have no control. Once the unconscious is open to suggestion, you and your therapist can more easily change the way you perceive problems—and promote new ways of responding to them.

Although "trances" may sound like psychological hocus-pocus, they are neither mysterious nor unfamiliar to most of us. We have all daydreamed or become lost in a novel. Sometimes we concentrate so deeply on a problem that we drive right past our exit on a highway. In all such cases, we are in a sort of trance—a state of "focused concentration" in which we are neither fully awake nor fully asleep. We have blocked out all distractions so that we can think exclusively on a particular subject, memory, problem, or sensation.

The concept of using trances to alleviate ills, both physical and mental, has recurred throughout the history of medicine. The ancient Greeks and Egyptians induced trance-like states to cure what we would call anxiety and hysteria. The Druids called trances "magic sleep." Native Americans and Africans recognized the hypnotic effect of drumming and dancing.

Modern hypnotherapy got a false start in the 18th century, when Austrian physician Franz Anton Mesmer propounded his theory of "animal magnetism." Believing that illness was a result of imbalance in the body's magnetic forces, he insisted that he could restore balance—and thus cure diseases—by transferring magnetism from his body to his patients. He endeavored to achieve this by waving iron rods, magnets, and his hands in front of his subjects and using "soothing words" to induce a trance. His influential contemporaries branded him a charlatan, and his magnetic theory was soon discarded.

Interest in the healing potential of the trance was later resurrected by James Braid, an English ophthalmologist, who coined the term "hypnosis," after the Greek word for sleep. To induce a trance, Braid simply stared at his subjects intently. Although he realized he could implant ideas in his subjects while they were in this deep, relaxed state, he could not explain why this was so.

Hypnosis remained in vogue until the late 19th century, and Freud used it in his early work. It then fell out of favor once again, resurfacing in the 1950s when Milton Erickson began experimenting with it for the treatment of both mental and physical ailments. By 1955 the British Medical Association had approved hypnotherapy as a valid medical treatment; the American Medical Association (AMA) followed suit in 1958. Today, the therapy is so widely accepted that the American Society of Clinical Hypnosis, a professional association of physicians, psychologists, and dentists, boasts 4,300 members.

While there seems to be little doubt that hypnosis provides lasting benefits for many of those who try it, no one is quite certain of the reason. Some scientists speculate that it prompts the brain to release chemicals called enkephalins and endorphins, natural mood-altering substances that can change the way we perceive pain and other physical symptoms. The majority, however, feel that it acts through the unconscious, the part of the mind responsible for involuntary reactions ranging from blood pressure and heart rate to hunger. Normally, these reactions are beyond our control. Hypnotherapy seems to put them under our power.

Whatever the truth of the matter, it's clear that when you are in a relaxed, trance-like state, you are receptive to suggestions that can help you react differently to negative situations, turn your attention away from harmful or unpleasant stimuli such as pain, discourage unwanted behavior, and even change your pulse rate or body temperature. The technique can also put you in touch with memories that may explain the origins of current problems and habits. Once you understand why you act a certain way, proponents suggest, you're in a better position to change the way you respond. Your mind can focus on productive solutions and hopefully overcome negative reactions.

One of hypnotherapy's greatest benefits may be its ability to reduce the effects of stress. Many physicians and psychologists believe that the mind has a direct impact on physical well-being. According to this theory, tension, anxiety, and depression can undermine immunity and compromise your health, while a positive attitude can reinforce the immune system, enabling it to better fight infections, toxins, and other invaders. Hypnosis can allay stress by putting you into a relaxed state, offering positive suggestions, and ridding the mind of negative thoughts. As tension in your muscles—and even your blood vessels—recedes, the theory goes, your circulation then improves, and your entire body feels healthier.

Who Should Avoid This Therapy?

Hypnosis is considered safe no matter what your condition.

What Side Effects May Occur?

Many people avoid hypnotism for fear of losing control to the therapist. They take showbiz stunts, with audience members clucking like chickens or bawling like babies, as genuine examples of hypnotic power.

Fortunately, the truth of the matter is that the hypnotist is never in control. A hypnotic suggestion works only if you accept it, and the therapist cannot make you do something you would not do consciously, something that goes against your moral code or religious beliefs, for example. The practitioner's goal is to help you use your own mind to solve problems, rather than give you the answers.

How to Choose a Therapist

Although legally, anyone can practice hypnotherapy without either special training or a license, it is important to make sure your hypnotherapist is a professional—most are physicians or psychologists—with a thorough training in psychotherapy. Also make sure he or she has experience in treating your particular condition.

To find such a therapist, ask your physician for a reference or contact one of the following organizations. (See addresses and telephone numbers on page 164.)

- American Council of Hypnotist Examiners
- American Institute of Hypnotherapy
- American Society of Clinical Hypnosis
- International Medical and Dental Hypnotherapy Association
- Milton H. Erickson Foundation
- National Guild of Hypnotists

Before beginning therapy, it's also a good idea to spend an hour or so with the practitioner to determine whether you have a good rapport.

When Should Treatment Stop?

If you turn out to be among the 10 percent who can't be hypnotized, or find that you are only marginally susceptible, you may want to move on to other alternatives, such as biofeedback or acupuncture.

See a Conventional Doctor If . . .

Although hypnosis can provide symptomatic relief in a wide variety of illnesses, it can't cure any physical disorder and should never be used as a replacement for conventional treatment. Seek standard medical care first, and use hypnosis as an adjunct.

Likewise, even though it works with the mind, hypnosis is not the best choice for many psychological problems, which are now known to be caused by chemical imbalances in the brain. It is not recommended, for instance, as a treatment for psychosis, severe depression, or antisocial behavior.

Resources

ORGANIZATIONS

American Council of Hypnotist Examiners
1147 East Broadway, Suite 340
Glendale, CA 91205
Phone: 818-242-5378

The American Institute of Hypnotherapy
1805 East Garryn Ave., Suite 100
Santa Ana, CA 92705
Phone: 714-261-6400

The American Society of Clinical Hypnosis
2200 East Devon Ave., Suite 291
Des Plaines, IL 60018
Phone: 708-297-3317

International Medical and Dental Hypnotherapy Association
4110 Edgeland, Suite 80
Royal Oak, MI 48073
Phone: 248-549-5594
(800-257-5467 outside Michigan)

Milton H. Erickson Foundation
3606 North 24th St.
Phoenix, AZ 85016
Phone: 602-956-6196

The National Guild of Hypnotists
P.O. Box 308
Merrimack, NH 03054
Phone: 603-429-9438

FURTHER READING

The Alternative Medicine Handbook. Barrie R. Cassileth, PhD. New York: W. W. Norton & Company, Inc., 1998.

Applied Hypnosis. Benjamin Wallace. Chicago, IL: Nelson-Hall, 1979.

Hypnosis. H.B. Gibson. New York: Taplinger Publishing Company, 1980.

Juice Therapy

Consider This Therapy For

High in concentrated nutrients, fruit and vegetable juices are ideal for keeping your immunity high and fighting off colds, flu, and other infections. Enthusiasts claim that juice therapy can also lower blood pressure, remedy skin disorders, and relieve digestive problems, though the evidence for these benefits is less than conclusive. In addition, juice therapy is a favorite aid in "detoxification" regimens, and is often used during elimination diets to detect the cause of an allergy.

How the Treatments Are Done

Extracting the juice from fruits and vegetables yields a liquid that's rich in sugars, starches, enzymes, vitamins, and minerals, but low in mass—in other words a concentrate that contains almost all the nutrients of the plant without the fibrous cell walls that originally contained them. The juices are used in two ways: as a supplement to a normal diet, or as a substitute for solid food (a "juice fast"). Most treatments are do-it-yourself, although the oversight of a physician is occasionally required.

There are a variety of juice therapy combinations. Indeed, the growing number of juice recipe books reflects the increasing popularity of this type of therapy. Since juices are mostly water, they can be mixed in ways you'd rarely attempt with solid foods. For example, combining fruits and vegetables is common in juice therapy, although it's unwise to mix acidic juices, such as lemon or orange, with other types of juice. The acids can curdle some liquids, and are best when juiced and consumed alone.

Almost all fruits and most vegetables can be juiced. (A few vegetables—asparagus, broccoli, cauliflower, and squash—yield bitter juices that, for many people, aren't worth the benefits they provide.) The fastest and easiest way to extract juice from any of these products is with a commercial juice machine. Those on the market today typically use one of two mechanisms:

Centrifugal Force: This type of machine cuts fruits and vegetables into tiny pieces and then spins them at high speeds. The liquid is extracted by centrifugal force in much the same way that water is wrung from clothes during the spin cycle of your washing machine.

Triturator: This juice machine chews and rips the vegetables and fruits into a wet mass. The liquid is then squeezed out by a hydraulic press or some other mechanical pressure. Because this process exposes the pulp to less air and thus keeps more nutrients intact, some juice aficionados consider the triturator to be superior. However, it is also slower, larger, more complex, and higher priced.

Enthusiasts recommend drinking juice as soon as it's made, since raw, unpreserved juice is highly perishable. Any contact with light, heat, or air starts an oxidation process that will eventually break down many of the nutrients. Nevertheless, you can store juice for up to two days if you keep it as cold as possible—35 to 38 degrees Fahrenheit—without freezing it. Juice therapists also recommend using a dark, sterile, pre-chilled bottle to store any juice that contains riboflavin (vitamin B$_2$).

JUICE SUPPLEMENTS

When combined with other dietary regimens, juice therapy can be used to augment athletic training, or simply improve overall health. Keep in mind, however, that juicing a fruit or vegetable removes its fiber. Juices therefore cannot be used as a substitute for whole fruits or vegetables, but only as a low-fat supplement to a balanced diet.

A typical supplementary juice regimen calls for 3 to 4 eight-ounce glasses per day, taken throughout the day.

JUICE FASTS

Juice therapists advocate juice-only fasts to cleanse and rejuvenate the body. Such fasts are also a good way to detect an unsuspected food allergy. If you experience a major improvement in chronic symptoms during a juice fast, chances are they were caused by an item in your regular diet. Reintroducing your favorite foods one at a time after the fast should quickly identify the culprit.

Juices can also provide at least some nutrients if you are unable to keep solid food down—for example, if you're undergoing cancer chemotherapy or have a severe illness. They are especially good for convalescents because they are easier to consume and digest than solids, yet still provide the much-needed nutrition.

Juice fasts typically last for 2 to 5 days. Juice advocates often recommend them for general health improvement twice a year, in spring and fall.

What Treatment Hopes to Accomplish

Juice serves as a valuable nutritional supplement in the treatment of all manner of debilitating illnesses, from cancer to AIDS. However, it's important to remember that it's not a magic cure-all. It won't do any more for you than a similar supply of vitamins and minerals from any other source. It lacks the fiber, fat, and protein needed to maintain energy and preserve optimum health. And it won't necessarily give you any more quick energy than you'd get from iced tea or cola.

Juice therapy has a lore all of its own, some of it true, some of it not.

- Carrot juice, rich in vitamins and minerals, is a favorite among advocates, but despite claims to the contrary, it won't boost energy, and combining it with beet juice doesn't stimulate the liver.
- Green juices, those made from green vegetables, are said to heal, stabilize, and calm frayed nerves, but they are not a source of long-term energy.
- Wheatgrass juice, made from kernels that have sprouted to resemble grass, is another favorite, often recommended to

detoxify the body, flush the liver, and purify the blood. There is, however, no evidence to support such claims, nor is there any reason to believe that it will remedy degenerative disorders such as Parkinson's disease.

Juice advocates also focus on the many antioxidants and phytochemicals that show a promising role in the prevention of cancer. Foods such as cabbage, kale, broccoli, cauliflower, garlic, onions, leeks, shallots, oranges, grapefruit, and lemons are especially rich in these compounds. Juice from these sources can provide you with a concentrated mixture of unique nutrients that can't be obtained from commercial supplements.

Who Should Avoid This Therapy?

Juice fasts provide minimal calories and little fat or protein. They are not recommended during pregnancy or while breastfeeding, and they are also unwise for infants, young children, and the elderly.

Certain health problems can make it necessary to avoid or limit intake of particular juices. For example, you should obviously avoid the juice of any fruit or vegetable to which you may have an allergy. If you have a problem with sugar, you'll need to dilute sugary juices such as carrot and beet with low-sugar juices such as celery. And if you have diabetes or suffer from hy-poglycemia, you should always take fruit juices with food.

What Side Effects May Occur?

Although, in general, there are no side effects from juice therapy, certain medical conditions such as diabetes may be aggravated by excessive intake of certain juices. It's also possible for a juice such as grapefruit to interact badly with certain prescription drugs such as Crixivan, Halcion, Lexxel, and Neoral. If you have chronic health problems or are currently undergoing treatment, it's wise to check with your doctor before undertaking juice therapy.

Avoid including excessive amounts of tomato and citrus juices in your regimen. Because they are highly acidic, they could conceivably upset the body's natural acid-base (pH) balance. Remember, too, that the juice of a food to which you're allergic can be just as upsetting as the original source.

How to Choose a Therapist

There are no special certification requirements for physicians who prescribe juice therapy. Any medical doctor should be able to help you with recommendations for most any health problem. However, if you are seeing a specialist for a particular ailment, it's best to consult this physician first.

You may also want to consider consulting a naturopathic physician, since these doctors tend to be especially experienced in juice therapy. The American Association of Naturopathic Physicians in Seattle maintains a referral database of naturopathic physicians who practice juice therapy throughout the United States. (See "Resources" below.)

When Should Treatment Stop?

Juice supplementation can last a lifetime. Juice fasts, however, should be limited to no more than 2 weeks at a time. No matter how many juices you include in the regimen, it will still lack many of the elements of a balanced diet. A protracted diet of juice alone will damage, rather than improve, your health.

See a Conventional Doctor If . . .

While juice can boost overall health and resistance, it can't cure any serious chronic disease. For example, cabbage juice may relieve the symptoms of an ulcer, but it won't cure one. (For that, you'll typically need a course of antibiotics and antacids.) Seek standard medical treatment for any long-term problem, and use juice only as an adjunct to regular therapy.

Likewise, juice therapy may help the body overcome an infection, but it won't kill any germs by itself. If an infection hangs on or gets worse, your best bet for getting rid of it is probably a prescription drug. Don't delay seeing a conventional doctor. Some uncontrolled infections can quickly become life-threatening.

Resources

ORGANIZATIONS

American Association of Naturopathic Physicians
2366 Eastlake Ave., Suite 322
Seattle, WA 98102
Phone: 206-323-7610

FURTHER READING

Juice It Up! Pat Gentry and Lynne Devereux. The Cole Group, 1991.

Juicing for Good Health. Maureen Keane. Pocket Books, 1992.

The Complete Juicer. Lionel Martinez. Running Press, 1992.

Juice Fasting and Detoxification. Steve Meyerowitz. Sprout House, Inc., 1996.

The Complete Book of Juicing. Michael Murray. Prima Publishing, 1992.

The Juicer Book II. Joanna White. Bristol Publishing Enterprises, Inc., 1992.

Light Therapy

Consider This Therapy For

Light has several well-proven uses in medicine. Regular sessions with a light box are an excellent remedy for the "winter depression" known as seasonal affective disorder. Ultraviolet light is frequently used in the treatment of psoriasis. Natural light is a potential remedy for jaundice in newborns. And, for all of us, sunlight is a leading source of vitamin D.

The list of ailments that light will NOT cure is, unfortunately, much longer. Despite claims to the contrary, there is no scientific evidence that light—colored or otherwise—will cure cancer, arthritis, menstrual problems, Alzheimer's disease, high blood pressure, headaches, hyperactivity, or AIDS. There is also little reason to believe that light will reduce stress, cure jet lag, relieve insomnia, improve fertility, speed healing, boost immunity, reduce cholesterol levels, increase the amount of oxygen in the blood, or stimulate the thyroid gland.

How the Treatments Are Done
SEASONAL AFFECTIVE DISORDER

Bright light therapy is the treatment of choice for seasonal affective disorder (SAD). The "white" lights used in these treatments match the radiation you would get from natural sunlight shortly after sunrise or before sunset, but do not contain any ultraviolet wavelengths.

Most people take the treatments at home, although some receive therapy in an office or clinic. If you are being treated by a therapist, you may be asked to lie on a couch under a lamp that emits at least 2,500 lux of illumination—about half the brightness of full sunlight. To receive any benefit from this therapy, you must keep your eyes open during the entire session.

For home treatments, you'll probably be advised to buy a light box. Most of these devices measure approximately 2 feet by 2 feet and enclose a full-spectrum

or bright white light that is angled toward your face. While most of these lights are 2,500 lux, some may be as bright as 10,000 lux. If you do not wish to purchase a light box, you can use any high-intensity fluorescent lamp that does not emit ultraviolet rays.

Place the box on a table or other flat surface where it is level with your eyes. You should sit about 18 inches from the box, facing the light source, but never looking directly at the bulb. (Some manufacturers recommend that you sit farther away. Be sure to read the directions on your box.) During the treatment session, you can read, eat, work, watch television, or perform other activities, as long as you remain facing the light with your eyes open. (If you need to move around during the sessions, you might want to buy a light visor powered by rechargeable batteries.) Never wear sunglasses or goggles during treatment.

Treatment Time: Ranges from 15 minutes to 3 hours, depending on the brightness of the light source. If you use a 2,500-lux source, you'll need 2 hours per session. A 5,000-lux light requires 30 to 90 minutes; a 10,000-lux source, 25 to 45 minutes.

Treatment Frequency: Therapy usually begins in the fall and lasts until early spring. It is best to have your sessions in the early morning or at dusk. One session per day is usually sufficient, although some therapists recommend twice-daily sessions for the first few days, or until your condition improves. You can probably take an occasional day off without any problem.

OTHER CONDITIONS

If you are receiving light therapy for skin conditions such as psoriasis or vitiligo, your doctor will probably give you a drug called psoralen 1 or 2 hours before your session. During therapy, your entire body will be exposed to ultraviolet light. A series of 30 sessions is usually required over a period of 10 weeks. (A similar approach to skin cancer, using light-activated drugs, is currently under investigation.)

For jaundice in newborns, intense full-spectrum light (or sunlight) is the recommended treatment. Full-spectrum lights, which are now being installed in many offices, factories, and other workplaces, have also been recommended for ailments ranging from migraines to premenstrual syndrome, but have yet to be conclusively proven effective for anything but jaundice.

For a wide variety of other conditions, ranging from pain to glandular problems, some physicians advocate treatments with colored light. There's no scientific proof that such treatments will work, but if you decide to experiment, you'll have several options. In one form of therapy, the practitioner directs light at a specific part of your body with a quartz-tipped "crystal flashlight."

In another, you sit under a bulb that diffuses colored light around you. Treatments dubbed "syntonic optometry" employ specialized machines such as a Lumatron® to flash colored light into your eyes at the rate of 2 to 16 beams per second.

If you are being treated with a Lumatron, each session will last approximately 25 minutes. The time needed for other forms of light therapy varies widely. For localized pain, one practitioner recommends 2 five-minute applications of red light to the site, followed by 10 to 15 seconds of light on the area around it. You'll receive 2 or 3 treatments daily for the first week, then twice daily sessions for a second week.

What the Treatment Hopes to Accomplish

Light has been used as a medicine for millennia. In the 6th century BC, Charaka, an Indian physician, treated a number of diseases with sunlight. Hippocrates and other ancient Greek physicians had their patients recuperate in roofless buildings, where they could soak up the rays of the sun. By the 1890s, European sanatoriums were prescribing incandescent electric "light baths" to treat many physical and psychological conditions, and Niels Finsen, a Danish physician, was using ultraviolet light to treat tuberculosis.

Light therapy as we know it today appeared in the 1980s, when doctors realized that people deprived of light sometimes developed symptoms such as depression, lethargy, inability to concentrate, and difficulty sleeping. Researchers speculated that the problems stemmed from a disruption of the patient's circadian rhythm, an internal 24-hour "dark-light cycle clock" that governs the timing of hormone production, sleep, body temperature, and other functions.

Circadian rhythm is regulated by the pineal gland, which, in turn, is controlled by the presence or absence of external light. During the first hours of darkness, the pineal gland produces the hormone melatonin, a substance that promotes sleep and, according to some researchers, may even strengthen the immune system. When you disturb the circadian rhythm by sleeping during the day, traveling across time zones, or getting insufficient exposure to light, your health begins to suffer. The two most striking examples of the phenomenon are jet lag and seasonal affective disorder (SAD).

SAD strikes 4 to 6 of every 100 people, most of them women over 20 years of age, although children also develop the disorder. The victims, who usually live in northern climates, generally feel fine during the spring, summer, and early fall, when the days are long, but become sleepy, gain weight, crave carbohydrates, and grow unhappy as the days get shorter. Some develop insomnia, lose their sex drive, grow irritable and moody, and find it impossible to complete tasks. Children may become hyperactive

or have problems learning and concentrating.

To reset the body's internal clock, researchers tried giving SAD patients regular doses of full-spectrum or bright white light from late autumn to early spring. They speculated that the extra light would suppress overproduction of melatonin (the suspected cause of SAD) and keep the melatonin cycle "in time with the real world." This theory was never substantiated, but the success of the treatments—for whatever reason—was indisputable.

Other experiments with light therapy have not, unfortunately, worked out as well. Light has been tried for a wide variety of ailments, but with little documented success. For example, one Israeli study claimed to show that a light-tipped probe inserted into the nasal passages of allergy patients could provide at least partial relief of symptoms. The study, however, did not meet critical physicians' demands for scientific proof. Similarly, use of light therapy to cure certain types of cancer is still awaiting conclusive validation.

Support is also lacking for the theory that colored light can eliminate problems in different parts of the body—for example, that flashing opaque white or violet light can reduce stress and relieve pain; or that red light can remedy ailments ranging from endocrine problems to depression, impotence, headaches, stomachaches, and diabetes. Colored-light therapies such as syntonic optometry have never been scientifically verified. Although the colored beams striking the eyes are supposed to regulate various body functions by stimulating corresponding areas of the brain, there's no evidence that this actually occurs.

There's disagreement, too, over exactly how such therapies might work. When light enters the eye, brightness- and color-sensitive cells in the retina convert it to electrical impulses that travel up the optic nerve to the brain. According to one theory, these impulses stimulate the hypothalamus, the region of the brain that regulates such automatic functions as sleep, body temperature, digestion, moods, sexual function, and the immune system. Other theories suggest that light may affect other parts of the brain, such as the cerebral cortex, which governs creativity, learning, and memory; the cortex, which governs movement; and the brain stem, which controls balance. Critics of light therapy point out that none of the theories have been scientifically verified, and dismiss the whole issue.

Scientists also reject the claim that too much artificial light and too little natural light prevents the body from absorbing adequate nutrients. (Advocates of light therapy charge that sunglasses, windows, and pollution are reducing our exposure to the full spectrum of natural sunlight, and that indoor lighting—usually about 500 lux—is insufficient to compensate for the loss of the 50,000 lux supplied by sunlight.) Al-

though it's clear that exposure to sunlight increases the body's supply of vitamin D—a necessity for healthy teeth and bones—critics say that its benefits stop there.

Who Should Avoid This Therapy?

Light therapy is not advisable if your skin or eyes are highly sensitive to light. Avoid it, too, if you have any type of manic-depressive disorder.

If you are taking any medications, you might want to check with your doctor or pharmacist before beginning light therapy. A wide variety of drugs can increase your sensitivity to light.

What Side Effects May Occur?

Overexposure to ultraviolet rays can cause skin cancer and may contribute to premature aging of the skin. Other possible side effects of light therapy may include a "hyper" feeling, mild headache, trouble sleeping, sore eyes, and other eye problems.

If you are taking light therapy for skin cancer, you may find that the dye often used in these treatments increases your sensitivity to sunlight.

How to Choose a Therapist

Light therapy for skin problems should be performed only by a board-certified dermatologist. Seasonal affective disorders can usually be treated on a do-it-yourself basis at home. For the more speculative forms of light therapy, information and referrals are available from the organizations listed under "Resources." Each specializes in a specific form of treatment:

- *College of Syntonic Optometry* offers referrals to optometrists who use optometric phototherapy.
- *Dinshaw Health Society* provides information on self-treatment with color therapy.
- *Environmental Health & Light Research Institute* supplies information on full-spectrum lighting.
- *Society for Light Treatment and Biological Rhythms* can give you information on SAD and sleep problems.

When Should Treatment Stop?

If you develop any serious side effects, stop treatment immediately and see your physician.

See a Conventional Doctor If . . .

If you think you have SAD, see a physician skilled in diagnosing and treating this condition before undergoing light therapy. He can rule out the possibility that you have clinical depression, a serious—and potentially life-threatening—condition that can be easily remedied with modern medications, but won't respond to light.

Also check with your doctor before starting light therapy if you have:

- An eye disorder, such as glaucoma, cataracts, or retinal detachment

- Any sort of depression that lasts the entire year, even if it gets worse in winter
- A rash and fever (You may have an infection such as measles or chicken pox.)

Resources

ORGANIZATIONS

College of Syntonic Optometry
1200 Robeson St.
Fall River, MA 02720-5508
Phone: 508-673-1251

Dinshaw Health Society
100 Dinshaw Dr.
Malaga, NJ 08328
Phone: 609-692-4686

Environmental Health & Light Research Institute
16057 Tampa Palms Blvd.,
Suite 227
Tampa, FL 33647
Phone: 800-544-4878

Society for Light Treatment & Biological Rhythms
10200 West 44th Ave., Suite 304
Wheat Ridge, CO 80033-2840
Phone: 303-424-3697

FURTHER READING

Let There Be Light. Darius Dinshaw. Malaga, NJ: Dinshaw Health Society, 1985.

Healing with Color and Light. Theo Gimbel. New York: Simon & Schuster, Inc., Fireside Books, 1994.

Light: Medicine of the Future. Jacob Liberman. Santa Fe, NM: Bear & Co, Publishing, 1993.

Health & Light. John Ott. Old Greenwich, CT: The Devin-Adair Co., 1988.

Macrobiotic Diet

Consider This Therapy For

This Oriental-style vegetarian diet is low in fat, emphasizes whole grains and vegetables, and restricts fluids. These are some of the same dietary principles that have been found to help prevent heart disease. Low-fat high-fiber diets are also believed to play a role in preventing some types of cancer. And the macrobiotic emphasis on fresh, nonprocessed foods may prove helpful in dealing with certain food allergies and chemical sensitivities.

Despite these benefits, few mainstream nutritionists endorse a strict macrobiotic diet. The selection of foods is so limited, they warn, that you can easily develop significant nutritional deficiencies. They add that while a macrobiotic diet may indeed reduce your risk of heart disease and cancer, it will not *cure* any specific disorder—including cancer.

How the Treatments Are Done

The macrobiotic diet is based not so much on Western nutritional principles as on elements of ancient Chinese philosophy. It is a nutritional attempt to balance the "complementary opposites" known as "yin" and "yang"— forces that the Chinese believed must be kept in harmony to achieve good health. These forces are woven into every aspect of life. Yin is said to be expansive, while yang is contractile; yin is cold, yang is hot; yin is wet, yang is dry; yin is slow, yang is fast; yin is passive, yang is aggressive; yin is sweet, yang is salty; yin is loose, yang is tight; yin is dark, yang is light.

To the extent that these qualities are reflected in food, the macrobiotic dietary regimen strives to bring them into balance. Certain foods are said to be very yin, others very yang, and some in-between. The most balanced foods in the yin/yang continuum (though not necessarily in nutritional science) are brown rice and whole grains. Hence these foods constitute the foundation of the macrobiotic diet.

To this foundation, the macrobiotic regimen adds foods reflecting different degrees of yin and yang, selected in accordance with the individual's dietary needs and temperament. In practice, this usually works out to a diet consisting of:

50 to 60 percent whole grains. Grains include brown rice, barley, millet, oats, corn, rye, wheat, and buckwheat.

25 to 30 percent fresh vegetables. Especially recommended are cruciferous vegetables (members of the cabbage family) and other dark green and deep yellow vegetables. They should be grown organically, and locally if possible. Macrobiotic advocates recommend lightly steaming or boiling them, or sautéing them with a small amount of vegetable oil. For purposes of the macrobiotic diet, vegetables fall into three categories:

—*Eat frequently:* cruciferous vegetables, including arugula, bok choy, broccoli, cabbage, cauliflower, collards, kale, kohlrabi, mustard greens, radishes, rutabaga, turnips, turnip greens, and watercress; Chinese cabbage, dandelion, onion, daikon, orange squashes, pumpkin

—*Eat occasionally:* celery, iceberg lettuce, mushrooms, snow peas, string beans

—*Avoid:* potatoes, tomatoes, eggplant, peppers, asparagus, spinach, beets, zucchini, avocado

5 to 10 percent beans, soy-based products, and sea vegetables. In this category, tofu (soy bean curd) is a favorite. Sea vegetables to consider include wakame, hiziki, dombu, noris, arame, agar-agar, and Irish moss.

5 to 10 percent soups. Miso soup, a broth made with soy bean paste, is a popular choice. Also permissible are soups made with vegetables, grains, seaweed, or beans.

Occasional treats: One to three times a week, a serving of seeds, nuts, fruits, or fish is considered acceptable.

Advocates suggest emphasizing local, in-season foods and avoiding processed, refined products. Completely proscribed are meat, poultry, dairy products, eggs, and warm drinks, all of which are considered too "yang" for consumption. Also to be avoided (because they are extremely "yin") are sweets and sugar, alcohol, coffee, caffeinated tea, and strong spices.

What Treatment Hopes to Accomplish

Proponents assert that the balance and harmony of the macrobiotic diet and lifestyle create the best possible conditions for health. They claim that the diet yields many positive health effects, including a general sense of well-being; and some studies do confirm that people on the diet have a decreased risk of heart disease and some forms of cancer.

However, claims that the diet can reverse cancer or AIDS (or generally strengthen the immune system) are based on isolated reports that have yet to be confirmed by scientific tests. The National Institutes of Health's Office of Alternative Medicine is studying the macrobiotic approach to cancer, but for now there's no concrete evidence that it's particularly effective.

Who Should Avoid This Therapy?

While a moderate approach to macrobiotics is not likely to cause harm and may promote health, extreme macrobiotic diets (often little more than brown rice and grain) lead to deficiencies that are especially damaging in children and pregnant women. Choose a more balanced approach to nutrition during pregnancy and a youngster's early years.

What Side Effects May Occur?

Vitamin and mineral deficiencies are a distinct possibility, particularly with the extreme versions of the diet. Studies of children consuming a macrobiotic diet revealed growth retardation in 6- to 18-month-olds, lack of energy, and deficiencies of protein, vitamin B_{12}, vitamin D, calcium, and riboflavin. Researchers also found that the breast milk of mothers on a macrobiotic diet contained abnormally low levels of vitamin B_{12}, calcium, and magnesium.

Another study links macrobiotic diets with an increase in iron-deficiency anemia, noting that impaired psychomotor development due to iron deficiency has been reported in infants fed a macrobiotic diet. Researchers have also linked macrobiotic infant diets with an increase in rickets, a disease of weakened bones and skeletal deformities associated with vitamin D and calcium deficiencies.

How to Choose a Therapist

Cookbooks, special food items, and macrobiotic cooking classes are available in most health food stores. Many cities have "East-West Centers" which give courses in macrobiotic cooking and philosophy. Tuition can cost more than $1,000 per week, with additional charges for personal counseling sessions.

The leading proponent of macrobiotic beliefs in the United States is Michio Kushi, who teaches the macrobiotic way of life at the Kushi Institute, near Boston, Massachusetts. In California, the George Ohsawa Macrobiotic Foundation publishes books and magazines about macrobiotics, and offers classes in macrobiotic cooking.

When Should Treatment Stop?

Discontinue or moderate a macrobiotic diet if you develop any symptoms of nutritional deficiency. (For telltale signs, see the section below.)

See a Conventional Doctor If . . .

Although a macrobiotic diet may possibly stave off heart disease and cancer, it's unlikely to cure them. If you suspect either problem (or any other serious disease) do not attempt to forego conventional treatment. Check with a mainstream doctor, for instance, if you have any of these signs or symptoms of cancer: changes in bowel or bladder habits, sores that don't heal, obvious changes in a mole or wart, unusual bleeding or discharge, a new lump or thickening in your breast or elsewhere, difficulty swallowing or frequent indigestion, or a bothersome cough or hoarseness.

The lack of animal protein in the macrobiotic diet is especially apt to cause a deficiency of vitamin B_{12} unless you include unfermented soy products fortified with B_{12}. This, in turn, can lead to anemia, which is typically signaled by loss of appetite, diarrhea, numbness, tingling of the hands and feet, paleness, shortness of breath, fatigue, weakness, and sore mouth and tongue. See a doctor if any of these problems appear.

It's also worth a trip to the doctor if you develop any symptoms of general nutritional deficiency. These include fatigue, muscle and joint pain, poor concentration, irritability, or susceptibility to infections.

Resources

ORGANIZATIONS

Kushi Institute
Becket, MA 01223
Phone: 800-975-8744

George Ohsawa Macrobiotic Foundation
1999 Myers St.
Oroville, CA 95965
Phone: 916-533-7702

FURTHER READING

Pocket Guide to Macrobiotics. Carl Ferre. Crossing Press, 1997.

Essential Ohsawa: From Food to Health, Happiness to Freedom. Carl Ferre and George Ohsawa. Avery Publishing Group, 1994.

An Introduction to Macrobiotics: A Beginner's Guide to the Natural Way of Health. Carolyn Heidenry. Avery Publishing Group, 1992.

Aveline Kushi's Complete Guide to Macrobiotic Cooking. Aveline Kushi and Alex Jack. Warner Books, 1989.

The Cancer Prevention Diet: Michio Kushi's Macrobiotic Blueprint for the Prevention and Relief of Disease. Michio Kushi and Alex Jack. St. Martin's Press, 1994.

Diet for a Strong Heart: Michio Kushi's Macrobiotic Dietary Guidelines for the Prevention of High Blood Pressure, Heart Attack, and Stroke. Michio Kushi and Alex Jack. St. Martin's Press, 1987.

The Macrobiotic Way: The Complete Macrobiotic Diet & Exercise Book. Michio Kushi, et al. Avery Publishing Group, 1993.

American Macrobiotic Cuisine. Meredith McCarty. Avery Publishing Group, 1996.

The Macrobiotic Brown Rice Cookbook: Delicious and Wholesome Grain-Based Dishes. Craig and Ann Sams. Inner Traditions International Ltd., 1993.

Magnetic Field Therapy

Consider This Therapy For

This hotly debated form of therapy is usually prescribed to relieve pain—primarily muscle and joint pain, but occasionally headaches, carpal tunnel syndrome, and other types of pain as well. Among its many applications are muscle strains; sprains of the spine, neck, or limbs; hip and joint pain; arthritis; phantom limb pain; fibromyalgia; osteoarthritis; persistent rotator cuff tendinitis; and chronic pelvic pain. In addition, magnetic fields are sometimes used to speed the healing of bone fractures, and some proponents even advocate magnets to relieve stress, combat infections, and prevent seizures.

The numerous studies that have been conducted on the efficacy of magnets have typically yielded quite contradictory results. Proponents announce favorable findings, only to find themselves debunked in subsequent trials. They usually respond that the follow-up studies failed to properly employ the precise magnetic devices responsible for initial success.

How the Treatments Are Done

The devices employed in this form of therapy range from small, simple magnetic discs to large, sophisticated magnetic field generators capable of producing high-intensity magnetism. The larger machines are typically used to treat bone fractures and pseudoarthrosis (a false joint at the site of an unknit fracture).

For pain management, small magnetic discs are usually taped to the body over the areas that radiate the pain, known as the pain trigger points. Magnets used for this type of therapy typically generate a field measured at 350 to 500 gauss, or about 10 times the strength of a typical refrigerator magnet. To hold the magnet in place, many people find sports bandages, headbands, elastic bandages, or Velcro more comfortable and less confining than tape.

To relieve stress and insomnia, some practitioners advocate magnetic blankets and beds. These devices produce a much stronger field in order to compensate for the loss of potency caused by their greater distance from the skin. For example, in such conditions, a 4,000 gauss magnet is needed to deliver 1,200 gauss to the patient.

Although all magnets have two poles—positive (south) and negative (north)—they vary drastically in size and strength. If you plan to try a magnet for pain relief, your best bet is to purchase a therapeutic magnet from a reputable medical vendor who will allow you to use it on a trial basis. Magnets delivering between 300 and 500 gauss are considered safe for home use.

Treatment Time: Depending on the severity of the pain, the magnet may be left in place for as little as 3 minutes or as long as several days.

Treatment Frequency: Varies with the nature and severity of the condition. Often the magnet is applied several times per day for several days or weeks at a time. Many people use this therapy at the first sign of a recurrence of pain.

What Treatment Hopes to Accomplish

The rationales for magnetic field therapy are as controversial as the treatment itself. Here are some of the leading theories.

Pain Relief. Some advocates ascribe the therapy's purported benefits to its affect on the nervous system, which depends on electrical charges to deliver its signals. Others say that magnets exert a pull on charged particles within bodily fluids, thereby promoting the flow of blood to the damaged joints or muscles, boosting levels of oxygen and nutrients, and ultimately relieving pain.

(Advocates warn that these results are often difficult to achieve without the guidance of a professional trained in magnetic field therapy. To be effective, they say, the magnetic field and the target bodily fluids must be at right angles, creating what is known as the "Hall Effect." This, they say, makes proper placement of the magnet a crucial part of therapy.)

It remains to be seen whether either of these theories is valid. One fact, however, is certain: Magnets will not cure the underlying cause of muscle or joint pain, and once the devices are removed, the pain may return.

Stress. Some proponents say that a negative magnetic field applied to the top of the head has a calming, sleep-inducing effect. Since stress is a factor in a wide range of ailments, they say the therapy can be beneficial as an adjunct in virtually any circumstance. (The treatments cannot, however, be relied on to remedy the problem.)

Infections. A few advocates of magnetic therapy go so far as to say that negative magnetic fields can destroy bacteria, fungal, and viral infections. However, there's no definitive proof of such an effect, and mainstream physicians warn against any attempt to substitute magnets for traditional antibiotics.

Central Nervous System Disorders. Some magnetic therapy practitioners have reported that placing small ceramic neodymium or iron oxide magnets upon patients' heads can relieve seizures, panic attacks, and hallucinations without disturbing mental alertness. There have been no formal clinical trials, however, to validate this contention.

Because magnetic therapy is a noninvasive, drug-free form of treatment, physicians who prescribe it claim it's one of the safest long-term remedies available—much more effective, they say, than aspirin or other over-the-counter medications. Fans of this therapy even argue that treatment outcomes are more predictable than most traditional approaches.

Who Should Avoid This Therapy?

Anyone with a cardiac pacemaker or defibrillator should completely avoid magnetic fields. It's also wise to forego this type of therapy during pregnancy. If you find that you have an allergy to the metal in the magnets, use only devices encased in hypo-allergenic plastic.

What Side Effects May Occur?

Side effects are generally considered unlikely. However, some practitioners have reported slight cases of dizziness when magnetic therapy devices were used near a carotid artery (the carotids are the two main arteries in the neck). Feelings of light-headedness have also been reported when the devices were used for more than 24 hours.

Some patients experience an increase in the intensity of the pain during the first few treatments; others notice a warming sensation due to expansion of the tiny blood vessels in the area over which the device is placed. The most common complaint, however, is a skin rash or irritation that often develops from the adhesive used to attach the magnets to the skin. To alleviate this discomfort, many physicians recommend protective barrier products that can be applied to the skin prior to the tape. Vitamin E creams can also be used to soothe skin irritated by adhesives.

Practitioners of this form of therapy recommend a number of additional precautions:

- Never use a magnetic bed for more than eight hours.
- Wait at least 60 minutes after meals before applying magnets to the abdomen. Earlier application is said to interfere with normal contractions in the digestive tract.
- Remember that the magnetic devices will stick to other metal products, possibly causing injury. Be cautious, for example, when removing a pan from the stove while wearing a device on your wrist.
- Be careful to keep the devices

away from anyone wearing a pacemaker or defibrillator.

How to Choose a Therapist

There are no training programs in this form of therapy, and no certification or credentials for its practitioners. To assure yourself of competent care, your best course is to seek a physician skilled in pain management. Such doctors can provide a range of treatment options, including psychological and physical rehabilitation once the pain is under control.

Although the treatments are usually administered at home, you'll need the advice of an experienced practitioner when starting therapy, since proper placement of the magnets is considered very important. It's also best to remain under the supervision of a qualified health care professional until your condition has resolved.

See a Conventional Doctor If . . .

Even its advocates do not recommend magnetic therapy for immune system disorders, digestive problems, fevers, kidney failure, liver failure, impotence, or any life-threatening disorder. In fact, whatever the problem, your best course is to seek conventional diagnosis and treatment first, seeking symptomatic relief through magnetic therapy only if other alternatives fail.

Remember, for relief of pain you now have an astonishing array of possibilities at your disposal, ranging from conventional medications to bodywork, acupuncture, hypnosis, and biofeedback. With so many promising options to be tried, magnetic field therapy can safely be considered a last resort.

Resources

ORGANIZATIONS

Bio-Electro-Magnetics Institute
2490 West Moana Lane
Reno, NV 89509-3936
Phone: 702-827-9099

FURTHER READING

Alternative Medicine: The Definitive Guide. The Burton Goldberg Group. Future Medicine Publishing, Inc., 1994.

Biomagnetic Handbook. William Philpott and Sharon Taplin. Enviro-Tech Products, 1990.

Cross Currents. Robert O. Becker, MD. Jeremy P. Tarcher, Inc., 1990.

Dr. Rosenfeld's Guide to Alternative Medicine. Isadore Rosenfeld, MD. Random House, 1996.

Magnetic Field Therapy. Robert Allen Walls. Inner Search, Inc., 1995.

Massage Therapy

Consider This Therapy For

Massage isn't capable of curing any serious or life-threatening medical disorders, but it can provide welcome relief from the symptoms of anxiety, tension, depression, insomnia, and stress, as well as back pain, headache, muscle pain, and some forms of chronic pain. It's also frequently recommended for the treatment of minor sports injuries and repetitive stress injuries, and for the enhancement of physical conditioning. Some people find that it even relieves such digestive disorders as constipation.

How the Treatments Are Done

There are dozens of specialized massage techniques in use today, including several that are discussed under separate headings in this book (see Hellerwork, Reflexology, and Rolfing). However, the most widespread variation builds upon the five basic strokes of Swedish massage:

- *Effleurage:* Slow, rhythmic, gliding strokes, usually in the direction of blood flow toward the heart, for example, from wrist to shoulder. Usually the massage therapist uses the whole hand (palm and fingers), gradually applying an increasing amount of pressure. Variations of effleurage involve strokes applied with the fingertips, heel of the hand, or knuckles.
- *Petrissage:* Kneading, pressing, and rolling muscle groups. The massage therapist will take hold of the tissue and alternately tighten and loosen his grasp.
- *Friction:* Steady pressure or tight circular movements across muscle fibers without moving across the skin, often used in areas around joints.
- *Percussion (Tapotement):* Drumming hand movements on broad areas of the body, particularly

the back. Techniques include *beating* with the side of loosely clenched fists; *cupping* or striking with the fingertips and heel of the hand; *hacking*, rapid chopping motions with the edge of the hand; and *clapping*, using the flattened hand to clap rapidly over fleshy areas.

Vibration and Jostling: Vibration entails rapid movements by the therapist to transmit an oscillating action to the patient; mechanical vibrators are also used for this purpose. Jostling requires rapid shaking of a muscle back and forth, usually for a brief period.

You may also encounter some specialized techniques employed for specific purposes. These include:

Neuromuscular Massage: Also known as trigger point therapy, this technique applies concentrated finger pressure to painful areas in muscles called trigger points.

Deep Tissue Massage: Slow strokes and deep finger pressure on areas of the body suffering from chronic muscle tension or areas that simply ache or feel contracted. Deep tissue massage is especially effective with tense areas such as stiff necks or sore shoulders.

Sports Massage: This rapidly expanding field, popular among both professional athletes and fitness enthusiasts, focuses on the use of massage to assist training, prevent injury, and aid healing in case of soreness or injury. It is used both before

and after exercise, as well as in the treatment of sports injuries such as sprains, strains, and tendonitis.

Manual Lymph Drainage: This rhythmic pumping form of massage stimulates the movement of lymph fluid through the lymph vessels. It is used to treat lymphedema, a side effect of any surgery in which the lymph nodes are removed or of radiation administered in the area of the lymph nodes.

The length of massage sessions varies, but a full-body massage generally takes an hour.

What Treatment Hopes to Accomplish

Massage is nothing more than a systematic manual application of pressure and movement to the soft tissue of the body— the skin, muscles, tendons, ligaments, and fascia (the membrane surrounding muscles and muscle groups). It encourages healing by promoting the flow of blood and lymph, relieving tension, stimulating nerves, and stretching and loosening muscles and connective tissue to keep them elastic.

Before physical exercise, massage helps get blood moving to assist in the warm-up. Massage after a workout has been shown to reduce the waste products (lactic and carbonic acid) that build up in muscles after exercise and cause cramping and discomfort. There is also some scientific evidence to support claims that massage enhances the immune system and aids recovery from soft tissue injuries by increasing blood circulation to injured areas. Some studies indicate that massage can even reduce blood pressure.

The healing powers of massage have been recognized since antiquity. In the 5th century BC, the Greek physician Hippocrates wrote that his colleagues should be experienced "in rubbing . . . for rubbing can bind a joint that is too loose, and loosen a joint that is too rigid." Various forms of massage were also employed by the ancient Chinese, Egyptians, and Romans. However, the technique as we know it today didn't appear until the late 19th century when Per Henrik Ling, a Swedish gymnast, formulated the principles of Swedish massage.

In addition to its general health benefits, massage has shown value for a variety of special problems in a host of recent medical studies:

- In premature infants, massage therapy was found to enhance weight gain and shorten hospital stays.
- When given massage, babies of HIV-positive mothers achieved greater weight gain and superior performance than babies in a control group that received no massage.
- Massage was shown to promote relaxation and alleviate pain and anxiety in hospitalized cancer patients.
- Massage reduced anxiety and lowered stress hormone levels in children with asthma, resulting in fewer asthma attacks.

- In a group of depressed teenage mothers, massage therapy helped relieve anxiety and depression.
- Mothers who were massaged during labor experienced less agitation, faster delivery, and less postpartum depression than those in a control group.
- On-site massage at a downsizing company was found to yield significant reductions in employee anxiety.
- After massage, a group of patients with chronic fatigue syndrome had lower anxiety and depression scores, and lower levels of the stress hormone cortisol, than did the members of a control group.
- Slow-stroke back massage in hospice patients was found to lower blood pressure, heart rate, and skin temperature.
- After daily massages for a month, a group of men with HIV infection had improved immune function and decreased anxiety.

Who Should Avoid This Therapy?

Generally, massage is not advised for anyone with an infectious skin disease, a rash, or an unhealed wound. It's also wise to avoid it immediately after surgery, or if you're prone to blood clots. Circulatory ailments such as phlebitis or varicose veins preclude the use of massage, and it should never be performed directly over bruises, inflamed or infected injuries, areas of bleeding or heavy tissue damage, or at the sites of recent fractures or sprains.

Massage is not recommended for cancer patients immediately after chemotherapy or radiation therapy. While there is no evidence that it actually prompts cancer to metastasize to other parts of the body, the theoretical possibility exists. Avoid massage over any known tumor, and in any area with a recent surgical incision.

Forego massage in the abdominal area for at least two hours after eating—and if you have an abdominal hernia, avoid it completely. Abdominal massage should also be strictly avoided during the first three months of pregnancy; during this period, massage of the legs and feet is also inadvisable. Indeed, it's best to consult your obstetrician before any massage during pregnancy.

Finally, if you suffer from panic attacks or have a history of sexual abuse, you may find that hands-on therapies such as massage just aren't right for you.

What Side Effects May Occur?

Massage can aggravate existing swelling (edema). The pressure that massage exerts on the skin can be painful for someone who has a nerve injury.

How to Choose a Therapist

It's important to make sure your therapist is properly qualified. The best evidence of this is membership in the American Massage Therapy Association (AMTA). Membership means that the therapist has graduated from a training program approved by the Commission on Massage Training Accreditation/Approval, holds a state license that meets AMTA certification standards, has passed an AMTA membership examination, or has passed the National Certification Examination for Therapeutic Massage and Bodywork. Licensing of massage therapists is now required in 25 states, and an increasing number of states are adopting the National Certification Exam. A national list of trained massage therapists is available from the AMTA. You can also check with a local school of massage for the names of qualified nearby therapists.

When Should Treatment Stop?

While the pressure of some massage techniques may cause momentary discomfort, pain should not persist throughout the session. If it continues, stop the treatment immediately.

See a Conventional Doctor If . . .

If your symptoms fail to improve—or get worse—see your doctor. Ongoing consultation with a physician is a good idea in any event.

Resources

ORGANIZATIONS

American Massage Therapy Association (AMTA)
820 Davis St., Suite 100

Evanston, IL 60201-4444
Phone: 847-864-0123

Touch Research Institute (TRI)
University of Miami School of
Medicine
Coral Gables, FL 33124
Phone: 305-284-2211

FURTHER READING

Hands-On Healing: Massage Remedies for Hundreds of Health Problems. John Feltman (ed). Rodale Press, 1991.

Mosby's Fundamentals of Therapeutic Massage. Sandy and Sandra Fritz. Mosby-Year Book, 1995.

The Complete Body Massage: A Hands-On Manual. Fiona Harrold and Sue Atkinson (photographer). Sterling Publishing, 1992.

Loving Hands: The Traditional Art of Baby Massage. Frederick Leboyer. Newmarket Press, 1997.

The Art of Touch: A Massage Manual for Young People. Chia Martin and Sheila Mitchell (photographer). Hohm Press, 1996.

The New Guide to Massage; A Guide to Massage Techniques for Health, Relaxation and Vitality. Carole McGilvery and Jimi Reed. Lorenz Books, 1998.

The Complete Illustrated Guide to Massage: A Step-By-Step Approach to the Healing Art of Touch. Stewart Mitchell. Element Books, Ltd., 1997.

The Complete Guide to Massage. Susan Mumford. Penguin Books, 1996.

Meditation

Consider This Therapy For

The calming mental exercises of meditation are a proven antidote for stress, tension, anxiety, and panic. Meditation is also a scientifically verified way to reduce high blood pressure and relieve chronic pain. Many people find it helpful for headaches and respiratory problems such as emphysema and asthma.

How the Treatments Are Done

Meditation is a deliberate suspension of the stream of consciousness that usually occupies the mind. Its primary goal is to induce mental tranquillity and physical relaxation. There are many different approaches to meditation, each with its own specialized techniques. However, all have a few requirements in common:

- A quiet environment where you won't be disturbed
- A comfortable position, usually sitting in a straight-backed chair
- A point of focus for your mind

Most people take lessons in meditation, but it's possible to teach yourself, using books or videos and applying some basic principles. At the outset, whatever the form of meditation, you need to wear comfortable clothes and assume a sitting position. Most people choose to sit in a straight-backed chair, although some find it comfortable to sit in the classic meditating position, cross-legged on the floor. Either way, the spine should be vertical. Slow, rhythmic breathing is a necessity in all forms of meditation, although each approach has a different way of achieving this. As you sit quietly and breathe rhythmically, you must focus on something—it may be your own breathing; or an image such as a religious symbol, a flower, or a candle; or a word or phrase repeated rhythmically. This word or phrase is called a mantra.

Many people prefer to keep their eyes closed during meditation, to avoid visual distractions and enhance concentration. Some people use soothing music. Try to stay as still as possible throughout the meditation period and let your attention, as much as possible, be passive. If you catch your mind wandering, try to refocus on the image or mantra you're using. Most people find that, as they gain practice, their random thoughts diminish, and the meditative state becomes more natural and instinctive.

Approaches to meditation fall into three major categories:

Transcendental Meditation (TM). This is the most common form of meditation in the western world. It involves mental repetition of a mantra, usually a Sanskrit sound provided by the instructor. TM practitioners sit upright in a straight-backed chair with their eyes closed, and meditate for 15 to 20 minutes twice a day, morning and evening. A nonreligious off-shoot of TM has been developed by Dr. Herbert Benson of Harvard University, with the sole goal of achieving the relaxation response that TM is known to trigger.

Mindfulness Meditation. An outgrowth of a Buddhist tradition called *vipassana*, this form of meditation focuses on the present moment. A favored technique in mindfulness meditation (shared with other forms) is the body scan, in which you move your focus through the body, from the tips of the toes to the top of the head, paying particular attention to any areas that cause pain or suffer from a medical problem (for example, the lungs for asthma, the pancreas for diabetes, the heart for heart disease). The body scan is usually done while lying down.

Breath Meditation. This technique calls for concentration on respiration, the process of inhaling and exhaling. In other respects it is similar to TM and other forms of meditation.

No matter which approach you adopt, each session typically takes 15 to 20 minutes, once in the morning and again in the evening. Advocates recommend scheduling your sessions for the same times each day, before rather than after eating.

What Treatment Hopes to Accomplish

By relaxing the body and calming the mind, meditation seeks to alleviate the harmful effects of tension and stress—factors that are known to aggravate a number of medical conditions. Although meditation has its roots in Eastern religious practices, its health benefits are independent of its spiritual aspects. Each practitioner can bring his or her own beliefs and world view to the meditative experience.

Meditation has measurable effects on the pattern of electrical impulses flowing through the brain. Studies with an electroencephalograph (EEG) show that it boosts the intensity of the alpha waves associated with quiet, receptive states to levels not even seen during sleep. Other studies show increased synchronization of brain waves between the two hemispheres of the brain during meditation, lower levels of stress hormones, and improved circulation. Levels of lactic acid, a potential by-product of tension and anxiety, drop after meditation. When practiced for an extended period of time, meditation has also been found to reduce oxygen consumption, slow the heart rate, and bring down blood pressure.

Devotees of meditation often claim that it improves their memory and other mental abilities, protects them from disease, and reduces their use of alcohol and drugs. Some studies have found that long-standing practitioners (those who've been meditating for several years or more) tend to make fewer doctor's visits than non-meditators. Other studies have found that meditation can reduce or reverse cardiovas-cular disease; improve the ability to cope with chronic illness; reduce anxiety, panic, and fear of open spaces; and relieve mild depression, insomnia, tension headache, irritable bowel syndrome, and premenstrual syndrome. One study of mindful meditation found that it reduced the rate of relapse in those with emotional disorders. Meditation has even been found to increase the longevity of healthy older adults.

Pain relief is another of meditation's more successful applications. While it can't completely eliminate discomfort, it does help people cope by reducing their tension and anxiety. For instance, the deep breathing exercises taught in childbirth classes are a form of meditation that helps women cope with the pain of labor and delivery.

Who Should Avoid This Therapy?

Some people may be temperamentally unable to achieve the tranquillity of meditation, and unsuccessful attempts may actually aggravate their stress and anxiety. Meditation can also prove counterproductive for people who are working on strengthening ego boundaries, releasing powerful emotions, or working through complex relationship problems.

What Side Effects May Occur?

For a few people, meditation can provoke the very problems it's supposed to defeat: fear, anxiety, confusion, depression, and self-doubt. During the first 10 minutes of meditation, as you unwind into a state of deep relaxation, it's possible for unsettling thoughts to pop up, disrupting relaxation. The problem is most common among beginners, but occasionally crops up in the more experienced.

How to Choose a Therapist

There is no licensing or certification procedure for teachers of meditation, and no central directory of practitioners. The transcendental meditation method has a number of "universities" around the country, run by the Maharishi Vedic Education Development Corporation. However, if you want to avoid the expense of a "university education," there are plenty of other options available. Some hospitals, clinics, or private practices maintain relationships with meditation instructors and may be able to refer you to one. Holistic health centers can also provide referrals, as can many of the books on the market. Look for someone who is experienced, and whose personality and approach you feel comfortable with.

When Should Treatment Stop?

If you find that meditation is *increasing* your anxiety or depression, or that it just doesn't feel right, it's a good idea to stop. (Some people find one approach more comfortable than another, so you might want to try another technique before giving up on meditation entirely.)

If, on the other hand, meditation yields the tranquillity and relaxation for which it's intended, it can be continued for a lifetime.

See a Conventional Doctor If . . .

Although meditation can provide significant relief from anxiety and stress-related conditions such as high blood pressure, it's more of a coping tool than a curing tool. See a conventional doctor for any continuing medical symptoms—such as headaches, shortness of breath, fatigue, or chronic pain—that may have prompted you to try meditation.

Resources

ORGANIZATIONS

Insight Meditation Society
1230 Pleasant St.
Barre, MA 01005
Phone: 508-355-4378

Institute for Noetic Sciences
475 Gate Five Rd., Suite 300
Sausalito, CA 94965
Phone: 415-331-5673

Maharishi Vedic Universities
Call 800-888-5797 for the university closest to you.

Siddha Yoga Meditation Center
South Fallsburg, NY 12779
Phone: 918-434-2000

Omega Institute
260 Lake Dr.
Rhinebeck, NY 12572
Phone: 800-944-1001

The Vipassana Meditation Center
P.O. Box 24
Shelburne Falls, MA 01370
Phone: 413-625-2160

FURTHER READING

Creating Health: How to Wake Up the Body's Intelligence. Deepak Chopra. Houghton Mifflin Co., 1995.

Thoughts Without a Thinker. Mark Epstein. BasicBooks, 1995.

The Art of Meditation. Joel S. Goldsmith. HarperCollins Publishers, 1990.

Active Meditation: The Western Tradition. Robert R. Leichtman, Carl Japikse. Ariel Press, 1990.

How to Meditate: A Guide to Self-Discovery. Lawrence Leshan. Bantam Books, 1984.

Basic Meditation (101 Essential Tips). Naomi Ozaniec. Dorling Kindersley Publishers, 1997.

Breath by Breath: The Liberating Practice of Insight Meditation. Larry Rosenberg and David Guy. Shambhala Publications, 1998.

Breath Sweeps Mind: A First Guide to Meditation Practice. Jean Smith, (ed). Riverhead Books, 1998.

Myotherapy

Consider This Therapy For
This specialized form of deep muscle massage is said to quickly relieve virtually any sort of muscle-related pain. Examples include strains, sprains, back pain, headache, repetitive motion disorders, fibromyalgia, shoulder pain, carpal tunnel syndrome, sciatica, and temporomandibular joint disorder. Also remedied by myotherapy are many conditions caused by muscle spasms, including certain types of foot and leg pain, incontinence, and abdominal pain.

Although mainstream physicians regard myotherapy as a plausible approach to treatment, it has only one major advocate: Bonnie Prudden, the person who originated it. It's also worth remembering that, despite an impressive collection of successful case studies, myotherapy has never been validated through controlled clinical trials.

How the Treatments Are Done
Expect your first visit to a myotherapist to last about 90 minutes. The therapist will begin by taking an extensive history. You'll probably be questioned about your birth (birth trauma is believed to underlie some types of muscle pain in both baby and mother), past and current occupations, sports, accidents, injuries, and presence of diseases.

The therapist will then evaluate your muscle strength and flexibility, searching for the "trigger points" that myotherapists blame for most types of muscle pain. To relieve the problem, the therapist will apply pressure to each trigger point for about 5 to 7 seconds, using his fingers and hands. This pressure will be painful, but is likely to provide almost immediate relief from at least some of the pain that led you to seek therapy. It can also result in a virtually instant increase in the mobility of tightly contracted muscles. Finally, the therapist will stretch the affected muscles and show you a set of corrective stretching exercises to do at home.

Subsequent sessions will last about 1 hour. They usually focus on eradicating the trigger points, reevaluating corrective exercises, and teaching you how to prevent pain through self-help myotherapy and exercises. The average patient needs 5 sessions, and few require more than 10. After the treatments are finished, you'll need to do exercises on a daily basis to prevent spasms—and accompanying pain—from returning.

What Treatment Hopes to Accomplish

The trigger points that myotherapy seeks to eliminate are nothing more than damaged, tender spots in the muscles. When these irritable points are "fired" by physical or emotional stress, they throw the surrounding muscle tissue into painful spasms. Repeated spasms can keep the muscle tight and foreshortened, not only causing pain but also interfering with function, posture, and balance. If the cycle of spasms and pain continues long enough, the muscles will become permanently shortened.

Trigger points are thought to be the remnant of a trauma such as the physical stress of birth (either giving birth or being born), accidents, injury, or repetitive stress. They can lie dormant for years, then be activated by substance abuse, age, or disease.

It's not clear why a few seconds of pressure is enough to correct a trigger point. Bonnie Prudden, the technique's originator, believes that the pressure denies oxygen to the spot, causing the muscle to relax. Physicians, however, respond that lack of oxygen is often the *cause* of a cramp. Whatever the truth of the matter, once the point is relaxed, myotherapists use exercises to reeducate the foreshortened muscle back to its original, relaxed position, allowing it to once more function normally. According to Prudden, this combination of trigger-point pressure and corrective exercise cures pain of muscular origin 95 percent of the time.

Myotherapy is an offshoot of the trigger-point injection therapy developed by Janet Travell, MD, the White House physician under President John F. Kennedy. Travell treated trigger points by injecting them with saline and the anesthetic drug procaine. While working with Desmond Tivy, another physician interested in trigger point injection, Bonnie Prudden found that simply pushing on a trigger point in a patient's stiff neck was sufficient to loosen it up. After similar results with two patients who had a sore elbow and shoulder, respectively, Prudden began refining the technique that was to become myotherapy.

Myotherapy is so simple that almost anyone can learn it; therapists usually train patients and family members to do it themselves. The trigger points are easy to find because they're relatively painful. You simply press each muscle with your finger at one-inch intervals until you hit a tender spot. You must then continue the pressure until it becomes painful, releasing it as soon as the pain begins. Once the point has released, simple exercises serve to keep the muscle relaxed.

Although myotherapy has never been scientifically validated, it did receive a sort of ad hoc trial over a 5-year period at a General Motors assembly plant. There, the medical director gave myotherapy to 1,000 workers with muscle injuries or other muscle-based pains. He reported a greater than 90 percent success rate, including symptom relief, elimination of lost work time, and reduction of medical costs for x-rays and physical therapy. The majority of patients required only one treatment.

Who Should Avoid This Therapy?

If you have any condition that could be aggravated by deep pressure, it's best to avoid this therapy. For example, if you have fragile blood vessels due to leukemia, you should probably seek another form of therapy. It's also wise to avoid pressure on a tumor, a recent fracture, or a surgical incision.

What Side Effects May Occur?

Pressure on the trigger points is temporarily painful. Bruising is also an occasional problem.

How to Choose a Therapist

It makes sense to seek out someone trained by the inventor of this form of therapy. A "Certified Bonnie Prudden Myotherapist" receives 1,300 hours of training during a 9-month course at the Bonnie Prudden School for Physical Fitness and Myotherapy in Tucson, Arizona. Certified therapists must also pass a board examination given by the Bonnie Prudden Pain Erasure clinic, and must receive an additional 45 hours of training every 2 years to maintain certification. The school has been licensed by the state of Arizona. In some states, myotherapists must obtain a massage therapy license.

To use a Certified Bonnie Prudden Myotherapist, you will probably need written clearance from your doctor (an MD or DO), your chiropractor, or, in the case of temporomandibular joint disorder, your dentist. (In some states, clearance from a physical therapist is sufficient.) To find a certified therapist, call 800-221-4634 or check the school's website at http://www.bpmyo.com.

When Should Treatment Stop?

Myotherapy almost always works very quickly. Therapists can usually tell after one treatment whether the method will help. If it does not seem to be effective, the therapist will probably refer you to a physician who can check for a non-muscular cause of the problem.

After completing the treatments, you'll need to continue corrective exercises at home. They may be needed indefinitely, depending on your particular problem. At age 84, Bonnie Prudden still does them every day.

See a Conventional Doctor If . . .

For anything other than muscle-related pain, you'll need to see a standard physician. For example, if your back pain is due to a spinal tumor or your headache is caused by a subdural hematoma, myotherapy is not going to help. Other conditions that clearly require standard care are a fracture, tuberculosis, or an aneurysm.

For some conditions, it makes sense to see a conventional doctor and a myotherapist at the same time. The myotherapist can provide symptomatic relief of pain while the doctor treats the underlying disease.

Resources

ORGANIZATIONS

Bonnie Prudden Pain Erasure
7800 E. Speedway
Tucson, AZ 85710
Phone: 800-221-4634;
520-529-3979
Web: http://www.bpmyo.com

FURTHER READING

Myotherapy: Bonnie Prudden's Complete Guide to Pain-Free Living. Bonnie Prudden. New York: The Dial Press, 1984.

Pain Erasure the Bonnie Prudden Way. Bonnie Prudden. New York: Evans & Company, Inc., 1980.

Naturopathic Medicine

Consider This Therapy For

More of a philosophical approach to health than a particular form of therapy, naturopathic medicine offers a wide variety of natural, noninvasive remedies for an array of troubling minor ailments. Some naturopathic recommendations, such as certain dietary modifications and the use of selected vitamins and food supplements, have been shown in scientific studies to confer lasting health benefits, and have been wholeheartedly adopted by conventional medicine. (Natural childbirth and acupuncture also fall into this category.) Other naturopathic prescriptions, such as detoxifying enemas and the use of homeopathic medicines, lack any scientific support.

Naturopathy offers a wealth of mostly harmless and possibly helpful approaches to a healthier diet and lifestyle. Many of its tenets, such as a diet high in fruits, vegetables, and whole grains, are now standard recommendations for those hoping to reduce the risk of cancer, heart disease, and obesity. Its noninvasive physical therapy techniques offer significant relief from a variety of muscle and joint complaints.

Be selective, however, in adopting naturopathic recommendations. Heat treatments and hydrotherapy, for instance, are not necessarily the most effective way to treat an infection. And the various "detoxifying" regimens advocated in naturopathy are even more suspect. There is neither evidence of any "toxic build-up" to be dealt with, nor proof that the regimens could eliminate one if it existed.

How the Treatments Are Done

Naturopathic practitioners range from physicians to massage therapists, and their approach to diagnosis varies accordingly. Among all practitioners, evaluation of diet and lifestyle is considered crucial. However, if your practitioner has a high level of medical expertise, diagnosis may also involve laboratory analysis, allergy testing, x-rays, and a physical exam.

Recommendations for treatment may include any of the following, depending on your symptoms and the practitioner's experience and philosophy:

Homeopathic Remedies: Preparations containing an extremely diluted amount of a substance that causes the symptoms, prescribed on the assumption that "like cures like."

Herbal Medicines: Whole herbs or standardized extracts, prescribed as mild, natural alternatives to synthetic medications.

Dietary Supplements: Vitamins, minerals, enzymes, and other food substances, recommended as a natural boost to health and resistance.

Dietary Restrictions: Vegetarianism or elimination of certain food categories (such as dairy products), recommended to relieve sensitivity reactions and clear the body of toxins. Dietary advice often includes instruction on "proper combining" of groups.

Physical Medicine: Manipulation of muscles, bones, and the spine, and physiotherapy using water, heat, cold, ultrasound, and exercise, employed to relieve a broad array of ailments.

Stress Reduction: Counseling, hypnotherapy, biofeedback, and other methods, employed to heal physical damage from stress.

Detoxifying Regimens: Fasting, using enemas, or drinking large amounts of water in an effort to purify the body.

Naturopaths typically recommend an assortment of these approaches in an attempt to boost your natural defenses (the immune system), restore good health, and prevent disease.

What Treatment Hopes to Accomplish

Naturopathy endeavors to cure disease by harnessing the body's own natural healing powers. Rejecting synthetic drugs and invasive procedures, it stresses the restorative powers of nature, the search for underlying causes of disease, and the treatment of the whole person (emotional, genetic, and environmental influences included). It takes very seriously the medical motto "first, do no harm."

Naturopathic medicine began as a quasi-spiritual "back to nature" movement in the 19th century. Reacting against the often misguided medical practices of the day and the disease, dirt, and degradation caused by the Industrial Revolution, the European founders of naturopathy advocated exposure to air, water, and sunlight as the best therapy for all manner of ailments, and recommended spa treatments such as hot mineral baths as virtual cure-alls.

In the late 19th and early 20th centuries, naturopathy evolved and grew enormously, rivaling conventional medicine in popularity. Benedict Lust, a German doctor who emigrated to the U.S. in 1892, founded the health food store as we know it, and crystallized the focus of naturopathy on diet and nutrition as the chief route to health. During this period, health-food faddism rivaled that of the present day, with influential practitioners like Dr. Kellogg (of cereal-company fame) insisting that meat and other "unnatural" foodstuffs were wreaking untold havoc on human health.

With the rise of increasingly sophisticated drugs and advanced medical technology after World War II, naturopathy fell from favor (with a hearty push from organized medicine). Grains and herbs seemed like mere snake oil in the brave new world of antibiotics and polio vaccines. Science reigned supreme until the 1960s, when the discovery of unsuspected side effects from DDT, thalidomide, and other high-tech wonders reminded Americans that "better living through chemistry" sometimes had short-comings of its own.

Meanwhile, a new and more scientifically minded crop of naturopathy advocates, including nutrition writer Adele Davis and vitamin C researcher Linus Pauling, helped bring fresh respectability to the idea that nature still held healing powers. This new breed was quick to adopt the research techniques of "conventional" medicine to prove the effectiveness of age-old remedies like herbs and newer options such as vitamin pills. Placebo-controlled, double-blind clinical trials, in which neither the doctor nor the patient knew who was getting genuine treatment and who was getting a fake, soon became common not only for drugs, but for diet as well. As the results accumulated, it became clear that our choice of food can indeed have significant impact on our health.

How well does naturopathy work? That depends on the aspect of naturopathy in question. Organized medicine, which ignored nutrition for decades, now swears by low-fat, high-fiber diets to prevent a host of diseases that plague industrialized societies such as ours. Mainstream doctors are also gaining new respect for certain antioxidant vitamins, such as vitamin E, as potential bulwarks against disease, and some are even acknowledging the effectiveness of certain herbs (such as St. John's Wort for depression).

On the other hand, many time-honored tools in the naturopathic toolbox have little or no scientific basis. The naturopathic notion that illness arises from vaguely defined "toxins" in the body that must be purged through fasting, enemas, sweating, and water consumption has never been verified through clinical research. Likewise, many popular food supplements, as well as the megadose use of vitamins, have so far failed to show definitive effects—while a few have even proved harmful. Naturopathic use of "natural" hormone preparations can also be dicey, since the potency of these products can vary to dangerous degrees.

The vegetarian diet—a mainstay of the naturopathic lifestyle—is also subject to question. It is not necessarily a "perfect" diet, according to the latest scientific research, especially if it contains large amounts of high-fat foods such as cheese. While a vegetarian diet is less likely to boost cholesterol (and will almost certainly provide more fiber), mainstream nutritionists continue to recommend a diet that contains modest amounts of meat, pointing out its nutritional benefits, such as healthy amounts of iron.

Other naturopathic ideas about nutrition are on equally shaky footing. There's no evidence, for example, to support the contention that certain types of foods should never be combined. Scientists also question the heavy emphasis that many naturopaths lay on food allergies as a purported source of countless vague symptoms. And they warn that the naturopathic tendency to eliminate dairy products can result in an unbalanced diet deficient in calcium.

Who Should Avoid This Therapy?

For the most part, naturopathy focuses on gentle treatments that do no harm, and most people can undertake this type of therapy without undue worry. However, drastic dietary restrictions can undermine good health and should generally be avoided, especially by the very young, the elderly, and those with a medical condition (such as diabetes) that requires special dietary modifications. If a dietary recommendation seems extreme, your wisest course is to first seek the approval of a registered dietitian or a conventional physician knowledgeable about nutrition.

What Side Effects May Occur?

Potential adverse effects of most naturopathic therapies are few and mild. Nevertheless, "natural" does not invariably equal "safe." Some herbal preparations can be quite toxic, and excessive fasting or use of enemas can upset the body's balance of fluid and minerals, leading to potentially dangerous consequences such as irregular heartbeat. The greatest hazard, however, is that using naturopathic therapies without any conventional advice could allow a serious medical condition to go undiagnosed and unchecked.

How to Choose a Therapist

Although various naturopathic remedies are offered by other health care providers, including chiropractors, nutritionists, holistic nurses, and massage therapists, if you want the complete package, you need to seek out an ND (Doctor of Naturopathic Medicine). Such practitioners have completed four years of graduate-level training at a naturopathic medical college. (There are currently three accredited colleges in the U.S.: Bastyr College in Seattle, Washington; National College in Portland, Oregon; and Southwestern College in Tempe, Arizona.) A referral directory is available from The American Association of Naturopathic Physicians (see "Resources" on page 197).

In the 11 states where they are currently licensed, naturopathic physicians must pass either a national or state-level board examination. Their scope of allowable practice varies from state to state, but generally conforms to their training in the types of therapies described above. Some states also grant certification in specialties such as natural childbirth or acupuncture. There are now about 1,500 NDs practicing in the U.S., but that number (which is minuscule compared to the number of MDs) is expected to double in the next five years based on current enrollment in naturopathic colleges.

NDs frequently refer to themselves as "general practice family physicians" or "primary care doctors." They are also fond of pointing out that the naturopathic curriculum actually offers more hours of basic biological science than do leading medical schools such as Johns Hopkins and Stanford. But beware: According to mainstream MDs, such claims can be misleading. They charge that, despite the use of scientific-sounding terminology, most naturopathic research consists largely of isolated case studies and untested theories. It's best, they say, to avoid naturopaths who try to impress you with elaborate explanations, and ones who claim to know as much about medicine as any MD.

When Should Treatment Stop?

Given the broad range of therapies under the umbrella of naturopathy, no general guideline applies. Dietary modifications to reduce the risk of chronic disease or control food allergies, for example, may need many months to make a significant difference, whereas therapy for an acute condition such as an infection or minor injury should reasonably be expected to produce much faster results. Use common sense, and consult the appropriate profiles in this book for more detailed advice on what to expect from specific types of therapy.

See a Conventional Doctor If . . .

Appealing as the idea may be, nature doesn't have the cure for all our medical problems. Although naturopathic physicians have considerable medical training, they are not necessarily qualified to diagnose and treat urgent or potentially life-threatening conditions. (Responsible naturopathic physicians refer such cases to more appropriate medical specialists.) If you have symptoms that may indicate a serious disease, consult a regular physician as well as a naturopathic practitioner.

Resources

ORGANIZATIONS

The American Association of Naturopathic Physicians
601 Valley St., Suite 105
Seattle, WA 98109
Phone: 206-298-0125
Web: http://www.naturopathic.org

FURTHER READING

The Encyclopedia of Natural Medicine. Michael Murray, ND, and Joseph Pizzorno, ND. Rocklin, CA: Prima Publications, 1991.

Neural Therapy

Consider This Therapy For

Neural therapy relies on anesthetic injections to clear up "electrical interference" causing problems elsewhere in the body. It enjoys its greatest popularity in Germany, where it is typically used to treat chronic pain.

Claims for this unusual therapeutic approach do not stop with pain, however. Advocates will tell you that it's effective in the treatment of hundreds of conditions, many of which defy other forms of therapy. In fact, proponents say that the people most likely to benefit are those who've failed to respond to chiropractic, acupuncture, or physical therapy. It's also recommended if surgery or nerve block treatments fail. Among the wide array of conditions for which it's advocated are:

- Allergies, hay fever, headache, migraines, sinusitis;
- Arthritis, back pain, chronic pain, whiplash;
- Asthma, emphysema;
- Arteriosclerosis, circulatory disorders;
- Bladder dysfunction, prostate disorders, kidney disease;
- Gallbladder disease, heart disease, liver disease, skin diseases, ulcers;
- Colitis, menstrual cramps, hemorrhoids;
- Depression, dizziness;
- Ear problems, glaucoma, inflammatory eye disease;
- Hormonal imbalance, thyroid disease;
- Muscle injuries, postoperative recovery, and sports injuries.

While some European studies seem to indicate that neural therapy works as well as a placebo (fake treatment), there is no scientific proof that it works any better.

How the Treatments Are Done

Neural therapists believe that a disruption in the "energy flow" at one point in the body can cause disease at another. Like devotees of acupuncture, they argue that if interference develops at a given point along one of the "meridians" through which vital energy flows, a problem will crop up at a corresponding point elsewhere in the body. Other likely sites of interference include tense, tender "trigger points" in the muscles, glands, scars, and nerves.

Because finding the supposed point of interference is crucial to successful treatment, neural therapists begin with a careful patient history. You'll probably be closely questioned about previous physical injuries, as well as any surgery or illnesses you've had. Scars will receive particular attention on the theory that if one of them cuts across an acupuncture meridian, it can be expected to impact the corresponding acupuncture site, as well as adjacent joints. For example, a nasty scar from gallbladder surgery might be the source of problems in the shoulder. Neural therapists are especially suspicious of scars that haven't faded with time, or seem to be pulling the surrounding skin, or feel hard.

If the therapist decides that a scar is the culprit, he will inject it with an anesthetic such as procaine or lidocaine. Otherwise, he'll give the injection in an acupuncture point, trigger point, or nerve. If the exact site of interference cannot be pinpointed, he will give an injection in the general area under suspicion, then adjust the location according to your response. He'll use a similar approach if the suspected area is too sensitive to tolerate injections.

Injections are not always recommended. In some cases, the therapist may conclude that an electrical imbalance stems from nothing more than metal eyeglass frames, jewelry, or dental fillings. Removing the offending object or replacing the fillings with plastic is then thought to be all that's necessary to cure your condition.

Treatment Time: Location of the ideal injection site occupies most of the visit. The injection itself takes seconds.

Treatment Frequency: There is no set number of treatments. Some patients improve following a single injection; others require several. If improvement occurs at all, it will usually be seen by the sixth treatment.

You'll be asked to keep a log of any unusual changes that occur in the two days following each injection. The therapist will use these notations as a guide for determining subsequent treatments. If multiple injections are deemed necessary, they are typically given twice a week.

What Treatment Hopes to Accomplish

Neural therapists lack a complete explanation of the way the treatments work. Although the goal is to correct "interference fields" in the body's electrical circuitry and thereby restore normal energy flow, it's not clear why an injection of anesthetic would accomplish this. The interference fields themselves have never been scientifically demonstrated; the energy flow that they are thought to disrupt is also an unproven supposition, and the anesthetic wears off in a couple of hours.

Interference fields are thought to develop at the site of a trauma. Accidents, surgery, and dental procedures are all considered leading culprits. The site can remain dormant long after the initial trauma, until another injury or stress triggers negative electrical activity. For example, if a person experiences significant weight gain, a scar could become stretched. Strain on the scar could then provoke an energy blockage that leads to problems in a linked site elsewhere in the body.

To neural therapists, inflammation or infection at one location—particularly in the mouth—strongly suggests the possibility of a problem elsewhere in the body. Therapists also suspect an energy blockage if a condition has failed to respond to other treatments, or has been aggravated by them. Other tip-offs of a purported energy blockage are the appearance of complaints on only one side of the body, or a series of illnesses in rapid succession without complete recovery.

Neural therapy is not recommended for any sort of structural abnormality, and it obviously cannot correct any genetic disorders or relieve problems stemming from malnutrition. It is also considered ineffective once a chronic condition such as kidney disease has caused severe damage, and it won't remedy emotional and psychiatric disorders. It is usually performed in conjunction with more conventional forms of treatment or when other methods fail.

Who Should Avoid This Therapy?

Neural therapy won't cure cancer, and could actually make it worse. It is believed to stimulate the lymph system, which is often the route through which cancer cells spread. Avoid this therapy if you have any form of cancer.

You should also forego neural therapy if you have diabetes, since the injections could interfere with day-to-day efforts to maintain stable insulin levels. Kidney failure and myasthenia gravis are other conditions that preclude neural therapy. Avoid it, too, if you are taking morphine or drugs that regulate the heartbeat, many of which are chemically similar to the local anesthetics injected during the neural therapy. People who have clotting problems such as hemophilia, or who are taking drugs that thin the blood, should also avoid this therapy.

If you are allergic to local anesthetics, you obviously cannot be injected with such drugs and thus cannot receive neural therapy.

What Side Effects May Occur?

No side effects have been reported in people who are suitable candidates. Make sure, however, that you have none of the conditions that preclude this form of treatment. If you do, the consequences could be severe.

How to Choose a Therapist

It's much easier to find a neural therapist in Europe or South America than in the United States. Your best course is to contact The American Academy of Neural Therapy for a referral (see "Resources" below).

When Should Treatment Stop?

Treatments rarely last longer than 6 weeks. If you obtain no relief within this period, you should consider another form of therapy.

See a Conventional Doctor If . . .

Your best course is to use neural therapy as a supplement to standard medical care. If you are using it in place of mainstream treatment or after conventional methods have failed, consider returning to your doctor if you fail to see improvement. If the condition gets *worse*, see a doctor without fail.

Resources

ORGANIZATIONS

The American Academy of Neural Therapy
1468 South Saint Francis Dr.
Santa Fe, NM 87501
Phone: 505-988-3086

National Chronic Pain Outreach Association
7879 Old Georgetown Rd.,
Suite 100
Bethesda, MD 20814
Phone: 301-652-4948

American Chronic Pain Association
P.O. Box 850
Rocklin, CA 95677
Phone: 916-632-0922

FURTHER READING

Facts About Neural Therapy According to Huneke. A Brief Summary for Patients. Peter Dosch, MD. Heidelberg: Karl Haug International, 1985.

Matrix and Matrix Regulation Basis for an Holistic Theory in Medicine. Alfred Pischinger, MD. Heidelberg: Karl Haug International, 1991.

Neurolinguistic Programming

Consider This Therapy For

This form of treatment seeks to replace counterproductive reactions that hamper the healing process with beneficial ones that boost it. Proponents say that it can ease pain, speed recovery from injury, combat allergies, and even enhance the immune system.

Unfortunately, despite a number of enthusiastic testimonials, there's no solid evidence that this type of therapy really makes a difference. If you try it, you'll have to take it on faith that it works. There's no question that psychological reactions do have physical impact on the body, so the therapy's effectiveness remains a genuine, if unproven, possibility.

How the Treatments Are Done

The theory behind this form of treatment is that people who are ill—particularly those with chronic disorders—become victimized by their own negativity. This process ultimately changes their self-perceptions and even their identity. They begin to think of themselves primarily in terms of their disease. When someone becomes "a diabetic," rather than "a person with diabetes," the disease has taken over. The more you identify with your condition, say neurolinguistic therapists, the less likely you'll be able to overcome it.

At the outset, therefore, your therapist will seek to detect any ingrained, unconscious attitudes that may be interfering with your body's natural healing abilities. As you describe the symptoms and health problems that have spurred you to get treatment, he'll attempt to analyze the underlying meanings of your words. Have you unconsciously despaired over your recovery? If so, you may reveal it in the *way* you describe your illness. The therapist will also look for clues in your facial expressions and body language, and even in the amount of moisture on your lips or eyes or subtle changes in your skin color.

Drawing on the clues he uncovers, the therapist will then attempt to help you modify your outlook and reactions in order to break the self-reinforcing cycle of negativity. The goal is to break the psychological hold that your illness has established and eliminate the preconceived notions that limit your progress. Neurolinguistic therapy attempts to accomplish this by training you to approach your problems in a new and better way, replacing negative thoughts with positive images.

Do you foresee only more and more illness as you look ahead? The therapist will use a technique called "guided imagery" to replace this potentially self-fulfilling prophecy with a more beneficial vision of your future health. This image of a happier, healthier outcome will eventually, it's hoped, prompt your mind (and your body) to deal more effectively with your disorder.

Neurolinguistic programmers begin and end each session with what they call an "ecology check." This is a sort of progress report in which the therapist seeks to evaluate what you think you're capable of accomplishing, what you're actually doing, and how you're going about it. These findings help the therapist keep your treatment in harmony with your basic values and beliefs, and serve to maintain balance in your family, social, and professional relationships. Repeating this check at the beginning and end of each session helps keep the therapy on target.

Treatment Time: There is no set limit on the length of a session.

Treatment Frequency: This is largely determined by your needs and your response to therapy.

What Treatment Hopes to Accomplish

The goal of this form of therapy is to reprogram your automatic mental and physical responses, replacing debilitating patterns with reactions that promise to combat your illness. By teaching you to substitute more positive thoughts and images for the previously negative thinking and imagery, Neurolinguistic practitioners hope to remove the psychological roadblocks that obstruct the body's natural healing mechanisms.

Can "the power of positive thinking" really cure illness? Those who endorse neurolinguistic programming suggest that the brain begins to respond in kind to more positive images and behavior patterns—just as it did to negative ones. This, in turn, is said to stimulate the body's immune system, thus improving your chances of healing.

Researchers have been able to demonstrate that an image and the underlying reality do, in fact, have similar effects on the brain. However, they've been unable to show that positive imagery shortens or alleviates any kind of serious disease.

Who Should Avoid This Therapy?

Neurolinguistic programming may aid in *recovery* from a serious injury or life-threatening illness, but you need conventional treatment first. Don't undertake this form of therapy for any serious medical problem without first seeing a doctor.

What Side Effects May Occur?

No side effects have been reported.

How to Choose a Therapist

The organizations listed under "Resources" on page 203 may be able to help you locate a practitioner in your area. When contacting a practitioner, however, remember that not everyone certified in neurolinguistic programming has been trained in the physical healing aspects of the discipline. Check to make sure the practitioner feels capable of dealing with your problem.

When Should Treatment Stop?

You may need substantial training in order to break ingrained habits of response and adopt a more beneficial approach to your condition.

However, if you see no improvement after a sincere effort, you'd probably be well advised to try another form of therapy.

See a Conventional Doctor If . . .

While neurolinguistic programming can give your attitude a boost, improve your approach to life, and promote relaxation, there is still no evidence that it can cure any disease or disorder. Many of its advocates regard it as nothing more than a helpful adjunct to conventional treatment—and, at least until further evidence is in, that's probably the best attitude to take. Certainly, if you develop any serious illness, your first stop should be a standard physician.

Resources

ORGANIZATIONS

Dynamic Learning Center
P.O. Box 1112
Ben Lomond, CA 95005
Phone: 408-336-3457
Fax: 408-336-5854

NLP Comprehensive
2897 Valmont Rd.
Boulder, CO 80301
Phone: 303-442-1102

Western States Training Associates
2290 East 4500 South, Suite 120
Salt Lake City, UT 84117
Phone: 801-278-1022
Fax: 801-278-1088

FURTHER READING

Beliefs: Pathways to Health and Wellbeing. Robert Dilts, Tim Hallbom, and Suzi Smith. Portland, OR: Metamorphous Press, 1990.

Introducing Neuro-Linguistic Programming: The New Psychology of Personal Excellence. J. O'Connor and J. Seymour. London: Mandala (HarperCollins), 1990.

Orthomolecular Medicine

Consider This Therapy For

For the better part of the 20th century, we've been taking vitamin and mineral supplements to eliminate deficiencies. Ortho-molecular medicine takes this idea one step further, holding that larger than usual doses of certain nutrients can actually prevent or cure disease. Although there's still considerable debate over specific dosages and their therapeutic effects, the basic principle is now firmly established and widely accepted. Two of America's greatest scourges—heart disease and high blood pressure—can both be held at bay by high-dose nutrients, and advocates insist that many other chronic conditions, including diabetes and schizophrenia, can be helped as well.

How the Treatments Are Done

With certain vitamins, it's possible to boost your intake to therapeutic levels simply by altering your diet. For instance, you can easily get 400 micrograms of heart-healthy folic acid by increasing your consumption of green leafy vegetables and fresh fruits.

However, the only way to get medicinal doses of many other nutrients is to take supplements. This is true of vitamin E. For most people, it's also true of vitamin B_6, even though it's plentiful in whole-grain cereals and breads, beans, and nuts. Likewise, therapeutic levels of calcium are hard to achieve without taking a supplement.

What Treatment Hopes to Accomplish

HEART DISEASE

Mainstream medical experts have long held that reducing the amount of animal fat in the diet can reduce your risk of heart disease. Now they are beginning to recognize that large doses of vitamin E have a similar protective effect. While the Recommended Dietary Allowance for the vitamin is only 30 international units (IU) daily, several large surveys have linked higher doses of vitamin E—at least 200 IU—with lower rates of cardiovascular disease. Even better, the Cambridge Heart Antioxidant Study (CHAOS for short) discovered that 400 to 800 IU of vitamin E slashed the number of non-fatal heart attacks among heart disease patients by 50 percent in the first year of treatment.

Another nutrient with strong links to heart health is folic acid, a member of the vitamin B family. Scientists first began to suspect its impact when they noticed high levels of homocysteine in children suffering from a severe form of hardening of the arteries that's usually found only in older adults. Homocysteine is suspected of damaging blood vessel walls, and further investigation revealed that the kids lacked adequate amounts of an enzyme needed to clear it from the blood. As it turns out, this enzyme requires folic acid to do its job.

Additional research found that many adults also have higher than normal levels of homocysteine in the blood, and that they too are at greater risk of heart disease. The investigators found that a daily dose of between 0.5 and 5 milligrams of folic acid could bring homocysteine levels under control. But would this alone protect them from heart disease?

The question remained unanswered until Dr. Eric Rimm and his associates at Harvard University conducted a study of over 80,000 nurses. Rimm discovered that, as the women increased their intake of folic acid and vitamin B_6 (another vitamin involved in homocysteine metabolism), their risk of heart attack declined. The risk was lowest in women who were getting more than 400 micrograms of folic acid and more than 3 milligrams of vitamin B_6 in their daily diet (more than twice the Recommended Dietary Allowances). The evidence was so compelling that, in an April 1998 editorial, the prestigious New England Journal of Medicine concluded that all Americans should take 400 micrograms of folic acid a day.

The bottom line: To maximize your chances of escaping heart disease, many experts now recommend that you not only follow a low-fat diet, but also supplement it with 400 IU of vitamin E, 3 milligrams of vitamin B_6, and 400 micrograms of folic acid per day.

HIGH BLOOD PRESSURE

There is accumulating evidence that an increase in your mineral intake can be an effective remedy for mild hypertension. Clinical studies have found that, for people with a deficiency, extra calcium can lower high systolic blood pressure readings by as much as 13 points, and reduce diastolic readings to some extent as well. (Systolic blood pressure is the force against the artery walls during each beat of the heart. Diastolic readings give the pressure while the heart is at rest.) Calcium supplements have proven especially effective for people who are salt-sensitive—that is, those whose blood pressure goes up when they eat too much salt.

Similarly, a recent study entitled Dietary Approaches to Stop Hypertension (DASH) linked deficiencies in calcium, magnesium, and potassium with higher blood pressure readings, and found that merely boosting intake to recommended levels is sufficient to lower systolic and diastolic readings by 11.4 and 5.5 points respectively in people with high blood pressure. This modest increase in mineral intake produces the same results as a standard high blood pressure medication. Recommended Daily Allowances of the minerals are 1,000 milligrams of calcium, 400 milligrams of magnesium, and 3,500 milligrams of potassium.

When taking calcium supplements, it's important to boost your intake of vitamin D as well, since without enough of this vitamin, the calcium you take won't be absorbed into the bloodstream. For example, when older women take calcium supplements to forestall the brittle-bone disease osteoporosis, they are usually advised to take as much as 800 IUs of vitamin D daily—twice the standard recommendation.

SCHIZOPHRENIA

This calamitous and still unexplained mental disorder sparked the first experiments with high-dose nutrient therapy. Indeed, when Linus Pauling, PhD, coined the word "orthomolecular," he was referring to the schizophrenia treatments pioneered by Abram Hoffer, MD. Believing that large doses of niacin, vitamin C, and other nutrients might relieve the disease, Hoffer conducted controlled trials in which neither the patients nor the doctors knew who was getting real vitamins and who was taking fakes. Although patients with established cases of the disease were unaffected, those in its early stages showed dramatic improvement.

Although subsequent trials by other researchers failed to confirm Hoffer's results, his proponents charge that the later trials either were poorly planned or failed to include early-stage patients. At this point, the majority of mainstream physicians still regard the treatments as unproven, even though many patients swear by them.

DIABETES

Years ago, when doctors first learned how to feed seriously ill patients intravenously, the early

IV formulas did not include trace amounts of chromium, an essential nutrient. Many of these patients mysteriously developed a diabetes-like disorder which, as it turned out, was a direct result of a chromium deficiency. Since then, researchers have found that daily intake of 200 micrograms of chromium picolinate can provide significant relief from diabetes, reducing the patient's need for insulin and oral diabetes drugs. A Chinese study found that between 200 and 1,000 micrograms a day improved blood sugar levels, serum cholesterol, and total metabolic control of the disease.

Although conclusive proof is still lacking, chromium picolinate may have other benefits as well. It has been prescribed for obesity, insomnia, depression, acne, and fatigue, and some advocates say it can even promote longevity.

HIGH CHOLESTEROL

A form of the B-complex vitamin niacin has long been an accepted remedy for high cholesterol levels. Dubbed nicotinic acid, and prescribed under the brand names Nicolar and Nicobid, it's taken in doses of 250 to 500 milligrams per day.

Who Should Avoid This Therapy?

Almost everyone can increase their vitamin/mineral intake to therapeutic levels without fear of harmful consequences. However, if you are taking the blood-thinning drug warfarin (Coumadin), you should avoid vitamin E supplements unless your doctor approves. Some reports suggest that the vitamin may cause bleeding under such circumstances. Another precaution: Vitamin E may interact with iron, so it's probably best not to take them at the same time of day.

What Side Effects May Occur?

Vitamin E. Even large doses of vitamin E are relatively safe, and most adults can handle up to 1,000 IU with little or no harmful effects. There have been a few scattered reports of fatigue and weakness among persons taking 800 IU a day, but the symptoms cleared up as soon as the supplements were stopped.

Folic Acid. While 400 micrograms of folic acid is considered safe for most people, larger doses can pose a problem for the elderly, who frequently suffer from a deficiency of vitamin B_{12}. Folic acid can hide the signs of this deficiency which, left unchecked, can progress to irreversible nerve damage. To eliminate the danger, simply take B_{12} supplements along with the folic acid.

Folic acid can also pose a problem for people taking an antiseizure medication such as Dilantin or phenobarbital. Each of these drugs causes a folic acid deficiency that needs to be remedied. However, a return to normal folic acid levels will increase the amount of drug needed to prevent seizures. To sidestep this problem, doctors now prescribe the drugs and folic acid together. If you're not already taking this combination, you'll need to see your doctor for a dosage adjustment when you begin taking the supplement.

Niacin. The high doses of niacin used in the treatment of schizophrenia (usually several grams a day) pose a slight risk of liver damage. It's best to take them under the supervision of a physician who will have regular liver function tests performed. If you have diabetes, you also face the possibility of an increase in blood sugar levels when taking niacin.

Unlike regular niacin, the nicotinic acid form has a variety of potential side effects, including darkening of the skin or urine, diarrhea, dry skin, eye disorders, flushing, gout, headache, indigestion, irregular heartbeat, itching, low blood pressure, low urine output, muscle pain, tingling, ulcers, vomiting, warts, and yellow skin and eyes.

Chromium. Doses of as much as 1,000 micrograms a day (5 times the maximum recommended allowance) have failed to produce side effects in major clinical trials. Nevertheless, there have been a few isolated reports that suggest some very minor degree of risk. Among the reported reactions were "disturbed thinking" and mental slowness. One woman taking 600 micrograms a day suffered chronic kidney failure. Another developed kidney and liver problems after taking 1,200 to 2,400 micrograms a day for 5 months.

Also, if you have diabetes, don't forget that chromium supplements can decrease the need for insulin or oral medication, and could lead to an unhealthy drop in blood sugar levels unless your medication dosage is reduced. All the more reason to check with your doctor when you begin taking chromium.

How to Choose a Therapist

Orthomolecular therapy is offered by a wide variety of health care practitioners, ranging from physicians and psychiatrists to nurses and nutritionists. Some belong to organizations like the Society of Orthomolecular Health Medicine or the International Society for Orthomolecular Medicine. Others may have no organizational affiliation, but may have studied under a specialist in the field.

There are several steps you can take to assure yourself that a practitioner is reputable. First, if you're dealing with a doctor or nurse, you can check with your state board of licensing to make certain that he or she has a valid license to practice. (In some states, nutritionists must also be licensed.) You can also check with the board regarding the practitioner's education and credentials, and can find out if any complaints have been lodged against him.

You may also want to ask the practitioner for some references. Ideally, you should aim to talk with patients who've had the same health problem you're currently facing. Ask them how well the treatments worked, and whether they suffered any side effects. Remember, though, that a few positive testimonials won't guarantee that the treatment is always effective. Try to read up on it if you have any doubts.

When Should Treatment Stop?

There's no reason to discontinue vitamin/mineral supplements unless side effects set in. If you do begin to develop unexpected symptoms, alert the practitioner immediately, and check with your regular doctor as well.

See a Conventional Doctor If . . .

It's wise to continue seeing your regular doctor while undergoing orthomolecular therapy, especially if you are also receiving conventional treatments. A number of prescription drugs interact with vitamins and minerals, and the higher the doses, the more likely an interaction will be. To guard against problems, make sure the orthomolecular practitioner knows about your prescriptions, and that your doctor knows about the supplements you're taking.

Resources

ORGANIZATIONS

Society of Orthomolecular Health Medicine
2698 Pacific Ave.
San Francisco, CA 94115
Phone: 415-922-6462

International Society for Orthomolecular Medicine
16 Florence Ave.
Toronto, Ontario,
Canada M2N 1E9

International and American Associations of Clinical Nutritionists
5200 Keller Springs Rd.,
Suite 102
Dallas, TX 75248
Phone: 972-250-2829

FURTHER READING

Nutritional Influences on Illness, Second Edition. Melvyn Werbach, MD. Tarzana, CA: Third Line Press, 1992.

Orthomolecular Nutrition, Revised Edition. Abram Hoffer, MD, and Morton Walker. New Canaan, CT: Keats Publishing, Inc., 1978.

Osteopathic Medicine

Consider This Therapy For

Born over a century ago from the belief that displaced bones, nerves, and muscles are at the root of most ailments, osteopathy has long since merged into the medical mainstream. Most practitioners still use osteopathic manipulative treatment to correct harmful "obstructions" in at least a few selected patients, but they also stand ready to provide all other forms of medical care. The majority of osteopathic physicians (DOs) enter family practice, and you can use them the same way you'd use any other family physician.

Although originally used to treat virtually all forms of disease, osteopathic manipulation *per se* is now considered useful primarily for musculoskeletal disorders such as back and neck pain, joint pain, sciatica, sports injuries, repetitive stress injuries, and some types of headache.

How the Treatments Are Done

A visit to a DO is much like one to an MD. The doctor will begin by asking you for your complete medical history. Since DOs pride themselves on their "holistic" approach to patients, he may also spend some time discussing your physical condition and lifestyle. You'll then be asked to undress for a complete physical examination.

An osteopathic physical covers all the concerns addressed in a standard medical exam. However, because of osteopathy's emphasis on the musculoskeletal system, it typically includes a slightly more intensive structural exam. During this portion of the physical, the DO will assess your posture, spine, and balance, use his hands to palpate your back, legs, and arms, and check your joints, muscles, tendons, and ligaments.

If you need laboratory tests, x-rays, or other diagnostic procedures, the DO will order them, just as an MD would. As with any other physician, the tests may be conducted in the doctor's office or at an outside lab or hospital. When the results of the tests are in, the DO will make a diagnosis, then establish a treatment plan. He will write prescriptions for medicines you may need, or refer you to an osteopathic or other specialist, if required.

For most disorders, the treatment offered by an osteopathic physician is essentially the same as what you'd receive from an MD, including prescription medicines and surgery as needed. However, for problems involving bones, muscles, tendons, tissues, and the spinal column, many DOs employ osteopathic manipulative treatment (OMT). This form of therapy ranges from light pressure on the soft tissues to high-velocity thrusts on the joints. In its most typical form, it calls for little more than gentle manipulation of the joints and spine.

To many people, manipulative treatment seems like a specialized type of massage. Others erroneously compare it with chiropractic adjustment, which focuses exclusively on realignment of joints. Although a few DOs (roughly 6 percent) still use manipulative treatment on a majority of their patients, most undertake it only a quarter of the time—or less. Younger DOs tend to use it least of all.

Treatment Time: Osteopathic physicians claim to spend more time with each patient than their

MD counterparts. However, there are no firm statistics to support this assertion. For practical purposes, you can expect a visit to be as long as one to a medical doctor—30 to 60 minutes the first time, 20 to 30 minutes thereafter.

Treatment Frequency: As in other forms of care, there is no set frequency for treatment by an osteopathic physician. If you are receiving manipulative treatment, however, you may require 3 to 6 sessions in all.

What Treatment Hopes to Accomplish

Osteopathic medicine began as an outgrowth of conventional U.S. medicine in the late 1800s, a period when the causes of disease were still unknown and most treatment consisted of crude surgery or the use of drugs to control obvious symptoms. Disenchanted with the persistent failure of these techniques, Civil War physician Andrew Taylor Still devised a kinder, gentler approach based on his belief that all disease was related to disorders in the muscles and joints.

Still was convinced that structural problems in the spinal column can affect the nerves that radiate out to the various organs, and that this is the true cause of disease. He called these problems "osteopathic lesions" ("osteo" for bone and "pathic" for diseased), and devised osteopathic manipulations to treat them. These treatments, he believed, could break up obstructions in the circulatory system, allowing the blood to flow freely and the nerves to resume their normal function. With proper balance restored, the body could then exert its own natural healing powers. In 1892, Still founded the American School of Osteopathy to teach these precepts.

From these beginnings, osteopathic medicine diverged from the predominant form of medical practice for several decades, relying less on surgery or drugs and more on manipulation, nutrition, and lifestyle. Then, as scientists learned more about the genuine causes of disease, Still's original theories were gradually downplayed, ultimately to be abandoned by many DOs. In the 1940s, osteopathy began edging back into the mainstream, and by 1972 osteopathic physicians were licensed to practice in all 50 states, often enjoying full hospital privileges alongside their MD brethren. Today, osteopathy is definitely on the rise. The number of DOs has increased 50 percent in the last decade alone. By the year 2000, the U.S. will have 45,000 DOs in practice.

Osteopathic physicians, like other physicians, must earn a four-year undergraduate degree emphasizing the sciences, take the Medical College Admissions Test (MCAT) for admission to medical school, undergo four years of medical education, and complete required residency training. Specialization in a specific area of practice, such as internal medicine, surgery, pediatrics, radiology, or pathology, may require from two to six years of additional training. Both DOs and MDs must pass state licensing exams. Both can be found in licensed hospitals, and both are eligible for membership in the American Medical Association.

DOs, however, undergo a completely separate course of training in the 19 medical schools and 200 teaching hospitals approved by the American Osteopathic Association (AOA). In addition to conventional medical training, they receive instruction in "hands-on" osteopathic diagnosis and osteopathic manipulative treatment. Most DOs ultimately enter primary care practice, specializing in the areas of family medicine, internal medicine, obstetrics/gynecology, and pediatrics. However, a few can be found in every other medical specialty as well.

Who Should Avoid This Therapy?

Any problem that would prompt you to consult an MD can also be taken to a DO. You should avoid osteopathic manipulation, however, if you have bone cancer, a bone or joint infection, or the brittle-bone disease osteoporosis. It's also best to forgo manipulation if you've had spinal fusion or suffer from a prolapsed disk.

What Side Effects May Occur?

DOs offer the full range of standard medical treatments, and side effects depend entirely on the approach the doctor selects. Osteopathic manipulative treatment itself has no potential side effects

other than temporary soreness for a day or two after therapy.

How to Choose a Therapist

If you are seeking an osteopathic physician as your primary-care provider, begin by looking for a board-certified practitioner. Referrals from other physicians or your local medical association can help point you in the right direction. Arrange an initial appointment to see if you are comfortable with the DO's personality and style of practice. Be wary of any doctor who presents manipulation as a cure-all; most reputable DOs use it only for problems of musculoskeletal origin. And be especially suspicious of a doctor who offers craniosacral therapy, an offshoot of osteopathy that has no proven benefits (see the separate profile in this book).

When Should Treatment Stop?

As you would with any physician, you should discuss your progress with your DO. If a particular treatment isn't working, he can try another approach or provide you with a referral to a specialist.

If you're receiving osteopathic manipulative treatment, you'll probably need a number of sessions, although pain due to muscle spasm may vanish after a single treatment.

See a Conventional Doctor If . . .

From the majority of DOs, you're likely to get the same care that you'd receive from an MD. As with any physician, however, a second opinion is always in order if you become dissatisfied.

Resources

ORGANIZATIONS

American Osteopathic Association
142 East Ontario St.
Chicago, IL 60611
Phone: 312-280-5800

American Academy of Osteopathy
3500 De Pauw Blvd., Suite 1080
Indianapolis, IN 46268
Phone: 317-879-1881

FURTHER READING

The D.O.'s: Osteopathic Medicine in America. Norman Gevitz. Baltimore, MD: Johns Hopkins University Press, 1991.

Foundations of Osteopathic Medicine. Robert C. Ward and Barbara E. Peterson. Baltimore, MD: Williams and Wilkins, 1997.

Osteopathic Medicine. Chicago, IL: American Osteopathic Association, 1996.

Oxygen Therapy

Consider This Therapy For

The little nasal prongs and masks that provide patients with extra oxygen are a common sight in hospitals. Use of supplemental oxygen is also common among people with chronic lung diseases such as emphysema. But the more exotic forms of oxygen therapy discussed here seek to do far more than simply boost the body's oxygen supply. Their goal is to cure diseases ranging from gangrene to AIDS.

Only one of them has any proven value. Known as hyperbaric oxygen therapy, it is the primary mode of treatment for gas embolisms (dangerous air bubbles in the bloodstream), the "bends" (a type of gas embolism that occurs when a deep-sea diver surfaces too quickly), carbon monoxide poisoning, and smoke inhalation. It is also generally accepted as supplementary treatment for burns, gangrene, radiation injuries, chronic bone infections, compromised skin grafts, non-healing wounds, destructive soft tissue infections, exceptional blood loss, and crush injuries.

Two other forms of oxygen therapy—employing ozone and oxygen peroxide, respectively—have been touted as cures for cancer, a variety of infections, and many other problems. To date, there is no scientific evidence that they work.

How the Treatments Are Done

HYPERBARIC OXYGEN

"Hyper" means increased; "baric" means pressure. During hyperbaric oxygen therapy, patients inhale 100 percent oxygen (versus 21 percent in the air we breathe) under pressures of up to two atmospheres (pressure at sea level is described as "one atmosphere"). The most common environment for this treatment is a specially designed, air-tight chamber used for one person only. In a multi-place chamber—a room or series of rooms—a group of people may receive treatment simultaneously.

In a single-place chamber, the patient lies down; in multiplace chambers, the patients may sit. Treatment occurs in three phases: *compression,* when pure oxygen is released into the chamber; *treatment,* when pressure is slowly increased to the prescribed level; and *decompression,* when pressure is slowly returned to normal. Patients are usually awake during the procedure. Patients who are uncomfortable in close, cramped spaces may find the single-place chamber anxiety-provoking. In such cases, a mild sedative may be given before treatment.

Treatment Time and Frequency:
The length and frequency of treatments depend on the patient's illness. For example, the standard recommendation for smoke inhalation is five 90-minute treatments followed by a review by a physician outside the treatment team to determine whether additional sessions are needed. Treatments for soft tissue injuries or tissue damaged by radiation therapy may require 2 hours in the chamber once a day for several weeks. Some chronic conditions may require therapy sessions on a long-term basis.

OZONE THERAPY

Ozone (O_3) is a molecule of oxygen (O_2) with an extra atom attached. Proponents of ozone therapy claim that the extra atom assures higher oxygen levels in the blood and tissues after normal oxidation begins stripping the atoms away.

Ozone in the upper atmosphere absorbs certain forms of radiation, protecting us from its harmful effects. In the lower atmosphere, however, it can irritate the eyes and lungs and aggravate respiratory problems. For therapeutic purposes, it's taken in a variety of ways that avoid inhalation. Among the more common:

- by ingesting it in water instilled with the gas
- by applying a mixture of olive oil and ozone directly to the skin
- by a process in which blood is withdrawn from the body, mixed with ozone, and injected back into a vein (known as major autohemotherapy) or a muscle (known as minor autohemotherapy)
- by blowing the gas into a body cavity such as the vagina, rectum, or eardrum (known as insufflation)
- by circulating the gas around a limb that has been wrapped in a bag (known as "limb-bagging")

The "ozone machines" offered by various manufacturers will not suffice for this type of therapy. In fact, it should be administered only by an experienced practitioner, since excessive oxidation can be damaging.

Treatment Time and Frequency:
The number and length of

treatments depend on the practitioner's approach to ozone therapy and the condition for which it is being administered. One treatment plan recommends sessions twice a week for 15 to 30 minutes. Practitioners who use ozone therapy to treat patients with HIV recommend treatments twice daily.

HYDROGEN PEROXIDE THERAPY

Most people know hydrogen peroxide as the liquid you buy at the drug store for disinfecting scrapes and cuts. It forms when ozone comes into contact with water: the extra oxygen atom attached to the ozone molecule breaks off and combines with a water molecule (H_2O) to create hydrogen peroxide (H_2O_2). It exists in the atmosphere, in raw fruits and vegetables, even in mother's milk. In the human body it serves to activate the immune system, and is produced in areas such as the large intestine to prevent bacteria from growing out of control.

Hydrogen peroxide is manufactured in different strengths or grades for different purposes. For example, the liquid at the drug store is 3 percent hydrogen peroxide. In manufacturing, a solution of 30 percent hydrogen peroxide is used to wash transistors before assembly. Cheese, eggs, and whey food products are washed in 35 percent "food grade" hydrogen peroxide, which is also used to kill microorganisms in food storage products such as aluminum foil.

Advocates of "hydrogen peroxide therapy" usually recommend using food grade, 35 percent hydrogen peroxide, which can be purchased in some health food stores or by mail. They advise bathing in a diluted solution, gargling with it, spraying it over the body, or soaking injured body parts in it. Some practitioners inject the diluted solution directly into the bloodstream.

Treatment Time and Frequency: Daily or weekly treatment recommendations are common, depending on the condition. For chronic ailments, hydrogen peroxide therapy may be recommended on a long-term basis. IV hydrogen peroxide therapy may take as long as 3 hours to administer.

What Treatment Hopes to Accomplish
HYPERBARIC OXYGEN

Hyperbaric oxygen has been used for more than a century to treat the effects of decompression sickness. When a diver surfaces too quickly, bubbles of gas develop in the bloodstream and threaten to disrupt circulation to vital organs. The pressurized atmosphere in the hyperbaric chamber reduces the size of these bubbles so that they can pass through the circulatory system without blocking the arteries.

Used as an antidote for carbon monoxide poisoning, hyperbaric oxygen treatment floods the body with oxygen to force the carbon monoxide out. The high pressure within the chamber helps speed oxygen to the tissues where it's needed for vital body functions.

Hyperbaric oxygen also has an antibacterial effect. To anaerobic bacteria (bacteria that live without oxygen) exposure to it is poisonous. In addition, since much of the body's immune system is oxygen-dependent, high oxygen levels can give a boost to the cells that fight off infection, particularly deep in the tissues. Hyperbaric oxygen can also compensate for disrupted circulation, helping to reduce swelling and promote tissue recovery following burn or crush injuries.

Other applications are still considered experimental. Some plastic surgeons recommend hyperbaric treatment to hasten healing after the operation. Migraine pain, memory loss from dementia or Alzheimer's disease, and multiple sclerosis are other conditions for which the therapy is considered potentially beneficial. In some animal studies and limited clinical studies, hyperbaric oxygen has shown promise for treatment of stroke.

OZONE AND HYDROGEN PEROXIDE

Oxygen plays a key role in every cellular process. It supports the immune system, destroys toxic substances, fuels metabolism, and promotes new cell growth. Proponents of oxygen therapy (also called hyperoxygenation, superoxygenation, or oxidative therapy) contend that ozone and hydrogen peroxide, with their extra atoms of oxygen, are more efficient than ordinary O_2 for fighting disease and repairing injury. They argue that increased oxidation in the body can neutralize toxic substances and kill invading microorganisms; and they advocate oxygen therapy for everything from infections to chronic fatigue. Even a partial list of the conditions they cite includes such circulatory diseases as gangrene, dementia, and stroke; such respiratory diseases as asthma, chronic bronchitis, and pneumonia, and such infectious diseases as herpes, candidiasis, and AIDS.

Although the theory underlying use of these compounds may seem reasonable, their effectiveness has never been verified in clinical trials. Ozone, for instance, has been found to inactivate the AIDS virus in laboratory tests, but when given to patients, has failed to work any improvement. Speculation that high oxygen levels could cure cancer have also proven baseless. The U.S. Food and Drug Administration (FDA) has found no evidence of any medical benefits from industrial-strength hydrogen peroxide, and has banned any claims to the contrary. Neither hydrogen peroxide therapy (or the solutions used for it) nor ozone therapy (and the machines used to make and dispense the gas) is approved or regulated by the FDA.

Despite its detractors in the United States, oxygen therapy is widely used abroad. Proponents hint darkly that a "medical Mafia" has blocked its adoption in this country, favoring more lucrative pharmaceuticals over such cheap, readily available remedies as ozone and hydrogen peroxide. Whatever the truth of the matter, there's still no reliable evidence supporting their use. So for any condition with a clinically proven remedy, they have to be considered an experimental last resort.

Who Should Avoid This Therapy?

HYPERBARIC OXYGEN

Avoid these treatments if you have a seizure disorder, emphysema, a high fever, or an upper respiratory infection. Do not undergo them if you have a severe fluid build-up in the sinuses, ears, or other body cavities. Forego them if you've had surgery for optic neuritis, or have ever had a collapsed lung. Avoid them, too, if you are taking doxorubicin (Adriamycin), cisplatin (Platinol), disulfiram (Antabuse), or mafenide acetate (Sulfamylon).

Pregnancy was once considered a contraindication for hyperbaric therapy. However, it's now deemed acceptable if a condition will cause long-term damage to the mother or fetus. For example, the treatments are given to pregnant women with carbon monoxide poisoning, which is toxic to both mother and child.

OZONE AND HYDROGEN PEROXIDE

According to practitioners who use and study ozone therapy, the treatments should never be given to anyone with a hemorrhage—including a menstruating woman—because ozone can increase bleeding. For the same reason, ozone should be avoided by those with thrombocytopenia, a condition characterized by a lack of blood platelets that can lead to easy or profuse bleeding.

Ozone therapy should not be given in cases of acute alcohol intoxication. It should also be avoided if you have a transplanted organ or any sort of prosthesis or metal or silicone implant. Do not undertake the treatments if you are pregnant, have recently had a heart attack, or suffer from hyperthyroidism. And avoid them if you are sensitive to ozone.

Hydrogen peroxide is officially contraindicated for internal use. Never drink it or take it rectally; it can cause nausea and vomiting, and inflame the intestinal tract. If you are allergic or sensitive to this compound, you should avoid external contact as well.

What Side Effects May Occur?

HYPERBARIC OXYGEN

Seizures, a result of the direct effect of oxygen on the brain, are the most serious side effect associated with hyperbaric therapy. The risk is estimated at one in 5,000. Every chamber is equipped with a quick-release mechanism. If a seizure occurs, the oxygen will be immediately released and the seizure will subside.

Minor side effects include popping of the ears similar to that experienced in a descending aircraft. Sinus pain, earache, and headache are other possible side effects. In fact, pain may occur in any body cavity where air can get in but can't get out. For example, dental pain may occur if a filling has trapped air beneath it. In rare cases, pressurized oxygen may rupture an eardrum.

OZONE AND HYDROGEN PEROXIDE

Ozone is highly irritating to the lungs and can be fatal when inhaled directly. When administered by injection, it can cause phlebitis (vein inflammation), poor circulation, chest pain, shortness of breath, fainting, coughing, flushing, heart irregularities, or bubbles in the bloodstream. When given rectally, it can inflame the lower intestinal tract. It is also highly irritating and drying to vaginal membranes.

Hydrogen peroxide, when given by injection, may cause faintness, fatigue, headaches, and chest pain.

How to Choose a Therapist
HYPERBARIC OXYGEN

Hyperbaric oxygen chambers are very expensive, and are usually found only in large hospitals and medical centers. They are often operated by the emergency medicine department, although internists and anesthesiologists are frequently involved with hyperbaric treatment and research.

To get insurance coverage for the therapy, you'll need a prescription from a board-certified physician. The treatments themselves are usually administered by a technician working under a physician's supervision. Technicians are often retired undersea divers and Navy medical personnel with experience in handling gas under pressure. Nurses involved with hyperbaric medicine are known as baromedical nurses. Both nurses and technicians in this field must earn certification.

One good way to determine if your prescribing physician is trained and knowledgeable about hyperbaric medicine is to ask if he's a member of the Undersea and Hyperbaric Medical Society (UHMS). Membership ensures that the physician is practicing according to guidelines for the ethical use of hyperbaric medicine. You can double-check with the society to make sure your physician is a member; the society also provides free information about the specialty.

The UHMS is in the process of developing a certification examination for physicians. Presently, the society offers continuing education courses in hyperbaric medicine through the American Medical Association, and issues credits for completing the training. (In some states, a physician must have completed 60 hours of training to qualify for reimbursement.) The Society approves conditions for which hyperbaric medicine may be recommended. It reviews published data in the field yearly and adds or withdraws approvals based on the latest medical evidence.

OZONE AND HYDROGEN PEROXIDE

These treatments are offered by selected physicians and naturopaths (practitioners who are trained in naturopathic medicine), among other health care providers. The Medical Society for Ozone Therapy, located in Stuttgart, Germany, certifies and trains many practitioners, as well as publishing research on the topic.

When Should Treatment Stop?

Stop hyperbaric oxygen treatments immediately if you experience side effects or fail to see any improvement. Guidelines for treatment duration and frequency are available from UHMS. Hyperbaric treatments are expensive; ethical practice of this treatment option should follow the UHMS guidelines.

If you decide to pursue either hydrogen peroxide or ozone therapy, suspend treatment if you see no improvement or your condition deteriorates. Walk away, too, if the practitioner makes any recommendations that you feel are counterproductive or threatening to your health.

See a Conventional Doctor If . . .

Do not rely solely on these therapies for any life-threatening condition such as cancer or AIDS. The stakes are too high, and the evidence too low, to make their use advisable.

Additionally, because ozone and hydrogen peroxide are unapproved, unregulated forms of therapy, and may be offered by quacks as well as serious practitioners, you need to take the following extra precautions:

- Check with your personal physician before undertaking therapy.
- Make sure the treatments won't interfere with any medications you're taking, or aggravate any other conditions you may have.
- Remember that you have a right to a second opinion. Seek one immediately if you suspect you're receiving a sales pitch.
- Check the practitioner's credentials with nearby hospitals and local professional associations.
- Be wary of any practitioner who tries to sell you supplies.

Resources

ORGANIZATIONS

Medical Society for Ozone Therapy
Klagen Furtestrasse 4
D-7000 Stuttgart 30, Germany

Undersea and Hyperbaric Medical Society
10531 Metropolitan Ave.
Kensington, MD 20895
Phone: 301-942-2980
Web: www.uhms.org

FURTHER READING

Dr. Rosenfield's Guide to Alternative Medicine. Isadore Rosenfield, MD. New York: Random House, 1997.
The Use of Ozone in Medicine, First English Edition.

Siegried Rilling and Renate Viebahn. Heidelberg: Haug Publishers, 1987.

National Council Against Health Fraud. Website at www.ncahf.org

Quackwatch. Website at www.quackwatch.com

Qigong

Consider This Therapy For

The exercises typical of this well-known Chinese discipline can reduce stress and anxiety, while improving overall physical fitness, balance, and flexibility. By alleviating tension, they may also combat insomnia and relieve certain types of headache.

In traditional Chinese medicine, however, qigong (pronounced "chee-gong") is credited with much more. Proponents claim it has cured cancer, heart disease, AIDS, arthritis, and asthma. They also recommend it for migraines, hemorrhoids, constipation, diabetes, high blood pressure, menstrual problems, prostate trouble, impotence, and pain. Some say it even corrects nearsightedness and farsightedness.

Unfortunately, while advocates cite case studies to support these claims, there are no large, scientifically organized clinical trials to back them up. Although qigong can undoubtedly improve fitness and general well-being, there's currently no reason to believe that it will prevent or cure any serious disease.

How the Treatments Are Done

Officially, qigong seeks to stimulate the flow of *qi* (the elemental life force of Chinese medicine) along the invisible channels, or meridians, that are thought to course throughout the body. This can be achieved through internal qigong, the do-it-yourself exercises now familiar in the West, or external qigong, a form of psychic therapy available only from a qigong master.

External qigong is almost impossible to find in the U.S. However, the instruction in the internal variety is now widely available. There are at least 3,000 variations, ranging from simple movements that coordinate breathing and calisthenics to complex exercises aimed at altering such vital bodily functions as heart rate and brain wave frequency.

Internal qigong can be practiced by anyone—healthy or sick, young or old. The exercises, which can be easily adapted to your physical capabilities, can be performed walking, standing, sitting in a wheelchair, or even lying down, if necessary.

You can teach yourself qigong by following instructions in the many training manuals available in bookstores and libraries. Videotapes are also available for those who want to go it alone. However, many experts warn that, even though the exercises seem simple, it's wise to start with professional instruction, either one-on-one, or in a group. Classes are often offered at local YMCAs, community fitness centers, and hospitals.

Wear loose, comfortable clothing and flexible shoes (no sneakers) when you exercise. Do not eat or drink anything, especially alcoholic beverages, within 90 minutes of your qigong sessions. Some practitioners suggest you avoid sexual intercourse for at least one hour before and after exercising; others don't seem to think this is necessary.

It is important to approach qigong with an optimistic attitude, proponents say. It's also important to try to do your best, even if it seems difficult. For example, if you are told to hold your breath, hold it as long as possible. If you are supposed to remain in one position, do it as long as you can. If your arm or leg wants to change positions, let it go naturally. If you find you cannot follow all three aspects of an exercise—visualizing, moving, and breathing—at the same time, concentrate first on visualization.

Qigong exercises can be performed in any order. Repeat each one 6 times when you start, and increase the repetitions when you feel you are ready. Do not rush, and do not expect immediate results.

Your teacher will begin with simple movements. To attain the greatest benefit, you must follow his or her instructions exactly. The opening position prepares your mind and body to "enter a qigong state." The remainder of the exercise (moving and breathing) is supposed to stimulate the flow of *qi*.

You may be asked to stand with your legs apart and breathe from the diaphragm while you move your arms and legs in a specific way. Or you may have to sit and roll objects between your palms, or simply walk slowly. You may also be taught meditation techniques. Here are a few typical exercises:

Child Worships the Buddha (said to strengthen the legs, "lighten" the body, and relieve stress).
1. Stand with legs apart. Open your arms and inhale deeply.
2. Bring your hands together in front of you and raise your left leg.
3. Rest your left leg on your right knee. Breathe out and, at the same time, gently bend your right leg.
4. Hold the position, then return to the starting position and repeat.

Directing vital life energy to internal organs.
1. Rub your hands together.
2. Place your right hand on the lower right edge of your rib cage (the area of the liver) while you visualize your liver receiving *qi*.
3. Place your left hand on the lower left side of your ribs (the area of the spleen and pancreas), while visualizing these organs receiving *qi*.
4. Move your hands in a circle, while breathing deeply and relaxing. Try to feel heat passing through the surface of your skin and penetrating these organs, making them work more efficiently.

5. Hold your hands over the organs and continue feeling the heat.
6. Exhale while visualizing *qi* circulating from the center of your body to your arms and hands and then into other organs.
7. Move your palms to cover your naval and breastbone. As you rub them, visualize the *qi* pouring into your naval, heart, and thymus, improving their functioning.
8. Move your palms down to your lower back and rub the area. Visualize your kidneys and adrenals receiving *qi* and working better, as above.

Breathing to increase energy.
1. Sit (or stand) with eyes closed or slightly open, shoulders relaxed, head centered above shoulders, and hands palm up with fingertips pointing toward each other approximately two inches below your navel.
2. As you slowly breathe in, raise your hands to the lower edge of your breastbone. Take three short puffs of breath to fill your lungs, raising your hands with each puff until they reach the level of your armpits. Hold.
3. Turn your palms face-down. Lower your hands to your navel while exhaling slowly. Exhale three additional puffs to empty your lungs. Hold.
4. As you inhale, visualize the *qi* building up inside your pelvic and abdominal cavities. Continue visualizing as you exhale.

Spontaneous movement (said to produce an immediate sensation of *qi*).
1. Stand with your feet apart or sit in an armless chair.
2. Wiggle your fingers, shake and rock your body.
3. Breathing more deeply, shake your arms, then your head, and finally your shoulders.
4. Relaxing your jaw, sigh or make another sound as you exhale.
5. Exaggerate or prolong the movements, shift your weight from foot to foot, make more sounds, make up your own routine.

The external variety of qigong, as practiced in China, requires none of the foregoing activities. Instead a qigong "master" endowed with plentiful *qi* imparts life force to the patient. To transmit the *qi*, the master may wave his hands above the person's body, touch him, or press down on specific points. The extra *qi* is said to balance the patient's own life force, thus promoting healing.

In China, such masters have their own medical association, and many hospitals use their services for routine treatment. In the early 1980s, Lu Yan Fang, a Beijing scientist, discovered that the hands of the masters emitted low frequency sound waves that were 100 times more powerful than those of normal people, and 1,000 times stronger than the elderly or ill. She then built a machine (the Infratonic QGM) to replicate this sound and found that it seemed to reduce pain.

Today, the Infratonic QGM is used in the Far East, parts of Europe, Mexico, and Argentina. In the U.S., it's available as an FDA-approved "massage device" that's frequently used to treat pain.

Treatment Time: If you are exercising at home between formal classes or private lessons, your sessions should last for approximately 30 minutes. People with certain medical problems may have to exercise for longer periods.

Treatment Frequency: Classes or professional instruction are usually scheduled twice a week. On all other days, exercise both morning and evening on your own.

What the Treatment Hopes to Accomplish

The practice of qigong dates back at least two thousand years. Many ancient cultures felt that a supernatural or physical "energy flow" regulated the functioning of their bodies and of the world around them. In China, manipulation of this flow to improve health was gradually formalized in such medical disciplines as acupuncture, acupressure, and qigong.

The philosophical foundations of qigong stipulate that the vital energy *qi* flows along meridians that link the internal organs with the fingers or toes and more than 100 acupuncture points on the head, spine, and other parts of the body. It's believed that illness results from an imbalance of *qi*—when more accumulates in one place than another. The meditation, visualization, breathing, and movement exercises of qigong seek to restore balance, breaking down blockages in the flow of *qi* and reestablishing a healthy supply to diseased or distressed parts of the body.

Although *qi* itself is undetectable, modern proponents of traditional Chinese medicine maintain that manipulating this force with qigong results in a variety of physical benefits, including reductions in heart rate and blood pressure, dilation of the blood vessels, and enhanced oxygenation of the tissues. The exercises are said to have a beneficial effect on the nerves that regulate the pain response. By increasing the flow of lymphatic fluid, they are thought to improve the efficiency of the immune system. And by improving circulation, they are said to speed elimination of toxic substances from the body, improving general health.

Some adherents claim that qigong moderates the function of the hypothalamus, pituitary, and pineal glands, as well as the fluid surrounding the brain and spinal cord, to decrease pain, increase immunity, and improve mood. Others say that it increases the amount of disease-fighting white blood cells in the blood, promotes the production of enzymes and other substances needed for digestion, and improves the oxygen supply by increasing the lung's capacity to absorb this vital substance.

While such effects could indeed promote better health, critics in the West demand scientific proof that they actually occur. They'd also like to see definitive proof that qigong has actually cured any illness. Although there are many Chinese studies that seem to prove its powers, it has never been subjected to the kind of rigorous tests that Western therapies routinely undergo. (In such trials, a real treatment must outperform a fake, and neither the patients nor the doctors know who receives which.)

Although the actual extent of its powers remains to be seen, even critics of qigong admit that it can enhance fitness and promote healthy relaxation. And, though the reasons remain a mystery, many conventional physicians in this country admit that they have treated patients whose health has improved after they've adopted qigong.

Who Should Avoid This Therapy?

Because qigong may thin the blood and increase circulation, you should forego it during periods when bleeding could become a problem—for instance after a tooth extraction or injury, or when suffering from internal bleeding. The exercises should also be suspended during pregnancy. And it's best to avoid them completely if you have a tendency to dizziness or are suffering a severe mental or emotional disturbance.

What Side Effects May Occur?

The gentle exercises of qigong are unlikely to cause any adverse reactions.

How to Choose a Therapist

You can often find qualified instructors teaching qigong courses in adult education programs, community centers, YMCAs, and hospitals. A local acupuncturist or practitioner of traditional Chinese medicine may also be able to give you a referral.

If none of these resources are able to help you, the following organizations may know of practitioners and classes in your area. (See addresses and telephone numbers in "Resources" below):

American Foundation of Traditional Chinese Medicine
Healing Tao Center
Health Action

When Should Treatment Stop?

Used as a health and fitness regimen, regular qigong exercise can be a lifelong practice.

See a Conventional Doctor If . . .

Because the jury is still out on qigong's curative powers, you should still check with your doctor whenever you develop serious symptoms of any sort.

Resources

ORGANIZATIONS

American Foundation of Traditional Chinese Medicine
505 Beach St.
San Francisco, CA 94133
Phone: 415-776-0502

China Healthways Institute
115 North El Camino Real
San Clemente, CA 92672
Phone: 800-743-5608

Health Action
243 Pebble Beach
Santa Barbara, CA 93117
Phone: 805-682-3230

East-West Academy of the Healing Arts
450 Sutter St., Suite 916
San Francisco, CA 94108
Phone: 415-788-2227

Qigong Institute
561 Berkeley Ave.
Menlo Park, CA 94025
Phone: 650-323-1221

Qigong Universal
2828 Beverly Blvd.
Los Angeles, CA 90057
Phone: 213-487-2672

The Healing Tao Center
P.O. Box 1194
Huntington, NY 11743
Phone: 516-367-2701

World Natural Medicine Foundation
College of Medical Qi Gong
9904 106 St.
Edmonton, AB T5K IC4 Canada
Phone: 403-424-2231

FURTHER READING

Books:
The Complete System of Self-Healing: Internal Exercises. Stephen T. Chang. San Francisco, CA: Tao Publishing, 1986.
Chi Kung, the Ancient Chinese Way to Health. Paul Dong and Aristide H. Esser, MD. New York: Paragon House, 1990.
Encounters with Qi: Exploring Chinese Medicine. David Eisenberg and Thomas Lee Wright. New York: Penguin, 1985.
The Most Profound Medicine. Roger Jahnke. Santa Barbara, CA: Health Action Books, 1990.
Chi Kung: Cultivating Personal Energy. James MacRitchie. Longmead, Shaftesbury, Dorset, UK: Element Books, 1993.
Miracle Healing from China: Qigong. Charles T. McGee and Effie Poy Yew Chow. Coeur d'Alene, ID: Medi Press, 1994.
Qigong for Health: Chinese Traditional Exercise for Cure and Prevention. Masaru Takashashi and Stephen Brown. Tokyo and New York: Japan Publications, 1986.

Magazines:
Qigong Magazine.
Pacific Rim Publishers, Inc.
P.O. Box 31578
San Francisco, CA 94131
Phone: 800-824-2433

QI: The Journal of Traditional Eastern Health & Fitness
P.O. Box 221343
Chantilly, VA 22022
Phone: 800-787-2600

Reconstructive Therapy

Consider This Therapy For

With a series of injections into the joints, reconstructive therapy endeavors to speed healing of torn, damaged, injured, pulled, or weak joints, ligaments, tendons, and cartilage. It is typically given to treat degenerative arthritis, low back pain, bursitis, tennis elbow, or carpal tunnel syndrome.

How the Treatments Are Done

Treatment programs typically begin with a thorough diagnosis of the problem, including an orthopedic, neurological, and—in some instances—osteopathic musculoskeletal exam. The doctor will also order x-rays or an MRI (magnetic resonance image), as well as laboratory tests.

The injections are made directly into the damaged area. They are typically supplemented with amino acid mixtures, B-complex vitamins, and minerals to further stimulate growth of healthy connective tissue. Patients are advised to avoid caffeine, alcohol, and nonsteroidal anti-inflammatory drugs (NSAIDs), such as Advil and Motrin.

Treatment Time: After the initial diagnostic work-up, sessions are usually brief.

Treatment Frequency: Once per week. About 12 to 30 injections are usually needed to bring a joint back to full strength and function; and some severe conditions may require multiple injections during the same visit. You should begin to notice marked improvement after the first six weeks, when new tissue has begun to develop. The ultimate length of treatment depends upon the severity of the problem and how well the body responds. Treatments can continue for a few months to as much as a year.

What Treatment Hopes to Accomplish

Reconstructive therapy relies on natural irritants to mobilize the healing process in a damaged joint. The injections typically contain the local anesthetic lidocaine and an irritant such as sodium morrhuate (a purified derivative of cod liver oil), dextrose, phenol, minerals, or other natural substances.

According to the therapy's proponents, the injected solution prompts blood vessels in the area to dilate and triggers a migration of healing cells known as fibroblasts into the damaged tissue. Once there, the fibroblasts produce collagen, a structural protein needed for the formation of such connective tissues as ligaments, tendons, and cartilage. These regenerated tissues serve to stabilize and cushion the joint, thus enhancing its strength and endurance and alleviating pain.

Although it is the pain of a damaged joint that sparks most patients to seek therapy, practitioners of reconstructive therapy are careful to point out that the treatments are not merely painkillers. Instead, they ease pain by remedying its cause—in this case worn-down cartilage or torn ligaments and tendons. As healthy new tissue grows, the pain diminishes, until finally it disappears altogether.

Although not yet widely used in the United States, reconstructive therapy has been validated in several clinical trials. For example, in a series of studies conducted in the 1980s at the University of Iowa the researchers found that reconstructive treatments increased tendon and ligament size by 35% to 40%; increased strength in those areas by as much as 40%; and more firmly attached the tendons to the bone. A later study at a clinic in California documented moderate to marked improvement in 88% of the chronic low back pain patients who received treatment.

Also known as sclerotherapy, prolotherapy, and proliferative therapy, reconstructive therapy appeals to many people as an alternative to surgery and drug treatments. Advocates boast that it's not only more effective than surgery in many instances, but provides relief at a fraction of the cost. And unlike drugs, they add, the treatment is permanent. Once the injections are finished, no further treatments of any type should be required.

Who Should Avoid This Therapy?
Before beginning treatment, check with both your own physician and the doctor giving the injections to make sure that you're not susceptible to an allergic reaction. Also make certain that any medications you must take won't conflict with the treatments.

What Side Effects May Occur?
When performed correctly, reconstructive therapy carries a low risk of side effects. However, some patients experience an allergic reaction to the injections, often resulting in stiffness, pain, swelling, and redness at the injection site.

Some pain can also be expected after the first two or three injections, due to the development of a controlled microinflammatory condition. Pain is particularly likely if several injections are given in a single session. To provide relief, the doctor will probably recommend Tylenol, Tylenol with Codeine, or ice packs, since nonsteroidal antiinflammatory drugs (NSAIDs) can interfere with the formation of new tissue. The pain typically subsides within a few hours.

Other reactions include nausea and headache, usually ending within a few days after treatment. There is also a minor risk of infection and hemorrhage.

How to Choose a Therapist
Due to the risk of side effects, you should make certain that the physician offering the injections has undergone specialized training in the necessary techniques. Reconstructive therapy is not taught in medical school; but postgraduate education and certification

is offered by both the American Association of Orthopedic Medicine and the American Osteopathic Academy of Sclerotherapy.

Keep in mind, however, that although reconstructive therapy has been practiced for more than 40 years, it is still relatively new to the United States. There are less than 100 physicians who offer it in the U.S. and even fewer who practice it in Canada. To find the nearest practitioner, you may need to turn to the *Alternative Medicine Yellow Pages*, available at your local library. On the Internet, you can find a listing of physicians offering these services by searching under "reconstructive therapy."

These resources can provide you with basic information about the available practitioners. However, you may also want to check with potential therapists regarding their backgrounds, training, qualifications, and success rates. Because there is usually some pain associated with the injections, you should ask about the doctor's protocols for pain management.

When Should Treatment Stop?

Although many patients begin to notice improvement within the first week of treatment, it may take two or three injections to produce noticeable results if swelling is present.

By the sixth injection, you should experience improvement no matter what the situation. If you don't, treatment should be suspended while the doctor attempts to find out what's interfering with therapy. In otherwise healthy individuals, an irritant such as the injections should almost immediately jolt the body's healing mechanisms into action. Failure to respond implies a hidden medical problem capable of defeating the healing mechanism.

See a Conventional Doctor If . . .

Most people turn to reconstructive therapy only after traditional drug treatments and surgery have failed. If the reconstructive approach also meets with failure, you'll need to explore other options—perhaps bodywork or osteopathy—or return to conventional treatment. Certainly, if treatment failure leads to detection of another, unsuspected medical problem, conventional measures may well be required.

Resources

ORGANIZATIONS

American Association of Orthopedic Medicine
90 South Cascade Ave.,
Suite 1230
Colorado Springs, CO 80903
Phone: 719-475-0032

American Osteopathic Academy of Sclerotherapy
107 Maple Ave.
Wilmington, DE 19809
Phone: 302-792-9280

FURTHER READING

Alternative Medicine: The Definitive Guide. The Burton Goldberg Group. Future Medicine Publishing, Inc., 1994.

Pain, Pain Go Away. William J. Faber, DO. Ishi Press International, 1990.

Reflexology

Consider This Therapy For

Is the foot a microcosm of the entire body? Reflexologists say it's true—and press on various "reflex points" along the foot to relieve symptoms elsewhere in the body. Although they don't promise to cure the underlying cause, they do believe that their technique can alleviate a wide variety of stress-related problems, as well as headache (both tension and migraine), premenstrual syndrome, asthma, digestive disorders, skin conditions such as acne and eczema, irritable bowel syndrome, and chronic pain from conditions· such as arthritis and sciatica. Reflexology is also sometimes used for neurological symptoms, such as those seen in multiple sclerosis.

Although a number of small research studies seem to show that reflexology can help with problems such as headache and bladder control, there have been no major clinical trials to verify its theoretical underpinnings. It is recommended, even by its advocates, only as an adjunct to conventional therapy.

How the Treatments Are Done

Unlike massage, which involves a generalized rubbing motion, reflexologists use their hands to apply pressure to specific points of your foot. Typically, you remain fully clothed, sitting with your legs raised or lying on a treatment table. The reflexologist may powder your foot or use lotion to make manipulating it easier.

After gently massaging your foot, the reflexologist will begin applying pressure to the reflex points thought to correspond to your health problems. He will treat first one foot, and then the other; some believe it is more effective to start with the left foot. No instruments are required, but some practitioners use devices such as rubber balls to apply some of the pressure. If you have foot problems, such as severe calluses or corns, the therapist may refer you to a podiatrist for treatment. Although most reflexologists work only with the feet (a few work with the hands), they do not treat foot disorders.

You can learn to do reflexology for yourself, as well, by having your practitioner demonstrate the techniques appropriate for your problem.

Treatment Time: Sessions typically last from 30 to 60 minutes.

Treatment Frequency: Treatments are usually given once a week, at least initially. After the first few weeks, they may be scheduled less frequently.

What Treatment Hopes to Accomplish

You're likely to see a chart in the reflexologist's office showing the parts of the body that correspond to the various zones of the foot. Reflexology teaches that the toes correspond to the head and neck, the ball of the foot to the chest and lungs, the arch to the internal organs, the heel to the sciatic nerve and the pelvic area, and the bone along the curving arch of the foot to the spine. The right side of the body is reflected in the right foot, the left side in the left foot.

The idea that manipulating the feet can improve health is far from new. Ancient pictographs show Egyptians massaging their feet, while old texts and illustrations show that the Chinese, Japanese, and Indian people all worked on their feet to combat illness. However, the current scheme linking various parts of the foot with specific parts of the body got its start in the early 1900s, when Dr. William H. Fitzgerald developed a system he called "zone therapy." In the 1930s, Eunice Ingham, a nurse and physiotherapist who used zone therapy, refined the system, identifying especially sensitive areas she called "reflex points" and creating a map of the body as represented on the feet.

The original zone therapy was used only for pain, but Ingham found that alternating pressure on several points could achieve other therapeutic effects as well. In 1938, she published a book describing her theories. Ingham's nephew, Dwight Byers, continued her work, and is now considered the leading authority in the field.

In its early years, reflexology was thought to work in much the same way as traditional Chinese acupuncture. Practitioners maintained that a life force, or vital energy, flows along channels from the feet to all the organs of the body, and that any blockage in the flow will eventually lead to disease. Stimulation of reflex points in the foot could, they believed, break up blockages in the flow farther along the channel.

Today, many reflexologists have come up with other explanations for the therapy's effect. Some say that manipulation of the feet reduces the amount of lactic acid in the tissues while releasing tiny calcium crystals, accumulated in the nerve endings of the feet, that hold back the free flow of energy to corresponding organs. Others speculate that pressure on the reflex points may trigger the release of endorphins, chemicals in the brain that naturally block pain. Some practitioners ascribe the therapy's benefits to a relaxation response that opens the blood vessels and improves circulation. Others credit a detoxifying effect, suggesting that manipulation dissolves crystals of uric acid that settle in the feet.

While none of these explanations—from the life force to the release of endorphins—has been scientifically verified, reflexology appears to produce satisfactory results for a surprising number of people. It's accepted around the globe, with more than 25,000 practitioners worldwide.

Who Should Avoid This Therapy?

As an adjunct to other forms of treatment, reflexology is generally considered quite safe. However, if you have a foot injury or clots, thrombosis, phlebitis, ulcers, or any other vascular problems in your lower legs, you should discuss reflexology with your doctor first.

Be sure to let the reflexologist know if you have a pacemaker, gallstones, or kidney stones, since he will need to avoid stimulating certain points in the feet. And if you're pregnant, make a point of discussing the treatments with both your obstetrician and the reflexologist, since some evidence suggests that vigorous stimulation of the feet may induce uterine contractions.

What Side Effects May Occur?

There are no known side effects.

How to Choose a Therapist

Reflexology is offered by many types of practitioners, including chiropractors, podiatrists, nurses, and massage therapists. No licensing is required for reflexology itself, although many states require anyone offering massage therapy to obtain a license.

Your best bet is to find a practitioner who has been trained or certified by one of the organizations listed below. They can help you locate a skilled practitioner in your area.

When Should Treatment Stop?

Reflexology treatments may be continued as long as you find them beneficial.

See a Conventional Doctor If . . .

Reflexology is not a substitute for regular medical care. You'll need to see a doctor for a reliable diagnosis of the symptoms for which you're seeking treatment, and for any new symptoms that appear.

Resources

ORGANIZATIONS

American Reflexology Certification Board and Information Service
P.O. Box 620607
Littleton, CO 80162
Phone: 303-933-6921

International Institute of Reflexology
P.O. Box 12642
St. Petersburg, FL 33733
Phone: 813-343-4811

Reflexology Association of America
4012 South Rainbow Blvd.
Las Vegas, NV 89103

FURTHER READING

Better Health with Foot Reflexology. Dwight C. Byers. Ingham Publishing, 1991.

Hand and Foot Reflexology. Kevin and Barbara Kunz. Prentice Hall, 1992.

Feet First: A Guide to Reflexology. Laura Norman. Fireside, 1988.

Reflexology: Art, Science and His-

tory. Christine Issel. New Frontier, 1993.

Reflexology for Good Health: Mirror for the Body. Anna Kaye and Don Matchan. Wilshire Book Company, 1982.

Rolfing

Consider This Therapy For

The vigorous deep-tissue massage known as Rolfing isn't aimed at any specific injury or ailment. Instead, it promises to relieve stress, improve mobility, and boost energy, thus improving your general well-being.

Although not devised for this purpose, it has, however, helped people with chronic back pain, whiplash, and other spinal problems.

How the Treatments Are Done

The deep massage techniques employed in Rolfing seek to loosen and relax the fascia—the membranes that surround the muscles. (Rolfers believe that the fascia toughen and thicken over time, subtly contorting the body and throwing it out of healthy alignment.)

To break up knots in the fascia and "reset" the muscles, Rolfers apply slow, sliding pressure with their knuckles, thumbs, fingers, elbows, and knees. The treatments are not mild and relaxing—indeed, they can cause a degree of pain. However, practitioners view this temporary discomfort as a sign that the treatment is achieving the changes necessary to bring the body back into proper alignment.

Before beginning the treatments, your therapist will take a full medical and personal history, and evaluate your posture and body structure for signs of tension and misalignment. The treatments themselves are performed while you lie or sit on a massage table or floor mat. You'll probably be asked to synchronize your breathing with the therapist's manipulations. You may also be required to move your arms and legs in certain ways.

During each session, the Rolfer will concentrate on a different set of muscles, starting with those nearest the surface and moving on to those deep within the body. To maximize the benefits of treatment, the therapist may also teach you self-help exercises known as "movement integration."

Treatment Time: Sessions usually last 60 to 90 minutes.

Treatment Frequency: The standard Rolfing Structural Integration Program consists of 10 weekly sessions.

What Treatment Hopes to Accomplish

Rolfing is the creation of Ida Rolf, a biochemist and physiologist who established the Rolf Institute for Structural Integration in 1970. She believed that, for optimum health, the body must be in alignment with gravity: Any deviation from the norm requires extra energy for movement and imposes unnecessary strain on the muscles. She contended that, as the muscles work to compensate over the passing years, the fascia surrounding them tend to bunch up and harden, creating even more strain. Ultimately, she said, the cumulative stress can interfere with normal breathing and impair circulation, digestion, and the nervous system.

The treatments she developed do seem to make a difference. Although research is limited, a controlled study conducted by the Department of Kinesiology at UCLA found that people who underwent Rolfing demonstrated a greater range of motion. They were able to move more easily, smoothly, and energetically. Their posture was improved, and they were able to maintain this posture more comfortably—in other words, they could stand in a given position without straining themselves to hold that position.

Researchers at the University of Maryland obtained similar results. They found that Rolfing resulted in greater physical strength, less stress, and enhanced nervous-system response. This study also noted an improvement in subjects who had curvature of the spine. Children with cerebral palsy benefited from Rolfing, as did people with whiplash and chronic back pain.

Who Should Avoid This Therapy?

Don't undertake Rolfing if you have cancer; there is a theoretical possibility that the manipulations could encourage the spread of malignant cells. Rolfing is also ill-advised for people with rheumatoid arthritis and other inflammatory conditions.

What Side Effects May Occur?

While the treatments have no lasting side effects, they sometimes prove painful. They are also said to occasionally release suppressed memories of severe emotional anguish.

How to Choose a Therapist

Authentic Rolfing therapists are certified by the Rolf Institute for Structural Integration, where they must complete seven months of classroom training in the procedure. There are several hundred individuals trained in Rolfing worldwide, and the Institute can give you the names of those nearest you.

When Should Treatment Stop?

The standard regimen is 10 weekly sessions. Be suspicious of suggestions that treatment should be prolonged.

See a Conventional Doctor If . . .

Any new or aggravated symptoms are a signal to check with your regular doctor. Remember that Rolfing is not intended to remedy any serious illness or injury.

Resources

ORGANIZATIONS

Rolf Institute for Structural Integration
205 Canyon Blvd.
Boulder, CO 80302
Phone: 303-499-5903
Web: http://www.rolf.org

FURTHER READING

Rolfing: The Integration of Human Structures. Ida P. Rolf. New York: Harper and Row, 1977.

Sound Therapy

Consider This Therapy For

There's no question that sound has a major impact on all of us. Soft ballads soothe us, anthems stir us, heavy metal sends some of us into frenzies. It's no wonder, then, that doctors have adopted sound and music for a variety of therapeutic uses.

MUSIC THERAPY

Of all the sound therapies in use today, music is the most common. Music therapy can reduce heart rate, blood pressure, pain, and anxiety. In hospitals, it's used to alleviate pain (along with pain medication or anesthesia), improve patients' moods and counteract depression, promote movement during physical rehabilitation, calm or sedate, induce sleep, counteract fear, and reduce muscle tension. In nursing homes, it's used to boost the residents' level of physical, mental, and social functioning.

You're likely to encounter music therapy in a variety of situations. Among its many applications:

- Relieving anxiety before and after surgery.
- Reducing stress in the hospital's intensive care unit.
- Relaxing infants and children.
- Reducing chemotherapy-induced nausea and vomiting.
- Breaking the cycle of pain in people with chronic pain.
- Helping stroke patients and people with Parkinson's disease walk normally.
- Helping some women in labor to forego anesthesia.
- Reducing anxiety during flexible sigmoidoscopy, an uncomfortable, 5- to 10-minute procedure in which the lower colon and rectum are examined for potentially cancerous polyps.
- Reducing stress in healthy persons.

OTHER SOUND THERAPIES

The Tomatis Method. Employing specially modified auditory feedback in a broad range of frequencies, this approach is promoted for use in children with auditory processing problems, dyslexia, learning difficulties, attention deficit disorder, autism, and impaired motor skills. In adults, it has also been used to relieve depression, speed up foreign language training, improve communication skills, and enhance the skills of actors, musicians, and singers.

The Berard Method. This form of treatment uses electronically enhanced music to correct hypersensitive or distorted hearing. It is thought to be helpful for children with dyslexia, autism, attention deficit disorder, pervasive developmental delay, and central auditory processing disorder.

Spectral Activated Music of Optimal Natural Structure (SAMONAS). Another form of electronically tailored music, SAMONAS is intended to train the auditory system to process the full range of sound without distortion, hypersensitivity, or frequency loss. It is said to improve overall neurologic function, and is advocated for use in children with hypersensitive hearing, hearing loss, auditory processing problems, autism, developmental delays, attention deficit disorder, dyslexia, learning disabilities, cerebral palsy, and other disorders. Advocates say that singers, musicians, and individuals who "experience auditory discrimination problems or have difficulty expressing themselves verbally" should also consider this therapy.

Toning. This therapy, in which you're asked to repeat certain vowels is said to bring "new life energy" to "inhibited" or "unbalanced" parts of the body. It is advocated to release stress, improve the ability to listen, improve the speaking voice, and balance the mind and body.

There has been little if any scientific testing of these therapies, and the few available reviews are quite mixed. In addition, leading mainstream critics of alternative therapy warn that the more exotic types of sound therapy are highly susceptible to quackery. The treatments are unlikely to cause harm unless they are used as substitutes for proven therapies. However, they may not be very helpful either.

How the Treatments Are Done
MUSIC THERAPY

Music therapy ranges from listening to music to improvising tunes, writing songs, discussing lyrics, performing compositions, using music and imagery, and learning through music. Because music therapy is used in so many different ways, there is no one typical approach.

Music intended for relaxation should have about 70 to 80 beats per minute, similar to the heart rate. A faster beat may create tension. It should be low in pitch, since a high pitch also fosters tension. Volume should be kept low. High volume can cause pain.

When used to reduce anxiety, music should have a slow, steady rhythm, a low pitch, liberal orchestration, and relaxing melodies. Instrumental selections are considered more effective than vocal music, since patients may focus on words and their meaning rather than relaxing with the music.

OTHER SOUND THERAPIES

The Tomatis Method. Treatments are delivered by a machine called the Electronic Ear. This device is intended to simulate the stages of listening development. Special headphones equipped with a bone-conduction sensor deliver sound through a sophisticated stereo system. The sensor captures vibrations through the bone. Lower frequencies are filtered out, so that only the "proper" sounds are heard.

The Berard Method. The treatments employ a device known as the Ears Education and Retraining System (EERS). The system adjusts all sound frequencies so that they can be heard with the same clarity. The resulting music is "administered" through headphones for half an hour twice a day for 10 days. Treatment can be repeated every 6 months.

SAMONAS. The National Academy for Child Development, a private organization, provides individualized treatment plans for using this therapy at home. Patients listen to 6 or 7 SAMONAS compact discs 5 days a week, 15 to 60 minutes a day, for 4 to 7 months. Patients submit periodic progress reports. The CDs contain classical chamber music and nature sounds that have been spectrally activated, filtered, and modulated by something called an Envelope Curve Modulator.

Toning. This form of therapy requires you to stand with eyes closed and jaw relaxed while you vocalize extended vowel sounds.

What Treatment Hopes to Accomplish

MUSIC THERAPY

This form of therapy has been extensively studied, and has yielded a host of positive results. For instance, stroke patients who listened to music with imbedded metronome pulses for 30 minutes a day over a period of 3 weeks were able to walk with better stride, cadence, and foot placement than patients who did not receive the treatments. Similar improvement was seen in patients with Parkinson's disease. The researchers theorized that muscle activity that is synchronized to auditory rhythm becomes more regular and efficient.

Music therapy has also been used successfully during childbirth in at least one set of clinical trials. The mother and her partner were permitted to choose the type of music to be used during the various stages of labor and after delivery. About half the women who tried the technique did not require anesthesia.

In another study, a single, 30-minute music therapy session produced a significant increase in immune system function in 19 children being treated for cancer. A control group of 17 children who did not receive music therapy showed no significant change.

OTHER SOUND THERAPIES

The Tomatis Method. Developed about 40 years ago by French ear, nose, and throat specialist Alfred A. Tomatis, these treatments aim to repattern a child's hearing range and attention span, thus enhancing learning capacity. Eight small trials conducted in South Africa during the 1980s found that the treatments resulted in improved self-control, self-concept, and interpersonal relations, as well as higher achievement levels. However, a later clinical study found that, a year after therapy stopped, learning disabled children who were not treated with the Tomatis method showed better auditory discrimination than those who received it.

The Berard Method. This form of therapy originated with the French physician Guy Berard. The wide-spectrum music employed in the treatments can improve auditory discrimination in anyone suffering a deficit in this area, according to the Georgiana Institute, the method's primary U.S. proponent. Although the institute claims that nearly two dozen clinical studies have been conducted in the past 5 years, only one report has appeared in the medical press, and its conclusions were negative. The American Speech-Language-Hearing Association, the professional credentialing association for audiologists and speech language pathologists, has called for more testing before rendering judgment.

SAMONAS. Developed in Germany by physicist Ingo Steinbach, this system is said to train the auditory system to process sound without distortion, hypersensitivity, or frequency loss. Purported benefits include restored hearing, improved speech and language ability, and better concentration.

Toning. Somewhat like the mantras used in some forms of meditation, the vowel sounds uttered in this type of therapy are said to cause the brain waves to synchronize and balance within 3 to 5 minutes. This, in turn, is thought to promote a sense of physical and emotional well-being.

Who Should Avoid This Therapy?

All forms of sound therapy are considered safe for anyone.

What Side Effects May Occur?

Be careful to keep the volume low when using a sound therapy device. Otherwise, you might suffer hearing loss. No other side effects are likely.

How to Choose a Therapist

To find a reputable music therapist, contact the American Music Therapy Association (see "Resources" on page 237). This organization represents some 5,000 registered or certified music therapists who've completed a college program in the discipline. (Certified music therapists must also pass an examination conducted by the Certification Board for Music Therapists.)

Referrals to a practitioner of the Tomatis Method can be obtained from the Sound, Listening and Learning Center in Phoenix (see "Resources" on page 237).

To locate a practitioner of the Berard method contact the Georgiana Institute (see "Resources" below). This organization conducts seminars for audiologists, speech language pathologists, and psychologists interested in the technique.

SAMONAS therapy is available from the National Academy of Child Development (see "Resources" below). The academy creates an individualized program for each patient based on a medical and developmental history, voice analysis testing, and a telephone interview. It also trains "qualified professionals" in the SAMONAS method.

When Should Treatment Stop?

The Berard treatment typically "works or doesn't work" within a 10-day period. SAMONAS therapy generally lasts 7 months. Other treatments vary in length.

See a Conventional Doctor If . . .

Music and sound therapies should be used in addition to, not instead of, conventional medical treatment. Patients should always consult a conventional doctor.

Resources

ORGANIZATIONS

American Music Therapy Association, Inc.
8455 Colesville Rd., Suite 1000
Silver Spring, MD 20901
Phone: 301-589-3300
Fax: 301-589-5175
E-mail: info@musictherapy.org
Web: http://www.namt.com

American Speech-Language-Hearing Association
10801 Rockville Pike
Rockville, MD 20852
Phone: 800-638-8255
301-897-5700 (Voice)
301-897-0157 (TTY)
Fax: 301-571-0457
Web: http://www.asha.org

Georgiana Institute, Inc.
P.O. Box 10
Roxbury, CT 06783
Phone: 860-355-1545
Fax: 860-355-2443

National Academy for Child Development, Inc.
P.O. Box 380
Huntsville, UT 84317
Phone: 801-621-8606
Fax: 801-621-8389
E-mail: nacdinfo@nacd.org
Web: http://www.nacd.org/samonas.html

Sound, Listening and Learning Center
2701 East Camelback, Suite 205
Phoenix, AZ 85016
Phone: 602-381-0086

FURTHER READING

The Alternative Medicine Handbook. Barrie R. Cassileth, PhD. W.W. Norton & Company, 1998.

Tai Chi

Consider This Therapy For

More of a fitness regimen than a "therapy," tai chi is gaining popularity in the United States as an aid to good health, especially for older adults. This slow, graceful Chinese exercise program pays dividends in increased strength and muscle tone, enhanced range of motion and flexibility, and improved balance and coordination. In clinical trials, it has also shown an unquestionable ability to reduce blood pressure and heart rate.

Many who practice tai chi find that it also offers a variety of "quality of life" benefits such as improved concentration, an increased sense of well-being, decreased feelings of stress, more energy, improved posture, and better circulation. Derived from the martial arts, this low-intensity, low-impact form of exercise is especially well suited for those recovering from an injury; and because it's a weight-bearing exercise, it's also helpful for preventing the brittle-bone disease, osteoporosis.

How the Treatments Are Done

Tai chi exercises encompass a set of "forms." With names like "Grasping the Bird's Tail" and "Wave Hands Like Clouds," each form consists of a series of positions strung together into one continuous movement, including a set beginning and end. A single form may include up to 100 positions and may take as long as 20 minutes to complete. The forms can be performed anywhere at any time, but for maximum health benefits, tai chi experts recommend setting aside the same time every day. In China, tai chi is often performed in large groups as an early morning exercise.

To learn the forms, you'll need to attend classes with a tai chi instructor, typically someone who has mastered the Chinese martial arts. No special equipment is necessary, although comfortable loose-fitting clothing and flat shoes or socks are recommended. Some programs encourage participants to wear loose-fitting uniforms similar to those used in other types of martial arts programs.

In each weekly session, you'll be drilled in the positions that make up the various forms. You may find it hard to remember all the movements at first, but like ice skating and bike riding, they become easier with practice. The object is to achieve coordinated, fluid, whole-body movement, even though you may only move one part at a time.

You'll begin by assuming the basic tai chi position: standing with your feet parallel and shoulder-width apart, your knees bent slightly, your head slightly lifted, and your spine straight. Your shoulders should be somewhat rounded and your arms should hang loosely at your sides as you prepare to move into a position.

As you go through each sequence, your knees should remain slightly bent, with all movement originating from the waist. This area of the body located just below the navel is known as your "tantien." In Chinese philosophy, it's considered the center of the body's "chi" or vital energy. By focusing on this center as you practice the deep breathing and slow movements of tai chi, you can expect to experience a heightened awareness of your entire body.

In Bill Moyers' book *Healing and the Mind*, grand master Ma Yueh Liang describes five principles of successful practice:

First: Calm down. Think of tai chi only.
Second: Eliminate any exertion.
Third: Be consistent in movement and speed.
Fourth: Practice truly and precisely. Study the movements you make.
Fifth: Persevere. Practice for the same amount of time at the same hour each day.

Because you'll be practicing the same movements over and over again, tai chi may seem boring at first. However, for experienced tai chi practitioners, the forms become challenging. Some masters observe that while some people are quick to learn the basic movements of a form, their completed mastery can take a lifetime to achieve. To get the most from tai chi, say the experts, you must endeavor to be introspective, recognizing the stress and tension in your body, and working to release it.

Most people who practice tai chi say they feel they've had a "workout" after an hour-long session, even though they may have never raised a sweat. However, you're unlikely to feel the same type of fatigue you might expect from such exercises as jogging. Instead, you'll probably feel a sense of sustained energy and tension relief. Some practitioners claim that the flowing nature of tai chi so enhances the circulation that they feel warm and invigorated for the rest of the day.

Treatment Time: Classes take 60 minutes. An average tai chi form can be performed in 7 to 10 minutes, once it is mastered.
Treatment Frequency: Tai chi may be performed every day or periodically throughout the week. Daily practice is recommended.

What Treatment Hopes to Accomplish

Like other forms of traditional Chinese medicine such as qigong, tai chi is founded on a belief in *chi* (also spelled *qi*), a vital force thought to flow through the body along certain channels, or "meridians." It also reflects an attempt to harmonize the two opposing forces of yin and yang, universal principles that incorporate such polar opposites as male and female, light and dark, active and passive. All tai chi movements, for example, are pairs of opposites such as left and right or thrust and yield.

Practitioners of traditional Chinese medicine believe that tai chi improves health by breaking up blockages in the flow of chi, thus reestablishing balance in the body's supply of vital force. Western advocates of the discipline point out a number of less esoteric physical benefits. Especially for older adults, who face a decline in muscle strength, flexibility, and range of motion, tai chi offers all of the following:

- Its slow, deep breathing increases relaxation and concentration.
- Some of the basic movements—putting full weight on the lower leg, alternating from one leg to another, stepping backward and forward and from side to side—help to strengthen muscle and bone, while improving balance and thus preventing falls. (Nearly 30 percent of those over 65 sustain at least one fall. About half of these falls result in serious injuries, mostly fractures of the hip or wrist.)
- Moving the head, eyes, and body together helps to recalibrate the inner ear—the body's balance center.
- Natural extension of the body during tai chi helps encourage correct posture.
- Tai chi's low-intensity movements have an aerobic affect on the heart and vascular system.
- Focused attention on movements encourages mental alertness, while relaxing body and mind.

Researchers still aren't sure exactly which of these effects is responsible for tai chi's documented ability to reduce heart rate and blood pressure, but studies indicate that it's clearly more effective than ordinary aerobic exercise. One study also found that, among older individuals, mastering tai chi can reduce the risk of falling by nearly 50 percent.

Who Should Avoid This Therapy?

Tai chi is a safe and effective method of exercise and relaxation for most everyone, young or old, athletic or not. Although the exercises are generally performed while standing, and there is a lot of emphasis on shifting weight from one leg to another, the movements can be adapted to permit participation even by those using wheelchairs or walkers. The forms are flexible enough to allow each person to perform to his "personal best." An instructor may encourage a young athlete to flex deeply in the knees, for example, while suggesting that an elderly person perform only a partial equivalent of the movement.

What Side Effects May Occur?

There are no known side effects of tai chi.

How to Choose a Therapist

While many books and videos are available about tai chi, most advocates recommend taking a class with an experienced teacher who can help ensure that your movements and posture are correct.

Many tai chi classes are offered at community centers or health clubs. Instructors in these venues are typically experienced enough in the exercises to be able to teach them successfully. However, for training at a more advanced level, you'll need to seek out one of the tai chi masters who generally teach at a specialized school of tai chi. These individuals have practiced the exercises for many years, and must typically receive authorization from their own tai chi master before they begin to teach.

There is no national certifying organization for tai chi instructors, although even instructors at community centers are expected to adhere to a professional set of standards and ethics. When choosing an instructor, you'll therefore need to draw your own conclusions. Make your decision according to the following guidelines:

- Choose an environment that appears clean and safe, and one in which you feel you can learn.
- Ask how long the facility has been operating.
- Make sure the program and format meets your scheduling needs.
- Observe a class before joining or paying for it; watch and listen to the instructor:
  — Does he communicate clearly?
  — Does he embody the qualities you wish to learn and emulate?
  — Is he mindful of his students' individual abilities?
  — Does the class "feel good" to you?

- Ask about the instructor's credentials. Ideally, he should be experienced in all forms of tai chi, from the beginner's level to the advanced martial art form.

When Should Treatment Stop?

The health benefits of tai chi are associated with the exercise itself and won't persist if the practice is stopped. Tai chi is therefore best regarded as a lifelong preventive strategy to improve and maintain health while promoting relaxation and a calm outlook.

However, if for any reason the movements are painful or trigger an old injury, stop exercising and consult your doctor. You may also want to discuss the problem with your instructor to see if the exercise can be modified.

See a Conventional Doctor If . . .

Although tai chi promises to strengthen the heart and reduce high blood pressure, it is not a substitute for a doctor's care. When starting tai chi, you should not, for instance, discard your blood pressure medication until your doctor thinks it's safe to do so. In some cases, medication will still be needed, though perhaps at a reduced dosage.

If you are out of shape or have significant health problems, you should check with your doctor before starting the exercises. Be quick to check with your doctor, too, if symptoms of stress, depression, or pain continue to trouble you, or begin to get worse.

If you are using tai chi strictly as a relaxation exercise, you'll still need to see a doctor if you develop any physical problems such as sprains or strains. Although such injuries are highly unlikely, it is always possible that you may trigger an old injury or overexert your body.

Resources

ORGANIZATIONS

American Association of Acupuncture and Oriental Medicine
433 Front St.
Catasaugua, PA 18032
Phone: 610-226-1433

American Foundation of Traditional Chinese Medicine
505 Beach St.
San Francisco, CA 94133
Phone: 415-776-0502

East-West Academy of the Healing Arts
450 Sutter St., Suite 916
San Francisco, CA 94108
Phone: 415-788-2227

FURTHER READING

The Complete Tai Chi: The Definitive Guide to Physical and Emotional Self-Improvement. Master Alfred Huang. Charles E. Tuttle Co., 1993.

T'ai Chi for Beginners. Claire Hooten. The Berkeley Publishing Group, 1996.

Therapeutic Touch

Consider This Therapy For

A modern variation of the "laying on of hands," therapeutic touch is one of the most controversial forms of alternative therapy. Practitioners say that it heals by correcting imbalances in the energy field that emanates from the body, while mainstream critics respond that there's no evidence that such a field exists, or that it would have anything to do with health if it did.

In any event, proponents say therapeutic touch can heal wounds, relieve tension headaches, and reduce stress. According to Nurse Healers, the therapy's leading advocacy group, it also reduces pain and anxiety, promotes relaxation, and facilitates "the body's natural restorative processes."

Therapeutic touch is usually employed as a supplement to, rather than a replacement for, standard medical therapies. For example, it is sometimes used to relieve discomfort between scheduled doses of pain medication for hospitalized patients. It is also employed by hospice nurses to relieve pain in terminally ill patients, and to help the family accept the impending death of their loved one.

How the Treatments Are Done

Despite its name, therapeutic touch rarely involves physical contact between practitioner and patient. Instead, the therapist will move his or her hands just above your body.

You'll be asked to sit or lie

down before the procedure begins. No disrobing is necessary. The session is conducted in four steps:

Centering. The practitioner begins by "centering" himself—attaining a quiet, meditative state in which he's focused on and attuned to the patient's needs. Experienced practitioners can usually complete this process within a few minutes.

Assessment. The practitioner will then move his hands from head to foot along your body, holding them 2 to 4 inches away. This is done to assess the condition of the energy field that is thought to surround the body. Clues to the status of the field include feelings in the palms of the hands and "other intuitive or sensory cues" that signal areas of "congestion" or "blockage."

Treatment. Once he discovers a "blocked" area, the practitioner will move his hands in a flowing motion from the top of the location down and away from your body. This action is repeated until the practitioner no longer feels the blockage, or until you feel relief.

Evaluation. After you've had a chance to rest, the practitioner will ask you about your response to therapy and reassess your "energy field" to make sure that no blockages remain evident.

Some practitioners add another step to the treatment. Called energy transfer, it calls for the therapist to place one hand on your back, in the kidney area, and hold the other hand 2 to 3 inches from the corresponding location on your abdomen. He then visualizes energy passing from the hand on your back to the one held above you.

Treatment Time: Most sessions take 10 to 20 minutes; few exceed 30 minutes. Treatment stops when the practitioner no longer senses problems in the energy field, or feels you've had enough.

Treatment Frequency: The number of treatments needed varies according to the problem and the patient. A headache in an otherwise healthy person may require only one session; a person with a chronic illness may require multiple sessions. For frail, sick, and very young or very old patients, proponents recommend keeping the sessions short and conducting them more frequently.

What Treatment Hopes to Accomplish

Therapeutic touch was developed in the early 1970s by Dolores Krieger, PhD, RN, a professor of nursing at New York University, and Dora Kunz, a "natural healer." Krieger and Kunz first taught the technique to Krieger's graduate nursing students, and it remains primarily a nursing intervention today. It has been taught at more than 100 colleges and universities since the 1970s, and is currently offered in about 70 health care facilities nationwide.

All told, Krieger says she has taught the technique to more than 43,000 health care professionals and several thousand laypersons.

Controversy over therapeutic touch focuses on the "energy field" that its practitioners seek to balance. Krieger claims that the field can be sensed through "hand chakras," centers of consciousness posited in Indian mystical writings. As proof of the field's existence, other proponents cite images of an energy aura taken with Kirlian photography, a technique in which the hands are placed on film and a low-amp electrical current produces the picture.

Critics dismiss the entire energy theory as mystical, and ascribe any benefits of the technique to a positive psychological response to the care and attention provided by the practitioner. They argue that Kirlian images of the energy field are nothing more than the result of increased pressure or moisture. They also cite a recent study published in the *Journal of the American Medical Association* in which 21 self-described practitioners of therapeutic touch failed to detect energy from the nearby hand of an investigator when their view of the hand was blocked.

Advocates of therapeutic touch charge that the study was seriously flawed. They point out that the participants' credentials were never checked, that the number of participants was inadequate, and that one of the authors (a coordinator of the National Council Against Health Fraud's Task Force on Questionable Nursing Practices) was hopelessly biased. They add that therapeutic touch is not simply a mechanical manipulation of energy fields, but an act of compassion that requires personal interaction between patient and therapist.

Some proponents of therapeutic touch now speculate that mechanisms other than an energy field may be at work. In fact, Krieger herself states that the procedure conveys a "sense of deep peace that presages a rapid (2-to-4 minute) relaxation response," thus laying the groundwork for positive changes in the patient's immune system.

Whatever the explanation may be, a number of studies have detected genuine improvements following administration of therapeutic touch. In one trial, in which the patients didn't know whether or not they were being given the therapy, skin wounds healed significantly faster in those who received it. Another trial found that therapeutic touch effectively reduced headache pain, and a third investigation found that it reduced the time needed to calm hospitalized infants and toddlers after stressful experiences such as examinations and surgery.

Nevertheless, other studies have failed to show conclusive results. In one trial for postoperative pain, therapeutic touch reduced discomfort by only 13 percent, versus a 42 percent reduction afforded by standard pain medication. Researchers were forced to conclude that although the technique might reduce the need for drugs, it cannot be used to replace them. Likewise, the editor-in-chief of the *Journal of the American Medical Association* has admonished patients to "refuse to pay for this procedure until or unless additional honest experimentation demonstrates an actual effect."

Who Should Avoid This Therapy?

There are no medical conditions that preclude treatment with therapeutic touch. However, some people seem more susceptible to it than others. Among those best suited to it are pregnant women, newborns, children, older adults, and people with psychiatric disorders. Mainstream critics of the procedure warn everyone to avoid it, saying that there's no reason to believe that it will have any effect.

What Side Effects May Occur?

There have been reports of nausea and dizziness following the procedure, although it's unlikely that therapeutic touch was the cause. In addition, one expert warns that directing too much energy into a person's energy field can cause "discomfort and irritability."

How to Choose a Therapist

Look for a practitioner who has completed a workshop in therapeutic touch and has used the technique consistently for at least 1 year under the guidance of a mentor. Some practitioners hold continuing education credits granted by a state nursing association. Others have taken an invitational workshop offered by the procedure's developers, Krieger and Kunz. There is no formal certification program.

Nurse Healers, the procedure's leading advocacy group, offers a list of its roughly 1,500 members, but recommends checking the individual practitioner's background. If you are offered therapeutic touch at a health care facility, you might want to ask whether the organization follows Nurse Healers' policies and procedures.

When Should Treatment Stop?

Treatments can continue as long as your symptoms persist. However, if the therapy provides no relief, don't hesitate to seek an alternative.

See a Conventional Doctor If . . .

Since even proponents agree that therapeutic touch is not a replacement for conventional medical care, you should continue to see your doctor as necessary.

Resources

ORGANIZATIONS

Nurse Healers Professional Associates, Inc.
1211 Locust St.
Philadelphia, PA 19107
Phone: 215-545-8079
Fax: 215-545-8107
E-mail: nhpa@nursecominc.com
Web: http://www.therapeutic-touch.org

National Council Against Health Fraud
P.O. Box 1276
Loma Linda, CA 92354
Web: http://www.ncahf.org

FURTHER READING

The Therapeutic Touch. D. Krieger. Englewood Cliffs, NJ: Prentice-Hall, Inc., 1979.

Living the Therapeutic Touch: Healing as a Lifestyle. D. Krieger. New York: Dodd Mead & Company, 1987.

Reader's Guide to Alternative Health Methods. J. Zwicky, et al. Chicago, IL: American Medical Association, 1993.

Trager Integration

Consider This Therapy For

This light, gentle form of massage seeks to release deeply ingrained tensions, promoting a sense of relaxation and freedom. It appears to be especially helpful for people with chronic neuromuscular pain, including back problems and sciatica, and it has also been advocated for stress-related conditions, high blood pressure, strokes, migraine, and asthma. Proponents say that it can benefit patients with polio, multiple sclerosis, and muscular dystrophy as well.

How the Treatments Are Done

Also known as Tragerwork or the Trager Approach, this form of therapy has two components: bodywork conducted by the therapist and a set of movement exercises to be pursued between treatments.

Trager bodywork sessions are quite different from a run-of-the-mill massage. There's no oil, and no rubbing. Instead, the therapist enters a meditative state called "hook up," the better to sense areas of tension in the body. By rhythmically stretching tense muscles and rocking stiff joints, the therapist attempts to induce a feeling of lightness and freedom, inviting the patient to completely surrender muscular control. When he encounters an especially tense area, he relaxes his pressure instead of bearing down as he would during Rolfing or Hellerwork. For many, the net effect is an invigorating feeling of light, supple release.

The follow-up exercises, dubbed "mentastics" (for mental gymnastics), are designed to promote effortless motion. They range from simply shaking or swinging the hands or the feet to executing free, dance-like movements that enhance relaxation.

Treatment Time: A typical session lasts 60 to 90 minutes.

Treatment Frequency: There is no fixed schedule.

What Treatment Hopes to Accomplish

Like many other forms of bodywork, Trager Integration seeks to release the deeply rooted physical tensions that can build up over years of mental and physical trauma. It is one of the many outgrowths of the holistic medicine craze that swept California in the 1970s. Developed by Milton Trager, a physical therapist turned physician, it combines principles of physical therapy with precepts borrowed from Transcendental Meditation.

Trager therapists believe that the deeply relaxed feelings the technique induces can resonate through the nervous system, ultimately benefiting tissues and organs deep within the body. At least one clinical study has confirmed that the technique can indeed relieve pain. Another suggests possible benefits for people with lung problems. However, any other specific therapeutic effects have yet to be verified.

Who Should Avoid This Therapy?

The gentle massage and exercise of Trager Integration is unlikely to be harmful to anyone. Nevertheless, be sure to alert the practitioner if you have the brittle-bone disease osteoporosis or a tendency to clotting in the circulatory system (thrombosis).

What Side Effects May Occur?

No side effects are known.

How to Choose a Therapist

For authentic Tragerwork, you'll need a therapist trained and certified by the Trager Institute. This organization maintains a directory of its graduates, and can be contacted at the address below (see "Resources").

Currently there are nearly 1,000 certified therapists in practice worldwide.

When Should Treatment Stop?

Duration of treatment depends on the severity of your problem. Some athletes use regular sessions as a means of increasing their stamina.

See a Conventional Doctor If . . .

Remember that Trager therapists are typically not physicians. You should see a doctor for diagnosis of your problem before beginning therapy—and whenever your symptoms get worse.

Resources

ORGANIZATIONS

Trager Institute
33 Millwood
Mill Valley, CA 94941
Phone: 415-388-2688

FURTHER READING

Trager Mentastics: Movement as a Way to Agelessness. Milton Trager and Cathy Guadagno. Station Hill Press, 1995.

Vegetarianism

Consider This Therapy For

A meatless diet won't *cure* any ailments, but it may protect you from some. In particular, a typical vegetarian diet—low in fat, cholesterol, and calories—can reduce your blood cholesterol level, thus helping to lower your risk of heart disease. The vegetarian approach can also help you shed extra pounds—and keep them off. Vegetarians are less likely to develop diabetes and high blood pressure. And many of the compounds that scientists are isolating from vegetables may even protect against certain forms of cancer.

How the Treatments Are Done

Vegetarianism is, at bottom, a misnomer. Even the strictest vegetarians typically eat more than vegetables *per se*, indulging in fruits, nuts, beans, and just about anything else not derived from animals. Other vegetarians add dairy products and eggs. In practice, vegetarians fall into the following major categories:

- *Vegans,* the most dedicated vegetarians, eat exclusively plant products, and no meat, dairy, or fish products at all.
- *Lactovegetarians* also eat dairy products, but not eggs, meat, or fish.
- *Ovolactovegetarians* include both eggs and dairy products in the menu, but no meat or fish.

There are a number of individual variations on these themes. Some vegetarians (dubbed "fruitarians") eat only raw fruits, sometimes supplemented with vegetables and nuts. Others may be part-time vegetarians; or may eat no red meat, but include white meat such as chicken or fish in their diet. Some vegetarian diets restrict products such as alcohol, sugar, caffeine, or processed foods.

What Treatment Hopes to Accomplish

Although the benefits of a low-fat, high-fiber, vitamin-rich diet are not restricted to vegetarianism, the type of menu that vegetarians favor can promote health in a number of ways, reducing the risk of heart disease, liver and gallbladder disease, cataracts, and stroke. Many studies have found a link between reduced cancer rates and diets rich in fruits, vegetables, and grains; the American Cancer Society recommends five or more servings of fruits and vegetables and six or more servings of grain (bread, cereal, rice, pasta) daily.

As scientists delve into the specific components of the foods we eat, they are finding an array of so-called "phytochemicals" that protect good health and fend off disease. Plant products are especially rich in these compounds, and though you don't have to be a vegetarian to gain their benefits, it's clear that an all-vegetable diet is likely to provide them in greater than usual quantities. In addition to vitamins, minerals, and fiber, other beneficial compounds that you can gain from liberal helpings of vegetables include the following:

Sulforaphane, found in broccoli, has a role in neutralizing enzymes that may trigger cancer.
Glucobrassicin occurs naturally in all cruciferous vegetables (cabbage, broccoli, cauliflower, Brussels sprouts, Swiss chard, bok choy, and kale). This sub-

stance seems to help the body form indoles, a class of compounds that may have a role in preventing breast and other cancers.

Beta-carotene, found in orange or dark green vegetables, is an antioxidant that has been shown to reduce the risk of cancer and hardening of the arteries. Liberal intake of this substance may also discourage development of cataracts.

Other carotenoids found in dark green, leafy vegetables have been associated with a decreased risk of age-related macular degeneration, the most common cause of blindness in older adults.

Potassium has been linked to reduced risk of high blood pressure and stroke. Bananas, spinach, and potatoes are excellent sources of potassium. Beans, grapefruit, peppers, squash, grapes, and apples also contain significant supplies.

Phytate and protease inhibitors, both thought to have a role in cancer prevention, are found in beans. Beans are also an excellent source of fiber, and a high-fiber diet is associated with low cholesterol levels and a reduced risk of colon cancer.

Allicin is one of several ingredients in garlic and onions that seems to protect against heart disease by lowering cholesterol and blood pressure and discouraging blood clots. Allicin may also help prevent cancer.

Isoflavones, one of a set of compounds called flavonoids, has cancer-inhibiting properties.

Among the foods rich in isoflavones are green tea and soybean products such as tofu and tempeh.

Just as a vegetarian diet can promote health with the foods it includes, it may also prove beneficial through what it omits. An increasing body of evidence implicates excessive intake of meat and dairy products in a variety of ailments. One six-year study of women found that those who ate red meat every day had twice the risk of developing breast cancer as those who ate none. Similar results appeared in studies of heart disease and lung, colon, and prostate cancer. High-fat dairy products have long been regarded as leading contributors to heart disease, and to cancer as well. The high protein content in a meat-rich diet can aggravate kidney disease. Even rheumatoid arthritis is sometimes alleviated by a vegetarian diet.

All the health benefits of a diet high in fiber and low in fat are quite independent of any moral considerations. Ethical vegetarians reject meat because they believe no animal lives should be taken to satisfy human appetites. Certain religions—Hinduism in particular—also discourage consumption of meat. But for many people, religious or ethical concern for animals has no bearing on their choice of vegetarianism. For them, it's simply a matter of health.

Who Should Avoid This Therapy?

The American Dietetic Association has declared that vegetarian diets can be healthy and nutritionally complete when properly planned. However, it's unwise to be too restrictive with children under 2 years of age; they need liberal amounts of the essential fatty acids found primarily in meat. Likewise, during pregnancy and breastfeeding, it's advisable to consult a dietitian to make sure your vegetarian diet is as complete and balanced as possible.

What Side Effects May Occur?

With its limited selection of foods, vegetarianism poses a risk of several nutritional deficiencies. The greatest threat is a lack of vitamin B_{12}, which occurs naturally only in animal products. Inadequate supplies can cause anemia and raise homocysteine levels, increasing your risk of heart disease. Also at risk, especially in dark northern climates, is your supply of vitamin D, which comes from sunlight and fortified milk. The vitamin D-deficiency disease rickets has been found in young children on a vegetarian diet. To prevent such problems, most experts recommend that strict vegetarians supplement their diet with a daily multivitamin pill.

Under ordinary circumstances, a varied vegetarian diet supplies sufficient iron. However, if you're pregnant, have heavy menstrual bleeding, or suffer from iron deficiency, you may need to take a supplement. A strict vegetarian diet can also leave you short of the calcium needed to prevent the brittle-bone disease osteoporosis. Although some studies have found *increased* bone density in vegetarians, this finding may have been due to exercise rather than diet. If you've passed menopause and need liberal amounts of calcium, you may want to consider taking supplements of this mineral as well.

To maintain fully balanced nutrition, vegetarians must look for alternate sources of the nutrients that others get from meat, poultry, fish, eggs, and dairy products. While it was once thought that a vegetarian diet could not supply sufficient protein, it is now known that a combination of vegetable products can provide all the building blocks of protein that we need, including the eight essential amino acids the body can't manufacture on its own. To assure an adequate supply, however, you need liberal amounts of vegetable protein from sources such as beans and soy products. It's also important to get generous amounts of starches from whole grains, fruits, and vegetables; oils low in saturated fats; and nuts and seeds.

How to Choose a Therapist

Many people fashion vegetarian diets on their own, without professional consultation; and holistic health centers and health food stores can provide you with a wealth of information. However, if you have special requirements or a chronic medical condition, it's advisable to double-check your program with a registered dietitian or nutritionist.

When Should Treatment Stop?
Reconsider your diet at the first sign of vitamin deficiency (for symptoms, see the "Guide to Nutritional Therapy" in this book).

See a Conventional Doctor If . . .
See a doctor about the signs and symptoms of any significant health problem. While vegetarianism may promote good health, it doesn't guarantee it.

Resources
ORGANIZATIONS

American Vegan Society
P.O. Box H
Malaga, NJ 08328
Phone: 609-694-2887

Association of Vegetarian Dietitians & Nutrition Educators
3674 Cronk Rd.
Montour Falls, NY 14865
Phone: 607-535-6089

International and American Associations of Clinical Nutritionists
5200 Keller Springs Rd., Suite 102
Dallas, TX 75248
Phone: 972-250-2829

The North American Vegetarian Society
P.O. Box 72
Dolgeville, NY 13329
Phone: 518-568-7970

Vegan Action
P.O. Box 4353
Berkeley, CA 94704
Phone: 510-654-6297

Vegetarian Education Network
P.O. Box 3347
West Chester, PA 19381
Phone: 717-529-8638.

Vegetarian Resource Center
P.O. Box 38-1068
Cambridge, MA 02238
Phone: 617-625-3790

The Vegetarian Resource Group
P.O. Box 1463
Baltimore, MD 21203
Phone: 410-366-8343

FURTHER READING

The Ultimate Vegetarian Cookbook. Roz Denny. Smithmark Publishers, 1995.
Vegetarian Planet: 350 Big-Flavor Recipes for Out-of-This-World Food Every Day. Didi Emmons. Harvard Common Press, 1997.
Low-Fat & Luscious Vegetarian. Kristi Fuller, editor. Better Homes & Gardens Books, 1997.
1,000 Vegetarian Recipes. Carol Gelles. Macmillan, 1996.
The Health Promoting Cookbook: Simple, Guilt-Free, Vegetarian Recipes. Alan Goldhamer. Book Publishing Co., 1997.
The Moosewood Cookbook. Mollie Katzen. Ten Speed Press, 1992.
A Teen's Guide to Going Vegetarian. Judy Krizmanic. Puffin Books, 1994.

Diet for a Small Planet: 20th Anniversary Edition. Frances Moore Lappé. Ballantine Books, 1991.

Simple Vegetarian Pleasures. Jeanne Lemlin. HarperCollins Publishers, 1998.

The Garden of Earthly Delights Cookbook: Gourmet Vegetarian Cooking. Shea MacKenzie. Avery Publishing Group, 1995.

Becoming Vegetarian: The Complete Guide to Adopting a Healthy Vegetarian Diet. Vesanto Melina, et al. Book Publishing Co., 1995.

Vegetarian Times Complete Cookbook. Lucy Moll, editor. Macmillan, 1995.

Everyday Cooking With Dr. Dean Ornish: 150 Easy, Low-Fat, High-Flavor Recipes. Dean Ornish. HarperCollins, 1997.

The Essential Vegetarian Cookbook: Your Guide to the Best Foods on Earth. Diana Shaw, CN. Potter Publishers, 1997.

The First Book of Vegetarian Cooking: More Than 300 Recipes Combining Great Taste With Good Nutrition. Dionne Stevens. Prima Publications, 1996.

The New Vegetarian Epicure: Menus for Family and Friends. Anna Thomas. A.A. Knopf, 1996.

The High Road to Health: A Vegetarian Cookbook. Lindsay Wagner and Ariane Spade. Simon & Schuster Books, 1994.

Vegan Handbook: Over 200 Delicious Recipes, Meal Plans, and Vegetarian Resources for All Ages. Debra Wasserman and Reed Mangels, editors. Vegetarian Resource Group, 1996.

Yoga

Consider This Therapy For

The age-old set of exercises known in the West as "yoga" offers a significant variety of proven health benefits. It increases the efficiency of the heart and slows the respiratory rate, improves fitness, lowers blood pressure, promotes relaxation, reduces stress, and allays anxiety. It also serves to improve coordination, posture, flexibility, range of motion, concentration, sleep, and digestion. It can be used as supplementary therapy for conditions as diverse as cancer, diabetes, arthritis, asthma, migraine, and AIDS, and helps to combat addictions such as smoking. It is not, in itself, a cure for any medical ailment. But as part of the well-known Dean Ornish program of diet and exercise, it has contributed to the reversal of heart disease.

How the Treatments Are Done

Yoga exercises are usually conducted in group classes, although private instruction is also available in many areas. You should wear loose, comfortable clothing to the class, and should bring a "sticky" mat with you to prevent slipping during the exercises. No equipment is needed, although advanced students often use a strap to assist in leg stretches. Wall-mounted devices are sometimes available to help you maintain balance during difficult exercises. The exercises are almost always performed in bare feet.

A typical session includes

three disciplines: breathing exercises, body postures, and meditation. You may also be given advice on nutrition and lifestyle. Many proponents feel morning is the best time to practice yoga, but classes are offered throughout the day and evening. It's advisable to avoid eating for 1 hour before class.

Each session usually begins with a set of gentle warm-up exercises. The teacher will then ask you to focus on your breathing, and may take you through several breathing exercises. At the very least, you'll be asked to breathe through your nose, evenly through both nostrils. Then it's on to the yoga postures, a series of poses that typically must be held for periods of a few seconds to several minutes. Unlike the routine in calisthenics or weight training, you will not be asked to repeat postures more than three times, and some will be done only once.

Some of the postures, such as shoulder rolls or neck stretches, will probably be familiar to you, while others may seem extremely complicated or even contorted. Despite the difficulty of such postures, however, contortion for its own sake is never the point. Instead, the goal is to mildly stretch all the muscle groups in the body, while gently squeezing the internal organs. To balance the muscle groups, the postures follow a specific order.

As you assume the various postures, you'll be asked to move gently, without jerking or bouncing. Breathing techniques remain important. You'll need to focus on exhaling during certain movements and inhaling during others. Likewise, as you hold certain postures, you may be instructed to inhale through one nostril and exhale through the other. You'll be allowed to rest after every three or four postures, and at the conclusion of the exercises, there's usually a period of rest or meditation. You should remain comfortable throughout the session, and should leave with both body and mind relaxed.

Treatment Time: Classes usually last 45 minutes to an hour, but experts stress that even short sessions can be beneficial if you make them a regular routine.

Treatment Frequency: Classes may be taken once a week, or more often, as desired. Your teacher will probably ask you to practice new positions at home, and will encourage you to run through at least a portion of the yoga routine each day. Regular practice, even if brief, is recommended for the best results.

What Treatment Hopes to Accomplish

Although the yoga we know today is practiced mainly for its health benefits, it is rooted in Hindu religious principles some 5,000 years old. Derived from the Sanskrit word for "union," the term "yoga" refers to far more than exercise. In fact, it encompasses a variety of disciplines designed to ultimately bring its practitioners closer to God. *Dynana yoga*, for instance, seeks union through meditation, while *jnana yoga* entails the study of scriptures and *karma yoga* calls for selfless service to God and mankind.

The exercises we now call simply "yoga" are actually *hatha yoga*, a discipline intended to prepare the body for the pursuit of union with the divine while raising the practitioner's awareness of creation to a higher, keener state. Through controlled breathing, prescribed postures (called *asanas)*, and meditation, hatha yoga seeks to enhance the *prana*, or life force, that resides in the body and achieve a state of balance and harmony between body and mind. Each of these three disciplines contributes to the search for union in its own unique way:

Breathing. The life force *prana* is believed to enter the body through the breath, and much of hatha yoga is concerned with helping you control your breathing properly. Shallow, hurried breathing is believed to inhibit the life force, and affect mind and body adversely. Deep, slow breathing is encouraged.

Postures. Some yoga postures are intended to stretch and strengthen muscles, others to improve posture and work the skeletal system, while others aim to compress and relax the organs and nerves. The underlying purpose is to perfect the body, making it a worthy host for the soul.

Meditation. Meditation supplements and reinforces the disciplines of hatha yoga, focusing the mind and relaxing the body. Closely linked with focused breathing, it aims to produce a quiet, calm frame of mind. Many people find that it reduces stress and increases energy. The interplay of this and the other two facets of hatha yoga, and the quiet, considered repetition of each, is considered key to achieving yoga's benefits.

Despite its use of physical exercises, yoga is perhaps most closely related to the mind-body family of therapies, which includes meditation and biofeedback. Research shows that, like other mind-body practices, yoga produces measurable physiological changes in the body, including a decrease in the respiratory rate and blood pressure, and an alteration in brain-wave activity reflecting increased relaxation. Yoga has been shown to reduce stress and anxiety, both immediately and over time, and is often recommended to relieve the pain and anxiety of chronic illness. When practiced regularly, it promotes relaxation and enhances the sense of well-being. It also improves physical fitness and circulation, and some advocates say it improves memory. When combined with a low-fat diet and moderate aerobic exercise, it has been found to reverse the build-up of plaque in the coronary arteries—and the more it's practiced, the greater the improvement.

Although yoga's effects are unquestionable, scientists still don't know exactly how it produces them. Some speculate that, like other mind-body therapies, it works largely by relieving stress. Others suggest that it promotes the release of endorphins, the brain's natural painkillers. The Office of Alternative Medicine at the National Institutes of Health has several studies under way to clarify the matter. In the meantime, yoga continues to be practiced by some 6 million people in the United States.

Who Should Avoid This Therapy?

Avoid yoga completely if you've had a recent back injury or surgery. Check with your doctor first if you have arthritis, a slipped disk, heart disease, or high blood pressure. (Although yoga tends to relieve high blood pressure, certain postures must be avoided. Be sure to alert your instructor to the problem if you decide to proceed.)

Although some postures are not recommended during pregnancy, special classes are available for expectant mothers. Some experts also warn against strenuous postures during menstruation, and when you are ill with a cold or infection.

What Side Effects May Occur?

At the outset, you may suffer some stiffness while your body adapts to the postures. When done properly, however, yoga is not stressful or tiring, and any stiffness should be short-lived and minor.

How to Choose a Therapist

Each yoga instructor has his own style, and classes range from mildly taxing to extremely strenuous. To make sure you'll be comfortable with the teacher's approach, ask to observe a class before you sign up. You should select a program that will leave you rested and relaxed, not totally exhausted.

There are no standard certification or licensure requirements for yoga instructors. However, a number of reputable yoga schools do certify their graduates. You can check with the associations listed below for a list of recognized schools. Experts recommend that you look for an instructor who remains an active student himself, and who practices yoga daily.

When Should Treatment Stop?

You may continue yoga as long as it is helpful to you. Many people who find yoga beneficial continue to practice it for life.

See a Conventional Doctor If . . .

Yoga can alleviate a variety of chronic conditions, but it won't cure an acute medical problem. You should continue to see a doctor for regular check-ups and treatment.

Be sure to call the doctor immediately if the exercises cause any new symptoms, such as unusual headaches, muscle cramps, dizziness, or severe pain in your back, legs, or joints.

Resources

ORGANIZATIONS

American Yoga Association
3130 Mayfield Rd., W-301
Cleveland Heights, OH 44118
Phone: 216-371-0078

American Yoga Association
513 South Orange Ave.
Sarasota, FL 34236
Phone: 813-953-5859

International Association of Yoga Therapists
109 Hillside Ave.
Mill Valley, CA 94942
Phone: 415-383-4587

FURTHER READING

The American Yoga Association Beginner's Manual. Alice Christiansen. Fireside Books, 1987.

Back Care Basics: A Doctor's Gentle Yoga Program for Back and Neck Pain Relief. Rodmell Press, 1992.

The Complete Illustrated Book of Yoga. Swami Vishnudevananda. Harmony Books, 1980.

Yoga for Common Ailments. Robin Monro and Nagarantha and H.R. Nagendra. Fireside Books, 1991.

Yoga Journal, a publication of the California Yoga Teachers Association. For information, write to P.O. Box 12008, Berkeley, CA 94712, or phone 510-841-9200.

PART THREE

Guide to
Natural Medicines

Adonis

Latin name: Adonis vernalis
Other names: False Hellebore,
Ox-eye, Pheasant's Eye, Red
Morocco, Rose-a-rubie, Sweet
Vernal

A Remedy For
• Irregular heartbeat
• Weak heart

In Russian folk medicine, Adonis is used for treating water retention, cramps, fever, and menstrual disorders, but its effectiveness for these problems is unproven. Homeopathic uses for Adonis include heart conditions.

What It Is; Why It Works
Medicinal benefits derive from the dried, above-ground portion of the plant, collected during the flowering season. Compounds found in the plant include substances that boost the action of the heart muscle. Animal tests show a tonic effect on veins.

Legend has it that the plant sprang from the blood of the ill-fated Adonis, who was killed during a boar hunt. Found in Russia, Bulgaria, and Hungary, Adonis is one of the brightest and earliest spring plants, opening its anemone-like flowers during March. The plant is considered poisonous and is heavily protected in Germany.

Avoid If . . .
People taking digitalis-based drugs such as digoxin (Lanoxin) should avoid Adonis. It should also be avoided if you have a potassium deficiency.

Special Cautions
None are known.

Possible Drug Interactions
Adonis may enhance the efficacy—and side effects—of certain drugs, including:

Calcium supplements
Diuretics such as HydroDIURIL and Lasix
Laxatives

Quinidine (Quinaglute, Quinidex)
Steroid medications such as hydrocortisone and prednisone

Special Information If You Are Pregnant or Breastfeeding

No harmful effects are known.

How to Prepare

Adonis should be taken only in standardized powder form.

Typical Dosage

Adonis is taken orally. The usual daily dosage is 0.5 grams of standardized powder. The maximum single dose is 1 gram and the maximum daily dosage is 3 grams.

Adonis powder should be stored away from light and tightly sealed.

Overdosage

Although the drug is very potent if taken intravenously, the danger of an oral overdose is small.

Agrimony

Latin name: Agrimonia eupatoria
Other names: Church Steeples, Cocklebur, Liverwort, Philanthropos, Sticklewort

A Remedy For

• Diarrhea
• Skin inflammation
• Sore throat

What It Is; Why It Works

Agrimonia eupatoria, a small yellow flower with a pleasant fragrance and a tangy, bitter taste, is found in most temperate climates. Medicinal benefits are derived from the flowering portion of the plant, which is cut a few inches above the ground and dried.

The name "Agrimonia" comes from "argemone," the word given by the ancient Greeks to plants that healed the eyes. "Eupatoria" comes from the name of King Mithradates Eupator who was skilled in mixing herbal remedies. The Anglo-Saxons used Agrimony to heal wounds, bites, and warts, and the French still use it to treat sprains and bruises.

Avoid If . . .

There are no medical conditions that preclude the use of Agrimony.

Special Cautions

Because Agrimony contains tannins, use of larger than recommended doses could lead to constipation and other digestive problems.

Possible Drug Interactions

No interactions have been reported.

Special Information If You Are Pregnant or Breastfeeding

No harmful effects are known.

How to Prepare

The dried plant is ground into a powder and boiled to produce an extract.

Typical Dosage

Agrimony can be taken orally for diarrhea or inflammation of the mouth or throat or used externally for inflammation of the skin. The usual daily dosage is 3 grams (a little over one-half of a teaspoon) of herb or equivalent preparations.

Overdosage

No information on overdosage is available.

Alfalfa

Latin name: Medicago sativa
Other names: Buffalo Herb,
*   Lucerne, Purple Medic*

A Remedy For

• Appetite loss

Although Alfalfa has also been used as a treatment for diabetes, thyroid conditions, arthritis, and water retention, only its effect on appetite has been clinically verified.

What It Is; Why It Works

In Chinese and Indian medicine, Alfalfa has been used for digestive problems for thousands of years. It has gained popularity in the West recently for its apparent cholesterol-lowering effect. Discovery of an estrogen-like action in animal tests has also led to its use as a remedy for the symptoms of menopause. In addition, the plant is a good source of vitamins A, B_1, B_6, C, E, and K, as well as calcium, potassium, iron, and zinc.

As a grain product, Alfalfa is used primarily as animal fodder. Only the leaves—and sometimes the seeds—are used medicinally.

Avoid If . . .

At customary dosage levels, Alfalfa leaf poses no problems. However, overindulgence in Alfalfa seeds or sprouts could conceivably trigger systemic lupus erythematosus (SLE), a painful arthritis-like condition. Avoid the sprouts if you have SLE.

Special Cautions

Use of Alfalfa leaf requires no special precautions.

Possible Drug Interactions

No interactions have been reported.

Special Information If You Are Pregnant or Breastfeeding

No harmful effects are known.

How to Prepare

Alfalfa can be found in crushed-leaf form, and in tablets and capsules.

Typical Dosage

A dosage of 0.5 to 1 gram of Alfalfa leaf daily is sometimes recommended. Since potency of commercial products may vary, follow the manufacturer's directions whenever available.

Overdosage

No information on overdosage is available.

Aloe

Latin name: Aloe barbadensis
Other names: Barbados Aloe,
*   Cape Aloe, Curacao Aloe,*
*   Socotrine Aloe, Zanzibar Aloe*

A Remedy For
• Constipation

Aloe has also been used as a remedy for indigestion, worms, diabetes, hardening of the arteries, menstrual problems, infections, tumors, skin diseases, abdominal pain, water retention, and low back pain. Its effectiveness for these problems has not, however, been verified.

What It Is; Why It Works

Aloe has played a role in medicine since the 4th century BC, when ancient Greek doctors obtained it from the island of Socotra in the Indian Ocean. In the 10th century AD, its remedial powers were recommended to the British king Alfred the Great by the Patriarch of Jerusalem. Muslims who have made the pilgrimage to Mecca are entitled to hang an Aloe plant over their doors as a talisman against evil.

Aloe is a lily-like, succulent shrub with little if any stem. It produces about 25 fleshy, gray-green leaves in an upright, dense rosette. In Europe, Aloe is used almost exclusively as a digestive aid and laxative. Elsewhere, it's a popular ingredient in many skin preparations and cosmetics.

The medicinal agent is the dried juice of the leaves, which works by stimulating the colon. This action tends to reduce liquid absorption by moving food more quickly through the intestines. Aloe also kills bacteria and is effective against herpes simplex viruses.

Avoid If . . .

Because of its effect on the bowels, you should avoid Aloe if you have an intestinal obstruction, an acute inflammatory intestinal disorder such as Crohn's Disease, ulcerative colitis, appendicitis, or any abdominal pain of unknown origin. Not for children under 12.

Special Cautions

Aloe can cause abdominal pain or discomfort. If it does, reduce the dosage.

Do not take Aloe for more than 1 to 2 weeks without consulting a doctor. Long-term use can lead to potassium deficiency.

Possible Drug Interactions

Avoid combining Aloe with other medications that flush water and potassium from the body, including diuretics such as Diuril and Lasix, steroid drugs such as prednisone, and licorice root.

Potassium plays an important role in regulating the heart, so depleting it through long-term use of laxatives can affect the action of certain heart medications. The effects of drugs such as digitalis and digoxin (Lanoxin) may be increased. Drugs taken to steady the heartbeat could also be affected.

Special Information If You Are Pregnant or Breastfeeding

Do not take Aloe during pregnancy. Use caution when breastfeeding.

How to Prepare

Aloe is supplied as a powder and in various liquid forms.

Typical Dosage

Aloe is taken orally. The usual daily dosage is 20 to 30 milligrams. Use the smallest dose necessary to produce a soft stool. Don't take the entire daily dosage all at once; divide it into several smaller doses taken throughout the day.

Store away from light and moisture.

Overdosage

No information on overdosage is available.

Alstonia Bark

Latin name: Alstonia constricta
Other names: Australian Fever
Bush, Australian Quinine,
Devil Tree, Dita Bark, Fever
Bark, Pali-mara

A Remedy For

Although there's no formal evidence of its effectiveness, Alstonia Bark is sometimes taken to reduce fever. In the Far East, it is used for diarrhea and malaria. It has also been employed as a uterine stimulant and as a remedy for rheumatism.

What It Is; Why It Works

Alstonia Bark contains trace amounts of reserpine—an active ingredient in such high blood pressure medications as Diupres and Hydropres—but in quantities too small to be of any practical value. Aside from this slight antihypertensive effect, the bark is also said to combat spasms and relieve fever.

A 40-foot evergreen tree native to Australia, Alstonia takes its name from a Professor Alston who taught botany in Edinburgh. At one point, some experts considered Alstonia Bark better than quinine for treating malaria, but the herb has since fallen into disuse.

Avoid If . . .

Reserpine should be avoided during pregnancy, and by those with depression, stomach ulcers, or ulcerative colitis. Since Alstonia Bark contains a small amount of reserpine, you may wish to avoid it under these circumstances.

Special Cautions

Side effects are a slight possibility, due primarily to Alstonia's reserpine content. They could include nasal congestion, depression, fatigue, impotence, and slowed reaction time. Use caution when handling machinery or driving.

Possible Drug Interactions

Reserpine should not be combined with monoamine oxidase inhibitors such as Nardil or Parnate, alcohol and barbiturates, digitalis-based drugs such as Lanoxin, or quinidine products such as Quinaglute and Quinidex, levodopa (Sinemet), and many common flu remedies and appetite suppressants. You may wish to take similar precautions with Alstonia Bark.

Special Information If You Are Pregnant or Breastfeeding

Reserpine should be avoided during pregnancy or when breastfeeding. Due to its reserpine content, you should avoid Alstonia as well.

How to Prepare

Alstonia Bark may be used in the form of a powder, liquid extract, alcohol solution (tincture), or tea.

Typical Dosage

Tincture: 2 to 4 milliliters
Liquid extract: 4 to 8 milliliters
Tea: 15 to 20 milliliters (3 to 4 teaspoonfuls)

Overdosage

Symptoms of reserpine overdose include mental depression, heavy sedation, and a severe drop in blood pressure. If you suspect an overdose, seek medical attention immediately.

Angelica Root

Latin name: Angelica archangelica

A Remedy For

• Appetite loss
• Gas
• Indigestion

What It Is; Why It Works

Known in Europe since the 17th century, Angelica is the fleshy root of the wild celery plant. It stimulates production of digestive juices, improves the flow of bile into the digestive tract, and combats digestive spasms.

Don't confuse the European variety of this root with Chinese Angelica, or *Dong Quai*. The Chinese version is used as a remedy for menstrual problems and the symptoms of menopause, a tonic for anemia (loss of red blood cells), and a treatment for heart disease and high blood pressure.

European Angelica, on the other hand, was originally thought to be a cure for plague. Later, it was recommended for the common cold. Today, only its digestive uses are considered valid.

Avoid If . . .

No known medical conditions preclude the use of Angelica.

Special Cautions

Angelica increases sensitivity to sunlight. To avoid a sunburn, minimize your exposure to the sun while using this drug.

Possible Drug Interactions

No interactions have been reported.

Special Information If You Are Pregnant or Breastfeeding

No harmful effects are known.

How to Prepare

Crushed Angelica Root can be made into a tea, using one teaspoonful per cup. Allow the root to steep for 10 to 20 minutes. You may also find fluid extracts of Angelica, oil of Angelica, and solutions of Angelica in alcohol (tinctures of Angelica).

Typical Dosage

Angelica is taken orally. The usual daily dosage is:

Crushed Angelica Root: 4.5 grams (almost 1 teaspoonful)

Fluid extract of Angelica: 1.5 to 3 grams (about a half teaspoonful)

Angelica tincture: 1.5 grams (about a quarter teaspoonful)

Essential oil of Angelica: 10 to 20 drops

Strengths of commercial preparations may vary. Follow the manufacturer's labeling whenever available.

Overdosage

No information on overdosage is available.

Anise

Latin name: Pimpinella anisum

A Remedy For

- Appetite loss
- Bronchitis
- Colds
- Cough
- Fever
- Liver and gallbladder problems
- Sore throat
- Tendency to infection

Anise is also used for an upset stomach, but its effectiveness for this problem remains unproven.

What It Is; Why It Works

Anise is an expectorant that helps bring up phlegm. It's also a mild muscle relaxant, and shows antibacterial activity. It is well known for its ability to sweeten breath.

Originally from the Near East, the Anise plant is now grown in southern Europe, Turkey, central Asia, India, China, Japan, and Central and South America. The ripe fruit and dried seeds provide the plant's medicinal oil.

Avoid If . . .

Don't take this herb if you are allergic to Anise or its main ingredient, anethole.

Special Cautions

Anise poses no known risks when taken at customary dosage levels. There is a slight possibility that you could develop an allergic sensitivity to the herb.

Possible Drug Interactions

No interactions have been reported.

Special Information If You Are Pregnant or Breastfeeding

No harmful effects are known.

How to Prepare

Crushed Anise can be made into a tea. Preparations of essential oil of Anise can be used for inhalation.

Typical Dosage

When taken orally, the usual daily dosage is:

Dried Anise seed: 3 grams (a heaping half-teaspoonful)

Essential oil of Anise: 0.3 grams

Overdosage
No information on overdosage is available.

Arnica

Latin name: Arnica montana
Other names: Leopard's Bane,
Mountain Tobacco, Wolfsbane

A Remedy For
- Bruises, sprains, and dislocations
- Rheumatism
- Skin inflammation

Arnica has also been proven effective for the common cold, cough, bronchitis, fever, sore throat, and a tendency to infection. However, it is no longer recommended for these conditions due to its dangerous side effects. Modern use is limited to external applications.

Unproven uses in folk medicine include heart problems, chest pain, hardening of the arteries, severe uterine bleeding, fatigue, boils, insect bites, and inflamed veins.

What It Is; Why It Works
Arnica is found in Europe, southern Russia, and central Asia. The plant grows as high as 20 inches and produces aromatic, yellowish flowers.

Arnica exhibits antiseptic and pain-killing properties when applied to inflammations. Researchers have also found that, in animals, it increases the flow of blood to the heart muscle and reduces resistance in the veins.

Avoid If . . .
Do not take Arnica internally; an overdose can cause serious heart problems. External use is considered safe under all medical conditions.

Special Cautions
Repeated contact with Arnica, or cosmetics containing Arnica, can cause itching, blisters, ulcers, and dead skin. However, such side effects are unlikely when the herb is applied at standard potencies for limited periods of time.

Possible Drug Interactions
No drug interactions have been reported.

Special Information If You Are Pregnant or Breastfeeding
No harmful effects are known.

How to Prepare
Arnica is available in whole, cut, crushed, and powdered form. You may also find it available as an extract, an alcohol solution, a mouth rinse, an ointment, or an oil.

Typical Dosage
For external use only. Because the potency of commercial preparations varies, follow the manufacturer's instructions whenever available.

Overdosage
An overdose of Arnica can cause severe irritation of the digestive tract along with vomiting, diarrhea, and bleeding. It can also disrupt the heartbeat. If you suspect an overdose, seek emergency treatment immediately.

Artichoke

Latin name: Cynara scolymus

A Remedy For
- Appetite loss
- Liver and gallbladder problems

Although it has been proven effective only for the above problems, in folk medicine Artichoke is used to treat a variety of digestive problems, prevent the return of gallstones, and speed recovery during convalescence.

What It Is; Why It Works
Artichoke has been welcomed at the dinner table since the time of the ancient Greeks and Romans. For medicinal purposes, only the dried leaves are generally used. The root of the plant does not contain most of the plant's active ingredients.

Avoid If . . .
Because Artichoke stimulates the flow of bile, do not take this herb if you have a bile duct blockage.

Special Cautions
Take Artichoke with caution if you suffer from gallstones; you could develop painful spasms. You should also be aware that frequent contact with Artichoke occasionally leads to allergic reactions.

Possible Drug Interactions
If you react badly to Artichoke, you may also suffer a reaction to other plants in its family, including chrysanthemums.

Special Information If You Are Pregnant or Breastfeeding
No harmful effects are known.

How to Prepare
Artichoke is available as a dry powder and as pressed juice.

Typical Dosage
The customary dose is 500 milligrams of dry extract. Do not take more than 6 grams per day.

Store in well-sealed containers protected from light and insects.

Overdosage
No information on overdosage is available.

Asarabacca

Latin name: Asarum europaeum
Other names: Black Snakeroot, Canada Snakeroot, European Snakeroot, False Coltsfoot, Hazelwort, Heart Snakeroot, Indian Ginger, Southern Snakeroot, Vermont Snakeroot, Wild Ginger

A Remedy For
Asarabacca has shown promise as a remedy for asthma, cough, and bronchitis, but has yet to win official recognition as effective. It has also been used—without scientific validation—to induce vomiting, promote menstruation, trigger abortion, and relieve a variety of ailments, including eye inflammations, chronic sneezing, pneumonia, heart pain (angina), migraine, liver disease, and dehydration. In homeopathic medicine,

it is recommended for nervous problems.

What It Is; Why It Works

This plant has a peculiarly unflattering name: it is thought to be derived from the Greek words "ase" for "disgust" and "sarao" for "dirty." Worse yet, the Renaissance herbalist Culpeper wrote that "it is a plant under the dominion of Mars and therefore inimical to nature. This herb being drank, not only provokes vomiting, but purges downwards."

Despite this less than encouraging introduction, Asarabacca may well prove to be an effective remedy for bronchitis and bronchial asthma once additional tests have been conducted. Researchers have found that it loosens phlegm, calms bronchial spasms, and acts as a local anesthetic.

A tiny (1- to 4-inch high) shaggy-haired plant, Asarabacca is found from central Europe to western Siberia, and is cultivated in the U.S. Although the leaves have been used in folk medicine, only an extract of the root is recommended for use today.

Avoid If . . .

Take only the extract; use of the natural dried root is not advised. Not for children under 12.

Special Cautions

Be aware that a compound in Asarabacca root has caused liver cancer in mice.

Possible Drug Interactions

No interactions have been reported.

Special Information If You Are Pregnant or Breastfeeding

Since Asarabacca was once used to induce abortion, any use during pregnancy seems ill-advised.

How to Prepare

While obsolete in its natural form, Asarabacca can be found as a sneezing powder (20%) or as a purified dry extract in the form of coated tablets and pills.

Typical Dosage

For adults and children 13 and over, the usual dose of purified extract is 30 milligrams. Potency of commercial preparations may vary, so follow the individual manufacturer's directions.

Coated tablets and pills may be stored in brown glass, away from light, for up to 2 years.

Overdosage

Warning signs of overdose include burning of the tongue, stomach pain, diarrhea, skin rashes, and partial paralysis. If you suspect an overdose, seek medical attention immediately.

Ash

Latin name: Fraxinus excelsior

A Remedy For

- Colds
- Fever
- Rheumatism

Although its use has not been officially recognized, Ash is considered effective for these three problems. Preparations made from Ash leaves are also used for arthritis, gout, bladder disorders, constipation, and water retention. Preparations of the bark are taken as a tonic.

What It Is; Why It Works
Found in most parts of Europe, the Ash tree is valued primarily as a source of strong, flexible timber. The tree grows fast, reaching a height of up to 95 feet.

Fresh Ash bark appears to have pain-killing and anti-inflammatory properties.

Avoid If . . .
No known medical conditions preclude the use of Ash.

Special Cautions
No side effects have been documented.

Possible Drug Interactions
There are no known interactions.

Special Information If You Are Pregnant or Breastfeeding
No information is available.

How to Prepare
No information is available.

Typical Dosage
Strengths of commercial preparations may vary. Follow the manufacturer's labeling whenever available.

Overdosage
No information is available.

Asparagus Root

Latin name: Asparagus officinalis
Other name: Sparrow grass

A Remedy For
- Kidney and bladder stones
- Urinary tract infections

Only the below-ground stem and the roots of the plant have documented medicinal value, although the above-ground parts have also been used. In Asian medicine, Asparagus Root is given for cough, diarrhea, and nervous problems, but its effectiveness for these conditions remains unverified.

What It Is; Why It Works
Used in its wild form in ancient Greece and Rome, Asparagus is a natural diuretic that flushes out the kidneys and helps prevent the formation of kidney stones. A perennial with a woody root stock, Asparagus grows from 1 to 5 feet high. The female Asparagus plant is slimmer than the male, which is shorter and stockier. Although the plant's berries are thought to be poisonous, there is no proof of this.

Avoid If . . .
Do not take Asparagus Root if you have kidney disease.

Special Cautions
If you have a weak heart or poor kidneys, do not attempt to flush out the urinary system with Asparagus Root or other diuretics.

When using Asparagus, be sure to drink plenty of liquids.

Possible Drug Interactions
No interactions have been reported.

Special Information If You Are Pregnant or Breastfeeding
No harmful effects are known.

How to Prepare
Chopped Asparagus Root is used for teas.

Typical Dosage
Asparagus is taken orally. The usual daily dosage is 1 1/2 ounces to 2 2/3 ounces of the chopped stem and roots.

Strengths of commercial preparations may vary. Follow the manufacturer's labeling whenever available.

Overdosage
No information on overdosage is available.

Astragalus

Latin name: Astragalus membranaceus
Other names: Milk Vetch Root, Huang-qi (Yellow Leader)

A Remedy For
Astragalus boosts the immune system. It's taken for a variety of conditions that can benefit from improved resistance, including acquired immune deficiency syndrome (AIDS), burns and abscesses, chronic colds and flu, fatigue, night sweats, and loss of appetite. It's also taken to counter the toxic effects of cancer treatment and to relieve the symptoms of Alzheimer's disease. In Asian medicine, it's considered a remedy for asthma, arthritis, diarrhea, and nervousness.

What It Is; Why It Works
One of the most important herbs in Chinese medicine, Astragalus is a member of the bean family. Its yellow root (source of the Chinese name "Yellow Leader") contains polysaccharides that stimulate the immune system.

In test tubes, Astragalus has been found to increase the function of the immune system's T-cells, one of the body's key lines of defense against disease. Another study has shown that Astragalus may protect the heart from damage caused by the Coxsackie B virus.

Herbalists often combine Astragalus with other remedies to enhance their action.

Avoid If . . .
No known medical conditions preclude the use of Astragalus.

Special Cautions
Potential side effects include gas and loose bowel movements.

If you are considering using Astragalus as part of a cancer treatment regimen, remember that its value lies in aiding recovery from other therapies. By itself, it does not fight cancer.

When making Astragalus preparations, be sure to use *Astragalus membranaceus* only. Other plants in the Astragalus family, including the "locoweed" species found in the United States, are toxic when eaten by cattle.

Possible Drug Interactions

There are no known drug interactions with Astragalus.

Special Information If You Are Pregnant or Breastfeeding

Check with your doctor before taking Astragalus while pregnant or breastfeeding.

How to Prepare

Astragalus is available in capsule, tablet, and fluid extract form, and as dried root and prepared tea.

To make your own tea, boil 1 ounce of Astragalus root in 1 cup of water for 15 to 20 minutes.

In Chinese medicine, Astragalus is prepared by combining 1 part honey, 4 parts dried root, and a small amount of water in a wok or skillet, then simmering the mixture until the water evaporates and the herbs are slightly brown.

Typical Dosage

Capsules and tablets: Two or three 500-milligram pills 3 times a day

Alcohol solution (tincture): 3 to 5 milliliters (about one-half to 1 teaspoonful) 3 times per day

Strengths of commercial preparations may vary. Follow the manufacturer's labeling whenever available.

Overdosage

No information on overdosage is available.

Balsam

Latin name: Picea excelsa
Other names: Fir, Spruce, Norway Pine

A Remedy For

- Bronchitis
- Colds
- Cough
- Fever
- Nerve pain
- Rheumatism
- Sore throat
- Tendency to infection

What It Is; Why It Works

Picea comes from the Latin "pix" meaning "pitch." Balsam trees are found in northern and central Europe. Their medicinal property resides in the oil extracted from the needles, branch tips, or branches, and the fresh fir shoots.

All pines yield a certain amount of resin, obtained by tapping the trees. This is distilled to make oil of turpentine and rosin. The latter is used for treating violin bows and making sealing wax, varnish, oil paints, and resinous soaps. It was formerly used as "brewer's pitch" to seal the insides of beer casks. Both oil of turpentine and impure turpentine (known as tar) are used medicinally. Balsam is also used in the U.S. as an aroma for beer.

Used medicinally, Balsam exerts a decongestant and antibacterial action. Applied to skin, it improves local circulation.

Avoid If . . .

Avoid Balsam in any form if you have bronchial asthma or

whooping cough. Do not use it as a bath additive if you have a large skin injury or an acute skin disease, heart problems, unusually stiff muscles, or an infectious disease.

Special Cautions
Use of Balsam can aggravate bronchial spasms.

Possible Drug Interactions
No interactions have been reported.

Special Information If You Are Pregnant or Breastfeeding
No harmful effects are known.

How to Prepare
Balsam is available in oil, gel, emulsion, solution, and ointment forms.

Typical Dosage
Oral administration: 4 drops of Balsam oil on a lump of sugar or in a little water 3 times daily, not to exceed 5 to 6 grams (about 1 teaspoonful) daily

Inhalation: 2 grams (about one-half teaspoonful) of Balsam oil added to hot water several times daily

Skin application: Rub several drops of oil, lotion, or ointment into the affected area

Bath additive: Boil about 1 cup of oil with 1 quart of water; let stand for 5 minutes, then add to a full bath. Be sure to relax afterwards.

Store Balsam in a closed container.

Overdosage
No information on overdosage is available.

Balsam of Peru

Latin name: Myroxylon balsamum
Other names: Balsam of Tolu, Balsam Tree

A Remedy For
- Bronchitis
- Colds
- Cough
- Fever
- Hemorrhoids
- Sore throat
- Tendency to infection
- Wounds and burns

Balsam of Peru is used externally for infected and poorly healing wounds, burns, bedsores, frostbite, leg ulcers, bruises caused by artificial limbs, and hemorrhoids.

What It Is; Why It Works
Balsam of Peru is a resin extracted from incisions in the bark of the Peruvian Balsam tree. It is an antiseptic that combats bacteria, promotes wound healing, and kills parasites, especially scabies. When taken internally, it has an expectorant action, helping to loosen phlegm.

The tree is native to South and Central America. Despite its name, the drug's main source is San Salvador.

Avoid If . . .

There are no known medical conditions that preclude use of this medication.

Special Cautions

Whether taken internally or externally, large quantities of this medication can damage the kidneys.

Used externally, Balsam of Peru often causes skin reactions such as eruptions, ulcers, swelling, and red patches. Allergic reactions are also possible from internal use.

Because Balsam of Peru may increase your sensitivity to sunlight, minimize your exposure to the sun while using this medication.

Possible Drug Interactions

No interactions have been reported.

Special Information If You Are Pregnant or Breastfeeding

No harmful effects are known.

How to Prepare

Preparations are available for both external and internal use.

Typical Dosage

External preparations contain up to 20% Balsam of Peru. If the drug is to be applied over an extensive surface, use a product containing no more than 10% Balsam of Peru. Do not apply for more than 1 week.

For internal use, the typical dosage is 500 milligrams daily. Since potency of commercial preparation may vary, follow the

manufacturer's instructions whenever available.

Overdosage

No information on overdosage is available.

Barberry

Latin name: Berberis vulgaris
Other names: Jaundice Berry,
*   Mountain Grape, Pipperidge,*
*   Sow Berry*

A Remedy For

- Indigestion
- Liver and gallbladder problems
- Tendency to infection
- Urinary tract infections

Barberry's medicinal value has not been officially recognized. It is considered obsolete as a drug, and its use is discouraged. Nevertheless, the berries appear to be effective for boosting the immune system and combating urinary tract infections, while the root seems to serve as a remedy for indigestion and problems with the liver and gallbladder.

Barberry has been used for a variety of other problems as well, including enlarged spleen, diarrhea, tuberculosis, hemorrhoids, kidney disease, gout, arthritis, low back pain, malaria, and parasite infections. However, its effectiveness for all these conditions remains in doubt, and its use is not recommended.

What It Is; Why It Works

The berries of *Berberis vulgaris* are a source of vitamin C. They have also been shown to increase immune system activity, stimulate iron absorption, and flush excess water from the system.

Extracts from the root have been shown, in animal studies, to reduce blood pressure, increase the flow of bile, reduce fever, and relieve constipation. The root also appears to have some antibiotic properties.

Avoid If . . .
No known medical conditions preclude the use of Barberry.

Special Cautions
At customary dosage levels, Barberry poses no problems.

Possible Drug Interactions
No interactions have been recorded.

Special Information If You Are Pregnant or Breastfeeding
No information is available on the use of Barberry in pregnant or breastfeeding women.

How to Prepare
To make a tea from the berries, pour 5 ounces of hot water over 1 to 2 teaspoonfuls of whole or squashed berries, steep for 10 to 15 minutes, and strain.

For a tea from Barberry root, use 2 grams of drug per 250 milliliters (about 1 cup) of water.

Typical Dosage
Various extracts and alcohol solutions (tinctures) are available abroad. The recommended dosage of the tincture is 20 to 40 drops daily.

Since the strength of commercial preparations may vary, follow the manufacturer's labeling whenever available.

Overdosage
Signs of overdose include a mild stupor, nosebleeds, vomiting, diarrhea, and kidney irritation. If you suspect an overdose, seek medical attention immediately.

Barley

Latin name: Hordeum distychum
Other names: Pearl Barley, Pot Barley, Scotch Barley

A Remedy For
• Indigestion

Barley is also used as a remedy for diarrhea and inflammatory conditions of the stomach and bowels.

What It Is; Why It Works
Yes, common Barley does have healing properties, conferring a soothing effect on the digestive tract. The grain itself, with the husk removed, is the medicinal element. It can be made into a soothing and nutritional drink, and has been used to dilute cow's milk for very young children. Barley is also the source of malt extract and malt vinegar.

Avoid If . . .
No known medical conditions preclude the use of Barley.

Special Cautions
There are no known risks.

Possible Drug Interactions

No drug interactions have been reported.

Special Information If You Are Pregnant or Breastfeeding

No harmful effects are known.

How to Prepare

For medicinal purposes, Barley is usually taken as a malt extract.

Typical Dosage

There are no general recommendations on record. Follow the manufacturer's directions whenever available.

Overdosage

No information on overdosage is available.

Basil

Latin name: Ocimum basilicum
Other names: St. Josephwort,
* Sweet Basil*

A Remedy For

Basil and its essential oil are sometimes taken for fevers, colds, rheumatism, and indigestion. However, there is no evidence of their effectiveness, and because compounds in the oil have shown cancer-causing effects during animal experiments, their medicinal use is not recommended.

Basil oil has been used to treat wounds, bruises, and depression. The leaves have been used—again without validation—as an appetite stimulant, a remedy for gas, and a means of ridding the body of excess fluid. In Asian medicine, the leaves are also used to treat poor circulation, stomach cramps, bad breath, inflammations, clouded vision, earache, kidney disease, and ringworm.

What It Is; Why It Works

Windowsill gardeners beware: in past centuries it was believed that a sprig of Basil left under a pot would breed scorpions. Worse yet, one commentator tells of a man who spawned a scorpion in his brain after merely smelling the herb.

Modern research has failed to confirm the scorpion problem. However, lab tests do suggest a slight possibility that prolonged use of the herb during pregnancy could harm a developing baby. Suspicion over the herb's cancer-causing potential is also yet to be resolved. All told, there's reason to avoid taking large quantities of the herb on a regular basis, although an occasional dish of pesto won't do you any harm.

In India, believed to be the origin of Basil, the plant is very highly regarded indeed. It is dedicated to the gods Krishna and Vishnu, and a Basil leaf is laid on the breast of the dead as a token for entry to paradise.

Avoid If . . .

Regular medicinal use is not recommended for anyone. Pregnant or nursing women, infants, and toddlers should not take the herb at all.

Special Cautions

No side effects have been documented.

Possible Drug Interactions

No drug interactions have been reported.

Special Information If You Are Pregnant or Breastfeeding

Pregnant or nursing women should not take Basil in any form.

How to Prepare

Not recommended.

Typical Dosage

Not recommended.

Overdosage

No information on overdosage is available.

Bayberry

Latin name: Myrica cerifera
Other names: Candleberry,
  Tallow Shrub, Wax Myrtle,
  Waxberry

A Remedy For

Although there's no proof of its effectiveness, Bayberry is sometimes taken for cough and bronchitis, or applied externally for skin problems. In homeopathic medicine, it's prescribed for liver conditions and insomnia.

What It Is; Why It Works

A familiar shrub along the shores of New England, this plant is valued primarily for the wax from its berries. Harder and more brittle than beeswax, the wax is not only used in candles, but serves as the signature ingredient of the hair tonic, Bay Rum.

Both Bayberry wax and dried Bayberry bark are used medicinally. The bark is said to act as a stimulant and an astringent, drying and tightening the tissues. It also induces perspiration.

Avoid If . . .

No known medical conditions preclude the use of Bayberry.

Special Cautions

No hazards or side effects have been recorded.

Possible Drug Interactions

No interactions have been reported.

Special Information If You Are Pregnant or Breastfeeding

No harmful effects are known.

How to Prepare

Bayberry bark is available as a powder or liquid extract.

Typical Dosage

There are no standard guidelines. Follow the manufacturer's directions whenever available.

Overdosage

No information on overdosage is available.

Beans

Latin name: Phaseolus vulgaris

A Remedy For

- Kidney and bladder stones
- Urinary tract infections

Homeopathic practitioners recommend this herb for diabetes

and heart conditions. In folk medicine, it is used to increase urine flow and relieve diabetes.

What It Is; Why It Works
The Bean plant grows 1 to 2 feet high and when in bloom boasts white, pink, and lilac flowers. Only the crushed pods are used for medicinal purposes. They have a mild diuretic action, helping to flush excess water from the system.

The plant is believed to have originated in India, but now grows worldwide. Probably because of the pods' resemblance to the male reproductive organ, Beans were worshipped in ancient Egypt, and it was verboten to eat them. Today, Jewish High Priests cannot eat Beans on the Day of Atonement. In Italy, they are distributed to poor people on the anniversary of a death.

Avoid If . . .
No known medical conditions preclude the use of this herb.

Special Cautions
Large quantities of raw pods or beans can cause severe digestive distress. However, customary dosages of tea made from the pods produce no side effects.

Possible Drug Interactions
There are no known drug interactions.

Special Information If You Are Pregnant or Breastfeeding
No information is available.

How to Prepare
To make a tea, pour boiling water over 2.5 grams (about 1 1/2 teaspoonfuls) of crushed pods, steep for 10 to 15 minutes, and strain.

Typical Dosage
The usual daily dosage is 5 to 15 grams (about 3 to 10 teaspoonfuls).

Strengths of commercial preparations may vary. Follow the manufacturer's labeling whenever available.

Overdosage
A massive overdose of raw beans can cause vomiting, diarrhea, and stomach pain.

Bearberry

Latin name: Arctostaphylos uva-ursi
Other names: Arberry, Bearsgrape, Kinnickinick, Mealberry, Mountain Box, Mountain Cranberry, Sandberry

A Remedy For
• Urinary tract infections

What It Is; Why It Works
Bearberry has been used against urinary tract infections since the 17th century, and—despite the discovery of antibiotics—is still in use today. It contains a substance called arbutin which has proven antibacterial properties.

Bearberry works best when the urine is alkaline. To assure alkalinity, stick to a diet rich in fruits, vegetables (especially tomatoes), and fruit juices. Taking small doses of sodium bicarbonate will also help assure alkaline urine. The antibacterial effect of each dose of Bearberry lasts 3 to 4 hours.

Originally native to Spain, Bearberry has spread throughout Europe, Asia, and North America. There are two theories regarding its name: either that its awful taste makes it fit only for bears, or conversely, that bears are especially fond of it.

Avoid If . . .
Not for children under 12.

Special Cautions
Do not take this herb for extended periods without consulting your doctor. Protracted use can cause liver damage, particularly in children.

If you have a sensitive stomach, the herb can cause nausea and vomiting.

Possible Drug Interactions
While using Bearberry, avoid medications and foods that make the urine acid (for example, citrus fruits, cranberries, and blueberries).

Special Information If You Are Pregnant or Breastfeeding
Do not take this medication if you are pregnant or nursing.

How to Prepare
You can make a Bearberry tea from 2.5 grams (1 teaspoonful) of finely cut or coarsely powdered herb. Either mix it with 150 milliliters (two-thirds of a cup) of cold water and bring rapidly to a boil, or pour boiling water over it. Steep for 15 minutes, then strain.

Typical Dosage
Bearberry is taken orally. The usual dosage of the tea is 150 milliliters up to 4 times a day.

Strengths of commercial preparations may vary. Follow the manufacturer's labeling whenever available.

Overdosage
When taken in excessive amounts, Bearberry can inflame the lining of the bladder and urinary tract.

Belladonna

Latin name: Atropa belladonna
Other names: Black Cherry, Deadly Nightshade

A Remedy For
- Irregular heartbeat
- Liver and gallbladder problems
- Weak heart

Belladonna has been used in folk medicine as a remedy for stomach and abdominal pain, asthma, bronchitis, and muscular pain. Applied externally, it has been used for gout and ulcers. In medicinal plasters, it is currently used to combat intestinal and digestive spasms, excessive perspiration, and bronchial asthma.

In homeopathic medicine, Belladonna is considered a remedy for the bulging eyeballs that sometimes accompany an overactive thyroid, as well as a treatment for nerve pain and scarlet fever. Its effectiveness for these problems has not been scientifically verified.

What It Is; Why It Works

Belladonna interferes with the action of acetylcholine, one of the nervous system's chief chemical messengers. Belladonna acts primarily on the heart muscle and the smooth muscle in the digestive tract, relaxing it and relieving spasms. It also has a drying effect and, in high doses, can affect the brain, causing overexcitement and hallucinations.

Belladonna gained its name during the Middle Ages, when beautiful young women used it to dilate their pupils. Today, several common prescription medications, including Donnatal and Levsin, employ the active ingredients in Belladonna to relieve intestinal problems and other complaints.

Avoid If . . .

There are no known reasons to avoid Belladonna at recommended doses.

Special Cautions

Due to its effects on the brain and central nervous system, Belladonna can cause muscular tremor or rigidity. A variety of side effects—many of them dangerous—appear after an excessive dose (see "Overdosage" below).

Possible Drug Interactions

Belladonna can increase the side effects of the following drugs:

Amantadine (Symmetrel)
Quinidine (Quinaglute, Quinidex)

Tricyclic antidepressant medications such as Elavil, Pamelor, and Tofranil

Special Information If You Are Pregnant or Breastfeeding

No harmful effects are known.

How to Prepare

Belladonna leaves and flowering branch tips are collected in the wild from May to July. The roots of 2- to 4-year-old plants are dug up in mid-October to mid-November or shortly before the start of the flowering season. The dried plant material is available in powder and extract form.

Typical Dosage

BELLADONNA POWDER

The average single dose is 0.05 to 0.1 gram. The maximum dose is 0.2 gram. Take no more than 0.6 gram a day.

BELLADONNA EXTRACT

The average single dose is 0.01 gram. The maximum dose is 0.05 gram. Take no more than 0.15 gram a day.

Belladonna leaves, powder, and extract should be stored away from sources of direct light. Belladonna root can be stored for a maximum of 3 years in a well-sealed container protected from light and insects.

Overdosage

The following side effects are usually warning signs of overdose: red skin, dry mouth, abnormally fast heartbeat, prolonged or excessive pupil dilation, inability to focus, overheating due to reduced perspiration, difficult urination, and severe or persistent constipation. High doses lead to overexcitement and symptoms such as restlessness, compulsion to talk, hallucinations, delirium, and manic attacks followed by exhaustion and sleep.

Doses of 5 to 50 grams (about 1 teaspoon to 3 tablespoons) can prove fatal for adults. Much smaller doses are fatal in children. Death usually results from asphyxiation.

Bilberry

Latin name: Vaccinium myrtillus
Other names: Dyeberry,
Huckleberry, Trackleberry,
Whortleberry, Wineberry

A Remedy For
- Diarrhea
- Sore throat

Preparations of this herb's berries are taken for diarrhea, particularly diarrhea caused by inflammation of the intestines. They can also be used as a gargle for mild cases of sore throat.

The leaves of the plant are also used medicinally, although there is no evidence that they have any significant effect. They are sometimes taken for stomach upsets, infections of the urinary tract, rheumatism, diabetes, gout, and inflammation of the skin. The leaves are also occasionally used as a drying, tightening agent in rinses and solutions for washing out wounds.

What It Is; Why It Works
A dwarf shrub less than two feet high, the Bilberry plant is common to central and northern Europe, as well as Asia and North America. The name "Bilberry" is a corruption of "Bulberry," which comes from the Danish "bollebar," meaning "dark berry." In the United States, the plant is often called "Huckleberry," a corruption of "Whortleberry."

Avoid If . . .
No known medical conditions preclude the use of the berries. Use of the leaves is not recommended.

Special Cautions
At customary dosage levels, the berries pose no problems. The high tannin content of Bilberry leaf could possibly cause digestive problems.

Possible Drug Interactions
No interactions have been reported.

Special Information If You Are Pregnant or Breastfeeding
No harmful effects are known.

How to Prepare
To make a tea from the berries, place 5 to 10 grams (about 1 1/4 to 2 1/2 teaspoonfuls) of mashed berries in cold water, bring the mixture to a simmer for 10 minutes, then strain.

Although not recommended, Bilberry leaf tea can be prepared by pouring boiling water over 1 gram (about 1 3/4 teaspoonfuls) of finely cut leaves. Steep for 10 to 15 minutes, then strain.

Typical Dosage
The usual daily dose of the berry is 20 to 60 grams (about 1 to 2 ounces).

Overdosage
Sustained overdoses of Bilberry leaves can lead to malnutrition, low levels of red blood cells, and yellowing of the skin and whites of the eyes. If you choose to use the leaves, do not take large doses or use the herb on a continuing basis.

Birch

Latin name: Betula species
Other names: Silver Birch,
*   White Birch*

A Remedy For
• Kidney and bladder stones
• Urinary tract infections

In folk medicine, Birch leaves are also used, combined with other medications, to treat rheumatism, but their effectiveness for this purpose remains unverified. Birch tar is used to treat skin diseases, including scabies (a contagious disease caused by the itch mite).

What It Is; Why It Works
With its brilliant white bark, Birch has long been an object of admiration. Poets have written about its beauty and elegance. Its wood has been used for every-thing from boats to paneling. Young spring Birch leaves are sometimes found in salads, and are used as an ingredient in herb cheese.

Only the leaves of Birch are recommended for medicinal use. They relieve fever and help to rid the body of excess salt and water. Their ability to increase the flow of urine helps to wash harmful bacteria out of the urinary tract.

Avoid If . . .
No known medical conditions preclude the use of Birch leaves. Birch tar is an ingredient in several European ointments and liniments, but because it is thought to contain potentially cancer-causing compounds, it's best to avoid it.

Special Cautions
Birch leaves should not be used as a remedy for water retention if you have reduced heart or kidney function. When using Birch to flush out the urinary system, be sure to drink plenty of liquids (a minimum of 2 quarts per day).

Possible Drug Interactions
No interactions have been reported.

Special Information If You Are Pregnant or Breastfeeding
No harmful effects are known.

How to Prepare
Birch leaves may be made into a tea and the sap made into wine. Freshly pressed plant juices may also be taken.

Typical Dosage

Birch leaves are taken orally. The usual dosage is 2 to 3 grams (approximately one-half teaspoonful) of crushed Birch leaves several times a day.

Strengths of commercial preparations may vary. Follow the manufacturer's labeling whenever available.

Store in well-sealed containers protected from light and moisture.

Overdosage

No information on overdosage is available.

Bistort

Latin name: Polygonum bistorta
Other names: Adderwort,
    Dragonwort, Easter Giant,
    Oderwort, Osterick, Patience
    Dock, Red Legs, Snakeweed,
    Sweet Dock, Twice Writhen

A Remedy For

Although it has not achieved official recognition, Bistort root can be taken internally for diarrhea, used as a gargle for sore throat, or applied externally to treat wounds and burns. In Asian medicine, it's considered a remedy for epilepsy, fever, swollen glands, and tetanus.

What It Is; Why It Works

The name "bistort" (derived from the Latin "bi" for "twice" and "torta" for "twisted") refers to the characteristic double twist of the plant's rootstock. The old English name for the plant "Twice Writhen" is a literal translation.

The medicinal parts are the roots and underground stem. In times of famine, the roots, which contain large quantities of starch, can be roasted and eaten. Typically reaching a height of 3 feet, the plant is found throughout Europe, North America, and Asia.

Avoid If . . .

No known medical conditions preclude the use of Bistort.

Special Cautions

There are no side effects on record.

Possible Drug Interactions

No interactions have been reported.

Special Information If You Are Pregnant or Breastfeeding

No harmful effects are known.

How to Prepare

The powdered root can be made into a tea or mouthwash. An extract or ointment can be applied externally.

Typical Dosage

There are no standard recommendations.

Overdosage

No information on overdosage is available.

Bitter Orange

Latin name: Citrus aurantium
Other names: Bigarade Orange,
    Neroli

A Remedy For
- Appetite loss
- Indigestion

Only the peel has proven medicinal value, and only for digestive problems. However, in folk medicine the flower of Bitter Orange is also used—not only for gastric complaints, but also for problems ranging from nervousness and insomnia to gout and sore throat. In Asian medicine, the flower is used for poor appetite, chest and stomach pain, and vomiting—again without conclusive evidence of therapeutic effect. Homeopathic practitioners use both the peel and the flower as remedies for headache and pain.

What It Is; Why It Works
Bitter Orange comes from a flowering, fruit-bearing evergreen tree native to tropical Asia, but now widely cultivated in the Mediterranean region and elsewhere. The small, unripened fruit is a traditional flavoring in the liqueur Curaçao. The peel of the fruit, fresh or dried, soothes spasms in the digestive tract.

Avoid If . . .
No known medical conditions preclude the use of Bitter Orange.

Special Cautions
Frequent contact with the peel can cause skin irritation, including redness, swelling, and blisters. In light-skinned individuals, the drug may heighten sensitivity to sunlight.

Possible Drug Interactions
There are no known drug interactions.

Special Information If You Are Pregnant or Breastfeeding
There is no information available.

How to Prepare
Crushed Bitter Orange peel is available for use in teas. Alcohol solutions (tinctures) and liquid extracts may also be found.

Typical Dosage
Customary daily dosages are:

Crushed peel: 4 to 6 grams (about 1 teaspoonful)
Tincture: 2 to 3 grams (about one-half teaspoonful)
Extract: 1 to 2 grams (about one-quarter teaspoonful)

Strengths of commercial preparations may vary. Follow the manufacturer's labeling whenever available.

Overdosage
No information is available.

Black Cohosh

Latin name: Cimicifuga racemosa
Other names: Black Snake Root, Bugbane, Bugwort, Rattle Root, Richweed, Squaw Root

A Remedy For
- Menopausal disorders

Black Cohosh also is used for premenstrual discomfort and painful periods.

What It Is; Why It Works

Black Cohosh has an effect similar to the female hormone estrogen, which governs the menstrual cycle and declines after menopause. The herb was long used by Native Americans as a remedy for painful menstrual periods. It also has an anti-inflammatory, sedative effect. The medicinal part of the plant is the root, both fresh and dried.

Black Cohosh's scientific name, "cimicifuga," comes from two Latin words meaning "bug" and "flight," a reference to the fact that it is never attacked by leaf bugs. Black Cohosh is native to Canada and the United States, but is now cultivated in Europe as well.

Avoid If . . .

There are no known medical conditions that preclude the use of Black Cohosh.

Special Cautions

When taken at customary dosage levels, Black Cohosh poses no risks. Occasionally, it causes stomach discomfort.

Possible Drug Interactions

No interactions have been reported.

Special Information If You Are Pregnant or Breastfeeding

Because of the drug's hormone-like effect, check with your doctor before taking Black Cohosh during pregnancy or while breastfeeding.

How to Prepare

Black Cohosh can be taken in the form of the fresh or dried root, or as a liquid extract.

Typical Dosage

Black Cohosh is taken orally. The usual daily dosage is 40 milligrams.

Overdosage

Very high dosages (5 grams or about 1 teaspoonful of the root; 12 grams or about 2 teaspoonfuls of liquid extract) can cause vomiting, headache, dizziness, limb pains, and low blood pressure. If you suspect an overdose, seek medical attention immediately.

Black Mustard

Latin name: Brassica nigra
Other names: Brown Mustard,
  Red Mustard

A Remedy For

Applied externally, Black Mustard is used in the treatment of bronchial pneumonia and pleurisy. Homeopathic practitioners use it for runny nose, hay fever, and sore throat. Its effectiveness for these problems has not, however, been scientifically verified.

What It Is; Why It Works

Black Mustard's medicinal effects stem from a potent oil released when the powdered seeds are mixed with warm water. Dubbed allylisothiocyanate, this oil is strong enough to raise blisters where it touches the skin!

Mustard has been in use for well over 2,000 years. The ancient Greeks attributed its discovery to Aesculapius, the father of medicine—an indication of the high esteem in which it was held. The Romans ate mustard pounded and steeped in new wine. Later, the Saxons are believed to have used it as a condiment. Over the centuries, it has been recommended as a cure for epilepsy, a treatment for snake bites, and a tonic to "warm and quicken the spirits."

Avoid If . . .
Do not use Black Mustard if you have ulcers, vein problems, or kidney disease. Also, do not administer to children under the age of 6.

Special Cautions
Because mustard oil irritates mucous membranes, internal use can cause stomach problems and kidney irritation. Breathing the vapors of a mustard plaster can trigger sneezing, coughing, and asthma attacks, as well as eye irritation. Extended contact with the skin can lead to blisters, ulcers, and dead tissue. Remove mustard plasters after no more than 30 minutes.

Possible Drug Interactions
No interactions have been reported.

Special Information If You Are Pregnant or Breastfeeding
No harmful effects are known.

How to Prepare
To prepare a mustard plaster, combine 100 grams (about one-half cup) of powdered Black Mustard with lukewarm (but not hot) water and pack in a linen cloth.

Typical Dosage
For adults, leave mustard plasters on the chest for about 10 minutes; for children, limit the treatment to 3 to 5 minutes.

Overdosage
A moderate overdose can lead to vomiting, stomach pain, and diarrhea. Larger overdoses cause sleepiness, heart problems, breathing difficulties, and possibly even coma and death. If you suspect an overdose, seek medical attention immediately.

Black Root

Latin name: Leptandra virginica
Other names: Beaumont Root,
Bowman's Root, Culver's
Root, Oxadoddy, Physic Root,
Tall Speedwell, Tall Veronica,
Whorlywort

A Remedy For
• Constipation
• Liver and gallbladder problems

Black Root can also be used to induce vomiting.

What It Is; Why It Works
Black Root promotes perspiration, relieves gas, promotes bile flow from the gallbladder, and encourages movement of the bowels.

A perennial herb roughly 3½ feet in height, Black Root originated in the eastern United States, but now it grows in other areas as well. The root and fleshy underground stem are used medicinally. The fresh root is considerably more potent than the dried.

Avoid If . . .
No known medical conditions preclude the use of Black Root.

Special Cautions
At customary dosage levels, Black Root poses no risks.

Possible Drug Interactions
No interactions have been reported.

Special Information If You Are Pregnant or Breastfeeding
No harmful effects are known.

How to Prepare
The root is taken in powdered form.

Typical Dosage
There are no formal guidelines on record.

Overdosage
No information on overdosage is available.

Black Walnut

Latin name: Juglans nigra
Other names: Butternut, Lemon
  Walnut, Oilnut, White Walnut

A Remedy For
• Hemorrhoids
• Liver and gallbladder problems

Although its use has not been officially recognized, Black Walnut is considered effective for the above problems. In homeopathic medicine, it's used to treat headache, hepatitis, and skin conditions.

What It Is; Why It Works
Native to the forests of the United States, the Black Walnut tree grows over 90 feet high. Its bark and its root are used medicinally. Juglone, a compound isolated from Black Walnut, fights bacteria and worms, shows anti-tumor activity, and serves as a gentle laxative.

Avoid If . . .
No known medical conditions preclude the use of Black Walnut.

Special Cautions
At customary dosage levels, Black Walnut poses no problems.

Possible Drug Interactions
No drug interactions have been recorded.

Special Information If You Are Pregnant or Breastfeeding
No information is available.

How to Prepare
No information is available.

Typical Dosage
Strengths of commercial preparations may vary. Follow the manufacturer's labeling whenever available.

Overdosage

If you suspect an overdose, seek medical attention immediately.

Blackberry

Latin name: Rubus fruticosus
Other names: Bramble,
Dewberry, Goutberry,
Thimbleberry

A Remedy For
- Diarrhea
- Sore throat

Blackberry leaf has been found effective for diarrhea and mild sore throat. The root is sometimes taken to prevent water retention and swelling, but is not considered effective.

What It Is; Why It Works

Although the tannin in Blackberry leaves has a drying, tightening effect that can relieve diarrhea, researchers have failed to identify any other medicinal properties. Nevertheless, the flowers and fruit have long been invested with magical powers. Blackberry was believed to confer protection from "evil runes" and was used to cure snakebites. Merely sitting under a Blackberry bush was considered sufficient to cure rheumatism and boils.

Avoid If . . .

No known medical conditions preclude the use of Blackberry.

Special Cautions

At customary dosage levels, Blackberry poses no risks.

Possible Drug Interactions

No interactions have been reported.

Special Information If You Are Pregnant or Breastfeeding

No harmful effects are known.

How to Prepare

You can make crushed Blackberry leaf into a tea. Pour boiling water over 1.5 grams (about 2½ teaspoonfuls) of the herb, steep for 10 to 15 minutes, then strain. The solution can also be used as a mouthwash.

Typical Dosage

Blackberry leaf is taken orally. The usual daily dosage is 2 to 5 grams (about 1 to 3 tablespoonfuls) of the crushed herb.

Overdosage

No information on overdosage is available.

Blackthorn

Latin name: Prunus spinosa
Other names: Sloe, Wild Plum

A Remedy For
- Sore throat

Both the fruit and the flower of Blackthorn are used medicinally, but only the fruit is considered unquestionably effective—and only for inflammations of the mouth and throat. In folk medicine, Blackthorn is used as a laxative and a remedy for cramps, bloating, indigestion, and diarrhea. Homeopathic practitioners use it for nerve pain, urinary problems, weak heart, and nervous headaches.

What It Is; Why It Works

Blackthorn is a bulky, 10-foot-high bush with white flowers. Its bark was once thought to be a fever remedy, and its fruit is an ingredient in Sloe Gin. The plant is found in Europe and parts of Asia.

The fruit has a tightening, drying effect on mucous membranes such as those lining the oral cavity.

Avoid If . . .

No known medical conditions preclude the use of Blackthorn.

Special Cautions

When taken at customary dosage levels, Blackthorn poses no problems.

Possible Drug Interactions

No drug interactions have been reported.

Special Information If You Are Pregnant or Breastfeeding

No harmful effects are known.

How to Prepare

Blackthorn flowers can be prepared as a tea. Put 1 to 2 heaping teaspoons of crushed Blackthorn in boiling water, stir, steep for 5 to 10 minutes, then strain.

Typical Dosage

Blackthorn root: 2 to 4 grams daily as a mouth rinse

Blackthorn flower: 1 to 2 cups of tea during the day, or 2 cups in the evening

Store away from light and moisture. Do not keep for longer than 1 year.

Overdosage

No information on overdosage is available.

Bladderwrack

Latin name: Fucus vesiculosus
Other names: Black-tang,
    Cutweed, Kelpware, Quercus
    marina, Seawrack

A Remedy For

Bladderwrack has been used as a remedy for high cholesterol and hardening of the arteries, indigestion, excess weight, and insufficient thyroid, but its efficacy has not been scientifically verified.

What It Is; Why It Works

Bladderwrack is a type of seaweed supported by air bladders on the body of the plant. ("Fucus" is the Roman name for brown seaweed. "Vesiculosus" comes from the Latin "vesicula," meaning "little blisters.")

Most of the healing virtues of Bladderwrack seem to derive from its iodine content, which stimulates the thyroid gland. In the 19th century, Bladderwrack was used to promote weight loss by boosting thyroid activity.

Bladderwrack is often over a yard long. It is olive green when fresh and black/brown when dry. It is found on the Atlantic and Pacific coasts, and in the North Sea and the western Baltic.

Avoid If . . .
Because the amount of iodine in the plant is highly variable, its use is no longer recommended.

Special Cautions
High dosages of iodide (over 150 micrograms per day) can induce or worsen an overactive thyroid. Allergic reactions are also a possibility.

Possible Drug Interactions
No interactions have been reported.

Special Information If You Are Pregnant or Breastfeeding
No harmful effects are known.

How to Prepare
Not recommended.

Typical Dosage
Not recommended.

Overdosage
Warning signs of excessive thyroid stimulation include thyroid enlargement, rapid heartbeat, palpitations, nervousness, agitation, increased sweating, fatigue, weakness, insomnia, increased appetite, and weight loss.

Blessed Thistle

Latin name: Cnicus benedictus
Other names: Cardin, Holy Thistle, Spotted Thistle, St. Benedict Thistle

A Remedy For
• Appetite loss
• Indigestion

This herb is also used by nursing mothers to improve the flow of milk, although its effectiveness for this purpose has not been scientifically established.

What It Is; Why It Works
In Renaissance Europe, Blessed Thistle gained a reputation as a cure-all, and was even believed to have fought off the plague. The plant is praised for its medicinal powers in Shakespeare's *Much Ado About Nothing* and was recommended in early herbal treatises as a remedy for migraine and other headaches.

Despite its past popularity, Blessed Thistle is now considered genuinely useful only for digestive problems. It works by stimulating the production of saliva and digestive juices. The plant originated in southern Europe, but is now cultivated throughout the continent.

Avoid If . . .
No known medical conditions preclude the use of Blessed Thistle.

Special Cautions
It's possible to develop a sensitivity to Blessed Thistle that extends to similar plants such as

mugwort and cornflower. Outright allergic reactions are, however, quite rare.

Possible Drug Interactions

No drug interactions have been reported.

Special Information If You Are Pregnant or Breastfeeding

No harmful effects are known.

How to Prepare

To make a tea, pour boiling water over 1.5 to 2 grams of crushed Blessed Thistle and steep for 5 to 10 minutes. Drink 1 cup a half hour before meals.

Typical Dosage

The customary dosage is 1 cup of tea a half hour before meals, for a total of 4 to 6 grams of the herb daily.

Overdosage

No information on overdosage is available.

Bloodroot

Latin name: Sanguinaria canadensis
Other names: Coon Root, Indian Paint, Snakebite, Sweet Slumber, Tetterwort

A Remedy For

• Gingivitis

Once a popular cough medicine, Bloodroot is now valued primarily for its ability to prevent dental plaque and gum disease. An extract of the herb is found in many toothpastes and mouthwashes.

What It Is; Why It Works

Bloodroot contains a mixture of antimicrobial compounds that fight plaque-forming bacteria. Although these compounds serve as active ingredients in a variety of commercial formulations, use of Bloodroot itself is no longer recommended. Homemade preparations taken in excessive amounts can easily prove poisonous.

Bloodroot is native to the northeast U.S. and Canada, and was used as body paint by native Americans. As its name suggests, the root is dark red.

Avoid If . . .

No known medical conditions preclude the use of Bloodroot.

Special Cautions

Doses of 300 milligrams or more cause vomiting; in fact, the herb was once used for this purpose. Higher doses are poisonous.

Possible Drug Interactions

No interactions have been reported.

Special Information If You Are Pregnant or Breastfeeding

No harmful effects are known.

How to Prepare

Use only commercially produced formulations.

Typical Dosage

Follow the manufacturer's instructions.

Overdosage

Signs of significant overdose include vomiting, diarrhea, cramping, and collapse. If you suspect an overdose, seek medical attention immediately.

Blue Mallow

Latin name: Malva sylvestris
Other names: Cheeseflower,
   Mallow, Mauls

A Remedy For

• Bronchitis
• Cough

In folk medicine, Blue Mallow has also been used for stomach inflammation, bladder problems, and wounds. It has been proven effective, however, only for upper respiratory irritation.

What It Is; Why It Works

Blue Mallow is found in subtropical and temperate latitudes all over the world. A leafy plant growing up to 4 feet in height, it produces bright purple flowers with long dark stripes.

Blue Mallow soothes irritated membranes by coating them with a smooth, syrupy material. The leaves and flowers are both used medicinally—but only when the more effective Marshmallow is unavailable.

Avoid If . . .

No known medical conditions preclude the use of Blue Mallow.

Special Cautions

At customary dosage levels, Blue Mallow causes no problems.

Possible Drug Interactions

No drug interactions have been reported.

Special Information If You Are Pregnant or Breastfeeding

No harmful effects are known.

How to Prepare

To make tea from Blue Mallow flower, add 1.5 to 2 grams of crushed flowers to cold water and boil. Strain after 10 minutes.

For a tea from the plant's leaves, pour about two-thirds of a cup of boiling water over 3 to 5 grams (about 2 teaspoonfuls) of the herb and steep for 2 to 3 hours, stirring occasionally.

Typical Dosage

The usual dosage of both the flower and the leaf is 5 grams daily.

Overdosage

No information on overdosage is available.

Bog Bean

Latin name: Menyanthes
   trifoliata
Other names: Bean Trefoil, Bog
   Myrtle, Buck Bean, Marsh
   Clover, Moonflower, Water
   Shamrock, Water Trefoil

A Remedy For

• Appetite loss
• Indigestion

In homeopathic medicine, Bog Bean is used as a treatment for diabetes, headache, and urinary problems. Its effectiveness for such conditions has not, however, been verified.

What It Is; Why It Works
Found throughout the northern hemisphere, Bog Bean is an aquatic plant, up to 1 foot in height, with white or reddish-white flowers. It is called the Bog "Bean" because its leaves are similar to those on bean plants.

With a strong, bitter taste, Bog Bean works by stimulating production of saliva and gastric juices. The plant was once held in great esteem as a remedy for vitamin C deficiency (scurvy).

Avoid If . . .
Do not use Bog Bean if you have diarrhea or intestinal inflammation (colitis).

Special Cautions
At customary dosage levels, Bog Bean poses no problems.

Possible Drug Interactions
No drug interactions have been reported.

Special Information If You Are Pregnant or Breastfeeding
No harmful effects are known.

How to Prepare
To make a tea, put 0.5 to 1 gram (about 1 teaspoonful) of finely cut Bog Bean in boiling water (or in cold water rapidly brought to a boil), steep for 5 to 10 minutes, then strain.

Typical Dosage
Drink one-half cup of the tea, unsweetened, before each meal. The total daily dosage is 1.5 to 3 grams (about 1 1/2 to 3 teaspoonfuls).

Overdosage
No information on overdosage is available.

Boldo

Latin name: Peumus boldo

A Remedy For
- Appetite loss
- Liver and gallbladder problems

Boldo leaf is also used for indigestion and mild intestinal cramps, although its effectiveness for these problems remains unproven.

What It Is; Why It Works
Boldo is an aromatic evergreen shrub native to the west coast of South America, where it's used as a remedy for gonorrhea. It's now found in the Mediterranean mountains and the west coast of the United States as well.

Boldo stimulates production of digestive juices and bile, and eases spasms in the digestive tract.

Avoid If . . .
Do not use Boldo if you suffer from obstruction of bile duct or severe liver disease. If you have gallstones, check with your doctor before using this herb.

Special Cautions

When the leaf is taken in customary doses, no side effects are likely. However, oil of Boldo contains a high concentration of a toxin called ascaridiole, and should never be used.

Possible Drug Interactions

There are no known drug interactions.

Special Information If You Are Pregnant or Breastfeeding

There is no information available.

How to Prepare

Take only the crushed leaves.

Typical Dosage

The usual daily dosage is 4.5 grams (about 1 teaspoonful).

Strengths of commercial preparations may vary. Follow the manufacturer's labeling whenever available.

Overdosage

A massive overdose can cause paralysis. If you suspect an overdose, seek medical attention immediately.

Boneset

Latin name: Eupatorium perfoliatum
Other names: Agueweed, Crosswort, Feverwort, Indian Sage, Teasel, Thoroughwort

A Remedy For

Boneset is used primarily in homeopathic medicine, where it's recommended for fevers, flu, digestive problems, and liver disorders. Its effectiveness requires further confirmation.

What It Is; Why It Works

Indigenous to the eastern U.S., Boneset has long been a popular remedy among native Americans. It promotes perspiration and soothes inflammation. Laboratory tests suggest that it also has a positive effect on the immune system.

Avoid If . . .

No known medical conditions preclude the use of Boneset.

Special Cautions

Skin contact may cause an allergic reaction. Potential side effects include excessive sweating and diarrhea.

Possible Drug Interactions

No interactions have been reported.

Special Information If You Are Pregnant or Breastfeeding

No harmful effects are known.

How to Prepare

Boneset is generally found only in homeopathic preparations.

Typical Dosage

Follow the practitioner's instructions.

Overdosage

No information is available.

Boswellia

Latin name: Boswellia serrata
Other name: Salai Guggal

A Remedy For
• Rheumatism

Boswellia is used for a variety of inflammatory diseases, including bursitis, osteoarthritis, and rheumatoid arthritis.

What It Is; Why It Works
Boswellia serrata is a large tree native to India. When tapped, its trunk exudes a gummy resin that's been used in Indian medicine since ancient times. Boswellic acids, the active ingredients in the resin, have been found to have much the same effect as the nonsteroidal anti-inflammatory drugs (NSAIDS) typically prescribed for arthritis—but without the NSAIDS' irritating effect on the stomach.

Avoid If . . .
No known medical conditions preclude the use of Boswellia.

Special Cautions
It's best to have your doctor monitor your therapy. Side effects are rare, but can include diarrhea, nausea, and skin rash.

Possible Drug Interactions
No drug interactions have been reported.

Special Information If You Are Pregnant or Breastfeeding
No harmful effects are known.

How to Prepare
Boswellia is available as a standardized extract of the resin.

Typical Dosage
A common treatment program is 150 milligrams of the extract 3 times a day for 8 to 12 weeks.

Because strengths of commercial preparations may vary, follow the manufacturer's labeling whenever available.

Overdosage
If you suspect an overdose, seek medical attention immediately.

Brewer's Yeast

Latin name: Saccharomyces cerevisiae

A Remedy For
• Appetite loss
• Bronchitis
• Colds
• Cough
• Eczema, boils, acne
• Indigestion
• Sore throat
• Tendency to infection

Brewer's Yeast is typically used as a remedy for chronic forms of acne and boils, and as an appetite stimulant.

What It Is; Why It Works
Brewer's Yeast kills bacteria and promotes production of certain white blood cells. It has been used since antiquity, in all probability, both for the preparation of alcoholic beverages and as a medication.

Brewer's Yeast grows world-wide and is found extensively in the wild. It is, in fact, an independently living plant, but was not recognized as such until the 19th century. Its effectiveness as a health remedy was first confirmed in 1886.

Avoid If . . .

No known medical conditions preclude the use of Brewer's Yeast.

Special Cautions

If you are prone to migraine headaches, use Brewer's Yeast with caution; it can trigger migraines in susceptible people.

Large quantities of Brewer's Yeast can cause gas. In some people it prompts allergic-like reactions such as itching, eruptions, rashes, and swelling.

Possible Drug Interactions

Brewer's Yeast can trigger an increase in blood pressure if you take it with a drug classified as a monoamine oxidase (MAO) inhibitor, such as the antidepressants Nardil and Parnate and the Parkinson's disease medication Eldepryl.

Special Information If You Are Pregnant or Breastfeeding

No harmful effects are known.

How to Prepare

Brewer's Yeast is usually supplied as a dietary supplement.

Typical Dosage

Brewer's Yeast is taken orally. The usual daily dosage is 6 grams (about 1 teaspoonful).

Overdosage

No information on overdosage is available.

Broom

Latin name: Cytisus scoparius
Other names: Green Broom,
  Irish Broom, Irish Tops,
  Scoparium, Scotch Broom

A Remedy For

• Low blood pressure

Although Broom does have some effect on the heart, its value for conditions such as irregular heartbeat and weak heart has not been proven. Other unproven uses in folk medicine include water retention, heavy menstruation, hemorrhaging after delivery, hemophilia, sciatica, rheumatism, gout, gall- and kidney stones, liver disorders, enlarged spleen, respiratory conditions, snakebites, and as a blood purifier. In homeopathic medicine, the herb is used as a treatment for chest pain (angina), clogged arteries (arteriosclerosis), and tense or stiff muscles, but effectiveness has not been proven.

What It Is; Why It Works

The tough, dense, broom-like branches of this plant, which grows up to 6 feet in height, explain its name. Its medicinal benefit lies in the dried aerial parts. Active substances in the plant act to constrict blood vessels and raise blood pressure.

Avoid If . . .
Do not take Broom if you have high blood pressure or the heart irregularity called atrioventricular block.

Special Cautions
In large doses, Broom is poisonous (see "Overdosage" below). Use only at recommended dosage levels.

Possible Drug Interactions
Avoid using Broom if you are taking a drug classified as a monoamine oxidase inhibitor, such as the antidepressants Nardil and Parnate and the Parkinson's disease medication Eldepryl.

Special Information If You Are Pregnant or Breastfeeding
Do not use Broom if you are pregnant. It has a potentially abortive effect.

How to Prepare
A tea can be made from the leaves of the plant, or the drug can be taken as a liquid extract or alcohol solution (tincture).

Typical Dosage
The usual dosages are:

Tea: 1 cup 3 times daily
Liquid extract: 1 to 2 milliliters (about one-quarter of a teaspoonful) daily
Tincture: 0.5 to 2 milliliters daily

Store Broom protected from light and moisture.

Overdosage
Approximately 30 grams (2 tablespoonfuls) of Broom are sufficient to cause symptoms of overdose, including dizziness, headache, palpitations, prickling in the extremities, a feeling of weakness in the legs, outbreaks of sweat, sleepiness, pupil dilation, and other eye problems. If you suspect an overdose, seek medical attention immediately. Asphyxiation is a possibility.

Buchu

Latin name: Barosma species

A Remedy For
Buchu is used for urinary tract infections and prostate conditions, although its effectiveness for these problems has not be verified.

What It Is; Why It Works
Native to the Cape region of South Africa, Buchu has been used in Europe since the 16th century not only for urinary and prostate problems, but for gout and rheumatism as well. It is still popular in South Africa.

Buchu is a 6- to 9-foot bush with white and pink flowers. The leaves, which are the medicinal part, have a peppermint aroma. They are used as a flavoring agent in tea mixtures.

Avoid If . . .
No known medical conditions preclude the use of Buchu.

Special Cautions
The volatile oil extracted from the leaf can cause skin irritation. No other health hazards or side effects have been documented.

Possible Drug Interactions
There are no known drug interactions with Buchu.

Special Information If You Are Pregnant or Breastfeeding
No information is available.

How to Prepare
Extracts and alcohol solutions are sometimes available. The leaf can also be used for tea.

Typical Dosage
The customary dosage is 1 to 2 grams of the leaf.

Strengths of commercial preparations may vary. Follow the manufacturer's labeling whenever available.

Store the leaf in a sealed container away from heat, light, and moisture.

Overdosage
No information is available.

Buckthorn

Latin name: Rhamnus cathartica
Other names: Hartshorn,
  Highwaythorn, Ramsthorn,
  Waythorn

A Remedy For
• Constipation

Because it softens the stool, Buckthorn is used by people with anal fissures and hemorrhoids, and those who've recently undergone rectal surgery. It's also used as a cleansing agent prior to diagnostic exams. In folk medicine, it's used as a diuretic to flush excess water from the body.

What It Is; Why It Works
Buckthorn's potent laxative effect has been known since at least the 13th century, when Welsh physicians prescribed juice of Buckthorn for constipation. As recently as the late 19th century, syrup of Buckthorn was used as an overly powerful laxative for children. It is still used, with equal parts of castor oil, as a laxative for dogs.

There are three species of Buckthorn, all with similar laxative properties. The plant is found all over northern Africa, western Asia, and Europe, in the form of either a large, 9-foot-high bush or a small tree. The medicinal parts are the whole, ripe fruit, either fresh or dried.

Buckthorn works by stimulating the colon. This action tends to reduce liquid absorption by moving food more quickly through the intestines.

Avoid If . . .
Because of its effect on the bowels, you should avoid Buckthorn if you have an intestinal obstruction, an acute inflammatory intestinal disorder such as Crohn's disease, ulcerative colitis, appendicitis, or any abdominal pain of unknown origin. Not for children under 12.

Special Cautions

Buckthorn can cause abdominal pain or discomfort. If it does, reduce the dosage.

Do not take Buckthorn for more than 1 to 2 weeks without consulting a doctor. Long-term use can lead to potassium deficiency, intestinal dysfunction, heart problems, kidney disease, swelling, and bone problems.

Possible Drug Interactions

Avoid combining Buckthorn with other medications that flush water and potassium from the body, including diuretics such as Diuril and Lasix, steroid drugs such as prednisone, and licorice root.

Potassium plays an important role in regulating the heart, so depleting it through long-term use of laxatives can affect the action of certain heart medications. There could be an increase in the effect of drugs such as digitalis and digoxin (Lanoxin). Medications taken to steady the heartbeat could also be affected.

Special Information If You Are Pregnant or Breastfeeding

Consult with your doctor before using Buckthorn while pregnant or breastfeeding.

How to Prepare

Buckthorn can be prepared as a tea in two ways. You can pour boiling water over 4 grams (about 1 teaspoonful) of crushed Buckthorn, steep for 10 to 15 minutes, then strain. Or you can add 4 grams of Buckthorn to cold water, bring it to a boil for 2 to 3 minutes, then strain while still warm.

Typical Dosage

Buckthorn, in solid and liquid forms, is taken orally. The usual daily dosage is 20 to 30 milligrams. Take the minimum necessary to produce a soft stool. Since potency of commercial preparations may vary, follow the manufacturer's instructions whenever available.

Overdosage

Excessive doses can be poisonous. If you suspect an overdose, seek medical attention immediately.

Bugleweed

Latin name: Lycopus virginicus
Other names: Gypsywort, Sweet
*   *Bugle, Water Bugle, Virginia*
*   *Water Horehound*

A Remedy For
• Insomnia
• Nervousness
• Premenstrual syndrome (PMS)

Bugleweed is used in cases of mildly overactive thyroid, a condition which often leads to nervousness and insomnia. Bugleweed also relieves tension and pain in the breast.

What It Is; Why It Works

Bugleweed does its work by inhibiting the action of thyroid hormones and the reproductive hormones associated with the menstrual cycle. It also reduces levels of prolactin, the hormone that triggers breast milk production.

The herb is a creeping perennial that grows to about 2 feet in height and has a mint-like smell. It was discovered on the banks of streams in Virginia, but now grows throughout North America. A closely related plant called Gypsywort is found in Europe. Bugleweed's medicinal value lies in its fresh or dried above-ground parts collected during the flowering season.

Avoid If . . .
Do not use Bugleweed if you have thyroid insufficiency, if you are taking any thyroid medications, or if you will be undergoing any diagnostic tests that employ radioactive isotopes.

Special Cautions
High doses of Bugleweed can lead to enlargement of the thyroid gland. Suddenly stopping use of the herb can make the problem worse.

Possible Drug Interactions
Do not use Bugleweed if you are taking any thyroid medications.

Special Information If You Are Pregnant or Breastfeeding
No harmful effects are known.

How to Prepare
Bugleweed is available as a crushed dry herb, as a freshly pressed juice, and in liquid extract form. The dried herb may be used to make tea.

Typical Dosage
The best dosage of Bugleweed varies according to the patient's age and weight. The daily dosage for an adult usually lies between 1 and 2 grams of Bugleweed for tea. Liquid extracts should supply approximately 20 milligrams of the active ingredient.

Overdosage
No information on overdosage is available.

Bupleurum

Latin name: Bupleurum chinense
Other names: Hare's Ear,
  Thorowax Root

A Remedy For
Popular in Chinese medicine, this herb is considered a remedy for bloated stomach, pressure in the chest, chills, fever, indigestion, malaria, menstrual problems, nausea, uterine prolapse, and vertigo. Its effectiveness for these problems has not been scientifically verified; but clinical tests suggest that it might be effective in the treatment of flu and tuberculosis.

What It Is; Why It Works
The Chinese regard this herb as especially useful for reducing fever and relieving irritability. Only the root is considered medicinal.

Avoid If . . .
No known medical conditions preclude the use of Bupleurum.

Special Cautions
An excessive dose may cause nausea.

Possible Drug Interactions
No interactions have been reported.

Special Information If You Are Pregnant or Breastfeeding
No harmful effects are known.

How to Prepare
The root is available in Asian markets and some Western-style health food stores.

Typical Dosage
There are no standard guidelines on record. The root is often taken in herbal mixtures prepared by Chinese herbalists.

Overdosage
No information on overdosage is available.

Burdock

Latin name: Arctium lappa
Other names: Bardane, Beggar's Buttons, Cocklebur, Hareburr

A Remedy For
Burdock has been used to treat fevers and colds, urinary tract infections, and rheumatism, although proof of its effectiveness for these problems is lacking. Other unverified uses include treatment of digestive problems, water retention, eczema, and psoriasis. In Asian medicine, it's considered a remedy for deep skin infections, coughs, sore throats, and ulcers. Homeopathic practitioners also use it for skin conditions.

What It Is; Why It Works
Burdock is probably named for the tenacious burrs that stick to animals who feed on it. Sporting funnel-shaped crimson blossoms, the 3- to 5-foot high plant can be found throughout Europe, North Asia, and North America. It is mentioned in at least three of Shakespeare's plays: *As You Like It, King Lear,* and *Troilus and Cressida.*

In laboratory tests, Burdock root has exhibited antimicrobial activity. It also tends to moderate blood sugar levels. Although only the root is used today, the leaves were once used medicinally as well, apparently for their cooling, drying effect.

Avoid If . . .
No known medical conditions preclude the use of Burdock.

Special Cautions
There is a slight chance that contact with the skin will cause a reaction. No other side effects have been reported.

Possible Drug Interactions
There are no known drug interactions.

Special Information If You Are Pregnant or Breastfeeding
In large quantities, Burdock root may stimulate the uterus. Take with caution during pregnancy.

How to Prepare
Burdock root is available in dried and alcohol solution (tincture) form.

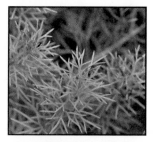

ADONIS: Adonis Vernalis

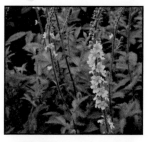

AGRIMONY: Agrimonia Eupatoria

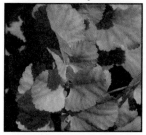

ALFALFA: Medicago Sativa

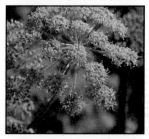

ANGELICA ROOT: Angelica Archangelica

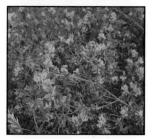

ANISE: Pimpinella Anisum

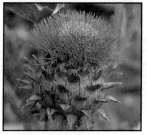

ARTICHOKE: Cynara Scolymus

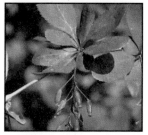

BARBERRY: Berberis Vulgaris

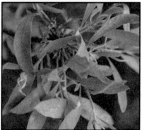

BAYBERRY: Myrica Cerifera

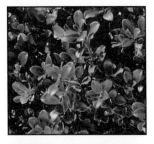

BEARBERRY: Arctostaphylos Uva-Ursi

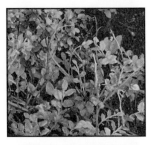

BILBERRY: Vaccinium Myrtillus

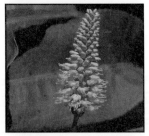

BISTORT: Polygonum Bistorta

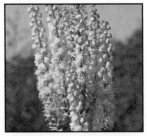

BLACK COHOSH: Cimicifuga Racemosa

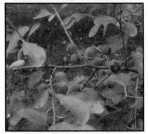

BLACKTHORN: Prunus Spinosa

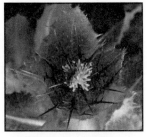

BLESSED THISTLE: Cnicus Benedictus

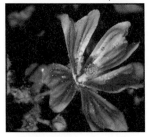

BLUE MALLOW: Malva Sylvestris

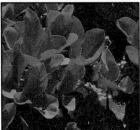

BOGBEAN: Menyanthes Trifoliata

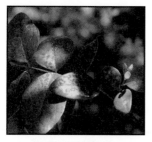

BOLDO: Peumus Boldo

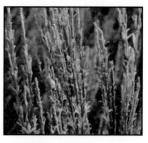

BROOM: Cytisus Scoparius

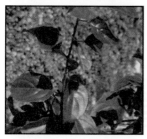

BUCKTHORN: Rhamnus Cathartica

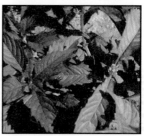

BUGLEWEED: Lycopus Virginicus

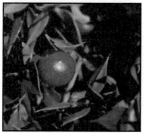

BUTCHER'S BROOM: Ruscus Aculeatus

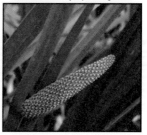

CALAMUS: Acorus Calamus

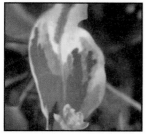

CAMPHOR: Cinnamomum Camphora

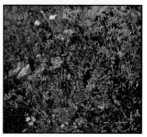

CARAWAY: Carum Carvi

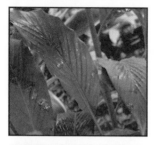

CARDAMOM: Elettaria Cardamomum

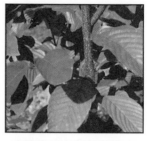

CASCARA: Rhamnus Purshianus

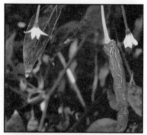

CAYENNE: Capsicum Annuum

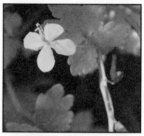

CELANDINE: Chelidonium Majus

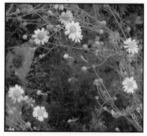

CHAMOMILE: Matricaria Chamomilla

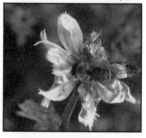

CHICORY: Cichorium Intybus

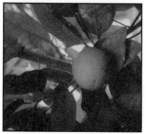

CHINA ORANGE: Citrus Sinensis

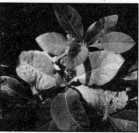

CINCHONA: Cinchona Pubescens

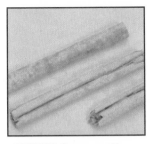

CINNAMON: Cinnamomum Verum

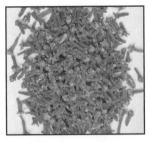

CLOVES: Syzygium Aromaticum

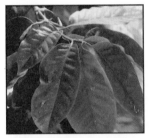

COFFEE CHARCOAL: Coffea Arabica

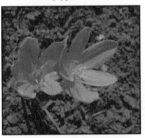

COLCHICUM: Colchicum Autumnale

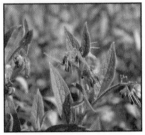

COMFREY: Symphytum Officinale

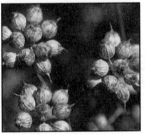

CORIANDER: Coriandrum Sativum

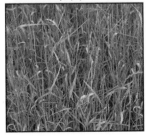

COUCH GRASS: Elymus Repens

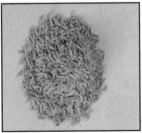

CUMIN: Cumimum Cyminum

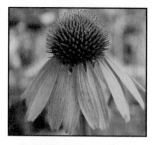

ECHINACEA: Echinacea Purpurea

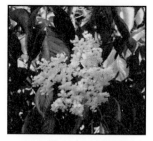

ELDER: Sambucus Nigra

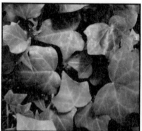

ENGLISH IVY: Hedera Helix

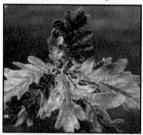

ENGLISH OAK: Quercus Robur

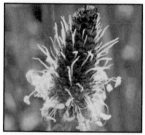

ENGLISH PLANTAIN: Plantago Lanceolata

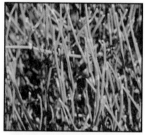

EPHEDRA (MA HUANG): Ephedra Sinica

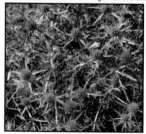

ERYNGO: Eryngium Campestre

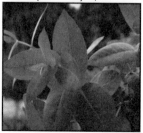

EUCALYPTUS: Eucalyptus Globulus

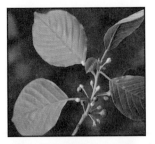 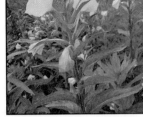

EUROPEAN BUCKTHORN: Rhamnus Frangula   **EVENING PRIMROSE:** Oenothera Biennis

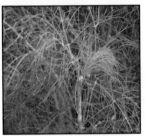 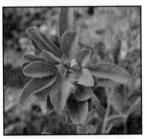

FENNEL: Foeniculum Vulgare   **FENUGREEK:** Trigonella Foenum-Graecum

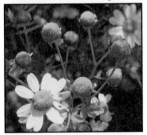 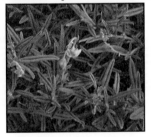

FEVERFEW: Tanacetum Parthenium   **FROSTWORT:** Helianthemum Canadense

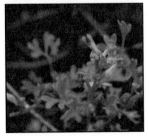 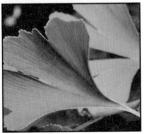

FUMITORY: Fumaria Officinalis   **GINKGO:** Ginkgo Biloba

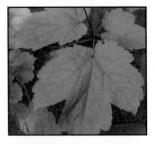

GOLDENSEAL: Hydrastis Canadensis

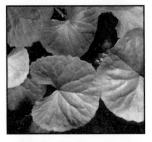

GOTU KOLA: Centella Asiatica

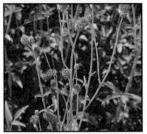

GREATER BURNET: Sanguisorba Officinalis

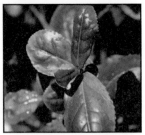

GREEN TEA: Camellia Sinensis

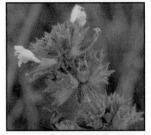

HEMP NETTLE: Galeopsis Segetum

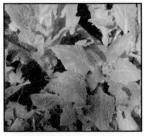

HENBANE: Hyoscyamus Niger

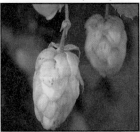

HOPS: Humulus Lupulus

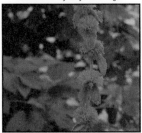

HOREHOUND: Marrubium Vulgare

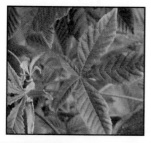

HORSE CHESTNUT: Aesculus Hippocastanum

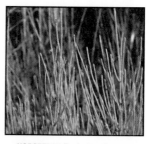

HORSETAIL: Equisetum Arvense

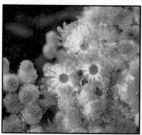

IMMORTELLE: Helichrysum Arenarium

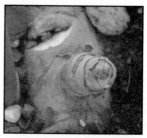

JAVANESE TURMERIC: Curcuma Xanthorrhizia

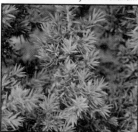

JUNIPER BERRY: Juniperus Communis

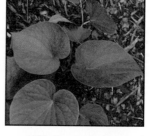

KAVA: Piper Methysticum

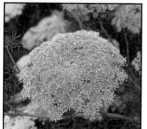

KHELLA: Ammi Visnaga

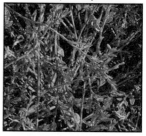

KNOTWEED: Polygonum Aviculare

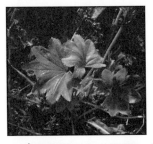 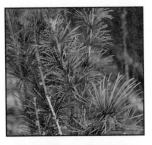

LADY'S MANTLE: Alchemilla Vulgaris

LARCH: Larix Decidua

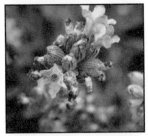 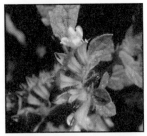

LAVENDER: Lavandula Angustifolia

LEMON BALM: Melissa Officinalis

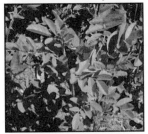 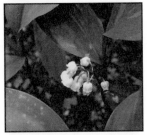

LICORICE: Glycyrrhiza Glabra

LILY-OF-THE-VALLEY: Convallaria Majalis

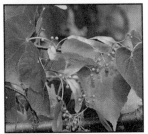 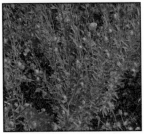

LINDEN: Tilia Cordata

LINSEED: Linum Usitatissimum

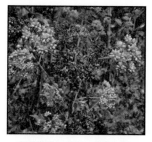

LOVAGE: Levisticum Officinale

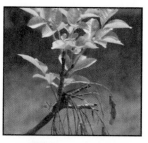

MANNA: Fraxinus Ornus

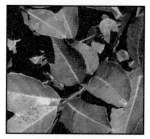

MATE: Ilex Paraguariensis

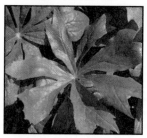

MAYAPPLE: Podophyllum Petaltum

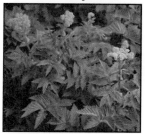

MEADOWSWEET: Filipendula Ulmaria

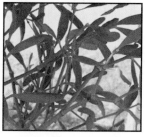

MISTLETOE: Viscum Album

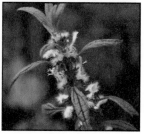

MOTHERWORT: Leonurus Cardiaca

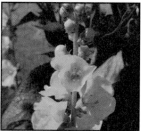

MULLEIN: Verbascum Densiflorum

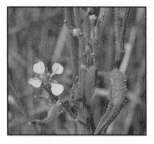

MUSTARD: Sinapis Alba

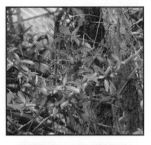

MYRRH: Commiphora Molmol

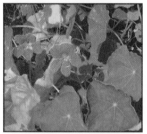

NASTURTIUM: Tropaeolum Majus

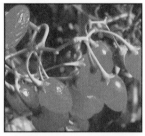

NIGHTSHADE: Solanum Dulcamara

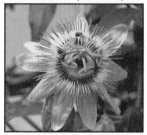

PASSION FLOWER: Passiflora Incarnata

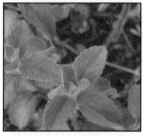

PEPPERMINT: Mentha Piperita

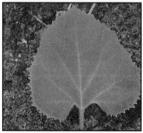

PETASITE: Petasites Hybridus

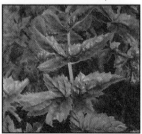

PIMPINELLA: Pimpinella Major

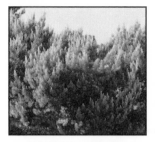

PINE OIL: Pinus Sylvestris

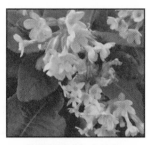

PRIMROSE: Primula Elatior

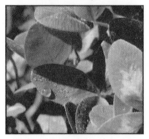

RED CLOVER: Trifolium Pratense

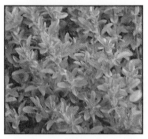

RESTHARROW: Ononis Spinosa

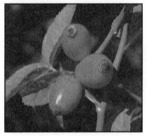

ROSE FLOWER: Rosa Centifolia

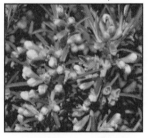

ROSEMARY: Rosmarinus Officinalis

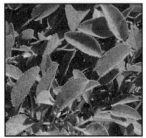

SAGE: Salvia Officinalis

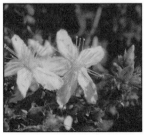

ST. JOHN'S WORT: Hypericum Perforatum

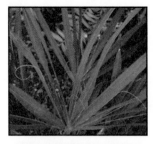

SAW PALMETTO: Serenoa Repens

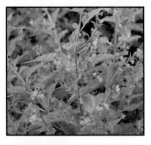

SCULLCAP: Scutellaria Lateriflora

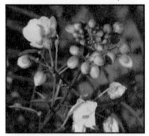

SENNA: Cassia Alexandrina

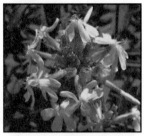

SOAPWORT: Saponaria Officinalis

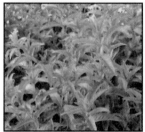

SPEARMINT: Mentha Spicata

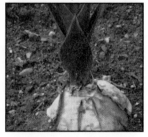

SQUILL: Drimia Maritima

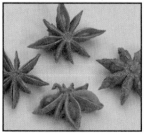

STAR ANISE: Illicium Verum

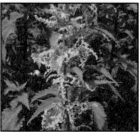

STINGING NETTLE: Urtica Dioica

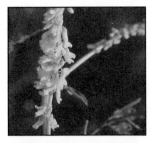

SWEET CLOVER: Melilotus Officinalis

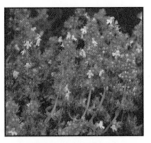

THYME: Thymus Vulgaris

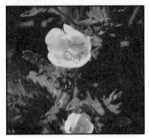

TORMENTIL: Potentilla Erecta

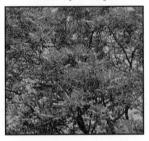

TREE OF HEAVEN: Ailanthus Altissima

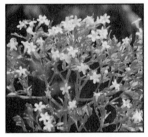

VALERIAN: Valeriana Officinalis

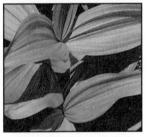

VERATRUM: Veratrum Album

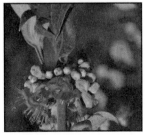

VITEX: Vitex Agnus-Castus

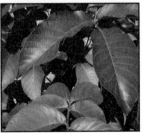

WALNUT: Juglans Regia

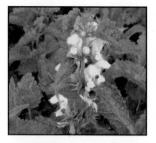

WHITE NETTLE: Lamium Album

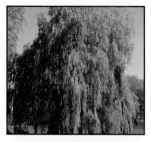

WHITE WILLOW: Salix Species

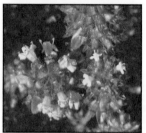

WILD THYME: Thymus Serpyllum

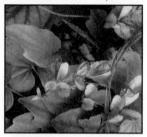

WILD YAM: Dioscorea Villosa

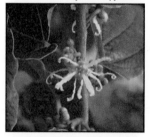

WITCH HAZEL: Hamamelis Virginiana

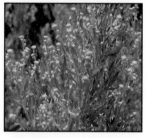

WORMWOOD: Artemisia Absinthium

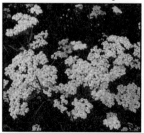

YARROW: Achillea Millefolium

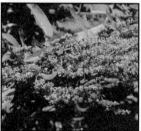

YELLOW DOCK: Rumex Crispus

Typical Dosage

Tincture: 2 to 4 milliliters (around one-half teaspoonful) daily

Dried root: 1 to 2 grams 3 times daily

Strengths of commercial preparations may vary. Follow the manufacturer's labeling whenever available.

Overdosage

No information on overdosage is available.

Butcher's Broom

Latin name: Ruscus aculeatus
Other names: Jew's Myrtle, Knee Holly, Kneeholm, Pettigree, Sweet Broom

A Remedy For
- Hemorrhoids
- Vein problems

What It Is; Why It Works

Used by ancient Greek physicians as a laxative and a diuretic for flushing excess water from the body, Butcher's Broom fell into disrepute until the 1950s, when a French scientist discovered two chemicals from the plant's underground stem that cause blood vessels to narrow and help reduce inflammation. Herbalists then began recommending the plant to treat the itching and burning of hemorrhoids (distended veins in the anal area). More recently it has been used to help treat lower leg discomfort, including cramps, pain, itching, and swelling, caused by pooling of blood in the veins.

A perennial evergreen, Butcher's Broom has tough stems and rigid leaves that make it useful for sweeping. Folklore tells us that bundles of Butcher's Broom were used to preserve hanging meat from mice, but more often the bundles were simply used to sweep butcher blocks clean. The plant grows throughout Europe, western Asia, and northern Africa.

Avoid If . . .

There are no known medical conditions that preclude the use of Butcher's Broom.

Special Cautions

In rare cases, stomach problems may occur.

Possible Drug Interactions

No interactions have been reported.

Special Information If You Are Pregnant or Breastfeeding

No harmful effects are known.

How to Prepare

Butcher's Broom can be made into a tea using 2 to 4 teaspoons of twigs or 1 to 2 teaspoons of fresh underground stem per cup of boiling water. Steep 10 to 20 minutes before drinking.

Typical Dosage

Butcher's Broom is taken orally. The usual daily dosage is sufficient extract to supply 7 to 11 milligrams of the active ingredients.

Strengths of commercial preparations may vary. Follow the manufacturer's labeling whenever available.

Overdosage
No information on overdosage is available.

Cabbage

Latin name: Brassica oleracea var. capitata

A Remedy For
Although some consider Cabbage juice a remedy for stomachache, ulcers, poor digestion, bronchitis, cough, and rheumatism, its effectiveness has not been formally recognized. In Asian medicine, Cabbage is also used to treat abdominal disorders, diarrhea, and skin diseases.

What It Is; Why It Works
Cabbage has been valued for its healing properties since the time of Christ. The 1st century healer Dioscorides recommended it for a variety of ailments, including diarrhea, snakebite, and worms. Today it's recognized for its ability to boost the stomach lining's resistance to gastric acids.

Originally cultivated in the Mediterranean region, the plant now grows in damp, temperate climates worldwide. Juice of the white Cabbage is the preferred medicinal product.

Avoid If . . .
No known medical conditions preclude the use of Cabbage juice.

Special Cautions
At customary dosage levels, Cabbage poses no risks.

Possible Drug Interactions
No drug interactions are known.

Special Information If You Are Pregnant or Breastfeeding
No harmful effects are known.

How to Prepare
Juice can be pressed from fresh chopped Cabbage, or purchased in prepared form.

Typical Dosage
As part of a bland diet: 1 quart daily
For stomachache: 1 teaspoonful before each meal

Overdosage
No information is available.

Cajuput Oil

Latin name: Melaleuca leucadendron
Other names: Paperbark Tree, White Wood

A Remedy For
• Rheumatism

Cajuput Oil eases the discomfort of rheumatism, pulled muscles or ligaments, sprains, bruises, muscle tension, slipped disk, low back pain, and sciatica.

What It Is; Why It Works
Cajuput Oil works by stimulating the circulation around the point of application. It also shows

antiseptic properties in laboratory tests.

The oil is distilled from the fresh leaves and twigs of a large tree native to Southeast Asia and the tropical regions of Australia. Historically, it has been used to help loosen phlegm and relieve spasms. It has a pleasant fragrance reminiscent of camphor and eucalyptus.

Avoid If . . .

No known medical conditions preclude the use of Cajuput Oil.

Special Cautions

Skin inflammation is a possibility. When using the oil on infants and small children, avoid the facial area. Application near the nose could cause throat spasms and interfere with breathing.

Possible Drug Interactions

No interactions have been reported.

Special Information If You Are Pregnant or Breastfeeding

No harmful effects are known.

How to Prepare

Available as a steam-distilled oil.

Typical Dosage

Follow the manufacturer's directions.

Overdosage

No information on overdosage is available.

Calamus

Latin name: Acorus calamus
*Other names: Cinnamon Sedge,
  Sweet Myrtle*

A Remedy For

• Indigestion

Although its use has not been officially recognized, Calamus is considered effective for indigestion. Applied externally, it's also used for rheumatism, chest pain (angina), and gum disease; and in Asian medicine, it's given for bronchitis, epilepsy, mental problems, and disorders of the mouth. Its value for these conditions has not, however, been proven.

What It Is; Why It Works

Calamus has been used medicinally since the time of the ancient Greeks, when it was prescribed for diseases of the eye. Native to India and North America, it now grows worldwide.

The medicinal part of the plant is its fleshy underground stem, which stimulates appetite and digestion while combating spasms, relieving gas, and calming the nerves. Used externally, it improves circulation.

Avoid If . . .

No known medical conditions preclude the use of Calamus.

Special Cautions

When used in moderation, Calamus presents no problems. Long-term use, however, should be avoided, since malignant tumors occurred in rats exposed to high doses of an oil found in a strain of Calamus.

Possible Drug Interactions
No interactions have been documented.

Special Information If You Are Pregnant or Breastfeeding
No information is available.

How to Prepare
Calamus oil and the powdered root are both used medicinally. Calamus can be prepared as a tea or used as a bath additive.

Typical Dosage
Bathing: Add 250 to 500 grams to the tub.

Strengths of commercial preparations may vary. Follow the manufacturer's labeling whenever available.

Calamus oil can be stored for up to 18 months. The powder should be used immediately.

Overdosage
No information is available.

Californian Poppy

Latin name: Eschscholtzia californica

A Remedy For
Californian Poppy has been proposed as a remedy for depression and anxiety, but its effectiveness for these disorders remains unconfirmed. Other unsubstantiated uses include insomnia, aches, agitation, bed-wetting, bladder and liver diseases, chronic mental and physical fatigue, nervous disorders, neuroses, mood swings, weather sensitivity, and migraine-type headaches.

What It Is; Why It Works
This bright yellow poppy reaches a height of 1 to 2 feet. Native to California, it is now cultivated in central Europe and southern France. It first came into medicinal use at the beginning of the 20th century as a remedy for sleep problems and pain, but is rarely recommended today.

Avoid If . . .
No known medical conditions preclude the use of Californian Poppy.

Special Cautions
No problems or side effects have been documented.

Possible Drug Interactions
No interactions have been reported.

Special Information If You Are Pregnant or Breastfeeding
No harmful effects are known.

How to Prepare
Californian Poppy is available in dried-herb and liquid-extract form. It can be made into a tea by combining 2 grams of the dried herb with 150 milliliters (about two-thirds cup) of water.

Typical Dosage
A customary dose of the liquid extract is 1 to 2 milliliters (about one-third teaspoonful). Because

potency of commercial preparations may vary, follow the manufacturer's directions whenever available.

Overdosage
No information on overdosage is available.

Camphor

Latin name: Cinnamomum camphora
Other name: Cemphire

A Remedy For
• Blood pressure problems
• Bronchitis
• Cough
• Irregular heartbeat
• Rheumatism
• Weak heart

In Asia, Camphor is also used for asthma, indigestion, inflammations, and muscle pain.

What It Is; Why It Works
Camphor is an active ingredient in such familiar over-the-counter remedies as Vicks VapoRub and Mentholatum ointment. Rubbed on the skin, Camphor stimulates circulation. Its inhaled vapors reduce bronchial secretions. When taken internally, it combats bronchial spasms, improves breathing, and promotes circulation.

In years past, cakes of Camphor were used as a moth-repellent. It was once popular as a remedy for stomach and bowel complaints, but fell out of favor due to the danger of overdose,

which can easily prove fatal. It was once believed to prevent infectious disease, a fallacy that probably sprang from its strong odor.

Camphor is an import from Japan and Taiwan, where it's distilled from the wood of the camphor tree, a large evergreen.

Avoid If . . .
There are no medical conditions that preclude the use of Camphor by adults, but Camphor salves should not be used on infants.

Special Cautions
External application of Camphor can cause skin irritation and even lead to poisoning through inhalation. Eczema (a skin inflammation) occasionally appears after application of oily salves containing camphor.

Possible Drug Interactions
No interactions have been reported.

Special Information If You Are Pregnant or Breastfeeding
No harmful effects are known.

How to Prepare
Camphor is used primarily in salves. However, solid and liquid preparations can be used for inhalation or taken internally.

Typical Dosage
For external use, concentrations of Camphor in salves should not exceed 25% for adults and 5% for children. When taken internally, the usual daily dosage is 30 to 300 milligrams.

Overdosage

As little as 1 gram can be lethal for a child. In adults, a dose of 20 grams can prove fatal. Symptoms of overdose, particularly in children, include intoxication, delirium, spasms, and breathing disturbances. If you suspect an overdose, seek medical attention immediately.

Caraway

Latin name: Carum carvi

A Remedy For

- Appetite loss
- Bronchitis
- Colds
- Cough
- Fever
- Liver and gallbladder problems
- Sore throat
- Tendency to infection

In folk medicine, Caraway has been used to improve lactation in nursing mothers, induce menstruation, and improve digestion. Its effectiveness for these purposes remains unproven.

What It Is; Why It Works

A familiar ingredient in cooking and liqueurs, Caraway is said to have originated in the Arab world. It once was recommended for girls with a pale complexion. It was also believed to confer a power of retention. An object containing it was supposedly protected from theft, and it was used to prevent lovers, fowl, and pigeons from straying.

Caraway is found in Europe, Siberia, the Caucasus, the Near East, the Himalayas, Mongolia, Morocco, and North America. The plant ranges from 1 to 3 feet in height and produces very small white or reddish flowers. Substances within the plant have been shown to improve digestion and combat certain bacteria.

Avoid If . . .

No medical conditions are known to preclude the use of Caraway.

Special Cautions

Large doses of Caraway oil taken for extended periods can cause kidney or liver damage.

Possible Drug Interactions

No interactions have been reported.

Special Information If You Are Pregnant or Breastfeeding

No harmful effects are known.

How to Prepare

To prepare Caraway tea, pour 150 milliliters (about one-half cup) of hot water over 1 to 2 teaspoons of Caraway, steep 10 to 15 minutes, and drain.

Typical Dosage

Caraway oil: The average dose is 2 to 3 drops on a sugar cube. Do not take more than 3 to 6 drops per day.

Caraway seeds: The average dose ranges from 1 to 5 grams. Do not take more than 6 grams per day.

Store Caraway protected from light and moisture in glass or metal containers.

Overdosage

No information on overdosage is available.

Cardamom

Latin name: Elettaria cardamomum

A Remedy For

- Appetite loss
- Bronchitis
- Colds
- Cough
- Fever
- Liver and gallbladder problems
- Sore throat
- Tendency to infection

In Asian medicine, Cardamom is used for asthma, stomach problems, hemorrhoids, and bad breath. However, its effectiveness for these ailments has not been proven.

What It Is; Why It Works

Cardamom improves the flow of bile out of the gallbladder and prevents viruses from multiplying. The parts of the plant used medicinally are the seeds and their oil. Cardamom is native to south India and Sri Lanka and is raised as a cash crop in Southeast Asia and Guatemala.

Cardamom has been used as a spice for centuries. It is referred to many times in *The Arabian Nights*. It became very popular early in the 20th century, when about 250,000 pounds were shipped each year to Britain alone. Today, Cardamom is used in cooking, as a health remedy, as a coffee flavoring in Egypt, and as an aromatic agent in perfume—especially in France and the United States.

Avoid If . . .

There are no known reasons to avoid Cardamom.

Special Cautions

Cardamom presents no problems under normal circumstances. However, if you have gallstones, it could trigger a painful attack due to its stimulative effect on the gallbladder.

Possible Drug Interactions

No interactions have been reported.

Special Information If You Are Pregnant or Breastfeeding

No harmful effects are known.

How to Prepare

Ground Cardamom seeds can be made into a tea. Cardamom can also be taken in an alcohol solution (tincture).

Typical Dosage

Cardamom is taken orally. The usual daily dosage is:

Ground Cardamom seed: 1.5 grams (about one-quarter teaspoonful)
Cardamom tincture: 1 to 2 grams

Overdosage

No information on overdosage is available.

Cascara

Latin name: Rhamnus purshianus

Other names: Bitter Bark, California Buckthorn, Cascara Sagrada, Chittem Bark, Dogwood Bark, Purshiana Bark, Sacred Bark, Sagrada Bark, Yellow Bark

A Remedy For

• Constipation

Because it produces quick, easy bowel movements with a soft or loose stool, Cascara is used by people with hemorrhoids or anal fissures (crack in skin near the anus). It is often recommended following anal or rectal surgery, and is used for bowel cleansing prior to bowel examinations and similar diagnostic tests.

What It Is; Why It Works

Native to the Pacific Northwest, Cascara probably earned the name "sacred bark" through its ability to relieve constipation so quickly. The medicinal bark is dried for one year before use in order to allow its naturally harsh ingredients to mellow.

The active ingredient in Cascara is found in several over-the-counter laxatives, including Doxidan and Peri-Colace. A strong, stimulant-type laxative, Cascara causes vigorous muscular contractions of the intestinal wall. This speeds passage of intestinal contents, leaving less time for liquid to be absorbed by the body and thus assuring a softer stool.

Cascara may be active against herpes simplex, the virus that causes cold sores and genital herpes. Research on this possibility is currently underway.

Avoid If . . .

Do not take Cascara if you have an intestinal obstruction, appendicitis, abdominal pain of unknown origin, or an inflammatory intestinal disorder such as ulcerative colitis, irritable bowel syndrome, or Crohn's disease. Not for children under 12.

Avoid the fresh rind of the Cascara plant. Taking it can lead to intestinal spasms and pain, bloody diarrhea, and kidney irritation.

Special Cautions

Cascara may cause cramping and nausea. Long-term use can deplete the body's stores of potassium and sodium, which are necessary for normal heart and muscle function. Chronic use may also cause kidney problems and fluid retention, irregular heart rhythms, bone deterioration, and laxative dependence. Do not use any stimulating laxative such as Cascara for more than 2 weeks without consulting your doctor.

Possible Drug Interactions

Because laxatives such as Cascara can cause fluid loss and potassium deficiency, you should not combine it with other potassium-depleting medications, including:

Thiazide diuretics such as HydroDIURIL

Steroid medications such as prednisone (Deltasone)

Licorice root

When potassium is low, certain heart medications may have a stronger effect. Be wary of laxatives such as Cascara while taking digoxin (Lanoxin) or a medication for heart irregularities.

Special Information If You Are Pregnant or Breastfeeding

Consult your doctor before using this medication.

How to Prepare

You can make a tea by pouring boiling water over 2 grams (about three-quarters of a teaspoonful) of finely cut Cascara. Steep for 10 minutes, then strain.

Typical Dosage

Cascara is taken orally. Use the smallest amount necessary to maintain a soft stool.

Cascara is available as crushed, powdered, or dry extracts and in various liquid forms. Strengths of commercial preparations may vary. Follow the manufacturer's labeling whenever available.

Overdosage

No information on overdosage is available.

Castor Oil

Latin name: Ricinus communis
Other names: Castor Bean,
    Mexico Seed, Oil Plant, Palma
    Christi

A Remedy For

• Constipation

Taken internally, Castor Oil is also used as a treatment for intestinal inflammation and worms. Powder from the Castor bean and leaves is applied externally to relieve skin inflammation, boils, abscesses, earache (otitis media), and migraine, although there's no proof of its effectiveness for these ailments. In Asian medicine, Castor Oil is used as a remedy for joint pain, dry stool, indigestion, facial paralysis, boils, and ulcers. Homeopathic practitioners prescribe it for digestive ailments.

What It Is; Why It Works

Castor Oil has been used as a laxative since antiquity. It's mentioned by the ancient Greek historian Herodotus, and beans from the Castor plant have been found in Egyptian tombs. The plant can be found from temperate latitudes to the tropics.

Castor Oil's laxative effect stems from its ability to prevent absorption of liquids from the intestinal tract. While the oil is relatively safe, the beans are extremely poisonous (as few as 12 can be fatal), and they should never be taken internally. They can cause severe fluid loss and lethal circulatory collapse.

Avoid If . . .

Don't take Castor Oil if you have nausea, vomiting, an intestinal blockage, appendicitis, severe inflammatory intestinal disease, or any abdominal pain of unknown origin. Not recommended for pregnant and nursing women and children under 12.

Special Cautions

Habitual use of Castor Oil discourages normal activity in the intestinal tract, leading to laxative dependence. Prolonged use can also result in an unhealthy depletion of minerals, particularly potassium. In rare cases, an allergic skin rash may develop.

Possible Drug Interactions

Potassium depletion due to habitual use can increase the body's sensitivity to certain heart medications, such as digitalis and digoxin (Lanoxin).

Special Information If You Are Pregnant or Breastfeeding

Do not use during pregnancy or while breastfeeding.

How to Prepare

Castor Oil is supplied commercially.

Typical Dosage

For acute constipation or worms, the dose is at least 10 grams (2 teaspoonfuls). Follow the manufacturer's directions whenever available.

Overdosage

An overdose will irritate the stomach, leading to queasiness, vomiting, cramps, and severe diarrhea. If you suspect an overdose, seek medical attention immediately.

Cat's Claw

Latin name: Uncaria tomentosa

A Remedy For

• Tendency to infection

Cat's Claw appears to give the immune system a boost, accounting for its popularity in the treatment of AIDS, cancer, viral diseases, and other infections. At this point, however, there's little hard evidence that it really does much good.

This herb also exhibits antiinflammatory properties, making it a candidate for treatment of arthritis, gastritis, ulcers, and inflammatory bowel disorders. Again, however, proof of its effectiveness is yet to be demonstrated.

In its native South America, Cat's Claw is a popular folk medicine for intestinal complaints, ulcers, arthritis, and wounds. Elsewhere, it has also been used for ailments ranging from asthma and diabetes to menstrual disorders, premenstrual syndrome, depression, acne, and hemorrhoids.

What It Is; Why It Works

A woody vine of up to 100 feet in length, Cat's Claw is found on trees in the rain forests of the Andes mountains, particularly in Peru. It earns its name from the sharp thorns on its stem.

In addition to its immune-stimulating and anti-inflammatory actions, Cat's Claw has antioxidant properties that could reduce the risk of hardening of the arteries and heart disease. Traditionally, the bark of the root was considered the medicinal part, but bark from the vine is now sold in its stead.

Avoid If . . .

Because Cat's Claw may cause the immune system to reject foreign cells, anyone with organ or tissue transplants should avoid it, as should those with autoimmune illnesses, multiple sclerosis, or tuberculosis. Cat's Claw should also be avoided during pregnancy, and is not for children under 2 years of age.

Special Cautions

Children over 2 and adults over 65 should begin with mild doses and increase the strength gradually if needed. Use by children for more than 7 to 10 days should be done only under the supervision of a doctor.

The only potential side effect is diarrhea.

Possible Drug Interactions

European herbalists avoid combining Cat's Claw with hormonal drugs, insulin, and vaccines. When it's taken in conjunction with other herbs, the dosage may need reduction.

Special Information If You Are Pregnant or Breastfeeding

Avoid Cat's Claw during pregnancy, and use it with caution, if at all, while breastfeeding.

How to Prepare

Cat's Claw is available as crushed bark, and in capsule, tablet, alcohol solution (tincture), and dry extract form. To prepare Cat's Claw tea, combine 1 gram of bark with 1 cup of water, boil for 10 to 15 minutes, allow to cool, and strain.

Typical Dosage

Tea: 1 cup of tea 3 times per day
Tincture: 1 to 2 milliliters up to 2 times per day
Dry extract: 20 to 60 milligrams per day

Since potency of commercial preparations may vary, follow the manufacturer's directions whenever available.

Overdosage

There is no information available.

Cat's Foot

Latin name: Antennaria dioica
Other names: Cudweed, Life Everlasting

A Remedy For

Cat's Foot is used to treat digestive problems and increase urine output, but there's no evidence that it's really effective.

What It Is; Why It Works

The bright red and white flowers of *Antennaria dioica* have been shown to ease spasms and increase bile flow—at least, to some degree—in animal tests. The possibility therefore exists for some minor value in the treatment of intestinal disorders.

The plant is nicknamed "Life Everlasting" because the cut flowers last up to a year before wilting. It is grown in Europe, Asia, and America as far north as the Arctic.

Avoid If . . .

No known medical conditions preclude the use of Cat's Foot.

Special Cautions

No harmful effects have been reported.

Possible Drug Interactions

No drug interactions have been documented.

Special Information If You Are Pregnant or Breastfeeding

No information is available.

How to Prepare

To make a tea, pour boiling water over 1 gram of finely cut Cat's Foot flower. Strain after 5 to 10 minutes.

Typical Dosage

There are no dosage recommendations on record.

Overdosage

No information is available.

Catechu

Latin name: Acacia catechu
Other name: Cutch

A Remedy For

Although of undetermined efficacy, Catechu is sometimes used as a sore throat remedy. Other uses include gingivitis, colitis, diarrhea, and bleeding. In Asian medicine, it is also recommended for diabetes, skin diseases, toothaches, and inflammation in the mouth.

What It Is; Why It Works

Catechu is extracted from the heartwood of a medium-sized Indian tree through a process of steam distillation. It is believed to have antiseptic and astringent qualities, fighting germs and drying the tissues. It is produced in India and Southeast Asia.

Avoid If . . .

No known medical conditions preclude the use of Catechu.

Special Cautions

At customary dosage levels, Catechu appears to present no problems.

Possible Drug Interactions

No interactions have been reported.

Special Information If You Are Pregnant or Breastfeeding

No harmful effects are known.

How to Prepare

Catechu is used in the form of an alcohol solution (tincture) which can be taken internally, used in a mouthwash, or painted directly onto inflamed tissues in the mouth.

Typical Dosage

Internally: 500 milligrams 3 times daily
Mouthwash: 20 drops per glass of lukewarm water

Overdosage

No information on overdosage is available.

Catnip

Latin name: Nepeta cataria
Other names: Catmint,
  Catswort, Field Balm

A Remedy For

Catnip is considered a useful treatment for fevers and colds, although its effectiveness has not been officially recognized. It is also used to ease cramps, and it is believed to have sedative properties that can remedy nervous disorders and migraine headache. Its calming effects, however, have yet to be scientifically verified.

What It Is; Why It Works

Regarded today as little more than a treat for the household cat, Catnip once enjoyed popularity as a kitchen and medicinal herb throughout England and France. And this common herb does, in fact, offer several medicinal benefits, including the ability to reduce fever, promote sweating, and relieve cramps. (Reports of a psychedelic effect from Catnip smoke are, however, inaccurate. They stem from confusion of the plant with cannabis.)

A perennial plant often reaching a 3-foot height, *Nepeta cataria* is native to Europe, and now grows wild in the United States as well. It has a pleasant, mint-like aroma. The leaves and tender shoots are considered medicinal.

Avoid If . . .

No known medical conditions preclude the use of Catnip.

Special Cautions

At customary dosage levels, Catnip appears to pose no risks.

Possible Drug Interactions

No interactions have been reported.

Special Information If You Are Pregnant or Breastfeeding

No harmful effects are known.

How to Prepare

To make tea, use 10 teaspoonfuls of Catnip per quart of water. Steep for 10 minutes.

Typical Dosage

Take 2 to 3 cups of tea daily.

Overdosage

No information on overdosage is available.

Cayenne

Latin name: Capsicum annuum
Other names: Chili Pepper,
  Paprika, Red Pepper

A Remedy For

- Muscular tension
- Rheumatism

Applied in a cream, Cayenne also relieves painful muscle spasms in the shoulder, arm, and spine areas, bursitis, the pain of shingles, phantom pain following amputation, and the pain of diabetic neuropathy.

Taken orally, Cayenne has also been used as a remedy for stomachaches, cramps, gas, indigestion, loss of appetite, diarrhea, alcoholism, seasickness, malarial fever, yellow fever, and other fevers, and has been taken as a preventive measure against hardening of the arteries, stroke, and heart disease. Its effectiveness for these purposes has not, however, been scientifically verified.

What It Is; Why It Works

Capsaicin, the active ingredient in Cayenne, depletes the chemical messengers that send signals through the pain-sensing peripheral nerves, thus deadening the sensation of pain even when its cause remains present. The effect builds up gradually, so capsaicin-containing creams must be applied regularly in order to provide relief.

A member of the same family that produces bell peppers, jalapeños, and paprika, Cayenne originated in Mexico and Central America, but today is cultivated in all warmer regions of the globe. In general, the hotter the pepper, the greater its medicinal value.

Avoid If . . .

No known medical conditions currently preclude the use of Cayenne, but you should avoid applying capsaicin creams to areas of broken skin.

Special Cautions

Limit external use of full-strength Cayenne to no more than 2 days, since longer use can cause skin inflammation, blisters, and ulcers. To avoid severe burning, keep all capsaicin-containing creams away from the eyes and mucous membranes; wash your hands thoroughly after each application.

When taken internally, Cayenne can cause diarrhea and cramps. High doses taken over extended periods of time may cause chronic stomach problems, kidney damage, liver damage, or nerve problems.

Possible Drug Interactions

No interactions have been reported.

Special Information If You Are Pregnant or Breastfeeding

Studies of Cayenne's effects during pregnancy have produced contradictory results. Until its safety is conclusively demonstrated, the wisest course while pregnant is to avoid its use.

How to Prepare

Cayenne is available in fresh and dried forms, as a liquid extract, and in creams and ointments containing 0.025% to 0.075% capsaicin.

Typical Dosage

Apply capsaicin cream 4 or 5 times daily. Allow 4 weeks for maximum benefit.

Since the potency of commercial preparations may vary, follow the manufacturer's directions whenever available.

Overdosage

An overdose of Cayenne can precipitate a drastic, life-threatening decline in body temperature. If you suspect an overdose, seek medical attention immediately.

Celandine

Latin name: Chelidonium majus
Other name: Tetterwort

A Remedy For
- Appetite loss
- Liver and gallbladder problems

Although its effectiveness has been conclusively verified for only the two problems shown above, Celandine is frequently used for a wide variety of other ailments, including stomach problems, intestinal polyps, breast lumps, chest pain (angina), cramps, asthma, hardening of the arteries, high blood pressure, stomach cancer, gout, and water retention. The fresh roots are sometimes chewed to relieve toothache, and a powder derived from the roots can be applied to ease tooth extraction. The herb has also been used for an assortment of skin conditions, such as rashes, scabies, and warts. In China, it is used to correct irregular menstrual periods.

What It Is; Why It Works
Celandine enjoys a long-standing reputation as a medicinal herb. The Roman scholar Pliny mentions its healing power, and we know that in the 14th century it was taken in liquid form as a blood tonic and was thought to sharpen sight and other senses. It was also used as an aid to wound healing, and was believed to be good for jaundice because of its vivid yellow flowers.

Only the above-ground parts of the plant have been tested for medicinal value. They exhibit mild pain-killing and sedative effects and appear to ease spasms of the internal organs. The plant may also inhibit the growth of cancers, combat infection, and boost resistance. Claims that it can reduce blood pressure and ease muscle tension require further testing.

Avoid If . . .
No known medical conditions preclude the use of Celandine.

Special Cautions
When taken in customary doses, Celandine poses no risks. Avoid contact with the eyes.

Possible Drug Interactions
No interactions have been reported.

Special Information If You Are Pregnant or Breastfeeding
No harmful effects are known.

How to Prepare
Celandine is supplied as a crushed herb and a powder, and in pills and liquids containing Celandine extract. To make Celandine tea, use 15 grams (1 tablespoonful) of crushed herb per quart of water. Steep the mixture for 15 minutes.

Typical Dosage
The usual daily dose of Celandine should supply 12 to 30 milligrams of its active ingredients.

This works out to roughly 2 to 4 grams of extract. If using Celandine tea, drink 3 cups daily between meals.

The strength of commercial preparations may vary. Follow the manufacturer's instructions whenever available.

Overdosage
It was once thought that Celandine could produce nausea, vomiting, bloody diarrhea, blood in the urine, and stupor, but recent studies offer no clear proof of this.

Centaury

Latin name: Centaurium umbellatum

Other names: Bitter Clover, Bitterbloom, Christ's Ladder, Feverwort, Wild Succory

A Remedy For
• Appetite loss

Although Centaury has been judged worthwhile only for poor appetite, it also has some effect against fever and is used for this purpose in homeopathic medicine. Other uses—all of doubtful effectiveness—include treatment of high blood pressure, kidney stones, diabetes, indigestion, and worms.

What It Is; Why It Works
This bitter-tasting plant is found in Mediterranean regions and as far north as Britain and Scandinavia. It is also cultivated in the United States. The medicinal parts of Centaury are the dried flowers, which grow purple to pink-red and occasionally white. A diminutive annual, the plant generally reaches a height of less than a foot.

Centaury works by stimulating production of saliva and digestive juices. It also has some effect on inflammation and fever. In medieval times it was recommended for snakebite and poisoning. Its name stems from Greek mythology, in which the centaur, Chiron, was said to have cured his wounds with the plant.

Avoid If . . .
Because Centaury tends to increase stomach acids, you should avoid it if you have an ulcer.

Special Cautions
At customary dosage levels, Centaury poses no particular risks.

Possible Drug Interactions
No drug interactions have been reported.

Special Information If You Are Pregnant or Breastfeeding
No harmful effects are known.

How to Prepare
Centaury is available in crushed, powdered, and liquid extract form.

To make a tea, pour 150 milliliters (5 ounces) of boiling water over 2 to 3 grams (about one-half teaspoonful) of crushed Centaury, steep for 15 minutes, and strain.

Typical Dosage

Crushed herb: 6 grams daily
Liquid extract: 1 to 2 grams daily
Tea: Half an hour before meals

The strength of commercial preparations may vary. Follow the manufacturer's directions whenever available.

Store away from light and moisture in a tightly sealed container.

Overdosage

No information on overdosage is available.

Chamomile

Latin name: Matricaria chamomilla

A Remedy For

- Appetite loss
- Bronchitis
- Colds
- Cough
- Fever
- Liver and gallbladder problems
- Skin inflammation
- Sore throat
- Tendency to infection
- Wounds and burns

Chamomile is also used internally to treat inflammation and spasms of the digestive tract.

What It Is; Why It Works

This traditional home remedy is native to Europe and northwest Asia, and now grows in North America and elsewhere as well. A small plant (8 to 16 inches in height), it sports little white and yellow flowers.

The entire flowering plant, or the flowers alone, may be used medicinally. It relieves inflammation and spasms, promotes wound healing, and fights bacteria.

Avoid If . . .

There are no known medical conditions that preclude the use of Chamomile.

Special Cautions

At customary dosages, Chamomile does not have side effects. However, a few people develop an allergy to the herb over time.

Possible Drug Interactions

No interactions have been reported.

Special Information If You Are Pregnant or Breastfeeding

No harmful effects are known.

How to Prepare

Chamomile tea: Pour 5 ounces (about one-half cup) of boiling water over 3 grams (about 3 teaspoonfuls) of Chamomile. Cover for 5 to 10 minutes and strain.

Chamomile compress: Pour 1½ cups of hot water over 2 teaspoonfuls of Chamomile. Cover, steep for 15 minutes, then strain. Soak a cloth in the lukewarm water and apply to the affected skin throughout the day.

Bath additive: Mix about 16 tablespoonfuls of Chamomile with 1 quart of water and add to the bath.

Chamomile ointments and gels may be used externally throughout the day.

Typical Dosage

The usual oral dosage is 10 to 15 grams (approximately 3 to 5 tablepoonfuls) daily.

Overdosage

No information on overdosage is available.

Chestnut

Latin name: Castanea sativa
Other names: Spanish Chestnut,
Sweet Chestnut

A Remedy For

Chestnut leaf is used as a remedy for poor circulation and upper respiratory disorders such as cough, sore throat, and bronchitis. In homeopathic medicine, it's prescribed for diarrhea, low back pain, and whooping cough. There is no evidence, however, that supports its effectiveness for any of these problems.

What It Is; Why It Works

Chestnut trees grow in northern, temperate regions near the coast. Once fed to the pigs in England, Chestnuts provide the French with the delicacy known as "marrons glacés." Although the Chestnut leaf is used as a remedy, there is no information on its medicinal actions, if any.

Avoid If . . .

No known medical conditions preclude the use of Chestnut.

Special Cautions

At customary dosage levels, Chestnut poses no threat.

Possible Drug Interactions

There are no known drug interactions with Chestnut.

Special Information If You Are Pregnant or Breastfeeding

No information is available.

How to Prepare

Chestnut is available in crushed-leaf and liquid-extract form.

To make a tea, pour boiling water over 5 grams (about 1 teaspoonful) crushed leaf and strain.

Typical Dosage

Doses of both the leaf and the liquid extract are typically 5 grams (1 teaspoonful).

Strengths of commercial preparations may vary. Follow the manufacturer's labeling whenever available.

Overdosage

No information is available.

Chickweed

Latin name: Stellaria media
Other names: Adder's Mouth,
Passerina, Satin Flower,
Starweed, Stitchwort, Tongue-
grass, Winterweed

A Remedy For

Chickweed has not gained official recognition as a remedy, but is sometimes taken for gout, joint stiffness, tuberculosis, and blood diseases. Applied externally, it's also used for psoriasis, eczema, and other skin diseases; wounds and burns; hemorrhoids; and eye inflammation.

What It Is; Why It Works
This long, heavily branched, creeping weed is found worldwide. Its popularity with birds probably accounts for its name. The above-ground portions of the plant are used medicinally, either fresh or dried.

Avoid If . . .
No known medical conditions preclude the use of Chickweed.

Special Cautions
No side effects or precautions have been documented.

Possible Drug Interactions
No interactions have been reported.

Special Information If You Are Pregnant or Breastfeeding
No harmful effects are known.

How to Prepare
For internal use, Chickweed can be made into a tea. For skin problems, it can be used as a bath additive or applied in a compress.

Typical Dosage
There are no general guidelines on record. Follow the manufacturer's instructions whenever available.

Overdosage
No information on overdosage is available.

Chicory

Latin name: Cichorium intybus
Other names: Hendibeh, Succory

A Remedy For
• Appetite loss
• Indigestion
• Liver and gallbladder problems

In Asia, Chicory has been used for headache, inflammations, sore throat, and skin allergies. It has also been used extensively for malaria, and in folk medicine, as a laxative for children. Its effectiveness for these uses has not been verified.

What It Is; Why It Works
As a vegetable, Chicory is mentioned by the ancient authors Horace, Pliny, Virgil, and Ovid. The blanched leaves can be used cooked and in salads. In France and Belgium, the roots are sliced, kiln-dried, roasted, ground, and added to coffee, imparting a slightly bitter taste and dark color.

For medicinal purposes, the leaves, the roots, and the entire plant—both fresh and dried—are all subject to use. Chicory works by increasing the flow of bile into the digestive tract.

Avoid If . . .
No known health conditions preclude the use of Chicory.

Special Cautions
At typical dosage levels, Chicory poses no hazards. A few people find that they are sensitive to skin contact with the herb.

Possible Drug Interactions
No interactions have been reported.

Special Information If You Are Pregnant or Breastfeeding
No harmful effects are known.

How to Prepare
To prepare Chicory tea, pour boiling water on 2 to 4 grams (about one-half to three-quarters teaspoonful) of dried Chicory, steep for 10 minutes, then strain.

Typical Dosage
The usual single dose is 2 to 4 grams of the herb in tea. The total daily dosage is 3 to 5 grams (up to 1 teaspoonful) of chopped Chicory.

Overdosage
No information on overdosage is available.

China Orange

Latin name: Citrus sinensis
Other names: Citrus Dulcis, Sweet Orange

A Remedy For
- Appetite loss
- Indigestion

What It Is; Why It Works
The outer peel of this particular variety of orange has a calming effect on the stomach.

Like other citrus trees, China Orange originated in Asia, but is now cultivated in subtropical regions worldwide. The plant was probably brought to Europe by Arab invaders.

Avoid If . . .
No known medical conditions preclude the use of China Orange.

Special Cautions
At customary dosage levels, China Orange poses no dangers.

Possible Drug Interactions
No drug interactions have been reported.

Special Information If You Are Pregnant or Breastfeeding
No harmful effects are known.

How to Prepare
Use only the fruit's outer rind; discard the white pith layer below it. The peel can be used fresh or dried.

Typical Dosage
China Orange is taken orally. The usual daily dosage is 10 to 15 grams (2 to 3 teaspoonfuls).

Overdosage
No information on overdosage is available.

Chinese Cinnamon

Latin name: Cinnamomum aromaticum
Other names: Bastard Cinnamon, Cassia, False Cinnamon

A Remedy For
- Appetite loss
- Bronchitis
- Colds
- Cough
- Fever
- Indigestion
- Sore throat
- Tendency to infection

This herb is also used to treat exhaustion and promote weight gain; and in Chinese medicine, it has been used for impotence, diarrhea, bed-wetting, rheumatism, testicle hernia, failure to menstruate, and symptoms of menopause. Its effectiveness for these conditions, however, remains unconfirmed.

What It Is; Why It Works
A common household spice, Chinese Cinnamon is cultivated in southern China, Vietnam, and Burma. The flowers, young twigs, and the bark of thin branches are all considered medicinal.

Researchers have found that the active agents in Chinese Cinnamon exhibit antibacterial properties, control the growth of fungi, boost immunity in animals, improve intestinal activity, and inhibit ulcers.

Avoid If . . .
No known medical conditions preclude the use of Chinese Cinnamon.

Special Cautions
No side effects are likely when this herb is used at customary dosage levels. However, some people develop a sensitivity to the herb.

Possible Drug Interactions
No interactions have been reported.

Special Information If You Are Pregnant or Breastfeeding
Chinese Cinnamon has a potentially abortive effect. Do not use it during pregnancy.

How to Prepare
Chinese Cinnamon is available as crushed bark, in solutions of alcohol, and as an essential oil.

Typical Dosage
Herb: The average dose is 1 gram (less than one-quarter teaspoonful). Take 2 to 4 grams daily.
Essential oil: 50 to 200 miligrams daily.

Store Chinese Cinnamon in cool, dry conditions in well-sealed containers.

Overdosage
No information on overdosage is available.

Chinese Foxglove Root

Latin name: Rehmannia glutinosa

A Remedy For
In China, this herb is often recommended for insomnia, restlessness, night sweats, chronic fever, and hot flashes. It's also consid-

ered a remedy for menstrual irregularity and uterine bleeding, especially after childbirth, and is taken for light-headedness, palpitations, stiff joints, low back pain, constipation, blurred vision, and hearing problems. Its effectiveness remains to be verified.

What It Is; Why It Works
In Chinese medicine, this thick, reddish yellow root is often cooked in wine and used as a tonic for the effects of aging. Its mode of action is unknown.

Avoid If . . .
People with digestive problems, especially those with a tendency to develop gas or bloating, should use Chinese Foxglove carefully; the cooked root can distend the abdomen and cause loose stools.

Special Cautions
Side effects may include diarrhea, nausea, and abdominal pain. To prevent these problems, Chinese herbalists frequently include in their Chinese Foxglove preparations an additive called "grains-of-paradise fruit."

Possible Drug Interactions
No interactions have been reported.

Special Information If You Are Pregnant or Breastfeeding
No harmful effects are known.

How to Prepare
Both the cooked root and the raw version can be found in Chinese pharmacies, Asian markets, and some Western health food stores.

Typical Dosage
There are no formal guidelines on record. Chinese medical practitioners often use Chinese Foxglove as part of various therapeutic combinations.

Overdosage
No information on overdosage is available.

Chondroitin

A Remedy For
- Osteoarthritis

Although many doctors demand further evidence, there's no longer any question that Chondroitin has provided relief to at least some arthritis sufferers. It is said to ease joint pain, reduce inflammation, and even repair the damaged cartilage that cushions the joints.

Because of its beneficial effect on connective tissue, Chondroitin has also been used to treat torn ligaments and tendons. And some advocates suggest that it can relieve the pain of gout, cure headaches, relieve respiratory ailments and allergies, hasten wound healing, prevent cancer, improve cardiovascular health, and stave off the effects of aging. For these many additional claims, however, there is still no solid scientific evidence.

What It Is; Why It Works
Chondroitin is a complex carbohydrate found in the connective tissue of all mammals. In the resilient cartilage that pads the

joints, Chondroitin acts like a magnet, drawing fluid into the tissues. This fluid plays two important roles: It attracts essential nutrients to the area, and it makes the cartilage spongier and better able to absorb shocks. Chondroitin also protects healthy cartilage from premature decline by preventing the production of certain enzymes that weaken connective tissue and defeating others that stop nutrients from reaching the cartilage.

Many researchers are convinced that Chondroitin strengthens the protein strands that make up connective tissue. There is also some evidence that, because it contains complex sugar molecules called glycosaminoglycans, it not only can reduce inflammation but can actually rebuild cartilage, especially if the tissue has not been totally destroyed. Chondroitin seems to play an active role in reducing the pain that often accompanies osteoarthritis; and, in some cases, it may even eliminate the need for surgery.

Although Chondroitin often works well on its own, it is most effective when combined with glucosamine sulfate. Advocates caution, however, that although this combination may help some people reduce their need for powerful painkillers such as nonsteroidal anti-inflammatories (NSAIDs), it will not work for everyone. It is also not guaranteed to restore complete mobility.

Avoid If . . .

Unless your doctor approves, do not give any preparation containing Chondroitin to children under 2 years of age.

Special Cautions

Children between the ages of 2 and 6 can usually take as much as 10 grams of Chondroitin per day without side effects.

Although Chondroitin contains sugar molecules, it is considered safe for diabetics.

Possible Drug Interactions

Consult your physician before taking Chondroitin if you are taking an anticoagulant drug such as Coumadin, or if you have a blood clotting disorder.

Chondroitin may interfere with the action of prescription and nonprescription drugs, herbal preparations, and nutritional supplements. If you are using any of these preparations, talk to your doctor before taking Chondroitin.

Special Information If You Are Pregnant or Breastfeeding

Do not take Chondroitin while pregnant or breastfeeding.

How to Prepare

Chondroitin sulfate capsules and Chondroitin sulfate/glucosamine sulfate combination capsules and tablets can be found in many health food stores or may be ordered by mail.

Typical Dosage

There are no standard dosage guidelines. Some advocates recommend 400 milligrams 3 times a day with meals. Others suggest doses ranging from 250 and

1,600 milligrams a day, depending on body weight.

For those using a combination of Chondroitin sulfate and glucosamine sulfate, a typical dosage recommendation is based on weight:

Less than 120 pounds: 800 milligrams Chondroitin, 1,000 milligrams Glucosamine
120 to 200 pounds: 1,200 milligrams Chondroitin, 1,500 milligrams Glucosamine
More than 200 pounds: 1,600 milligrams Chondroitin, 2,000 milligrams Glucosamine

You may adjust your dosage according to your response. If you are overweight or are taking a water pill (diuretic), you may need a larger dose of each supplement.

Overdosage
No information on overdosage is available.

Cinchona

Latin name: Cinchona pubescens
Other names: Jesuit's Bark, Peruvian Bark

A Remedy For
• Appetite loss
• Indigestion

Cinchona has many other uses, for the majority of which effectiveness is unconfirmed. In Asia it's taken for bacterial infections, chronic dysentery, fevers, and malaria. Homeopathic uses include gout, excessive irritability, and inflammation of the kidney. In folk medicine, it has also been used for fullness, gas, flu, enlarged spleen, muscle cramps, cancer, scrapes, and leg ulcers.

What It Is; Why It Works
Cinchona is an evergreen tree that grows 15 to 45 feet in height. It is named after the Countess of Cinchon, who first alerted Europe to the medicinal properties of the bark. It is native to mountainous regions of tropical America, but is cultivated elsewhere.

Cinchona is the original source of quinine, which in its purified form is used as a cure for malaria, the mosquito-borne plague of the tropics. In addition, quinine-based drugs such as Quinaglute and Quinidex are prescribed to control dangerous heartbeat irregularities.

For medicinal purposes, only the dried bark of 6- to 8-year-old trees has proven useful. Researchers have found that the unrefined bark stimulates production of saliva and gastric juices.

Avoid If . . .
There are no known medical conditions that preclude the use of Cinchona.

Special Cautions
If you have hemophilia or other bleeding problems, you should be aware that Cinchona can delay clotting. Quinine and quinine-based drugs have also been known to cause allergic skin reactions (eczema or itching). Remember, too, that when taken habitually or

used in excessive doses, Cinchona can be quite toxic. (See "Overdosage" below.)

Possible Drug Interactions
No interactions have been reported.

Special Information If You Are Pregnant or Breastfeeding
No harmful effects are known.

How to Prepare
Cinchona preparations range from dried bark to liquid extracts of varying potencies. You can make a medicinal tea by pouring boiling water over one-half teaspoonful of Cinchona and steeping it for 10 minutes.

Typical Dosage
Dried herb: 1 to 3 grams daily
5% liquid extract: 0.6 to 3 grams daily
20% extract: 150 to 600 milligrams daily

Because commercial preparations vary in potency, always be sure to follow the manufacturer's directions. Cinchona should be stored in a well-sealed container, protected from light and moisture.

Overdosage
Long-term use of Cinchona can lead to a build-up of the drug in the body, and hence to an overdose. Symptoms are primarily due to the bark's quinine content. As little as 3 grams (about one-half teaspoonful) of quinine can cause nausea, headache, a drop in body temperature, irregular heartbeat, buzzing in the ears, and hearing and visual disorders including deafness and blindness. Death comes with doses of 10 to 15 grams (about 2 to 3 teaspoonfuls) of quinine, which cause heart failure and asphyxiation.

If you suspect an overdose, seek medical attention immediately.

Cinnamon

Latin name: Cinnamomum verum

A Remedy For
- Appetite loss
- Bronchitis
- Colds
- Cough
- Fever
- Indigestion
- Sore throat
- Tendency to infection

Though its effectiveness for other uses is unconfirmed, Cinnamon is prescribed in homeopathic medicine for diarrhea, hemorrhage, and cancerous tumors. Additional Asian uses include heart problems, dental pain, and urinary problems. In folk medicine, Cinnamon is used internally for diarrhea in infants, chills, influenza, and worm infestation, and externally for cleaning wounds.

What It Is; Why It Works
A familiar ingredient in toothpaste, mouthwash, perfume, soap, lipstick, chewing gum, and cola drinks, Cinnamon is native to Sri

Lanka and southwest India. In the 18th century, the Dutch monopolized the Cinnamon trade, refusing to allow commercial farming until 1776 for fear that cultivation would destroy the valuable properties of the spice. Today, virtually all Cinnamon comes from cultivated trees.

The medicinal value of Cinnamon lies in the oil extracted from the bark and leaves. Substances in it have been shown to kill certain bacteria and fungi and to improve digestion. It is also an insecticide. This "true" form of cinnamon should not be confused with other varieties, such as Chinese cinnamon.

Avoid If . . .

There are no known medical conditions that preclude the use of Cinnamon.

Special Cautions

Be alert for unwanted effects. Cinnamon can cause a reaction in some individuals.

Possible Drug Interactions

No interactions have been reported.

Special Information If You Are Pregnant or Breastfeeding

Do not use Cinnamon while pregnant.

How to Prepare

You can prepare a tea by pouring boiling water over 0.5 to 1 gram (about one-eighth teaspoonful) of Cinnamon bark and steeping it for 10 minutes.

Typical Dosage

Crushed Cinnamon: 2 to 4 grams (about one-half teaspoonful) daily

Essential oil: 50 to 200 milligrams daily

Tea: 1 cup 2 to 3 times daily with meals

Liquid extract: 0.5 to 1 milliliter 3 times daily

Alcohol solution (tincture): Up to 4 milliliters (almost 1 teaspoonful) 3 times daily

Potency of commercial preparations may vary. Follow the manufacturer's instructions whenever available. Store away from light and moisture in a nonsynthetic container.

Overdosage

No information on overdosage is available.

Citronella

Latin name: Cymbopogon species
Other name: Lemongrass

A Remedy For

Citronella is sometimes used to treat indigestion, although its effectiveness remains to be proven. In Asian medicine, the herb is used for loss of appetite, gas, worms, and throat problems.

What It Is; Why It Works

Well known as an insect repellent, Citronella is often used as a fragrance in cheaper household soaps and scents. Medicinally, it acts as a mild astringent, tightening and drying the tissues. Lemongrass, a closely related species, has similar effects.

A native of the Asian tropics, Citronella grass is now cultivated in Central and South America and tropical regions of Australia as well.

Avoid If . . .
No known medical conditions preclude the use of Citronella.

Special Cautions
Salves containing Citronella have been known to cause an allergic reaction in rare cases. Do not inhale the vapors of Citronella oil, as this could cause lung problems.

Possible Drug Interactions
No interactions have been reported.

Special Information If You Are Pregnant or Breastfeeding
No harmful effects are known.

How to Prepare
The above-ground parts of the plant and its essential oil are both used medicinally.

Typical Dosage
There are no standard recommendations.

Overdosage
No information on overdosage is available.

Clivers

Latin name: Galium aparine
Other names: Barweed,
  Bedstraw, Catchweed, Goose
  Grass, Grip Grass, Hayruff,
  Hedge-burs, Scratchweed,
  Stick-a-back

A Remedy For
Clivers is sometimes used to treat urinary tract infections and skin disorders, but its effectiveness remains to be proven. Other unverified uses include ulcers, infected glands, kidney and bladder stones, bladder inflammation, difficult urination, swelling due to water retention, and breast lumps. In Asian medicine it's considered a remedy for stomach bloating, blood in the urine and other urinary problems, and deep-seated skin infections (carbuncles).

What It Is; Why It Works
This climbing, clinging plant, studded with thorny leaves, reaches a height of 2 to 5 feet. It grows wild throughout Europe, Asia, and North and South America. Known since the days of the Roman Empire, it is sometimes used as a coffee substitute and was formerly employed as a red coloring agent.

The dried above-ground parts of the plant are used medicinally. Its mode of action is unknown.

Avoid If . . .
No known medical conditions preclude the use of Clivers.

Special Cautions
At customary dosage levels, Clivers appears to pose no risks.

Possible Drug Interactions
No interactions have been reported.

Special Information If You Are Pregnant or Breastfeeding
No harmful effects are known.

How to Prepare
Clivers is taken as a tea, a juice, or an alcoholic extract, and can be applied externally for skin problems. To make a tea, add 4 teaspoons Clivers to 2 glasses of hot water.

Typical Dosage
For internal use, take the tea in sips throughout the day.

Overdosage
No information on overdosage is available.

Cloves

Latin name: Syzygium aromaticum

A Remedy For
• Bronchitis
• Colds
• Cough
• Dental pain
• Fever
• Sore throat
• Tendency to infection

In Asian medicine, Cloves are also used for stomach ailments, bad breath, and skin diseases, but their effectiveness for these purposes has not been confirmed.

What It Is; Why It Works
An extremely aromatic plant (the entire tree smells of Cloves), this familiar herb grows in tropical regions such as Tanzania, Madagascar, and Brazil. The medicinal element, oil of Cloves, is extracted from the plant's flower buds, leaves, and fruit. Boasting antibacterial, antifungal, antiviral, and pain-killing effects, it is used primarily as a local anesthetic, especially for toothache.

The Cloves found in the typical kitchen spice rack are flower buds picked at the embryo stage. (If picked when mature, they lose their pungency.) They appeared in Europe as early as the 4th century AD. In India and Indonesia, they are still smoked in cigarettes.

Avoid If . . .
No known health conditions preclude the use of Clove oil.

Special Cautions
In concentrated form, Clove oil can be irritating to mucous membranes. Allergic reactions, although rare, have been known to occur.

Possible Drug Interactions
No drug interactions have been reported.

Special Information If You Are Pregnant or Breastfeeding
No harmful effects are known.

How to Prepare
Cloves are used as a powder, ground herb, or whole herb.

Typical Dosage
A solution of 1 to 5% essential oil can be used as a mouthwash. Undiluted oil of Cloves is used for pain relief in dentistry.

Overdosage
No information on overdosage is available.

Cocoa

Latin name: Theobroma cacao
Other names: Cacao, Chocolate

A Remedy For
Cocoa is sometimes recommended for diarrhea, urinary tract infections, and liver and gallbladder disorders. However, there's little evidence of its effectiveness for these problems. Other unverified uses include diabetes and intestinal infections.

What It Is; Why It Works
It could have been a dream come true: The main ingredient in chocolate revealed as a medical necessity! Unfortunately, Cocoa's medicinal effects are actually quite limited. It does contain compounds that expand airway passages, dilate blood vessels, flush excess water from the body, strengthen the heartbeat, and relax the muscles. However, the amounts are too small for any practical effect.

Appropriately, the Latin name for Cocoa means "food of the gods." The more familiar "chocolate" is a corruption of the Mexican word for pounded Cocoa beans. The source of Cocoa, a small tree some 13 to 20 feet in height, is cultivated in tropical regions around the world.

Avoid If . . .
If you suffer from migraine, it's best to avoid chocolate. It carries compounds that can trigger attacks. Avoid it, too, if it sparks an allergic reaction.

Special Cautions
Cocoa contains significant amounts of caffeine, so overindulgence in chocolate products can lead to overexcitability, a racing pulse, and sleep disorders. In large amounts, Cocoa can also cause constipation.

Possible Drug Interactions
No drug interactions have been reported.

Special Information If You Are Pregnant or Breastfeeding
No harmful effects are known.

How to Prepare
Commercial food products abound.

Typical Dosage
Given Cocoa's lack of significant therapeutic effect, the best course is to seek an alternative.

Overdosage
No information on overdosage is available.

Coenzyme Q10

A Remedy For
• Weak heart

Like all heart medications, Coenzyme Q10 is not a cure. However, for some people suffering from congestive heart failure, irregular heartbeat, or angina, it may ease symptoms and improve cardiac function. Some doctors also recommend it after heart surgery to speed recovery with a minimum of permanent damage.

Some advocates contend that Coenzyme Q10 can stave off hardening of the arteries by discouraging the build-up of plaque on artery walls. Others suggest that it can boost the immune system, helping to prevent the spread of cancer. It has also been recommended for a host of additional disorders ranging from high blood pressure, diabetes, allergies, and fatigue to Alzheimer's disease, Bell's palsy, Huntington's disease, Ménière's disease, muscular dystrophy, and deterioration of the retina. However, its effectiveness for all such conditions has yet to be scientifically verified.

What It Is; Why It Works
Found in every cell in the body, Coenzyme Q10 plays a vital role in the production of energy, triggering the conversion of nutrients into a "fuel" for the cells to burn. This substance, called adenosine triphosphate (ATP), can't be stored in quantities sufficient to sustain optimum bodily functions for more than a few minutes. Stores must be continually renewed, making an ample supply of Coenzyme Q10 mandatory.

Adequate levels of the enzyme are particularly crucial for the heart because it's constantly in motion, burning twice as much energy as the other organs. If supplies of the enzyme decline, the action of the heart muscle will tend to weaken, reducing the amount of fresh blood the heart can pump out to the body. It is for this reason that some researchers regard a deficiency of the enzyme as an aggravating factor in conditions such as congestive heart failure.

Good dietary sources of Coenzyme Q10 include beef, pork, and lamb; certain types of fish and shellfish; vegetables such as broccoli and spinach; and vegetable oils. If you have a heart condition, however, you may want to consider a commercial supplement.

Avoid If . . .
No known medical conditions preclude the use of Coenzyme Q10.

Special Cautions
By itself, Coenzyme Q10 is not a sufficient treatment for any type of heart disease. It is generally employed as a supplement, rather than a replacement, for standard medical therapy. Do not attempt to substitute it for any of your regular prescriptions.

Possible Drug Interactions

No interactions have been reported.

Special Information If You Are Pregnant or Breastfeeding

Do not use Coenzyme Q10 while pregnant or breastfeeding.

How to Prepare

Coenzyme Q10 is available in capsule, tablet, softgel (gel cap), and chewable form. To improve its absorption, take it with some type of oil (olive oil is recommended) or fat (peanut butter, for example). It is also best to take your dosage with meals.

Store in a dry and cool place, away from light. Do not allow to freeze.

Typical Dosage

Dosage recommendations range from 30 milligrams to 400 milligrams daily, generally increasing with the severity of the problem. Large daily doses are typically divided into 2 or 3 smaller doses (for example, one 60 milligram tablet taken 2 times a day instead of a single 120 milligram tablet taken once).

If you are taking the enzyme for a heart condition, it may be 2 to 8 weeks before you notice any benefit, and you will need to continue taking the product to maintain any improvement.

Overdosage

Since Coenzyme Q10 is not toxic, experts say you may take large amounts without danger.

Coffee Charcoal

Latin name: Coffea arabica

A Remedy For

• Diarrhea
• Sore throat

When roasted until burned and blackened, then ground to a powder, coffee beans turn out to be an effective remedy for diarrhea and mild cases of sore throat.

Coffee prepared in the ordinary way fights physical and mental fatigue and is sometimes recommended for migraine headache. Homeopathy, under the theory of "like cures like," uses coffee as a *remedy* for nervousness and nerve pain.

What It Is; Why It Works

Caffeine, the active ingredient in coffee, is used to boost the action of a variety of prescription and over-the-counter painkillers, including Excedrin, Vanquish, Fiorinal, Fioricet, Esgic, Wigraine, and BC Powder. Caffeine has numerous physiological effects, serving to flush water out of the body, increase production of digestive juices, and stimulate the brain and nervous system. It also relaxes the walls of the blood vessels (except for vessels in the brain) and the airways in the lungs, while increasing the force of muscular contractions and, in higher concentrations, increasing the heart rate. In people who don't drink coffee, a single cup will cause a notable increase in blood pressure. (Regular coffee drinkers become immune to this effect.)

Caffeine begins to exert its stimulating effects within minutes, reaching maximum concentration in the blood between 15 and 45 minutes after it's taken. Significant amounts remain in the blood for 4 to 6 hours. Medicinal Coffee Charcoal does not, however, depend on caffeine for its effect. Instead, its therapeutic value lies in its ability to absorb liquid and dry out the tissues.

Coffee is believed to have originated in Ethiopia. (The name "coffee" is derived from Caffa, a region of Ethiopia.) It was introduced into Arab countries in the early 15th century, but did not reach Europe until the 16th century, appearing first in Constantinople, then spreading westward. London's first coffeehouse opened in 1652.

Avoid If . . .
Take caffeine with caution if you have a heart condition, kidney disease, an overactive thyroid, a disposition to convulsions, or a tendency to anxiety or panic attacks.

Special Cautions
Coffee Charcoal, when taken at customary dosage levels, has no side effects. Coffee in beverage form is a different matter. It can cause acid stomach, stomach irritation, diarrhea, and poor appetite; and sustained intake can lead to physical dependence. Withdrawal symptoms include headache and sleeping disorders. Drinking large amounts of steeped coffee over an extended period can also lead to a significant increase in levels of total and LDL ("bad") cholesterol. However, use of coffee filters largely eliminates this problem.

Possible Drug Interactions
Coffee Charcoal can interfere with the ability of the body to absorb medicines.

Special Information If You Are Pregnant or Breastfeeding
Many doctors recommend limiting coffee intake during pregnancy to 1 cup a day. There is some evidence that drinking 4 or more cups per day may slow the baby's development. Caffeine may also increase the risk of late first or second trimester miscarriage.

Caffeine intake while breastfeeding can cause sleep disorders in the nursing infant.

How to Prepare
Coffee Charcoal is taken in powder form.

Typical Dosage
The average individual dose of Coffee Charcoal is 3 grams (a heaping half-teaspoonful). Total intake per day should be 9 grams.

Store in a well-sealed container.

Overdosage
Sustained intake of 1,500 milligrams of caffeine daily (the equivalent of 15 cups of coffee) can lead to restlessness, irritability, sleeplessness, palpitations, dizziness, vomiting, diarrhea, loss of appetite, and headache. Higher doses lead to stiffness,

muscle spasms, and rapid, irregular heartbeat. The first signs of outright poisoning are vomiting and abdominal spasms. A lethal overdose is unlikely; it would be the equivalent of about 75 cups of coffee.

Cola Nut

Latin name: Cola acuminata
Other names: Bissy Nut, Gurru Nut, Kola Tree

A Remedy For
• Fatigue

In addition to its role as a remedy for mental and physical fatigue, Cola Nut is chewed to suppress hunger, thirst, morning sickness, and migraine, and is ground into compresses for wounds and inflammation.

What It Is; Why It Works
The source of Cola Nut's energizing effect is none other than common caffeine, which also tends to stimulate the digestive system, speed up the heart, and flush excess fluid from the body. The nut also contains a minute, medicinally useless amount of the asthma drug theophylline.

A native of tropical Africa, the Cola tree is an evergreen that grows to a height of 50 to 65 feet. In its homeland, its nuts are used as a condiment and an aid to digestion.

Avoid If . . .
Because Cola Nut stimulates production of digestive acids, avoid its use if you have a stomach or duodenal ulcer. Also, avoid giving large quantities of Cola drinks to children.

Special Cautions
Side effects are similar to those from coffee: difficulty falling asleep, excitability, restlessness, and stomach complaints.

Possible Drug Interactions
No interactions have been reported.

Special Information If You Are Pregnant or Breastfeeding
No harmful effects are known.

How to Prepare
Cola Nut is available as a dry extract, a fluid extract, an alcohol solution (tincture), and a wine.

Typical Dosage
The customary daily doses are:

Cola Nut: 2 to 6 grams
Cola extract: 250 to 750 milligrams
Cola liquid extract: 2.5 to 7.5 grams (about one-half to 1 1/2 teaspoonfuls)
Cola tincture: 10 to 30 grams (about 2 to 6 teaspoonfuls)
Cola wine: 60 to 180 grams (about one-quarter to three-quarters of a cup)

Because the strength of commercial preparations may vary, follow the manufacturer's instructions whenever available.

Store Cola Nut in sealed containers protected from light.

Overdosage

An overdose of Cola tea or drinks large enough to be dangerous is highly unlikely.

Colchicum

Latin name: Colchicum autumnale
Other names: Autumn Crocus, Meadow Saffron

A Remedy For

• Gout
• Mediterranean fever

Colchicum, which can be extremely poisonous, is used only for these two conditions—and primarily for gout. Mediterranean fever, a painful infection usually contracted from unpasteurized milk products or direct contact with farm animals, can be cured with a combination of antibiotics.

What It Is; Why It Works

Colchicine, the active compound in Colchicum, is one of the ingredients of ColBENEMID, a prescription medication for gout. Researchers do not know how Colchicine works, but it has proven effective both for relieving the pain of acute gout flare-ups and for reducing the frequency of attacks.

Colchicum takes its name from Colchis, the area in which the mythical witch Medea pursued her poisonous ways. The plant's flowers, seeds, and tubers are all medicinal, but are rarely used due to the danger of poisoning.

Avoid If . . .

Do not use during pregnancy (see "Special Information If You Are Pregnant or Breastfeeding" below).

Special Cautions

To avoid toxic effects, take Colchicum only at recommended dosage levels and for limited periods of time. Long-term use can cause kidney and liver damage, hair loss, nerve inflammation, muscle diseases, and bone marrow damage.

Possible Drug Interactions

No interactions have been reported.

Special Information If You Are Pregnant or Breastfeeding

Colchicine stops cell division, and can be harmful to a developing baby. Do not use the drug during pregnancy. Even Colchicum intake by the father can lead to abnormalities as the baby develops.

How to Prepare

Colchicum is available crushed or as a freshly pressed juice.

Typical Dosage

For an acute attack of gout, take an initial oral dose equivalent to 1 milligram of Colchicine, followed by 0.5 to 1.5 milligrams every 1 to 2 hours until the pain subsides. Do not exceed 8 milligrams of Colchicine per day and take no additional doses for at least 3 days.

For Mediterranean fever, should you choose to use Colchicum

rather than antibiotics, the dosage is the equivalent of 0.5 to 1.5 milligrams of Colchicine.

Overdosage

For adults, a dose of only 5 grams of Colchicum seeds can prove fatal. For a child, the lethal dose is 1 to 1.5 grams. A mere 200 milligrams of the active ingredient Colchicine is sufficient to cause death.

The first signs of poisoning appear 3 to 6 hours after intake of a toxic amount, when the victim develops a burning feeling in his mouth, has difficulty swallowing, and begins to experience intense thirst. After 12 to 14 hours, nausea and vomiting set in, accompanied by severe stomach pains, diarrhea, bladder spasms, blood in the urine, a fall in blood pressure, and, eventually, progressive paralysis. Death follows from exhaustion, asphyxiation, and circulatory collapse.

If you recognize any preliminary symptoms of overdosage, seek emergency medical treatment immediately.

Coltsfoot

Latin name: Tussilago farfara
Other names: Ass's Foot, British
Tobacco, Bullsfoot,
Coughwort, Donnhove,
Flower Velure

A Remedy For

Coltsfoot is an effective remedy for bronchitis, cough, and sore throat; but because it contains alkaloids that can damage the liver and cause cancer, its use is not recommended.

What It Is; Why It Works

Coltsfoot leaf has received official recognition as an effective medication for throat irritation. However, the dangers it poses make it an unwise choice. Preparations containing Coltsfoot flower should be avoided entirely.

The plant grows wild throughout most of Europe and much of Asia. It has spread to the mountains of northern Africa and has been introduced into North America. It has a slimy-sweet taste and gives off the smell of honey when the leaves are rubbed.

Coltsfoot works by coating the mucous membranes with a thick protective layer that fends off chemical and physical irritants.

Avoid If . . .

It's best to seek another remedy.

Special Cautions

Make sure that any preparation you take delivers no more than 1 milligram of toxic pyrrolizidine alkaloids and N-oxides on a daily basis.

Possible Drug Interactions

No drug interactions have been reported.

Special Information If You Are Pregnant or Breastfeeding

Be sure to avoid Coltsfoot while pregnant or nursing.

How to Prepare

To make a tea, add 1.5 to 2.5 grams of chopped Coltsfoot to boiling water, steep for 5 to 10 minutes, and strain.

Typical Dosage

The usual daily dosage of Coltsfoot leaf should not exceed 6 grams (about 1 heaping teaspoonful).

Overdosage

No information on overdosage is available.

Comfrey

Latin name: Symphytum officinale

Other names: Ass Ear, Black Root, Blackwort, Boneset, Bruisewort, Consolida, Consound, Gum Plant, Knitbone, Salsify, Slippery Root, Wallwort

A Remedy For

• Bruises, sprains, and dislocations

Applied in ointment form, Comfrey is considered an effective treatment for blunt injuries. The root portion of Comfrey is also used as a mouthwash and gargle for sore throat and gum disease.

Taken internally, the root has also been used as a remedy for stomachache, ulcers, rheumatism, chest congestion, diarrhea, and inflammation in the lining of the lungs; but its effectiveness for these problems is unconfirmed and internal use is not recommended due to the presence of dangerous, cancer-causing compounds.

What It Is; Why It Works

Comfrey has enjoyed a long-standing reputation for healing wounds and broken bones. Its very name, a corruption of the Latin "con firma," means "grow together." Similarly, the Latin name, "symphytum," is from the Greek "symphyo," meaning "to unite." In the early 20th century, allantoin, an active ingredient in Comfrey, was frequently prescribed as a remedy for wounds and ulcers.

There is considerable justification for this reputation. The allantoin in Comfrey stimulates reproduction of cells, thus promoting the formation of new tissue (callus) along the edges of a bone fracture. Other compounds in Comfrey effectively reduce inflammation and swelling.

Nevertheless, this herb—particularly the root—also contains toxic pyrrolizidine alkaloids that are known to cause cancer in animals while inflicting damage on the liver. Internal use of any part of the plant is therefore ill-advised; and the root should be avoided entirely.

Avoid If . . .

Do not use preparations containing Comfrey root. Ointments containing Comfrey leaf are considered safe when applied to unbroken skin for limited periods of time.

Special Cautions

Limit use of leaf-based Comfrey ointments to no more than 4 weeks.

Possible Drug Interactions

No interactions have been reported.

Special Information If You Are Pregnant or Breastfeeding

Never use any form of Comfrey during pregnancy or while breastfeeding.

How to Prepare

Use only commercially prepared ointments and creams.

Typical Dosage

In Europe, the German Federal Health Agency limits commercial preparations of Comfrey to amounts that supply no more than 1 microgram of toxic pyrrolizidine alkaloids per day when taken internally, or 100 micrograms per day when applied to the skin. In the United States, herbal preparations are not routinely monitored for potency, so there's no way to be certain that these limits are met. Follow the manufacturer's directions whenever available. When in doubt, use the ointment as sparingly as possible.

Overdosage

No information on overdosage is available.

Condurango

Latin name: Marsdenia condurango
Other name: Eagle Vine

A Remedy For

- Appetite loss
- Indigestion

What It Is; Why It Works

Condurango improves digestion by stimulating the production of saliva and digestive juices. It has also shown an ability to kill tumors in animals, and it was once thought to be a useful treatment for early cancers in humans. Its effectiveness against human cancer remains unconfirmed, however, and its former use as a treatment for stomach cancer has been discontinued.

The part of Condurango that is used in remedies is the dried bark of branches and the trunk of the tree.

Condurango grows on the western slopes of the Andes in Ecuador, Peru, and Colombia. The medicinal part of the tree is its dried bark.

Avoid If . . .

No known medical problems preclude the use of Condurango.

Special Cautions

When taken at customary dosage levels, Condurango presents no problems.

Possible Drug Interactions

No interactions have been reported.

Special Information If You Are Pregnant or Breastfeeding

No harmful effects are known.

How to Prepare

Condurango can be made into a tea. Add 1.5 grams (about one-quarter teaspoonful) of crushed Condurango to cold water and bring to a boil. Cool the tea, then strain.

Condurango also can be made into a medicinal wine. Add 50 to 100 grams (between one-quarter and one-half cup) of crushed Condurango to each liter of wine.

Take 1 cup of Condurango tea or 1 liquor glass of wine with each meal.

Typical Dosage

Condurango is taken orally. The usual daily dosage is:

Aqueous extract: 200 to 500 milligrams
Alcohol solution (tincture): 2 to 5 grams (about one-half to 1 teaspoonful)
Liquid extract: 2 to 4 grams
Crushed bark: 2 to 4 grams

Overdosage

No information on overdosage is available.

Coriander

Latin name: Coriandrum sativum

A Remedy For

- Appetite loss
- Indigestion

In folk medicine, Coriander has also been used to treat coughs, chest pains, bladder complaints, leprosy, rash, fever, diarrhea, headaches, mouth and throat disorders, bad breath, and childbirth complications; and in Asia, it is used for heartburn, diarrhea, hemorrhoids, measles, sore throat, rectal prolapse, and vomiting. Its effectiveness for these conditions remains unproven.

What It Is; Why It Works

Coriander has been used as an herbal remedy for centuries. In China, eating the seeds was thought to confer immortality. During the Middle Ages, Coriander was recommended as a treatment for anthrax and the epidemic illness St. Anthony's Fire.

The seeds and their oil are the medicinal part of the plant. The essential oil in Coriander stimulates digestive juices, relieves gas, and stops stomach and intestinal cramps. In laboratory experiments, it has shown an ability to kill bacteria and fungus.

The name Coriandrum comes from the Greek "koros," or "bug," a name given the herb because of the unpleasant smell of its unripe berries. When dried, however, the berries gain a pleasantly tangy odor; and Coriander is therefore used not only as a remedy, but also as a spice in candies, bread, and some alcoholic drinks, including gin. The related kitchen spice cilantro comes from the leaves of the coriander plant, but has a different flavor and is not used as a remedy.

Avoid If . . .

There are no known reasons to avoid Coriander.

Special Cautions

Coriander poses no known risks when taken at usual dosage levels. There is a slight possibility that you could develop a sensitivity to the herb.

Possible Drug Interactions

No interactions have been reported.

Special Information If You Are Pregnant or Breastfeeding

No harmful effects are known.

How to Prepare

A Coriander tea can be made by steeping 2 teaspoonfuls of crushed Coriander in 1 cup of boiling water for 15 minutes. Strain before drinking.

Typical Dosage

Coriander is taken orally. The usual dosage is:

Crushed Coriander seed: 1 gram 3 times daily
Coriander tea: 1 cup between meals
Coriander tincture (a solution of Coriander in alcohol): 10 to 20 drops after meals

Coriander should be stored in a sealed container in a cool, dark place.

Overdosage

No information on overdosage is available.

Corn Poppy

Latin name: Papaver rhoeas
Other names: Copperose, Corn Rose, Cup-Puppy, Headwark, Red Poppy

A Remedy For

Corn Poppy is sometimes used as a remedy for colds, coughs, and bronchitis, but conclusive proof of its effectiveness remains lacking. It is also used—again without validation—as a painkiller and sedative.

What It Is; Why It Works

Source of the familiar poppy seeds used in baking, the Corn Poppy grows in most temperate regions of the world. Its 4-inch scarlet or crimson flowers sit atop a 10- to 36-inch stem. The blossom—not the seed—is considered medicinal.

Avoid If . . .

No known medical conditions preclude the use of Corn Poppy.

Special Cautions

Although Corn Poppy presents no problems at customary dosage levels, there have been reports of poisoning in children who ate the fresh leaves and blossoms. Symptoms included stomach pain and vomiting.

Possible Drug Interactions

No interactions have been reported.

Special Information If You Are Pregnant or Breastfeeding

No harmful effects are known.

How to Prepare

To make a Corn Poppy tea, pour boiling water over 1.5 grams (about 2 teaspoonfuls) of crushed petals, steep for 10 minutes, then strain. If you wish, the tea may be sweetened with honey.

Typical Dosage

To loosen phlegm, drink 1 cup of tea 2 to 3 times daily.

Overdosage

No information on overdosage is available.

Cornflower

Latin name: Centaurea cyanus
Other names: Bachelor's
  Buttons, Bluebonnet

A Remedy For

Once used as a remedy for indigestion, fever, and colds, Cornflower has fallen into disfavor, perhaps because its effectiveness has never been demonstrated. Other unproven uses include treatment for menstrual disorders, vaginal yeast infections, water retention, liver and gallbladder complaints, eye inflammation, and eczema.

What It Is; Why It Works

Considered a weed by corn farmers, Cornflower infests fields worldwide. Although ineffective for most purposes, the dried flowers do show antibacterial activity in the laboratory.

Avoid If . . .

No known medical conditions preclude the use of Cornflower.

Special Cautions

Cornflower poses a slight possibility of an allergic reaction.

Possible Drug Interactions

There are no known drug interactions.

Special Information If You Are Pregnant or Breastfeeding

No information is available.

How to Prepare

The crushed dried flowers can be used to make tea.

Typical Dosage

Use 1 gram of Cornflower per cup of tea. Store away from light.

Overdosage

No information is available.

Couch Grass

Latin name: Elymus repens
Other names: Cutch, Dog-grass,
  Durfa Grass, Quack Grass,
  Quick Grass, Triticum, Twitch-
  grass, Witch Grass

A Remedy For

- Bronchitis
- Colds
- Cough
- Fever
- Sore throat
- Tendency to infection
- Urinary tract infections

Couch Grass is used as a homeopathic remedy for urinary tract conditions. In folk medicine, it has been used for bladder infections, urinary stones, gout, pain from rheumatism, chronic skin problems, and constipation. Its effectiveness for these problems has not been scientifically verified.

What It Is; Why It Works

Because Couch Grass is a diuretic, drawing water from the body, it is used to flush out the urinary tract during infections. It also has an antimicrobial effect, destroying or inhibiting the growth of germs. Its high mucilage content makes it useful as a cough remedy.

Although Couch Grass is generally considered a troublesome weed, it has been used for medicinal purposes for centuries. During the early 20th century, Couch Grass was used in France as a home remedy to soothe sore throats and to help "sweat out" illnesses. The medicinal part of the plant is its fleshy underground stem, collected in spring or autumn.

Avoid If . . .

You should not take Couch Grass if you have swelling caused by heart or kidney problems.

Special Cautions

Couch Grass presents no problems when taken at typical dosages. However, when using it to flush out the urinary tract, be sure to take it with plenty of fluids.

Possible Drug Interactions

No interactions have been reported.

Special Information If You Are Pregnant or Breastfeeding

No harmful effects are known.

How to Prepare

Crushed Couch Grass can be made into a tea. Pour 1 cup of boiling water over 3 to 10 grams (one-half to 2 teaspoonfuls) of the herb and steep for 10 minutes. Strain before drinking.

Couch Grass is also available as a liquid extract and an alcohol solution (tincture).

Typical Dosage

Couch Grass is taken orally. The usual daily dosage is 6 to 9 grams (between 1 and 2 teaspoonfuls).

Dried Couch Grass must be kept in an airtight container and protected from light and moisture.

Overdosage

No information on overdosage is available.

Cranberry

Latin name: Vaccinium macrocarpon

A Remedy For

• Urinary tract infections

Cranberry has long been recommended as a preventive measure against repeated urinary tract infections. It is also taken to prevent kidney stones and "bladder gravel."

What It Is; Why It Works

Cranberry prevents *E. coli*—the most common cause of urinary tract infections—from adhering to the wall of the bladder, making it difficult for infection to take hold. It will not, however, kill the bacteria once they're established.

Native to North America, the plant is cultivated in Cranberry bogs throughout New England and elsewhere. The medicinal part is the ripe fruit.

Avoid If . . .

No known medical conditions preclude the use of Cranberry.

Special Cautions

Remember that Cranberry will not cure an active urinary tract infection. For this, you need a course of antibiotics.

Possible Drug Interactions

No interactions have been reported.

Special Information If You Are Pregnant or Breastfeeding

Cranberry is considered safe for use during pregnancy and while breastfeeding.

How to Prepare

You can take concentrated tablets and capsules, or Cranberry juice. If taking the juice, choose pure, high-quality products, not Cranberry cocktail.

Typical Dosage

Capsule or tablet: 1 pill 2 to 4 times per day

Juice: 16 ounces (2 cups) per day

Since potency of tablets and capsules may vary, follow the manufacturer's directions whenever available.

Overdosage

No information is available.

Cumin

Latin name: Cumina cyminum

A Remedy For

• Indigestion

Although its use is not officially recognized, Cumin is considered an effective remedy for indigestion. It is also taken to relieve gas, diarrhea, and cramps; and in Asian medicine, it is used to induce milk production in breastfeeding mothers, relieve inflammation, and cure worm infestations. Its effectiveness for these other uses has not, however, been scientifically verified.

What It Is; Why It Works

A distinctive spice used in southwestern and Indian cuisine, Cumin is mentioned in the Bible and was used medicinally in Roman times, when ground Cumin was eaten with bread or wine. Today, Cumin is cultivated throughout the Mediterranean region and in Iran, Pakistan, India, China, the United States, and South America.

The seeds and their oil are both used medicinally. Laboratory studies have shown that powdered cumin has anti-infective effects and may inhibit blood clots.

Avoid If . . .

No known medical conditions preclude the use of Cumin.

Special Cautions

No special precautions are needed.

Possible Drug Interactions

Animal studies suggest that Cumin may prolong the effect of barbiturates such as phenobarbital.

Special Information If You Are Pregnant or Breastfeeding

Cumin is used in some cultures to induce abortion, so caution is advisable during pregnancy.

How to Prepare

Cumin can be taken internally or used externally. It can be used in the ground form or as a pressed oil.

Typical Dosage

Strengths of medicinal preparations may vary. Follow the manufacturer's labeling whenever available.

Overdosage

No information is available.

Damiana

Latin name: Turnera diffusa

A Remedy For

Damiana is thought to be a remedy for impotence, but its effectiveness remains unconfirmed. In homeopathic medicine, it's used for *female* sexual disorders.

What It Is; Why It Works

Although Damiana leaves are said to have antidepressant and aphrodisiac properties, researchers have not identified any real physiological effects. Harvested from a small shrub that grows in the region of the Gulf of Mexico, the Caribbean, and southern Africa, the herb is known in the U.S. as Mexican Damiana.

Avoid If . . .

No known medical conditions preclude the use of Damiana.

Special Cautions

No side effects or hazards have been documented.

Possible Drug Interactions

No interactions have been reported.

Special Information If You Are Pregnant or Breastfeeding

No harmful effects are known.

How to Prepare

No information is available.

Typical Dosage

There are no guidelines on record.

Overdosage

No information on overdosage is available.

Dandelion

Latin name: Taraxacum officinale
Other names: Blowball, Cankerwort, Lion's Tooth, Priest's Crown, Swine's Snout, Wild Endive

A Remedy For
- Appetite loss
- Indigestion
- Kidney and bladder stones
- Liver and gallbladder problems
- Urinary tract infections

In folk medicine, Dandelion is also used as a remedy for hemorrhoids, gout, rheumatism, eczema, other skin conditions, and diabetes. Its effectiveness for these problems has not, however, been verified.

In Asian medicine—again without verification—Dandelion is used to treat chronic ulcers, stiff joints, and tuberculosis. It is also used to induce milk production in nursing mothers and to soothe inflamed breast tissue.

What It Is; Why It Works
The stubborn and ubiquitous Dandelion has been used for medicinal purposes since the 10th century. It shows proven value as a diuretic, flushing excess water from the body. It also promotes the flow of bile and stimulates the appetite. Dandelion juice once enjoyed considerable popularity as a diuretic, laxative, and remedy for rheumatism.

Dandelion takes its name from the French "dent de lion," or "lion's tooth"—a reference to the toothed edges of its leaves. The entire plant is considered medicinal.

Avoid If . . .
Do not use Dandelion if you have an obstruction of the bowels or the bile duct. Check with your doctor before using Dandelion if you have any type of gallbladder problem.

Special Cautions
Chances of any sort of allergic reaction are remote, but Dandelion has been known to cause heartburn.

Possible Drug Interactions
No drug interactions have been reported.

Special Information If You Are Pregnant or Breastfeeding
No information is available.

How to Prepare
To make a tea, pour 1 cup of rapidly boiling water over 1 tablespoonful of finely cut Dandelion, steep for 15 minutes, and strain.

Typical Dosage
Tincture: 10 to 15 drops 3 times daily
Tea: 1 freshly made cup 2 times daily, morning and evening

Strengths of commercial preparations may vary. Follow the manufacturer's labeling whenever available.

Store away from light and moisture.

Overdosage
No information is available.

Delphinium Flower

Latin name: Delphinium consolida
Other names: Branching Larkspur, Knight's Spur, Lark Heel, Staggerweed

A Remedy For

Delphinium Flower is sometimes used as a remedy for urinary tract infections, appetite loss, and worms, although its effectiveness remains unproven.

What It Is; Why It Works

Delphinium is grown in Europe and the United States. The buds look like a dolphin, hence the name "delphin" or "delphinium." The flower is thought to have a diuretic action, flushing excess water from the system. In large quantities, it may prove poisonous.

Avoid If . . .

No known medical conditions preclude the use of Delphinium Flower.

Special Cautions

Do not overdo use of this herb. Fatal animal poisonings from Delphinium Flower are fairly common, although no poisonings among humans have been documented.

Possible Drug Interactions

There are no known interactions.

Special Information If You Are Pregnant or Breastfeeding

No harmful effects are known.

How to Prepare

Delphinium Flower is prepared as a tea.

Typical Dosage

The recommended average daily dose is 1.5 grams.

Overdosage

If you suspect an overdose, seek medical attention immediately.

Devil's Claw

Latin name: Harpagophytum procumbens
Other names: Grapple Plant, Wood Spider

A Remedy For

- Appetite loss
- Indigestion
- Liver and gallbladder problems
- Rheumatism

Although the effectiveness of Devil's Claw for other ailments remains unconfirmed, it has also been used for skin disorders, pain, and problems of pregnancy.

What It Is; Why It Works

Devil's Claw is native to south and central Africa. Its medicinal value lies in its fleshy roots, which are sliced, chopped, or pulverized while fresh. Once dry, they become extremely difficult to cut.

Researchers have found that the herb stimulates production of digestive juices. It also boosts production of bile, increases the appetite, fights inflammation, and relieves minor pain.

Avoid If . . .
Because the herb boosts production of stomach acid, you should avoid Devil's Claw if you have stomach or duodenal ulcers.

Special Cautions
Devil's Claw has been known to trigger an allergic reaction.

Possible Drug Interactions
No interactions have been reported.

Special Information If You Are Pregnant or Breastfeeding
No harmful effects are known.

How to Prepare
Devil's Claw is dried for use in teas and other preparations for internal use. To make a tea, combine 1 teaspoonful of chopped Devil's Claw with 300 milliliters (1¼ cups) of boiling water, steep for 8 hours, and strain. Take 3 times daily.

Typical Dosage
For loss of appetite, the usual daily dose is 1.5 grams (one-third of a teaspoonful).

For all other uses, the usual daily dose is 4.5 grams (1 teaspoonful).

Overdosage
No information on overdosage is available.

Dill

Latin name: Anethum graveolens

A Remedy For
- Appetite loss
- Bronchitis
- Colds
- Cough
- Fever
- Liver and gallbladder problems
- Sore throat
- Tendency to infection

Both Dill seed and Dill leaf have been used medicinally, but only Dill seed has been proven effective. It provides relief for all the conditions listed above, and is also used for upset stomach. In Asian medicine, it is used as a remedy for chest congestion, intestinal gas, bad breath, and skin diseases.

Dill leaf has been used for stomach and intestinal problems, kidney and urinary tract conditions, spasms, and sleep disorders, but its effectiveness for these conditions remains unproven.

What It Is; Why It Works
Dill is a familiar kitchen spice, best known as a flavoring for pickled cucumbers. The tiny seeds are extremely light: 1,000 of them weigh only 1 gram. They act medicinally by relieving spasms and blocking the growth of bacteria. The more potent oil of Dill is obtained from the seeds.

Dill's natural habitat includes the Mediterranean region, and the plant was well known in biblical times. In Matthew 23:23 it is mentioned by its original Greek name, Anethon. During the 1st century, Greek herbalist Dioscorides also used the Greek name. But by the 17th century, scholars were already calling it by the modern name "Dill."

Avoid If . . .

There are no known medical conditions that preclude the use of Dill.

Special Cautions

At usual dosage levels, Dill poses no health hazards. Contact with juice from the fresh plant, however, can make your skin react badly to sunlight.

Possible Drug Interactions

No interactions have been reported.

Special Information If You Are Pregnant or Breastfeeding

No harmful effects are known.

How to Prepare

Whole Dill seed can be made into a tea.

Typical Dosage

Dill is taken orally. The usual daily dosage is:

Dill seed: 3 grams
Oil of Dill: 0.1 to 0.3 grams (2 to 6 drops)

Overdosage

No information on overdosage is available.

Dong Quai

Latin name: Angelica sinensis

A Remedy For

Often referred to as the "female ginseng," Dong Quai has been used for thousands of years to treat menstrual problems such as PMS and relieve menopausal symptoms such as hot flashes. Chinese doctors also use it, for men and women alike, to treat high blood pressure, poor circulation, and anemia (loss of red blood cells).

What It Is; Why It Works

Contrary to some theories, Donq Quai is not, in itself, a replacement for estrogen, nor does it have any hormone-like effects on the body. Its ability to relieve menstrual difficulties is thought to stem from its power to quell spasms in the internal organs.

Chinese researchers have also found that Dong Quai stimulates production of the red blood cells that carry oxygen throughout the body, thus increasing energy and combating fatigue. Some scientists even claim that the herb contains an immune-boosting compound that could help prevent arthritis and cancer, although its effectiveness for such problems remains unproven.

A type of wild celery, Dong Quai should not be confused with its European cousin, *Anglica archangelica*, which is used primarily to relieve digestive problems. It is the Dong Quai root that's used medicinally. Look for moist specimens with a brown outer layer and a white cross section. Avoid dry roots and those with greenish-brown cross sections.

Avoid If . . .
No known medical conditions preclude the use of Dong Quai.

Special Cautions
If you are suffering from diarrhea or bloating, check with your doctor before using Dong Quai. Remember, too, that Dong Quai sometimes increases sensitivity to sunlight, particularly if you are fair-skinned. To avoid a sunburn when using this herb on an extended basis, limit your exposure to the sun.

Possible Drug Interactions
No interactions have been reported.

Special Information If You Are Pregnant or Breastfeeding
Dong Quai is not recommended for pregnant or nursing women.

How to Prepare
Dong Quai is available as crushed root, and in tablets, capsules, and alcohol solutions (tinctures).

To make a medicinal tea, use 1 teaspoonful of crushed root per cup of boiling water. Steep for 10 to 20 minutes.

Typical Dosage
Women often take 3 to 4 grams per day. Strengths of commercial preparations may vary, so follow the manufacturer's directions whenever available.

Overdosage
No information on overdosage is available.

Echinacea

Latin name: Echinacea species
Other names: Coneflower,
  Rudbeckia, Sampson Root

A Remedy For
- Bronchitis
- Colds
- Cough
- Fever
- Sore throat
- Tendency to infection

There are three types of *Echinacea: Echinacea purpurea, Echinacea pallida,* and *Echinacea angustifolia.* All are used to boost the immune system and fight infections, but only the purpurea and pallida varieties have been definitively proven effective. In general, the medicinal effects of the leaves are better documented than the effects of the roots.

In addition to the conditions listed above, the purpurea variety of Echinacea is considered an effective treatment for urinary tract infections and poorly healing wounds, skin ulcers, and burns. The root of *Echinacea purpurea* is used to reestablish the supply of white blood cells following cancer treatments, and to supplement other anti-infection drugs.

In folk medicine, the angustifolia variety of Echinacea is widely used for conditions such as wounds, burns, swelling of the lymph nodes, insect bites, stomach cramps, measles, gonorrhea, and snakebite. However, its effectiveness for these conditions has not been proven.

What It Is; Why It Works

As a natural buttress to immunity, Echinacea has become one of the hottest items in the current herbal renaissance—and its reputation is not unwarranted.

Researchers have found that the leaves of Echinacea purpurea speed the healing of wounds and boost the effectiveness of the immune system by increasing the number of white blood cells, spleen cells, and other disease-fighting agents such as T-helper cells and interleukin. In addition, Echinacea purpurea root has been shown to prevent the growth of bacteria and viruses.

Tests conducted on Echinacea pallida have shown that it too strengthens the body's defenses against disease; and extracts from the root have stopped the growth of viruses in the lab. Likewise, lab tests of Echinacea angustifolia have shown that it stimulates the immune system and will kill bacteria or prevent their growth.

Originating in North America, Echinacea was used by the Sioux tribe for snakebites, and by other Native Americans as a general antiseptic. It is now cultivated in the United States and Europe. Its taste is slightly sweet, then bitter, leaving a tingling sensation on the tongue.

Avoid If . . .

Because of Echinacea's effects on the immune system, you should not take this drug if you have multiple sclerosis, AIDS, tuberculosis, leukemia, and autoimmune diseases such as rheumatoid arthritis and lupus.

Do not take Echinacea injections if you have an allergy to the plant. Avoid them, too, if you have diabetes; they can upset the balance of the metabolism.

Special Cautions

You should not take Echinacea for longer than 8 weeks.

Echinacea does not have side effects when taken orally at customary dosage levels. However, when Echinacea extract is given intravenously it can lead to shivers, short-term fever, and very rarely an immediate allergic reaction.

Possible Drug Interactions

No interactions have been reported.

Special Information If You Are Pregnant or Breastfeeding

Do not take Echinacea purpurea injections if you are pregnant.

How to Prepare

Echinacea angustifolia root is often made into a tea. Pour boiling water over one-half teaspoonful of crushed root, steep for 10 minutes, and strain.

Typical Dosage

Echinacea pallida is usually taken orally. The daily dosage is 900 milligrams taken in a 50% alcohol solution (tincture).

The usual daily dosage of *Echinacea purpurea* leaf is 6 to 9 milliliters (about 1¼ to 1¾ teaspoonfuls) of expressed juice.

Echinacea purpurea root is taken in tincture form. The usual daily dosage is 30 to 60 drops taken 3 times a day.

If you are taking *Echinacea angustifolia* tea for a cold, drink a freshly made cup several times a day.

The potency and form of commercial preparations may vary. Follow the manufacturer's instructions whenever available.

If you are using the root, store it away from light, and do not crush until you are ready to make a preparation.

Overdosage

No information on overdosage is available.

Elder

Latin name: Sambucus nigra
Other names: Black Elder, Boor Tree, Bountry, Ellanwood, Ellhorn, European Alder

A Remedy For
• Bronchitis
• Cough

Elder is taken for symptomatic relief in all sorts of upper respiratory ailments. As an herbal compress, it is also used for swelling and inflammation; but its effectiveness for these problems remains unproven.

What It Is; Why It Works
The source of Elderberry wine (which is NOT medicinal), Elder is found throughout most of Europe. The plant is a tree or bush that reaches a height of over 20 feet, with strongly perfumed, yellowish-white flowers and black-violet berries that yield blood red juice. The bark, leaves, berries, and roots are all considered medicinal when harvested at the proper time.

Elder soothes coughs and inflammation by increasing bronchial secretions. It also noticeably increases sweating.

Avoid If . . .
No known medical conditions preclude the use of Elder.

Special Cautions
At customary dosage levels, Elder poses no risks.

Possible Drug Interactions
No drug interactions have been reported.

Special Information If You Are Pregnant or Breastfeeding
No harmful effects are known.

How to Prepare
To make Elder tea, simmer 3 to 4 grams (about 2 teaspoonfuls) of Elder flowers in two-thirds of a cup of boiling water for 5 minutes, then strain.

Typical Dosage
Drink 1 or 2 cups of the tea, as hot as you can stand, several times a day—especially in the afternoon and evening. Your total

daily dose should fall in the range of 10 to 15 grams.

Overdosage

No information on overdosage is available.

Elecampane

Latin name: Inula helenium
Other names: Elfdock, Horse-
*   Elder, Horseheal, Scabwort,*
*   Velvet Dock, Wild Sunflower*

A Remedy For

Elecampane is sometimes prescribed for bronchitis and cough, but because it can be severely irritating and allergenic, its use is not recommended.

The herb has a variety of other uses in folk medicine, although none has been scientifically validated. It is taken as a remedy for upset stomach, gas, gallbladder problems, water retention, and menstrual complaints. In Asian medicine it's also used for diarrhea, vomiting, and intestinal inflammation, and homeopathic practitioners recommend it for bronchial conditions.

What It Is; Why It Works

Elecampane has been known since the days of the Roman poet Horace. A perennial shrub some 2½ to 6 feet high, it is native to the temperate regions of Europe and Asia, and can now be found in China and the United States as well. Its Latin name "*Inula helenium*" echoes the many legends that associate the plant with Helen of Troy. (Your choice: It either sprang from her tears, or she was holding a branch of it when Paris stole her away.)

The active ingredients in Elecampane have shown an ability to reduce inflammation, kill bacteria and fungus, and loosen phlegm in the lungs. The portion of the plant used in remedies is the fleshy root, which has a strong odor and a pungent, bitter, tangy taste.

Avoid If . . .

No known medical conditions preclude the use of Elecampane.

Special Cautions

Use Elecampane with care, if at all. It is severely irritating to the lining of the nose, throat, stomach, and intestines, and frequently triggers an allergic reaction.

Possible Drug Interactions

No interactions have been reported.

Special Information If You Are Pregnant or Breastfeeding

No harmful effects are known.

How to Prepare

Elecampane can be made into a tea. Pour boiling water over 1 gram (about one-quarter teaspoonful) of the ground root, steep for 10 to 15 minutes, then strain. If you wish, sweeten the tea with honey.

Typical Dosage

To loosen phlegm, drink 1 cup of the tea 3 to 4 times daily.

Store in a cool, dark place. Do not use a plastic container.

Overdosage

Symptoms of overdose include vomiting, diarrhea, spasms, and signs of paralysis. If you suspect an overdose, seek medical attention immediately.

English Ivy

Latin name: Hedera helix
Other names: Common Ivy, Gum Ivy, True Ivy, Woodbind

A Remedy For

- Bronchitis
- Cough

Ivy has also been used, without proof of effectiveness, for a variety of other disorders. It has been taken internally for liver, spleen, and gallbladder disorders, gout, rheumatism, and inflamed lymph nodes. Externally, it has been used for ulcers, inflammation, burns, calluses, parasites, nerve pain, and inflamed veins.

What It Is; Why It Works

Despite its name, English Ivy is found throughout most temperate regions of the world. It is a creeping or climbing vine that can grow up to 45 feet long. The berries and leaves have a bitter taste.

The plant has an ancient history; it was highly regarded by the Greeks and Romans, who used its leaves in poets' laurels. Ivy was dedicated to Bacchus, the god of wine, and was often tied to the brow to prevent intoxication. As a direct outgrowth of that belief, English taverns used to display the sign of an Ivy bush over the door. Ivy is also used to decorate houses and churches at Christmas, although the practice was condemned by the early church as a pagan tradition.

English Ivy relieves bronchial spasms and has an expectorant action, helping to bring up phlegm.

Avoid If . . .

No known medical conditions preclude the use of English Ivy.

Special Cautions

When used at standard dosage levels, English Ivy presents no problems. However, some people develop allergic skin reactions to the leaves.

Possible Drug Interactions

No drug interactions have been reported.

Special Information If You Are Pregnant or Breastfeeding

No harmful effects are known.

How to Prepare

English Ivy can be taken as a crushed herb or a tea. The fresh leaves are used externally.

To prepare the tea, steep 1 heaping teaspoon of English Ivy in one-quarter cup of boiling water, then strain.

For external use, fresh leaves may be laid on festering wounds and burns. To prepare a soothing compress for rheumatism, boil 7 ounces of fresh leaves in 1 quart of water and allow to cool.

Typical Dosage

The customary oral dosage of the crushed herb is 300 to 800 milligrams per day. Ivy tea may be taken 3 times daily.

Overdosage

No information on overdosage is available.

English Oak

Latin name: Quercus robur
Other name: Tanner's Bark

A Remedy For

- Bronchitis
- Colds
- Cough
- Diarrhea
- Fever
- Skin inflammation
- Sore throat
- Tendency to infection

What It Is; Why It Works

English Oak has an anti-inflammatory effect, and also acts as an astringent, tightening and drying the tissues. The dried bark is the primary medicinal agent.

The English Oak grows very slowly, but to massive size. The tree is about 160 feet high with a broad, irregular, heavily branched crown and a trunk that divides into gnarled, strong, bent branches. The bark is deeply fissured, thick, and gray-brown. Oak bark from this and other species yields dye shades ranging from yellow to black. The tree is widespread in Europe, Asia Minor, and the Caucasus region.

The oak has been held sacred by many cultures including the Druids, Greeks, and Romans. The Round Table of the King Arthur legend was made from a single disk of oak.

Avoid If . . .

Do not use English Oak in whole-body baths if you have large, weeping skin inflammations or injuries, a fever or infectious illness, or a weak heart. Do not apply English Oak over large skin injuries.

Special Cautions

When taken at customary dosage levels, English Oak poses no serious risks. However, when taken internally, it sometimes causes digestive problems.

Possible Drug Interactions

English Oak can interfere with the absorption of a variety of alkaline substances, including morphine, quinine, nicotine, and caffeine.

Special Information If You Are Pregnant or Breastfeeding

No harmful effects are known.

How to Prepare

English Oak can be made into a tea. Place 1 gram (one-third teaspoonful) of finely cut or coarse, powdered English Oak in cold water, bring the water to a rapid boil, then strain.

For external use in a rinse, compress, or gargle, mix 20 grams (about 2 tablespoonfuls) of English Oak with 1 quart of water.

To prepare a bath additive,

pour 1 quart of boiling water over 5 grams (about 1²/₃ teaspoonfuls) of English Oak, then add to bath water.

Typical Dosage

For internal use, the usual daily dosage is 3 grams (about 1 teaspoonful) of finely cut or coarse powdered English Oak.

English Oak is occasionally included in tea mixtures, and in standardized preparations for digestive complaints. You may also find commercial bark extracts available for external use.

Overdosage

No information on overdosage is available.

English Plantain

Latin name: Plantago lanceolata
Other names: Buckhorn,
  Chimney-sweeps, Headsman,
  Ribwort, Ripplegrass,
  Soldier's Herb

A Remedy For

• Bronchitis
• Colds
• Cough
• Fever
• Skin inflammation
• Sore throat
• Tendency to infection
• Wounds and burns

English Plantain is used primarily for inflammation of the upper respiratory tract. In folk medicine, it has been used to stop bleeding.

What It Is; Why It Works

With a brush-like flower and pronounced ribs on the leaves, this 20-inch plant is widespread in the cool temperate regions of the world. The liquid extract and the pressed juice of the fresh plant exhibit proven antibacterial properties, as well as a tightening, astringent action.

Avoid If . . .

There are no known medical conditions that preclude the use of English Plantain.

Special Cautions

At standard dosages, use of this herb poses no problems.

Possible Drug Interactions

No drug interactions have been reported.

Special Information If You Are Pregnant or Breastfeeding

No harmful effects are known.

How to Prepare

To make a tea, pour boiling water over 2 to 4 grams (about one-half teaspoonful) of chopped herb, or put the herb in cold water and bring to a boil. Steep for 10 minutes, then strain.

English Plantain is also used in liquid extract, lozenge, and syrup form, and in many cough medications.

Typical Dosage

English Plantain can be taken orally or applied externally. The usual oral dosage is 3 to 6 grams (one-half to 1 heaping teaspoonful) daily.

Overdosage

No information on overdosage is available.

Ephedra (Ma Huang)

Latin name: Ephedra sinica

A Remedy For

• Bronchitis
• Cough

Ephedra is taken for mild respiratory disorders, including asthma, in adults and children over the age of 6. It is also used as a stimulant for the heart and for stimulation in general. In Asian medicine, the herb is taken for fever, swelling, and bone pain.

What It Is; Why It Works

Ephedra's value for respiratory problems derives from the calming effect it has on spasms in the bronchial walls. At the same time, Ephedra stimulates the nervous system, and boosts the rate and strength of heart contractions. It also tends to discourage the growth of bacteria.

Ephedra's effects have been known for over 4,000 years. The drug is well known in China, where it goes by the name Tsaopen-Ma Huang. Its active ingredient, ephedrine, is the main component in the familiar asthma remedy, Primatene Tablets. The drug is very potent and, because of its effect on the heart, can be very dangerous when taken in excessive amounts.

Ephedra grows mainly in Mongolia and the bordering area of China. The young branches and dried roots are the medicinal parts of the plant.

Avoid If . . .

Do not take Ephedra if you have high blood pressure, high pressure in the eyes (glaucoma), weakened blood vessels in the brain, prostate cancer, an overactive adrenal gland, or a thyroid disorder. In general, avoid Ephedra if you have any condition that makes you anxious or restless.

Special Cautions

Ephedra has numerous possible side effects, including sleeplessness, restlessness, irritability, headache, nausea, vomiting, urinary disorders, and rapid heartbeat. Higher doses can trigger a sharp rise in blood pressure and disrupt the rhythm of the heart.

Extended use can lead to tolerance and dependence, so that ever larger doses are required to obtain an effect. Because of these dangers, you should only take Ephedra for short periods.

Possible Drug Interactions

Combining Ephedra with a variety of other medications can lead to potentially serious problems. For example, when taken in combination with heart drugs such as digitalis or digoxin (Lanoxin), Ephedra is more likely to disturb the rhythm of the heart. Combining Ephedra with the blood pressure medication guanethidine (Ismelin) can dangerously exaggerate the herb's stimulative effects. A similar problem is possible when Ephedra is combined with drugs classified as MAŌ inhibitors, such as the antidepressants Nardil and Parnate and the Parkinson's disease medication Eldepryl. The combination of Ephedra and ergot-based drugs such as migraine remedies Ergomar and Wigraine can result in high blood pressure.

Special Information If You Are Pregnant or Breastfeeding

No harmful effects are known.

How to Prepare

Ephedra is available in crushed herb form, in alcohol solutions (tinctures), and as a liquid extract.

Typical Dosage

Potency of commercial preparations may vary, so be sure to follow the manufacturer's directions. General guidelines for adults are as follows:

Tea: Use 1 to 4 grams of crushed Ephedra; take 3 times daily.
Liquid extract: 1 to 3 milliliters (about one-quarter to one-half teaspoonful) 3 times daily.
Tincture (1:1): The usual single dose is 5 grams (1 teaspoonful).
Tincture (1:4): 6 to 8 milliliters (about 1 to 1½ teaspoonfuls) 3 times daily.

Overdosage

Doses of more than 100 grams (about 3 ounces) can be life-threatening. Symptoms of overdose include severe sweating, enlarged pupils, spasms, and increased body temperature. Death results from heart failure and suffocation.

If you suspect an overdose, seek emergency treatment immediately.

Eryngo

Latin name: Eryngium campestre
Other names: Sea Holly, Sea Holme, Sea Hulver

A Remedy For

Although this herb has been put to a variety of uses, its effectiveness has never been confirmed. The leaves and blossoms are taken for urinary tract infections, prostate problems, and bronchitis. The root is used for colds, coughs, bronchitis, bladder and kidney stones, kidney pain, kidney and urinary tract inflammation, difficulty urinating, water retention, and skin disorders.

What It Is; Why It Works

Eryngo has been used in medicine since at least the 1st century AD, when the Greek scholar Dioscorides recommended it as a cure for gas. Indeed, the herb's Latin name is thought to come from the Greek word "eruggarein," meaning to belch.

Researchers have found Eryngo leaves to have a mildly diuretic effect, flushing excess water from the body. The root has some minor ability to loosen phlegm and calm spasms.

A dwarf perennial bush growing no more than 2 feet high, Eryngo grows in most parts of

Europe, and in northern Africa and some parts of North America.

Avoid If . . .

No known medical conditions preclude the use of Eryngo.

Special Cautions

At customary dosage levels, Eryngo poses no risks.

Possible Drug Interactions

No interactions have been reported.

Special Information If You Are Pregnant or Breastfeeding

No harmful effects are known.

How to Prepare

Eryngo leaf is available in extract form, and the root can be taken as a tea, liquid extract, or alcohol solution (tincture).

To make tea from Eryngo root, use 1 level teaspoonful of ground root per cup of boiling water. Allow to steep until cold.

To make an Eryngo root tincture, soak 20 grams of ground root in 80 grams (about one-third cup) of 60% alcohol for a period of 10 days.

Typical Dosage

Eryngo is taken orally. The usual dosage is:

Tea: 3 to 4 cups daily
Tincture: 50 to 60 drops daily divided into 3 to 4 doses
Liquid extract: 2 to 3 grams (about one-half teaspoonful) daily

Overdosage

No information on overdosage is available.

Eucalyptus

Latin name: Eucalyptus globulus
Other names: Blue Gum,
Red Gum

A Remedy For

• Bronchitis
• Cough
• Rheumatism

Eucalyptus has a variety of other uses for which its effectiveness remains unproven. Among them are bladder, liver, and gallbladder conditions, whooping cough, fever, flu, hoarseness, asthma, diabetes, scarlet fever, measles, sinus conditions, loss of appetite, wounds, acne, bleeding gums, sore mouth, nerve pain, poorly healing sores, worms, gonorrhea, and digestive complaints. In Asia, it is also used for headache, bad breath, threadworm, and tuberculosis.

What It Is; Why It Works

Eucalyptus is the signature tree of Australia, but can now be found in subtropical regions throughout the world. With a distinctive silver-gray bark and twisted trunk, some species of Eucalyptus grow as high as a 12-story building.

The medicinal properties of Eucalyptus reside in its oil, which is extracted from the fresh leaves and branch tips, and is found in the dried leaves. It acts as a decongestant, loosens phlegm, and relieves spasms. Applied to the skin, the oil improves local circulation. In laboratory tests, the oil has shown an ability to kill bacteria and fungi.

Like the similar soothing agents menthol and camphor, Eucalyptus is found in several familiar over-the-counter remedies, including Listerine Antiseptic Mouthrinse, Mentholatum Cherry Chest Rub, and Vicks VapoRub.

Avoid If . . .

Do not take Eucalyptus if you have digestive problems, a disorder of the biliary duct, or liver disease. Do not apply preparations containing Eucalyptus oil to the face of an infant or small child; it could cause asthma-like symptoms or even death by asphyxiation.

Special Cautions

In rare cases, taking Eucalyptus can cause nausea, vomiting, and diarrhea. Poisoning, particularly of children, is possible with very small doses of Eucalyptus oil. (See the "Overdosage" section below.)

Possible Drug Interactions

No interactions have been reported.

Special Information If You Are Pregnant or Breastfeeding

No harmful effects are known.

How to Prepare

Eucalyptus can be found in various dry, semi-solid, and liquid preparations.

Typical Dosage

Eucalyptus oil: For internal use, the usual daily dose is 300 to 600 milligrams (a few drops). For external use, rub several drops into the skin.

Eucalyptus leaf: The average daily dose is 4 to 16 grams (about 1 to 3 teaspoonfuls), taken in small portions every 3 to 4 hours

Eucalyptus alcohol solution (tincture): The average daily dose is 3 to 4 grams (about one-half to three-quarters of a teaspoonful)

Eucalyptus tea: Drink a cup several times daily

The potency of commercial preparations may vary. Follow the manufacturer's instructions whenever available.

Store Eucalyptus in tightly sealed containers.

Overdosage

A few drops of Eucalyptus oil are sufficient to cause life-threatening poisoning in a child. Adults have been poisoned with only 4 to 5 milliliters (about 1 teaspoonful). Symptoms of overdose include a drop in blood pressure, circulation problems, collapse, and asphyxiation. If you suspect an overdose, seek emergency medical treatment immediately.

The leaf form of Eucalyptus is far less potent, and is unlikely to cause a problem.

European Buckthorn

Latin name: Rhamnus frangula
Other names: Arrow Wood,
  Black Alder, Frangula Bark,
  Persian Berries

A Remedy For
• Constipation

The ability to soften stool and ease its passage makes this herb especially helpful for people with hemorrhoids or cracks in the surface of the anus (anal fissures), as well as those who have undergone rectal surgery. It can also be used in preparation for diagnostic procedures and exploratory surgery.

What It Is; Why It Works
European Buckthorn takes the form of a large bush or weedy tree found throughout Europe, western Asia, Asia Minor, and North America. Only the bark—fresh or dried—is medicinal.

European Buckthorn works by stimulating contractions in the intestinal wall, thus accelerating passage of the contents. With less time for its liquid content to be absorbed through the intestinal wall, the stool tends to remain soft. European Buckthorn's laxative action is relatively mild, but an overdose can still prove poisonous.

Avoid If . . .
Do not take European Buckthorn if you have an intestinal obstruction, appendicitis, or an acute inflammatory disorder of the intestines, such as ulcerative colitis

or Crohn's disease. Not for children under 12.

Special Cautions
European Buckthorn can cause vomiting and cramps. Long-term use can deplete the body's potassium supply, and can lead to intestinal dysfunction, heart problems, kidney disease, swelling, and bone deterioration.

As with any laxative, do not take European Buckthorn for more than 1 to 2 weeks without your doctor's approval.

Possible Drug Interactions
If you have a heart condition, check with your doctor before using European Buckthorn; it can amplify the effect of certain heart medications.

Special Information If You Are Pregnant or Breastfeeding
Do not take European Buckthorn during pregnancy or while breastfeeding.

How to Prepare
European Buckthorn is available in a variety of dried and liquid extracts, and in crushed herbal form for use as a tea. To make tea, pour boiling water over 2 grams (about one-half teaspoonful) of crushed European Buckthorn, steep for 15 minutes, then strain. Alternatively, you can add 2 grams of the herb to cold water and let it stand for 12 hours at room temperature.

Typical Dosage
European Buckthorn is taken orally. The usual daily dosage of the refined active ingredient is 20

to 180 milligrams. Use the minimum amount required to produce a soft stool. Do not take the total daily dosage all at once; break it up into smaller doses taken throughout the day.

Store away from light and moisture.

Overdosage

Side effects such as vomiting and cramps could be signs of an overdose. Seek medical attention if you think an overdose has occurred.

Evening Primrose Oil

Latin name: Oenothera biennis
Other names: Fever Plant,
King's Cureall, Night Willow-
herb, Scabish, Scurvish,
Sun Drop

A Remedy For

• Premenstrual syndrome (PMS)
• Skin inflammation

Evening Primrose Oil is taken internally to relieve the itching, flaking, and inflammation of eczema and ease the symptoms of PMS. It is generally considered effective for these problems, though some controversy lingers. Of more dubious validity are claims that it will reduce hyperactivity in children and decrease cholesterol levels. In homeopathic medicine, it's prescribed—without scientific verification—for asthma, diarrhea, and whooping cough.

What It Is; Why It Works

Evening Primrose Oil is rich in gamma-linolenic acid, a compound that plays a role in the production of prostaglandins. These hormone-like substances sometimes work to reduce inflammation. It is through this anti-inflammatory action that Evening Primrose Oil is thought to work.

The Evening Primrose plant can be found throughout North America, most of Europe, and parts of Asia. In Britain, the flowers usually open between 6 and 7 PM, hence the name of the plant. In Germany, it's called "night candle" for the same reason.

In 1992, Oil of Evening Primrose was declared unsafe for human consumption by the Food and Drug Administration, and was, for a while, unavailable in the United States. However, it can now be purchased in capsule form at a variety of outlets.

Avoid If . . .

No known medical conditions preclude the use of Evening Primrose Oil.

Special Cautions

At customary dosage levels, no toxicity has been reported.

Possible Drug Interactions

No interactions have been documented.

Special Information If You Are Pregnant or Breastfeeding

No harmful effects are known.

How to Prepare

Evening Primrose Oil is typically supplied in 500-milligram capsules.

Typical Dosage

The usual recommendation is 1 to 2 capsules 3 times a day. Since potency may vary, follow the manufacturer's directions whenever available.

Overdosage

No information on overdosage is available.

Eyebright

Latin name: Euphrasia officinalis

A Remedy For

Eyebright has long been considered a remedy for eye inflammations, although its effectiveness has never been verified. Other unproven uses include the treatment of styes, tired eyes, functional eye disorders, coughs, and hoarseness. In homeopathic medicine, the herb is also recommended for inflamed prostate.

What It Is; Why It Works

Eyebright has been in use since at least the 14th century, when it was said to "cure all evils of the eye." An annual that reaches a height of about 1 foot, the plant produces white, bluish, or reddish-violet flowers. It can be found throughout Europe.

Avoid If . . .

No known medical conditions preclude the use of Eyebright.

Special Cautions

No problems or side effects have been documented.

Possible Drug Interactions

No interactions have been reported.

Special Information If You Are Pregnant or Breastfeeding

No harmful effects are known.

How to Prepare

Eyebright can be made into a tea by combining 2 to 3 grams (about one-half teaspoonful) of the finely cut herb with boiling water. Steep for 5 to 10 minutes, then strain.

Typical Dosage

Eyebright is usually applied externally in lotions, compresses, and eyewash. As an eye rinse, a 2% solution can generally be used 3 to 4 times a day. Since potency of commercial preparations may vary, follow the manufacturer's instructions whenever available.

Overdosage

No information on overdosage is available.

Fennel

Latin name: Foeniculum vulgare

A Remedy For

- Bronchitis
- Cough

Fennel syrup and Fennel honey soothe inflammations of the upper respiratory tract. Fennel is also a remedy for digestive problems, such as mild spasms in the stomach or intestines, a feeling of fullness, and intestinal gas; and in Asian medicine, it is used for anemia, bloating, heartburn, vomiting, diarrhea, hernia, skin diseases, and repeated bouts of intense thirst. Its effectiveness for these conditions has not, however, been scientifically verified.

What It Is; Why It Works

Fennel stimulates movement of food through the stomach and intestines; in higher doses it puts a stop to intestinal spasms. Lab experiments have revealed substances in Fennel that show an ability to dry up respiratory phlegm and destroy germs. The part of the fennel plant used medicinally is the dried seed and its oil.

Fennel first grew in the Mediterranean region, then spread to England, Germany, and Argentina. Today, it also grows in Iran, Iraq, and China. The plant's scientific name is from the Latin "foenum," which means "hay." This name evolved into "Fanculum" during the Middle Ages, later becoming "Fenkel," and finally "Fennel."

Avoid If . . .

Allergic reactions to fennel are very rare. If you have an allergy to celery, however, Fennel might also cause a reaction.

Special Cautions

When taken at usual dosage levels, Fennel poses no risks. However, preparations other than Fennel tea or the herb itself should not be given to small children. If you have diabetes, be sure to check the sugar content of any Fennel preparation you plan to take. Do not take Fennel for an extended period (several weeks) without consulting a doctor. Take Fennel oil preparations for no more than 2 weeks.

Possible Drug Interactions

No interactions have been reported.

Special Information If You Are Pregnant or Breastfeeding

If you are pregnant, avoid any Fennel preparation other than the herb itself or Fennel tea.

How to Prepare

Crushed or ground Fennel seed can be made into a tea.

Typical Dosage

Fennel is taken orally. The usual daily dosage is:

Fennel oil: 0.1 to 0.6 milliliters (about 2 to 12 drops)
Fennel seed: 5 to 7 grams (about 1 to 1 1/2 teaspoonfuls)

Overdosage

No information on overdosage is available.

Fenugreek

Latin name: Trigonella foenum-graecum
Other name: Bird's Foot

A Remedy For

- Appetite loss
- Indigestion
- Skin inflammation

Fenugreek is also used for upper respiratory inflammation and, applied externally, for boils, ulcers, hives, and eczema. In Asian medicine, it is considered a treatment for anorexia, beriberi, bronchitis, fever, hernia, impotence, and vomiting; but its effectiveness for these conditions has not been clinically verified.

What It Is; Why It Works

When used externally, Fenugreek has a soothing effect on the skin. Taken internally, it promotes healing, reduces blood sugar, and increases milk production. Researchers have been unable to pinpoint the active ingredient in the herb. However, it has recently aroused interest as a potential raw material for the production of steroids.

Fenugreek's medicinal benefits lie in the ripe, dried seeds. In use since the time of the ancient Greeks, it is still a common remedy in modern-day Egypt, where the seeds are soaked until they swell into a thick paste called "helba" that's used for fevers. Originally native to the Mediterranean region, the plant is now grown in southern France, Turkey, northern Africa, India, and China.

Avoid If . . .

No known medical conditions preclude the use of Fenugreek.

Special Cautions

When taken at customary dosage levels, Fenugreek poses little risk. However, repeated external applications sometimes trigger a skin allergy.

Possible Drug Interactions

No interactions have been reported.

Special Information If You Are Pregnant or Breastfeeding

No harmful effects are known.

How to Prepare

To make a Fenugreek tea, soak 0.5 grams (about one-eighth teaspoonful) of crushed seed in 1 cup of cold water for 3 hours. Strain before drinking. You can sweeten the tea with honey. Drink several times a day.

For external application, prepare a thick paste by mixing the powdered seeds with hot water.

Typical Dosage

When taken orally, the usual daily dosage is 6 grams (about 1 heaping teaspoonful) of crushed Fenugreek seed.

Overdosage

No information on overdosage is available.

Feverfew

Latin name: Tanacetum parthenium
Other names: Featherfoil, Midsummer Daisy

A Remedy For
• Migraine

Several clinical trials have shown that Feverfew reduces the frequency and severity of migraine headaches when taken in small amounts daily. It has no other scientifically verified effects, but has also been used for arthritis, allergies, cramps, indigestion, postnatal bleeding, painful menstruation, other gynecological disorders, and intestinal parasites. In folk medicine, it is regarded as a general tonic, tranquilizer, and "blood purifier." As a wash or rinse, it is used to prevent infection and reduce swelling from wounds and tooth extraction.

What It Is; Why It Works
Feverfew is a strongly aromatic perennial that originated in southeastern Europe and is now found all over Europe, Australia, and North America. Externally, it is also used as an insecticide and was formerly found in insect powders. Only the leaf is used medicinally.

Feverfew contains an active ingredient called parthenolide that seems to affect the release of serotonin—an important chemical messenger in the brain—while reducing the level of certain chemicals associated with inflammation, including histamines and prostaglandins. Its migraine-preventing effect takes 4 to 6 weeks to appear.

Avoid If . . .
No known medical conditions preclude the use of Feverfew. Not for use in children under 2 years.

Special Cautions
Potential side effects include edginess and upset stomach, but customary doses rarely cause any problem. Skin reactions due to contact with the herb are also a possibility.

Possible Drug Interactions
No interactions have been reported.

Special Information If You Are Pregnant or Breastfeeding
No harmful effects have been documented, but use of Feverfew during pregnancy is not recommended.

How to Prepare
Feverfew leaf is available in powder form, and in tablets and capsules. When purchasing pills, look for products containing at least 0.2 percent parthenolide.

To make a tea, combine 2 teaspoonfuls of Feverfew powder with 1 cup of water and steep for 15 minutes. To make a stronger solution for use as a wash or mouthwash, double the amount of Feverfew and steep for 25 minutes.

Typical Dosage

The recommended daily dosage of Feverfew is:

Leaf powder: 50 milligrams to 1.2 grams (up to about one-quarter teaspoonful)
Tea: 3 cups
Tablets and capsules: Follow the manufacturer's directions

Store the powder in a sealed container.

Overdosage

There is no information available.

Fig

Latin name: Ficus carica

A Remedy For

Figs are taken as a remedy for constipation, although a laxative effect has never been scientifically documented. In Asian medicine, Figs are recommended for infectious diarrhea and intestinal inflammation.

What It Is; Why It Works

The Fig is native to Asia Minor, Syria, and Iran. It is mentioned frequently in the Bible, and was held sacred by the Romans, who believed that Romulus and Remus, the founders of Rome, were suckled beneath the limbs of a Fig tree. By the time of the Roman historian Pliny, the Fig was considered so important that its export was outlawed. Today, it is grown in subtropical regions around the world.

Avoid If . . .

No known medical conditions preclude the use of the Fig.

Special Cautions

No side effects have been recorded.

Possible Drug Interactions

No interactions have been reported.

Special Information If You Are Pregnant or Breastfeeding

No harmful effects are known.

How to Prepare

Dried Figs may be used.

Typical Dosage

There are no recommendations on record.

Overdosage

No information on overdosage is available.

Fo-Ti

Latin name: Polygonum multiflorum
Other name: He-shou-wu

A Remedy For

- Constipation
- Hardening of the arteries
- High cholesterol

This popular Chinese herb may also boost the immune system. In traditional Chinese medicine, it is used to treat premature aging, weakness, vaginal discharges, numerous infectious diseases, chest pain (angina), and impotence.

Other unverified uses include dizziness, blurred vision, insomnia, nocturnal emission, deep skin infections, sores, abscesses, goiter and neck lumps, and sore knees and back.

What It Is; Why It Works

Fo-Ti is native to China, where it continues to be widely cultivated. It is also grown extensively in Japan and Taiwan. The unprocessed root—called white Fo-Ti—is sometimes used, but, more often, it is boiled in a special liquid made from black beans, upon which it is called red Fo-Ti.

Both animal and human studies have shown the root to be effective at lowering cholesterol levels and decreasing hardening of the arteries. The unprocessed root also possesses a mild laxative effect. The ingredients responsible for these properties are yet to be identified.

Avoid If . . .

Fo-Ti is usually not recommended for people with phlegm or diarrhea.

Special Cautions

The unprocessed root may cause mild diarrhea, flushing of the face, or digestive distress. Those who are particularly sensitive to Fo-Ti may develop a skin rash.

Possible Drug Interactions

No interactions with drugs have been reported, but some traditional sources say you should not take this herb with onions, chives, or garlic.

Special Information If You Are Pregnant or Breastfeeding

No harmful effects are known.

How to Prepare

Tea from processed Fo-Ti roots can be made by boiling 3 to 5 grams (about one-half to 1 teaspoonful) of Fo-Ti in 1 cup of water for 10 to 15 minutes. Fo-Ti tablets containing 500 kilograms apiece may also be found.

Typical Dosage

Tea: 3 or more cups per day
Tablets: 5 of the 500-milligram tablets 3 times daily

Since the strength of commercial preparations may vary, follow the manufacturer's instructions whenever available.

Overdosage

One warning sign of an excessive dosage is numbness in the arms or legs. If you suspect an overdose, call your doctor immediately.

Frostwort

Latin name: Helianthemum canadense
Other names: Rock-Rose, Sun Rose

A Remedy For

- Indigestion
- Skin inflammation

Although its use has not been officially recognized, Frostwort is considered effective for the two problems listed above. Homeopathic practitioners also recommend it for skin conditions.

What It Is; Why It Works

A native of the eastern United States, Frostwort is now grown in Europe as well. Its flowers, which bloom twice per season, are bright yellow with large petals.

The medicinal part of the plant is the leaf, which has a tightening, drying effect on the tissues.

Avoid If . . .

No known medical conditions preclude the use of Frostwort.

Special Cautions

No side effects have been recorded.

Possible Drug Interactions

No drug interactions have been documented.

Special Information If You Are Pregnant or Breastfeeding

No information is available.

How to Prepare

Frostwort is administered internally or externally as a liquid extract.

Typical Dosage

Strengths of commercial preparations may vary. Follow the manufacturer's labeling whenever available.

Overdosage

No information is available.

Fumitory

Latin name: Fumaria officinalis
Other names: Beggary, Earth Smoke, Vapor

A Remedy For

• Liver and gallbladder problems

In folk medicine, Fumitory has also been used for skin diseases, bladder inflammation, clogged arteries, arthritis, low blood sugar, and infections. Its effectiveness for these problems has not, however, been verified.

What It Is; Why It Works

Fumitory takes its name from the plant's blue-green color, which is reminiscent of smoke rising from the earth. According to ancient exorcists, the smoke from burning Fumitory had the power to ban evil spirits.

The plant's healing properties have been celebrated by physicians and writers from the ancient Greek Dioscorides to Chaucer. In the early 20th century it was still regarded as an excellent blood purifier.

Fumitory's medicinal value lies in the above-ground parts of the plant. It relieves spasms in the gallbladder, bile ducts, and gastrointestinal tract. It also stimulates the flow of bile.

Avoid If . . .

No known medical conditions preclude the use of Fumitory.

Special Cautions

At customary dosage levels, Fumitory seems to pose no risks.

Possible Drug Interactions

None are known.

Special Information If You Are Pregnant or Breastfeeding

No harmful effects are known.

How to Prepare

To make a tea, pour boiling water over 2 to 3 grams (about one-half teaspoonful) of Fumitory, steep for 20 minutes, and strain.

Typical Dosage

For relief of gallbladder complaints, drink 1 cup of warm tea before each meal. Your daily dosage should be a total of 6 grams (about 1 heaping teaspoonful).

Store Fumitory away from light and moisture.

Overdosage

No information on overdosage is available.

Galangal

Latin name: Alpinia officinarum
Other names: Catarrh Root,
  China Root, Chinese Ginger,
  Colic Root, India Root

A Remedy For

- Appetite loss
- Bronchitis
- Colds
- Cough
- Fever
- Indigestion
- Liver and gallbladder problems
- Sore throat
- Tendency to infection

In Asia, this herb is also used for arthritis, diabetes, diarrhea, and difficulty swallowing. However, its effectiveness for these problems has not been confirmed.

What It Is; Why It Works

Galangal has an exotic provenance. The name itself is an Arabic corruption of the Chinese word for ginger. The plant grows in India, Thailand, and southern China, and was probably introduced to the West by Arab or Greek physicians. Galangal has been used as a spice for over 1,000 years. In Russia, it's used as a flavoring for vinegar and the spirit "nastoika."

Galangal has several medicinal actions. It relieves spasms, combats inflammation, and fights bacteria.

Avoid If . . .

There are no known medical conditions that preclude the use of Galangal.

Special Cautions

No health risks or side effects following proper use of Galangal have been recorded.

Possible Drug Interactions

No interactions have been reported.

Special Information If You Are Pregnant or Breastfeeding

No harmful effects are known.

How to Prepare

Galangal may be used as a powder or drunk as a tea. It is also an ingredient in many so-called "Swedish herb" mixtures.

To make tea, pour boiling water over 0.5 to 1 gram (about one-eighth teaspoonful) of Galangal, steep for 10 minutes, and strain.

Typical Dosage
Drink 1 cup of tea one-half hour before meals. Use a total of 2 to 4 grams of the herb daily.

Overdosage
No information on overdosage is available.

Gamboge

Latin name: Garcinia hanburyi
Other names: Gummigutta,
  Gutta Gamba, Tom Rong

A Remedy For
• Constipation
• Indigestion

Although Gamboge seems effective for only the above problems, in Asian medicine it is used for diarrhea, hemorrhoids, inflammations, and ulcers. Homeopathic practitioners also prescribe it for diarrhea.

What It Is; Why It Works
Gamboge is usually combined with other constipation remedies, although it has a strong laxative effect of its own. A 50-foot tree native to Indochina and Sri Lanka, the plant's medicinal value lies in the resin extracted from its trunk. The remedy was first introduced in Europe by the Dutch in the mid-17th century.

Avoid If . . .
No known medical conditions preclude the use of Gamboge.

Special Cautions
Use with caution: as little as 200 milligrams of the drug can cause abdominal pain, ineffectual straining, and vomiting.
   Handle the powdered resin with care; it causes violent sneezing when inhaled.

Possible Drug Interactions
No drug interactions have been reported.

Special Information If You Are Pregnant or Breastfeeding
No harmful effects are known.

How to Prepare
Gamboge is available in powdered form.

Typical Dosage
There is no standard recommendation. Follow the manufacturer's directions whenever available.

Overdosage
A mere 4 grams (less than a teaspoonful) of this herb has been known to cause fatalities. If you suspect an overdose, seek medical attention immediately.

Garlic

Latin name: Allium sativum

A Remedy For
• Bronchitis
• Colds
• Cough

- Fever
- Hardening of the arteries
- Sore throat
- Tendency to infection

In folk medicine Garlic is also taken internally for high blood pressure, digestive ailments, menstrual pain, and diabetes, though its effectiveness for these problems is unproven. Also unverified is its ability to relieve corns, calluses, ear infections, muscle and nerve pain, and sciatica through external application.

What It Is; Why It Works

Garlic fights hardening of the arteries through its proven ability to lower cholesterol. It also has proven antibiotic properties and a mild anti-clotting effect on the blood.

Garlic has been used as a medicine and a food since the time of the Egyptian Pharaohs and the earliest Chinese dynasties. When Garlic cells are crushed, they release allicin, the active ingredient responsible for Garlic's characteristic odor. To be effective, Garlic preparations must smell of allicin.

Avoid If . . .

There are no known reasons to avoid Garlic when used at recommended dosages.

Special Cautions

If you are taking anti-clotting drugs or are preparing for surgery, check with your doctor before using Garlic.

Taking large quantities of Garlic may cause stomach problems, and will lead to bad breath and body odor. Although the problem is rare, frequent hand contact may cause eczema (itching and weeping rash).

Possible Drug Interactions

No harmful effects are known.

Special Information If You Are Pregnant or Breastfeeding

No harmful effects are known.

How to Prepare

Garlic oil: Crush the cloves using a Garlic press; stir into equal amounts of fatty oil and let stand for 48 hours. When finished, filter the oil preparation.

Solid Garlic extract: Chop bulbs and soak in alcohol for a while. Pour off liquid; allow alcohol to evaporate.

Aqueous (water) extract: Crush fresh bulbs in cold water using equal amounts of water and Garlic.

Fermented Garlic: Soak minced Garlic for a long period in a water-alcohol mixture.

Distilled preparations and tinctures (alcohol solutions) are also available.

Typical Dosage

The usual daily oral dosage is 4 grams (approximately three-quarters teaspoonful) of fresh Garlic or 8 milligrams of Garlic oil.

For external use, apply according to need.

Strengths of commercial preparations may vary. Follow the manufacturer's labeling whenever available.

Hang braided Garlic in a dry place to store.

Overdosage
No information on overdosage is available.

Gentian Root

Latin name: Gentiana lutea
Other names: Bitter Root,
Bitterwort

A Remedy For
- Appetite loss
- Indigestion

What It Is; Why It Works
This perennial grows over 4 feet high and produces yellow flowers. It is native to central and southern European mountainous regions, but is cultivated elsewhere as well. Because it is intensely bitter, it has been used in brewing. In fact, in certain mountainous regions, the root is used in the manufacture of spirits.

The medicinal parts are the dried, underground parts of the plant and the fresh, above-ground parts. Its name derives from Gentius, King of Illyria (180-167 BC) who discovered the plant's healing value. It was used in the Middle Ages as an antidote to certain poisons.

The plant works by stimulating the taste buds, which in turn prompt an increase in production of saliva and digestive juices.

Avoid If . . .
Do not use Gentian Root if you have stomach or duodenal ulcers.

Special Cautions
No health risks or side effects following proper use of Gentian Root have been recorded.

Possible Drug Interactions
No interactions have been reported.

Special Information If You Are Pregnant or Breastfeeding
No harmful effects are known.

How to Prepare
In addition to the dried herb, liquid extracts and alcohol solutions (tinctures) are available.

To make a Gentian Root tea, pour boiling water over 1 to 2 grams (about one-half teaspoonful) of chopped herb and allow to steep for 5 to 10 minutes. The tea may be sweetened with honey to improve its bitter taste.

Typical Dosage
The average single dose is 1 gram (about one-half teaspoonful). Limit daily use to 2 to 4 grams of the dried root or liquid extract, or 1 to 3 grams of the tincture.

Because the potency of commercial preparations may vary, follow the manufacturer's instructions whenever available. Store Gentian Root away from light.

Overdosage
No information on overdosage is available.

Gentiana

Latin name: Gentiana scabra

A Remedy For

Gentiana is used by Chinese herbalists as a treatment for hepatitis and other liver disorders, sexually transmitted diseases, vaginal discharge, inflammation of the pelvis, pain and swelling in the genital area, and seizures. Its effectiveness for these problems has not, however, been scientifically verified.

Like its European cousin Gentian Root (*Gentiana lutea*), this herb can also be used as a remedy for indigestion and poor appetite.

What It Is; Why It Works

The Gentian family of herbs contains amarogentin, possibly the most bitter of all known substances. Their extreme bitterness serves to stimulate the taste buds, causing increased production of saliva and digestive juices.

Among the oriental varieties of Gentian, *Gentiana scabra* is the most widely used. A long, thick yellow root, it can be found in Asian markets and in some western-style health food stores. In addition to its digestive action, it is believed to have an antibiotic effect and it is thought to be toxic to the parasite that causes malaria.

Avoid If . . .

Do not take Gentiana if you have diarrhea, acid indigestion, heartburn, or an ulcer.

Special Cautions

At customary dosage levels, Gentiana poses no risks.

Possible Drug Interactions

No interactions have been reported.

Special Information If You Are Pregnant or Breastfeeding

No harmful effects are known.

How to Prepare

Herbs in the Gentian family are usually taken as an alcohol solution (tincture) or a tea made from the dried, chopped root.

Typical Dosage

Tincture: Before each meal, sip a few drops dissolved in a small glass of water.

Tea: Take 25 milliliters (about 2 tablespoonfuls) 3 to 5 times a day.

Overdosage

No information is available.

German Sarsaparilla

Latin name: Carex arenaria
Other names: Red Couchgrass, Red Sedge, Sand Sedge, Sea Sedge

A Remedy For

German Sarsaparilla is often used to treat colds, fevers, urinary tract infections, and rheumatism, although there is no proof that it's effective. In folk medicine, it enjoys an even wider range of applications—all without clinical validation—including the prevention of gout and the treatment of skin conditions, venereal disease, liver disorders, diabetes, water retention, tuberculosis, gas, cramps, and menstrual irregularity.

What It Is; Why It Works
German Sarsaparilla is the dried underground stem of the sand sedge, a hardy marsh grass found along the North Atlantic and Baltic coasts of Europe. Sand sedge roots form a tight, thick mass that withstands erosion, making it a favored planting on the dikes of Holland and along the east coast of England.

Historically, German Sarsaparilla has been used primarily for skin conditions. However, Brazilians take it as snuff and use it to stupefy fish and kill insects. In veterinary medicine, it's given for mange and hoof-and-mouth disease.

Avoid If . . .
No known medical conditions preclude the use of German Sarsaparilla.

Special Cautions
There are no risks on record.

Possible Drug Interactions
No drug interactions have been reported.

Special Information If You Are Pregnant or Breastfeeding
No harmful effects are known.

How to Prepare
To make a tea, use 3 grams (a heaping half teaspoonful) of German Sarsaparilla per cup of boiling water. You can also make a cold solution using 2 teaspoonfuls per cup of water.

Typical Dosage
German Sarsaparilla is taken orally. The usual dosage is:

Hot tea: 1 cup daily
Cold solution: 1 cup 2 to 3 times daily

Overdosage
No information on overdosage is available.

Ginger Root

Latin name: Zingiber officinale

A Remedy For
• Appetite loss
• Motion sickness

Although its effectiveness has been verified for only the two problems listed above, Ginger Root is also taken to loosen phlegm, relieve gas, and tighten the tissues. Asian medicine employs it as a treatment for asthma, shortness of breath, water retention, earache, diarrhea, nausea, and vomiting; and homeopathic practitioners recommend it for sexual disorders as well.

What It Is; Why It Works
Valued primarily for the distinctive tang it lends to cuisine, Ginger Root also has proven medicinal effects. Its ability to prevent vomiting has been verified by clinical trial, and it has been shown to stimulate the

intestines and promote production of saliva, digestive juices, and bile. It also tends to boost the pumping action of the heart.

Native to Southeast Asia, Ginger was brought to Spain, and then America, by the Spanish in the 15th and 16th centuries. It is now commercially cultivated in tropical regions of the United States, India, China, and the West Indies. The plant is a creeping perennial that spreads underground. Only the root is medicinal.

Avoid If . . .

Although Ginger prevents vomiting, it should not be taken for morning sickness. People with gallstones should avoid it unless their doctor approves.

Special Cautions

At customary dosage levels, Ginger Root poses no problems.

Possible Drug Interactions

No drug interactions have been reported.

Special Information If You Are Pregnant or Breastfeeding

No harmful effects are known.

How to Prepare

Ginger Root is available in chopped and powdered form, and as a powdered extract.

To make a tea, pour boiling water over 0.5 to 1 gram (about one-quarter teaspoonful) of the chopped root, steep for 5 minutes, and strain.

Typical Dosage

To prevent vomiting, take 2 grams of powdered Ginger Root with a little liquid. For regular use, the usual dose is 2 to 4 grams (about 1 teaspoonful) of chopped root daily.

Overdosage

No information on overdosage is available.

Ginkgo

Latin name: Ginkgo biloba

A Remedy For

- Circulatory disorders
- Poor circulation in the brain
- Senility

Ginkgo is generally accepted as a remedy for minor deficits in brain function, such as those that occur with advancing age. It is used to improve concentration and combat short-term memory loss due to clogged arteries in the brain, and to treat dizziness, ringing in the ears, headache, and emotional hypersensitivity accompanied by anxiety. For people with intermittent circulation problems in the legs, it permits longer pain-free walks.

What It Is; Why It Works

Although the Ginkgo tree has been around for 200 million years, it's only during the last couple of decades that its true value has been recognized. Active compounds in Ginkgo extract improve circulation, discourage clot formation, reinforce the walls of the capillaries, and protect nerve cells from harm when deprived of oxygen. These ingredients also appear to have an antioxidant effect, sparing brain tissue from the damage caused by free radicals. Because the active ingredients are limited to minute quantities in natural Ginkgo leaves, only concentrated Ginkgo extract is really effective.

The Ginkgo tree grows over 100 feet high and can live for hundreds of years. Native to China, Japan, and Korea, it now grows worldwide, and is intensively cultivated in major plantations such as one in Sumter, South Carolina.

Avoid If . . .

If any Ginkgo Biloba preparation gives you an allergic reaction, avoid this drug.

Special Cautions

Use of Ginkgo can occasionally lead to side effects such as spasms, cramps, and mild digestive problems. On rare occasions, allergic skin reactions may occur.

Possible Drug Interactions

No interactions have been recorded.

Special Information If You Are Pregnant or Breastfeeding

Information is not available.

How to Prepare

Ginkgo extract is produced in liquid and solid forms, particularly as 40-milligram tablets. Tea made from Ginkgo leaves, as in traditional Chinese medicine, is too weak to be effective.

Typical Dosage

A total daily intake of 120 milligrams is usually recommended. Doses of up to 240 milligrams a day are taken by people with severe memory loss.

Strengths of commercial preparations may vary. Follow the manufacturer's labeling whenever available.

Overdosage

A massive overdose can reduce muscle tone, leading to severe weakness. If you suspect an overdose, seek medical attention immediately.

Ginseng

Latin name: Panax ginseng

A Remedy For
• Fatigue

The energizing effects of Ginseng are used to improve concentration, boost resistance, and combat weakness and debility. In Asian medicine, the herb is used as an aphrodisiac, and is considered a remedy for indigestion, heart problems, and urinary disturbances.

What It Is; Why It Works

Valued as a medicine in China for over 2,000 years, Ginseng was once held in such high esteem that only the emperor was allowed to collect it. It has traditionally been used by elderly Asians to boost physical and mental vitality. Only the root is medicinal.

The energizing ingredients in Ginseng are a set of compounds called ginsenosides. A second group of compounds called panaxanes appear to reinforce the immune system and help keep blood sugar levels under control.

Panax ginseng is native to China, but is also cultivated in Korea, Japan, and Russia. An almost identical plant, *Panax quinquefolius*, grows in the United States and was, in fact, exported to China during the 18th century.

Avoid If . . .
No known medical conditions preclude the use of Ginseng.

Special Cautions
At customary dosage levels, Ginseng appears to have no side effects. Overuse of the herb, however, can result in Ginseng abuse syndrome (see "Overdosage").

Possible Drug Interactions
There are no known interactions with Ginseng.

Special Information If You Are Pregnant or Breastfeeding
Because Ginseng's many active ingredients have not been tested in pregnant and nursing women, use during pregnancy is not recommended.

How to Prepare
To make a tea, pour boiling water over 3 grams of chopped root, steep for 5 to 10 minutes, and strain.

Typical Dosage
Root: 1 to 2 grams daily

Tea: Take 3 to 4 times daily for 3 to 4 weeks.

Standardized extracts are often taken at a rate of 100 to 200 milligrams daily.

Strengths of commercial preparations may vary. Follow the manufacturer's labeling whenever available.

Overdosage
Massive overdosage can lead to Ginseng abuse syndrome. Symptoms include sleeplessness, tight muscles, and water retention. If you suspect an overdose, seek medical attention immediately.

Glucosamine

A Remedy For
• Osteoarthritis

Although this natural remedy still inspires controversy, there is increasing evidence that Glucosamine does in fact relieve joint pain and inflammation for many arthritis sufferers, and that it may slow progression of the disease.

Because of its ability to reduce and—in some cases—completely eliminate the pain of osteoarthritis, some physicians and researchers feel Glucosamine might offer similar benefits for people suffering from rheumatoid arthritis, ankylosing spondylitis, spinal disk degeneration, tendinitis, bursitis, and physical injuries to the joints. There is even speculation that it could play a preemptive role, eliminating the development of osteoarthritis in people over 40.

What It Is; Why It Works

Glucosamine is a natural sugar produced by the body and found in certain foods. It plays an important role in the production, maintenance, and repair of cartilage, the white, smooth, rubber-like padding that covers the ends of bones and prevents them from rubbing against each other painfully as we move. It also helps form ligaments, tendons, and nails.

Glucosamine stimulates the production of glycosaminoglycans and proteoglycans, two essential building blocks of cartilage. In most cases, the joints produce sufficient Glucosamine to keep the cartilage in good repair, but if they fail to do so, it dries out, degenerates, cracks, and may even completely wear away. Left unprotected, the joints then become swollen, stiff, inflamed, tender, and painful—the condition known as osteoarthritis.

Advocates believe that by taking artificially synthesized Glucosamine sulfate supplements, osteoarthritis sufferers can "jump start" the natural production of Glucosamine by their own bodies. Combining Glucosamine with Chondroitin sulfate is thought to increase its effectiveness.

While Glucosamine has been used to treat osteoarthritis in Europe since the 1980s, its use in the United States has been confined mainly to arthritic animals. However, several scientific studies have recently supported its effec-

tiveness, and its popularity in this country is spreading quickly.

Avoid If . . .

No known medical conditions preclude the use of Glucosamine.

Special Cautions

Although Glucosamine may relieve your osteoarthritis, other treatments—such as a regular exercise program—remain just as important. If you have this condition, it's wise to keep in touch with your doctor for regular check-ups.

Unlike the potent nonsteroidal anti-inflammatory drugs (NSAIDs) usually prescribed for arthritis, Glucosamine does not produce serious side effects. You might, however, experience mild symptoms such as diarrhea, heartburn, indigestion, and nausea. Try taking the medication with food if it upsets your stomach (or if you have an ulcer). If this fails to eliminate the symptoms, check with your doctor.

Possible Drug Interactions

Glucosamine sulfate taken alone or in combination with Chondroitin does not interfere with NSAIDs, aspirin, or any other anti-inflammatory or analgesic medication. Indeed, there is some evidence that taking this supplement may help people reduce their use of these strong drugs.

Special Information If You Are Pregnant or Breastfeeding

Check with your doctor before taking Glucosamine while pregnant or breastfeeding.

How to Prepare

Glucosamine is available in three forms:

Glucosamine sulfate: This is considered the preparation of choice for osteoarthritis.

Glucosamine hydrochloride: This is the least expensive variety. It is used primarily for arthritic animals.

N-acetyl Glucosamine: This form delivers less of the active ingredient to the joints.

Glucosamine sulfate capsules and Glucosamine sulfate/Chondroitin combination capsules and tablets can be found in many health food stores and may also be ordered by mail.

Typical Dosage

There is no consensus on the ideal dosage of Glucosamine sulfate. Some doctors recommend 1,000 to 2,000 milligrams per day. Others suggest up to 3,000 milligrams a day, since they insist it is safe and produces no serious side effects.

For those using a combination of Chondroitin sulfate and Glucosamine sulfate, the typical dosage recommendation is based on weight:

Less than 120 pounds: 800 milligrams Chondroitin, 1,000 milligrams Glucosamine
120 to 200 pounds: 1,200 milligrams Chondroitin, 1,500 milligrams Glucosamine
More than 200 pounds: 1,600 milligrams Chondroitin, 2,000 milligrams Glucosamine

You may adjust your dosage according to your response. If you are overweight or are taking a water pill (diuretic), you may need a larger dose of each supplement.

Some people experience pain relief immediately. Nevertheless, it may take anywhere from 8 weeks to 6 months to repair damaged cartilage.

Overdosage

No information on overdosage is available.

Goat's Rue

Latin name: Galega officinalis
Other names: French Lilac,
Italian Fitch

A Remedy For

Although Goat's Rue is used as a flushing-out therapy for urinary tract infections, its effectiveness for this purpose remains unproven. Goat's Rue also contains a compound that theoretically lowers blood sugar levels—a potential boon to diabetics. However, the sugar-lowering effect has never been observed in practice and use of the herb is not recommended, given the seriousness of diabetes and the availability of a wide variety of effective alternatives.

What It Is; Why It Works

Goat's Rue is a strong, bright green shrub with numerous, erect, branched, hollow stems that grow 1½ to 3 feet high. It probably takes its name from the unpleasant odor it emits when bruised.

In the Middle Ages, Goat's Rue was taken during plagues, when its ability to promote perspiration was thought to have a protective effect. In 19th century France, it was used to increase milk yield in cows. It was also recommended in times past as a refreshing footbath for "persons tired with overwalking."

Goat's Rue grows wild throughout Europe and Asia. Only the above-ground parts of the plant are considered medicinal.

Avoid If . . .
No known medical conditions preclude the use of Goat's Rue.

Special Cautions
In moderate doses, Goat's Rue poses no documented risks. However, large quantities have been known to poison unwitting animals (see "Overdosage" below).

Possible Drug Interactions
No interactions have been reported.

Special Information If You Are Pregnant or Breastfeeding
No harmful effects are known.

How to Prepare
To make a Goat's Rue tea, pour boiling water over 2 grams (about one-half teaspoonful) of the crushed herb, steep 5 to 10 minutes, and strain.

Typical Dosage
Use is not recommended.

Overdosage
In sheep, an overdose has been observed to cause spasms, paralysis, and death through asphyxiation.

Goldenrod

Latin name: Solidago species

A Remedy For
- Kidney and bladder stones
- Urinary tract infections

Several species of Goldenrod are used to treat urinary infections and kidney and bladder stones. In folk medicine, the *Solidago virgaurea* species has been especially popular, and has been used to treat such diverse ailments as rheumatism, gout, diabetes, hemorrhoids, enlarged prostate, asthma, internal bleeding, enlarged liver, tuberculosis, mouth and throat infections, and festering wounds. Its effectiveness for these conditions remains unproven. In homeopathic medicine, Goldenrod is used for respiratory conditions and kidney pain.

What It Is; Why It Works
Because Goldenrod is a diuretic, drawing water from the body, it is used to flush out the urinary system during infections. It also provides limited action against spasms and inflammation.

The plant is found throughout North America, Europe, and some parts of Asia. For medicinal purposes, the above-ground parts of the plant are gathered during the flowering season and carefully dried.

The scientific name "Solidago" comes from the Latin term "solidare," meaning the plant that consolidates or makes whole.

Avoid If . . .

Do not take Goldenrod if you have chronic kidney disease. Do not use it to flush the urinary tract if you have swelling caused by heart or kidney problems.

Special Cautions

Goldenrod is unlikely to cause problems when taken at usual dosage levels, but be sure to drink lots of fluids while using it.

Possible Drug Interactions

No interactions have been reported.

Special Information If You Are Pregnant or Breastfeeding

No harmful effects are known.

How to Prepare

Crushed Goldenrod can be made into a tea, using 3 to 5 grams (1 to 2 teaspoonfuls) per 5 ounces of water. Steep for 15 minutes in water heated to just below boiling, then strain. You can have 1 cup, between meals, 2 to 4 times a day.

Typical Dosage

Goldenrod is taken orally as a tea, liquid extract, or alcohol solution (tincture). The usual dosage is:

Tea: A total of 6 to 12 grams (2 to 4 teaspoonfuls) of crushed herb daily

Liquid extract: 0.5 to 2 milliliters 3 times daily

Tincture: 0.5 to 1 milliliter 3 times daily

Store protected from light and moisture.

Overdosage

No information on overdosage is available.

Goldenseal

Latin name: Hydrastis canadensis
Other names: Eye Balm, Ground Raspberry, Indian Paint, Jaundice Root, Yellow Root

A Remedy For

Although not officially recognized as effective, Goldenseal is a popular remedy for canker sores, sore throat, and upper respiratory infections. It also has a long-standing history as a remedy for urinary tract infections, vaginal infections, and infectious diarrhea, and has also been used for indigestion and premenstrual syndrome (PMS), although it has never been formally tested for any of these ailments. Applied externally, it was once used to treat wounds and skin and eye infections. Homeopathic practitioners prescribe it for any type of inflammation.

What It Is; Why It Works

Goldenseal was introduced to the West by Native Americans, who used the root as a medicine and as a yellow stain for the face and clothing. Much of the plant's original habitat in the eastern U.S. has become the victim of deforestation. It is now cultivated in the Pacific Northwest.

The plant is a small herbaceous perennial that reaches a height of no more than a foot and produces small flowers and raspberry-like, inedible fruit. The plant has a bitter taste and a strong, disagreeable odor. Only the fleshy underground stem and roots are used medicinally.

Certain compounds in Goldenseal—particularly one called berberine—have antibiotic properties, attacking a variety of common germs. The herb also has mild laxative and anti-inflammatory effects.

Avoid If . . .

No known medical problems preclude the use of Goldenseal.

Special Cautions

If taken for an extended period of time, Goldenseal can cause digestive problems, constipation, nervous excitement, hallucinations, and delirium. Take it for no more than 3 weeks in a row, with a break of at least 2 weeks before resuming.

Possible Drug Interactions

No interactions have been reported.

Special Information If You Are Pregnant or Breastfeeding

Use of Goldenseal is not recommended during pregnancy or while breastfeeding.

How to Prepare

The powdered root is usually taken in tablet or capsule form. You may also find liquid extracts available.

You can make a strong Goldenseal mouthwash by combining 6 grams (about 2 teaspoonfuls) of the powdered root with 240 milliliters (1 cup) of water.

Typical Dosage

Goldenseal mouthwash may be used 3 to 4 times daily. When the herb is taken internally, the usual daily dose is 4 to 6 grams of powdered root or 4 to 6 milliliters of liquid extract.

Since potency of commercial preparations may vary, follow the manufacturer's directions whenever available.

Overdosage

Symptoms of overdose include vomiting, breathing difficulty, a slowdown in heart rate, and spasms ending in paralysis. If you suspect an overdose, seek medical attention immediately.

Gotu Kola

Latin name: Centella asiatica
Other names: Indian Pennywort,
 Marsh Penny, White Rot

A Remedy For

Although Gotu Kola has received no official recognition, a number of tests have confirmed its ability to speed the healing of wounds and burns. It is also a clinically proven remedy for symptoms of poor circulation in the veins of the legs.

Originally an Asian medicine, Gotu Kola is employed in the Far East for an extensive catalog of problems, including asthma, bronchitis, heart problems, dysentery, epilepsy, insomnia, jaundice, eye conditions, exhaustion, inflammation, high blood pressure, diarrhea, and problems with urination. In India, it's used for skin diseases, syphilis, muscle and joint problems, leprosy, dehydration, hysteria, and mental illness. There is, however, insufficient proof of its effectiveness for any of these conditions.

What It Is; Why It Works

Gotu Kola is a low-lying creeper found in swampy areas of the tropics and subtropical areas worldwide. The above-ground parts of the plant are considered medicinal. It is believed to work by regulating the growth of connective tissue and stimulating production of the protein needed in the healing of wounds.

In animal tests, Gotu Kola has shown a number of effects, including the ability to sedate, relieve depression, protect against ulcers, kill certain bacteria, and promote wound healing. Human trials have verified its ability to relieve pain, heaviness, and swelling in the legs. The jury is still out, however, on the practical value of these findings.

Avoid If . . .

No known medical conditions preclude the use of Gotu Kola.

Special Cautions

High doses have been known to cause nausea. Sedation and skin rash are also possibilities

Possible Drug Interactions

No interactions have been reported.

Special Information If You Are Pregnant or Breastfeeding

Use of Gotu Kola is not recommended during pregnancy or while breastfeeding.

How to Prepare

Gotu Kola is available in a wide variety of forms, including ointment, tablet, capsule, powder, extract, and drops.

To make a tea from the dried leaf, pour 150 milliliters (about two-thirds of a cup) of boiling water over 1 to 2 teaspoonfuls of crushed leaf and steep for 10 to 15 minutes.

Typical Dosage

In dried-leaf form, the usual dosage is 0.6 grams 3 times daily. For the tablet form, a typical recommendation is 3 to 6 of the 10-milligram tablets daily. However, the potency of commercial preparations varies, so you should follow the manufacturer's recommendations whenever available.

Overdosage

No information on overdosage is available.

Greater Burnet

Latin name: Sanguisorba officinalis
Other name: Garden Burnet

A Remedy For
- Menopausal disorders

Greater Burnet is taken internally to treat female disorders, such as heavy menstrual flow and hot flashes during menopause. It also is used in the treatment of intestinal inflammation, diarrhea, difficulty urinating, hemorrhoids, inflammation of leg veins, and varicose veins. In Asian medicine, it's considered a remedy for infectious diarrhea, nosebleed, and coughing up of blood.

Applied externally, it is used to treat wounds and boils, but its effectiveness for this purpose has not been scientifically confirmed.

What It Is; Why It Works

Greater Burnet was formerly in great demand to stop bleeding from wounds. In fact, its Latin name comes from "sanguis," for blood and "sorbeo," for stanch. Although it is still used as a remedy for bleeding, its effectiveness against the symptoms of menopause is more widely accepted. There have been no investigations into its exact mode of action.

The plant is widespread in the northern temperate regions of Europe, Asia, and North America. In addition to its medicinal applications, it is used as a vegetable and added to salads.

Avoid If . . .

No known medical conditions preclude the use of Greater Burnet.

Special Cautions

No risks or side effects are known.

Possible Drug Interactions

No interactions have been reported.

Special Information If You Are Pregnant or Breastfeeding

No harmful effects are known.

How to Prepare

Greater Burnet may be taken as a ground herb, extract, juice, or tea.

Typical Dosage

There are no formal guidelines on record.

Overdosage

No information is available on overdosage.

Green Tea

Latin name: Camellia sinensis
Other name: Chinese Tea

A Remedy For
- Diarrhea
- Indigestion
- Motion sickness

Although Green Tea has not been officially recognized as a medicinal agent, it is known to be effective against diarrhea and upset stomach. In Asian medicine, it is used to treat heart pain, dizziness, hemorrhoids, headache, excessive thirst, indigestion, and drowsiness. Homeopathic practitioners recommend it for headache, heart conditions, and insomnia.

What It Is; Why It Works

Green Tea contains caffeine, which stimulates the central nervous system, and tannins, which combat diarrhea. Taken in moderation, it has mild painkilling and stimulant effects. In excess, it can cause insomnia and digestive problems.

Green and black tea come from the same plant and differ only in their method of production. Green Tea is dried for a shorter time, and is heated sooner to prevent fermentation. Green Tea is produced in China and Japan; black tea comes from India, Sri Lanka, and Kenya. The plant is also cultivated in Indonesia, Turkey, Pakistan, Malawi, and Argentina.

Avoid If . . .

Take Green Tea cautiously, if at all, if you have a weak heart, kidney disease, an overactive thyroid, a susceptibility to spasms, or a tendency to anxiety or panic attacks.

Special Cautions

If you have a sensitive stomach, Green Tea may cause acid stomach, stomach irritation, and poor appetite. Intake of large quantities can lead to constipation or diarrhea. Adding milk to the tea will usually eliminate these side effects by reducing the potency of the tannins.

Possible Drug Interactions

Green Tea interferes with absorption of alkaline medications. If you are taking any medicines, check with your doctor before taking Green Tea.

Special Information If You Are Pregnant or Breastfeeding

Because of its caffeine content, you may want to restrict your intake of Green Tea during pregnancy. Although most studies show no harm to the developing baby, some evidence links slower fetal growth to daily intake of 400 milligrams or more of caffeine (6 or more cups of tea). Excessive caffeine intake may also increase the risk of late first or second trimester miscarriage.

Nursing mothers should drink little, if any, Green Tea because, like other beverages containing caffeine, it can cause sleep disorders in infants.

How to Prepare

When taking Green Tea for diarrhea, allow extra time for steeping. The longer Green Tea brews, the stronger its antidiarrheal effect.

Typical Dosage

There are no formal dosage guidelines.

Overdosage

Doses of 300 milligrams of caffeine (about 5 cups of tea) can cause restlessness, tremors, and exaggerated reflexes. The first signs of outright poisoning are vomiting and abdominal spasms.

It's impossible to drink enough

tea to be fatal. However, regular daily intake of excessive doses (1,500 milligrams of caffeine, or 25 cups of tea) will result in irritability, sleeplessness, irregular heartbeat, dizziness, vomiting, diarrhea, loss of appetite, and headache.

Guaiac

Latin name: Guaiacum officinale
Other names: Lignum Vitae, Pockwood

A Remedy For
• Rheumatism

Although judged effective only for symptomatic relief of rheumatism, Guaiac has a history of use as a treatment for syphilis, respiratory complaints, and skin disorders. It's also used in homeopathic medicine as a remedy for tonsillitis.

What It Is; Why It Works
Prepared from the wood of a tall evergreen that grows in Florida, the Antilles, Guyana, Venezuela, and Colombia, Guaiac wood shavings used to be sold under the name "lignum vitae." They play the unusual trick of turning green when exposed to air.

Both the shavings and an alcohol solution of the wood's resin are used medicinally. Researchers have found that the wood slows the growth of fungus. The tree's essential oil is considered a separate drug.

Avoid If . . .
No known medical conditions preclude the use of Guaiac.

Special Cautions
Although Guaiac presents no problems when taken at customary dosage levels, high doses can lead to inflammation of the stomach and intestines, intestinal pain, and diarrhea. Skin rashes have also been reported.

Possible Drug Interactions
No interactions have been reported.

Special Information If You Are Pregnant or Breastfeeding
No harmful effects are known.

How to Prepare
To make a tea, mix 1.5 grams of Guaiac shavings with 150 milliliters (5 ounces) of cold water, bring slowly to a boil, and strain after 15 minutes.

Typical Dosage
Guaiac shavings: 4 to 5 grams per day
Guaiac tincture: 20 to 40 drops per dose

Overdosage
No information on overdosage is available.

Guarana

Latin name: Paullinia cupana
Other name: Brazilian Cocoa

A Remedy For
• Fatigue

In homeopathic medicine, Guarana is used to treat headaches. There is, however, no evidence of its effectiveness for this problem.

What It Is; Why It Works

This exotic herb from the Amazon basin depends on plain old caffeine for its stimulating action. Among caffeine's many effects are a tendency to strengthen and speed up the heartbeat, relax blood vessels (except for those in the brain), and open bronchial tubes. Caffeine also discourages blood clots, stimulates the urinary system, and promotes production of digestive juices.

Guarana is an evergreen vine growing up to 30 feet long in the Amazon rain forest. Much like coffee beans, its seeds are peeled, dried, roasted, ground, and made into beverages. In Brazil, a fermented mixture of Guarana, cassava, and water has become a popular national drink. Although Guarana is an ingredient in some medicinal preparations, it is not itself used as a drug.

Avoid If . . .

In moderate amounts, Guarana poses no threat to a healthy adult.

Special Cautions

Especially if you are already getting caffeine from other sources, use Guarana with caution if you have a heart condition, kidney disease, an overactive thyroid, a tendency to spasms, or problems with anxiety or panic.

Possible Drug Interactions

No drug interactions have been reported.

Special Information If You Are Pregnant or Breastfeeding

Many doctors recommend limiting caffeine intake during pregnancy to the equivalent of 1 cup of coffee per day. Doses of over 400 milligrams a day (the equivalent of 4 cups of coffee) are suspected of stunting the baby's growth. Given the amount of caffeine in the typical Western diet, the wisest course is to completely avoid an extra source such as Guarana.

Excessive caffeine intake while nursing may cause sleeping disorders in the infant.

How to Prepare

Guarana can be taken as a powder or can be mixed with water or juice.

Typical Dosage

Amounts of Guarana delivering up to 400 milligrams of caffeine per day are considered harmless. This equals about 7 to 11 grams (up to about 2 teaspoonfuls) of the powder.

Overdosage

Early symptoms of Guarana overdose include difficult urination, vomiting, and abdominal spasms. If you suspect an overdose, seek medical attention immediately.

Guggul

Latin name: Commiphora mukul
Other names: Gugulipid, Gum Guggulu

A Remedy For

Guggul is taken to lower cholesterol levels and prevent hardening of the arteries. Several studies support its effectiveness, but conclusive proof has yet to appear.

What It Is; Why It Works

Guggul is a resin produced by the stem of the *Commiphora mukul* tree, a small, thorny plant that grows throughout India. Chemicals in the resin called guggulsterones are responsible for its favorable effect on cholesterol and triglycerides. They not only lower levels of LDL and VLDL—the "bad" cholesterols—but raise levels of the "good" cholesterol HDL. They also appear to reduce the stickiness of platelets in the blood, thus lowering the risk of dangerous clots.

Avoid If . . .

If you have liver disease, inflammatory bowel disease, or diarrhea, check with your doctor before using this medication.

Special Cautions

The unpurified resin can cause diarrhea, abdominal pain, loss of appetite, and skin rash. However, the purified extracts in use today are unlikely to cause anything more than mild abdominal discomfort.

Remember that it's important to have regular check-ups if you suffer from high cholesterol.

Possible Drug Interactions

There are no known drug interactions.

Special Information If You Are Pregnant or Breastfeeding

No harmful effects are known.

How to Prepare

The powdered resin is available in capsule form.

Typical Dosage

Dosage is based on guggulsterone content. A common recommendation is 25 milligrams of guggulsterones 3 times a day.

Because strengths of commercial preparations may vary, follow the manufacturer's labeling whenever available.

Overdosage

No information is available.

Gumweed

Latin name: Grindelia camporum
Other names: August Flower, California Gum Plant, Resinweed, Tar Weed

A Remedy For

- Bronchitis
- Cough

In homeopathic medicine, Gumweed is also used for stomach ulcers and disorders of the spleen. Its effectiveness for these problems has not, however, been scientifically verified.

What It Is; Why It Works

Gumweed is found in the southwest United States and Mexico. The plant is a small bush up to 3 feet high. The medicinal parts are the leafy branches, gathered during the flowering season.

In laboratory tests, Gumweed exhibits an antibacterial action.

Avoid If . . .

There are no known medical conditions that preclude the use of Gumweed.

Special Cautions

Stomach irritation and diarrhea are potential side effects.

Possible Drug Interactions

No drug interactions have been reported.

Special Information If You Are Pregnant or Breastfeeding

No harmful effects are known.

How to Prepare

Gumweed is prepared as a crushed herb for tea. You also may find extracts of Gumweed and solutions of Gumweed in alcohol.

Typical Dosage

Gumweed is taken orally. The usual daily dosage is:

Crushed Gumweed: 4 to 6 grams (about 1 teaspoonful)
Liquid extract: 3 to 6 grams

Because the potency of commercial preparations may vary, follow the manufacturer's instructions whenever available.

Overdosage

Large doses are said to be poisonous, but specific symptoms have not been recorded.

Gymnema

Latin name: Gymnema sylvestre
Other name: Gurmarbooti

A Remedy For

• High blood sugar

Although this Indian herb is now used primarily for Type 2 (adult-onset) diabetes, in the past it was also recommended for stomach problems, constipation, water retention, and liver disease. Its effectiveness for such problems is, however, doubtful.

What It Is; Why It Works

A tenacious climbing vine, Gymnema is native to the jungles of southern India. It has been clinically proven to reduce excessively high blood sugar levels, apparently by boosting the amount of insulin available to process sugar. It also exhibits cholesterol-lowering activity, although not to a degree that makes it useful.

Gymnema leaves, when chewed, have the unusual ability to block the taste of sweetness.

Avoid If . . .

No known medical conditions preclude the use of Gymnema.

Special Cautions

Without proper treatment, diabetes can lead to heart disease, kidney failure, blindness, and loss of limbs. It is not the sort of disease you want to treat on your own.

Gymnema has successfully controlled blood sugar levels for extended periods of time, but you may need additional medications—or even insulin—to maintain optimum health. If you've been diagnosed with diabetes and choose to take Gymnema, be sure to do so under your doctor's continuing care.

Possible Drug Interactions

No interactions have been reported.

Special Information If You Are Pregnant or Breastfeeding

No studies have been done on pregnant or breastfeeding women.

How to Prepare

Traditionally, patients have taken powdered Gymnema leaf. In recent research, a water-soluble extract has been used.

Typical Dosage

Powdered leaf: 2 to 4 grams per day
Extract: 400 milligrams per day

Strengths of commercial preparations may vary. Follow the manufacturer's instructions whenever available.

Overdosage

No information on overdosage is available.

Haronga

Latin name: Haronga madagascariensis

A Remedy For

- Appetite loss
- Indigestion
- Liver and gallbladder problems

What It Is; Why It Works

Used historically as a remedy for dysentery, Haronga is a small evergreen tree that grows up to 24 feet in height. It comes from Madagascar and East Africa and is widely distributed throughout tropical Africa.

Haronga's leaves and bark are used medicinally. They have been shown to stimulate digestive juices and kill certain bacteria. In animal tests, they have exhibited a protective effect on the liver.

Avoid If . . .

Do not use Haronga if you have a severe pancreas or liver disorder, gallstones, obstruction of the bile ducts, or other gallbladder problems.

Special Cautions

In large doses, Haronga can cause a harmful reaction to light. At typical dosage levels, however, this problem is unlikely.

Possible Drug Interactions

No interactions have been reported.

Special Information If You Are Pregnant or Breastfeeding

No harmful effects are known.

How to Prepare

Haronga leaves and bark are air-dried after collection. The medication is supplied in dry extract form.

Typical Dosage

The average dose of the dry extract is 7.5 to 15 milligrams daily.

Overdosage

No information on overdosage is available.

Hawthorn Leaf

Latin name: Crataegus species
Other name: Whitethorn

A Remedy For

- Angina
- Weak heart

Hawthorn Leaf is a useful preventive measure against angina (sharp chest pain caused by a shortage of oxygen in the heart muscle), and it's also recommended for mild cases of chronic heart failure.

What It Is; Why It Works

Hawthorn has come under intense scientific scrutiny in Europe, where researchers have found that it is capable of expanding the blood vessels and enabling more oxygen-rich blood to reach the muscles of the heart. This boosts the strength of the heartbeat and can slightly increase its speed. Hawthorn's vessel-dilating action also aids the heart by reducing resistance elsewhere in the circulatory system.

A dense, thorny shrub that grows 5 to 13 feet high, Hawthorn has been used to form hedgerows since at least the Middle Ages. The plant is found in the northern, temperate zones of Europe, Asia, and North America. Its flowers, leaves, and fruit are used medicinally.

Avoid If . . .

No known medical conditions preclude the use of Hawthorn Leaf.

Special Cautions

Hawthorn Leaf is useful only for long-term treatment. Although it can reduce the tendency to angina, it is very slow-acting and won't remedy an acute attack. It is notably free of side effects.

Possible Drug Interactions

No interactions have been reported.

Special Information If You Are Pregnant or Breastfeeding

No harmful effects are known.

How to Prepare

Hawthorn Leaf is available in liquid and dry extracts for oral intake. Although less reliable, the crushed herb may also be used.

Typical Dosage

The crushed herb is usually taken in doses of 1 gram, up to a total of 5 grams a day, for a minimum of 6 weeks. It should be stored in a tightly-sealed container protected from light.

Dosage of Hawthorn extract varies according to the potency of the product. Follow the manufacturer's directions.

Overdosage
No information on overdosage is available.

Heartsease

Latin name: Viola tricolor
Other names: Johnny-jump-up,
  Wild Pansy

A Remedy For
- Skin inflammation
- Warts

Warts and skin inflammation are the only disorders for which Heartsease has a demonstrable effect, but it has also been used for relief of eczema, acne, impetigo, female genital itching, and cradle cap in infants. It is taken internally for constipation and poor metabolism, and was once considered a remedy for respiratory and throat inflammation, whooping cough, and feverish colds.

What It Is; Why It Works
This little perennial, which grows to no more than a foot in height and sprouts a single yellow flower, is found throughout temperate Eurasia and is cultivated in Holland and France. Although now used mainly for unpleasant skin conditions, the flower was once a favored ingredient for love po-

tions, which presumably accounts for its name.

The entire plant is considered medicinal. It relieves inflammation and acts as an antioxidant. These properties have won it a place in many cosmetic formulas.

Avoid If . . .
No known medical conditions preclude the use of Heartsease.

Special Cautions
Used externally (and internally, for that matter) Heartsease poses no particular risks.

Possible Drug Interactions
No interactions have been reported.

Special Information If You Are Pregnant or Breastfeeding
No harmful effects are known.

How to Prepare
Heartsease is available in crushed and powdered form, for use in teas and compresses, and as a bath additive.

Typical Dosage
Heartsease is used primarily in compresses. If you plan to take it internally, use 1.5 grams (about one-quarter teaspoonful) per cup of water. Take 3 times daily.

Store Heartsease in well-sealed containers protected from light and moisture.

Overdosage
No information on overdosage is available.

Heather

Latin name: Calluna vulgaris
Other name: Ling

A Remedy For

Heather is sometimes recommended for prostate symptoms and other urinary problems, although proof of its effectiveness remains insufficient.

In folk medicine it is also used, without substantiation, for ailments of the kidneys and lower urinary tract, digestive disorders, cramps, diarrhea, liver and gallbladder disease, gout, rheumatism, respiratory complaints, insomnia, agitation, and wounds.

What It Is; Why It Works

Heather is thought to have a diuretic, flushing action that promotes urination. It is also believed to stimulate the flow of bile and inhibit the growth of germs, but none of these effects has been scientifically documented.

The many varieties of this dwarf, flowering shrub can be found across most of Europe, Russia, and Asia Minor, as well as on the Atlantic coast of North America. The entire above-ground part of the plant is considered medicinal.

Avoid If . . .

No known medical conditions preclude the use of Heather.

Special Cautions

At customary dosage levels, Heather poses no risks.

Possible Drug Interactions

No interactions have been reported.

Special Information If You Are Pregnant or Breastfeeding

No harmful effects are known.

How to Prepare

To make a tea, combine 1.5 grams (about one-third teaspoonful) of crushed Heather with 1 cup of water and boil for 3 minutes.

The herb can also be used in a bath; combine 500 grams (about 2 cups) of Heather with a few quarts of water. Boil, strain, and add to bath water.

A liquid extract is also available.

Typical Dosage

Tea: 3 cups daily between meals
Liquid extract: 1 to 2 teaspoons daily

Store Heather in well-dried, sealed containers.

Overdosage

No information on overdosage is available.

Hemp Nettle

Latin name: Galeopsis segetum

A Remedy For
- Bronchitis
- Cough

In folk medicine, Hemp Nettle has also been used to treat lung conditions and flush excess fluid from the body, but its effectiveness for such problems has not been scientifically established.

What It Is; Why It Works
Hemp Nettle is found in southern and central Europe. The plant grows 3 feet high, with large pale yellow flowers that are said to resemble a weasel's face. Its medicinal value lies in its ability to loosen phlegm. It also has an astringent, tightening effect on the tissues.

Avoid If . . .
There are no known medical conditions that preclude the use of Hemp Nettle.

Special Cautions
At customary dosage levels, Hemp Nettle poses no known danger.

Possible Drug Interactions
No drug interactions have been reported.

Special Information If You Are Pregnant or Breastfeeding
No harmful effects are known.

How to Prepare
To prepare a tea, pour boiling water over 2 grams (less than one-half teaspoonful) of crushed Hemp Nettle, steep for 5 minutes, then strain. The tea may be sweetened with honey.

Typical Dosage
Take the tea several times a day. The usual total daily dosage is 6 grams of the crushed herb.

Overdosage
No information on overdosage is available.

Henbane

Latin name: Hyoscyamus niger
Other names: Devil's Eye,
    Hogbean, Poison Tobacco,
    Stinking Nightshade

A Remedy For
• Liver and gallbladder problems

Only Henbane leaf has been deemed effective—and only for liver and gallbladder problems. However, the leaf is also taken for stomach and intestinal cramps, toothache, whooping cough, painful ulcers, and tumors, and oil from the leaf is used as a treatment for scar tissue. Henbane seed was once used as a vapor treatment for asthma and toothache.

In Asian medicine, Henbane leaf is considered a remedy for vaginal discharge, meningitis, scabies, and involuntary discharge of sperm, while the seed is used for epilepsy, toothache, and eye inflammation.

In homeopathic medicine, Henbane is prescribed for nervous conditions and stomach problems.

What It Is; Why It Works
Henbane contains hyoscyamine, the active ingredient in certain prescription drugs for spasms and cramps, including Cytospaz and Urised. Henbane fights cramps by relaxing the smooth muscles that line the internal organs,

especially those in the digestive tract. It also relieves muscle tremors and has a calming effect.

Henbane has been known for its wine-like sedative properties since the time of the ancient Greeks. Mentioned by Shakespeare, Marlowe, Gower, and Spenser, it is also one of the best known herbs in English literature. Still, it has never enjoyed much popularity as a medicine, perhaps because of its unpleasant side effects. Native to Europe and nearby regions of Asia and Africa, it now grows throughout the northern hemisphere.

Despite the sound of it, the name "Henbane" has no connection with poultry. Instead, it is a corruption of the 11th century Anglo-Saxon "Belene" or "Henbell," a reference to the bell-shaped flowers of the plant.

Avoid If . . .

Do not take Henbane if you suffer from rapid heartbeat, prostate cancer, glaucoma, fluid in the lungs, narrowing of the stomach or intestinal passages, or an enlarged colon.

Special Cautions

Use Henbane with great care; high doses are poisonous. Side effects, which become more likely as the dosage is increased, include impaired distance vision, heat build-up due to reduced sweating, and severe constipation.

Possible Drug Interactions

Henbane leaf can increase the severity of side effects from a number of prescription drugs. Be

cautious about combining Henbane with any of the following:

Amantadine (Symmetrel)
Antidepressants in the tricyclic category, including Elavil, Tofranil-PM, and Triavil
Antihistamines such as Benadryl
Drugs classified as MAO inhibitors, including the antidepressants Nardil and Parnate and the Parkinson's disease medication Eldepryl
Haloperidol (Haldol)
Major tranquilizers in the phenothiazine category, including Compazine, Stelazine, and Thorazine
Procainamide (Procanbid)
Quinidine (Quinaglute, Quinidex)

Special Information If You Are Pregnant or Breastfeeding

No harmful effects are known.

How to Prepare

Remedies usually are made from standardized Henbane powder.

Typical Dosage

The usual dose is 0.5 gram of standardized Henbane powder. Take no more than 3 grams per day.

Overdosage

A massive overdose poses the threat of suffocation, and can be lethal. The four warning signs of overdose are reddened skin, dry mouth, enlarged pupils, and a fast, irregular heartbeat. Early feelings of sleepiness are followed by restlessness, hallucinations, delirium, and hyperactivity, finally ending in exhaustion and sleep.

Severe poisonings are usually the result of recreational misuse of this herb. If you suspect an overdose, seek emergency medical assistance immediately.

Hibiscus

Latin name: Hibiscus sabdariffa
Other names: Guinea Sorrel,
   Jamaica Sorrel, Red Sorrel,
   Roselle

A Remedy For
Hibiscus flower is sometimes recommended for indigestion and loss of appetite, although its effectiveness for these problems has not been verified. Also unsubstantiated is its use as a remedy for colds, respiratory inflammation, phlegm, constipation, water retention, and circulation disorders.

What It Is; Why It Works
As herbal remedies go, Hibiscus is quite new to the scene. It wasn't until the 20th century that it began to appear in herbal tea mixtures. Hibiscus tea does have a laxative effect due to its high content of poorly absorbable fruit acids. Researchers have also found that extracts of Hibiscus leaf tend to relax the uterus and reduce blood pressure. None of these effects is pronounced enough to have won the herb a major following, however.

The Hibiscus plant, a small, bushy annual with spectacular red and yellow blooms, originated near the source of the Niger River in Africa, but is now grown worldwide. Only the blossom is used medicinally.

Avoid If . . .
No known medical conditions preclude the use of Hibiscus.

Special Cautions
No problems or side effects have been documented.

Possible Drug Interactions
No interactions have been reported.

Special Information If You Are Pregnant or Breastfeeding
No harmful effects are known.

How to Prepare
To make a tea, pour boiling water over 1.5 grams of crushed Hibiscus blossoms, steep for 5 to 10 minutes, then strain.

Typical Dosage
No recommendations are on record.

Overdosage
No information on overdosage is available.

Hollyhock

Latin name: Alcea rosea
Other names: Althea Rose,
   Malva Flowers, Rose Mallow

A Remedy For
Some people consider Hollyhock a remedy for bronchitis, cough, and indigestion, and it's taken for fever, sore throat, kidney inflammation, and menstrual problems

as well. Applied externally, it's used as a treatment for skin inflammation and ulcers. There is little evidence, however, that it will actually relieve any of these problems.

What It Is; Why It Works

From its origin in central Asia, Hollyhock has spread around the world. The plant is a tall ornamental that every two years produces showy groups of blood-red or purple flowers up to 4 inches in diameter. It's the dark purple blossoms that are considered medicinal. They have been used as a healing herb since at least the Middle Ages.

Avoid If . . .

No known medical conditions preclude the use of Hollyhock.

Special Cautions

At customary dosage levels, the flower poses no risks.

Possible Drug Interactions

No drug interactions have been reported.

Special Information If You Are Pregnant or Breastfeeding

No harmful effects are known.

How to Prepare

Hollyhock is prepared as a tea.

Typical Dosage

Follow the supplier's directions whenever available.

Overdosage

No information on overdosage is available.

Hops

Latin name: Humulus lupulus

A Remedy For

- Insomnia
- Nervousness

Although its only confirmed value lies in its use for edginess and insomnia, this herb has also been used to stimulate the appetite, increase the flow of digestive juices, and treat ulcers, skin abrasions, and bladder inflammation.

What It Is; Why It Works

Hops have long been associated with beer and ale, but the beverage originally called ale in English was made from fermented malt only, and contained no Hops. The use of Hops probably began in Holland in the early 14th century, and the resulting drink became known as "bier" or "beer." At first, there was much resistance to the use of Hops, which was regarded as a "wicked weed that would spoil the taste . . . and endanger the people."

The plant's medicinal value lies in a set of light yellow scales adjoining the fruit. Compounds in these scales have a sedative effect. Hop tea induces calm, and pillows stuffed with Hops assist sleep.

Avoid If . . .

No known medical conditions preclude the use of Hops.

Special Cautions

The fresh plant can occasionally

cause a reaction. However, when taken at customary dosage levels, Hops pose no problems.

Possible Drug Interactions

There are no known interactions.

Special Information If You Are Pregnant or Breastfeeding

No harmful effects are known.

How to Prepare

Hops are available in crushed and powdered form, and in commercial preparations for oral administration.

To make Hop tea, pour boiling water over the ground herb and steep for 10 to 15 minutes.

Typical Dosage

The usual single dose of Hops is 0.5 gram (about 1 heaping teaspoonful).

The strength of commercial preparations may vary, so follow the manufacturer's directions whenever available.

Store Hops protected from light and moisture.

Overdosage

No information on overdosage is available.

Horehound

Latin name: Marrubium vulgare
Other name: Houndsbane

A Remedy For

- Appetite loss
- Bronchitis
- Cough

- Indigestion
- Liver and gallbladder problems

In folk medicine, Horehound has also been used for whooping cough, asthma, tuberculosis, respiratory infections, lung inflammation, diarrhea, jaundice, painful menstruation, constipation, sores, and wounds. Its effectiveness for these conditions has not been confirmed.

What It Is; Why It Works

Horehound has been known throughout most of history. The Egyptians called it the Seed of Horus and used it as an antidote for certain poisons. They believed it had antimagical properties and that if it was put in a bowl of milk near a place infested with flies, it would kill them all.

Horehound was also a common remedy in ancient Rome, and may have been named after the ancient Italian town of Maria Urbs. Other authorities say the Latin name stems from the Hebrew "marrob," meaning bitter juice; it was one of the bitter herbs eaten at the feast of Passover. The plant is native to the Mediterranean region, but can now be found worldwide.

The entire flowering plant is considered medicinal when fresh; the flowering branches are medicinal when dried. Horehound stimulates digestive juices and production of bile by the liver. It also has an expectorant action, helping to loosen phlegm. Horehound tea is still regarded as an effective cure for colds in certain countries, and is commonly used in liqueurs and aperitifs.

Avoid If . . .
No known medical conditions preclude the use of this herb.

Special Cautions
When taken at customary dosage levels, Horehound poses no risks.

Possible Drug Interactions
No interactions have been reported.

Special Information If You Are Pregnant or Breastfeeding
No harmful effects are known.

How to Prepare
Horehound may be used internally or externally. It can be taken fresh or dried, as a powder, a juice, a liquid extract, or a tea. To prepare the tea, pour boiling water over 1 to 2 grams (about one-quarter teaspoonful) of Horehound, steep 10 minutes, and strain.

Typical Dosage
Fresh or dried herb: 4.5 grams (almost one teaspoonful) daily
Pressed juice: 30 to 60 milliliters (2 to 4 tablespoonfuls) daily
Liquid extract: 2 to 4 milliliters (about one-half teaspoonful) 3 times daily
Tea: Up to 3 cups daily

Overdosage
No information on overdosage is available.

Horse Chestnut

Latin name: Aesculus hippocastanum
Other names: Buckeye, Spanish Chestnut

A Remedy For
• Poor circulation in the veins

Only the seeds of the Horse Chestnut offer proven medicinal value, and only for symptoms of venous insufficiency, such as pain and heaviness in the legs, nighttime cramps in the calves, and itchy, swollen legs. However, the seeds are also used to treat painful injuries, sprains, bruises, swelling, and spinal problems.

The effectiveness of Horse Chestnut leaf needs additional documentation. However, some consider it effective for hemorrhoids, skin inflammation, premenstrual syndrome, and conditions affecting the veins, including phlebitis and varicose veins. In folk medicine, the leaf is used for cough, arthritis, and rheumatism.

Homeopathic practitioners use both the leaf and the seed for hemorrhoids, lower back pain, and varicose veins.

What It Is; Why It Works
Aescin, the active ingredient in Horse Chestnut seed, tones up the walls of the veins, thus improving the flow of blood back to the heart. It also relieves swelling by stopping excessive leakage through the walls of the capillaries (the tiny vessels that deliver blood to the tissues).

Avoid If . . .

No known medical conditions preclude the use of Horse Chestnut leaf or seed.

Special Cautions

In some people, Horse Chestnut seed causes side effects such as irritation of the digestive tract, reduced kidney function, and itching of the skin.

Possible Drug Interactions

There are no known drug interactions with Horse Chestnut.

Special Information If You Are Pregnant or Breastfeeding

No information is available.

How to Prepare

In Europe, Horse Chestnut seed is generally taken in the form of a dry extract containing up to 20 percent aescin.

The leaves can be used to make tea. Pour boiling water over 1 teaspoonful of finely cut leaves, steep for 5 to 10 minutes, then strain.

Typical Dosage

The recommended dosage of the seed extract is an amount delivering 30 to 150 milligrams of aescin daily. Since the strength of commercial preparations may vary, follow the manufacturer's instructions whenever available.

Overdosage

High doses of Horse Chestnut seed can be dangerous. Symptoms of overdose include diarrhea, enlarged pupils, loss of consciousness, reddening of the face, severe thirst, visual disturbances, and vomiting. If you suspect an overdose, seek medical attention immediately.

Horseradish

Latin name: Armoracia rusticana
Other names: Great Raifort, Mountain Radish, Red Cole

A Remedy For
• Bronchitis
• Cough
• Urinary tract infections

Horseradish has been used, without proven effectiveness, for a variety of other conditions. In folk medicine, it has been taken for influenza, digestive problems, gout, rheumatism, liver disease, and gallbladder disorders. Homeopathic practitioners use it for stomach cramps and all types of respiratory problems. It is also used externally for minor muscle aches.

What It Is; Why It Works

Horseradish is one of the five "bitter herbs" of the Jewish Passover feast. In ancient Rome, according to the historian Pliny, it was considered a medicine rather than a food. By the Middle Ages, however, it was widely used both medicinally and in cooking. Today it's prized primarily for the extra zing it lends to cooking.

A perennial plant that grows almost 4 feet high, Horseradish originated in the Volga-Don region of Russia, but has now spread throughout the world. Researchers have found that Horseradish discourages the growth of certain bacteria, improves circulation when applied to the skin, and restrains the growth of tumors. In animal tests it has been shown to relieve spasms.

Avoid If . . .

Because Horseradish can irritate the stomach lining and other mucous membranes, do not take it if you have stomach or intestinal ulcers. Also avoid it if you have kidney disease, and do not give it to children under 4.

Special Cautions

Aside from its impact on the digestive system, Horseradish presents no problems when used at customary dosage levels.

Possible Drug Interactions

No interactions have been reported.

Special Information If You Are Pregnant or Breastfeeding

No harmful effects are known.

How to Prepare

Horseradish root may be cut or ground and used fresh or dried. It may also be pressed for its juice.

Typical Dosage

For internal use, the usual daily dosage of fresh root is 20 grams (4 teaspoonfuls).

For external application, use ointments containing no more than 2% oils.

Overdosage

No information on overdosage is available.

Horsetail

Latin name: Equisetum arvense
Other names: Bottle-brush,
    Horse Willow, Paddock-pipes,
    Pewterwort, Scouring Rush,
    Shave Grass, Toadpipe

A Remedy For

• Kidney and bladder stones
• Urinary tract infections
• Wounds and burns

In folk medicine, Horsetail has also been used for tuberculosis, profuse menstrual bleeding, brittle fingernails, hair loss, water retention, rheumatic diseases, gout, swelling, fractures, frostbite, and nasal, pulmonary, and gastric bleeding. Its effectiveness for these problems has not, however, been confirmed.

What It Is; Why It Works

Horsetail gains its name from the bristly appearance of its jointed stems. Its ability to draw excess water from the body makes it useful for flushing bacterial infections and kidney stones from the urinary tract.

The plant is found throughout most of the northern hemisphere. Only stems collected during summer are medicinal.

Avoid If . . .

If you have water retention and swelling due to a weak heart or kidneys, do not use Horsetail.

Special Cautions

Consult a doctor before using Horsetail as a bath additive if you have a major skin disorder or eruptions of unknown origin, fever, an infectious disease, heart problems, or abnormal muscle tension.

Be sure to drink plenty of fluids while taking this herb.

Possible Drug Interactions

No interactions have been reported.

Special Information If You Are Pregnant or Breastfeeding

No harmful effects are known.

How to Prepare

To make a tea, mix 2 to 3 grams (about one-half teaspoonful) of crushed Horsetail with boiling water, boil for 5 minutes, then steep for 10 to 15 minutes and strain.

For external application in compresses, use 10 grams (about 2 teaspoonfuls) of crushed Horsetail per quart of water.

Typical Dosage

The customary daily dosage for internal use is:

Crushed Horsetail: 6 grams (about 1 heaping teaspoonful)
Liquid extract: 1 to 4 milliliters 3 times daily
Tea: Repeatedly during the day between meals

Store in a well-sealed container protected from light.

Overdosage

No information on overdosage is available.

Hyssop

Latin name: Hyssopus officinalis

A Remedy For

Hyssop is used as a treatment for fevers, respiratory ailments, intestinal inflammation, liver complaints, gallbladder problems, and poor circulation. For none of these disorders, however, has it been proven effective.

What It Is; Why It Works

Hyssop is among the oldest of medicinal herbs. Its healing powers are extolled in the Bible—"Purge me with Hyssop and I shall be clean"—and its name is derived from the ancient Greek for "holy herb."

Today Hyssop is still to be found in the liqueur Chartreuse, although its strong flavor obviates frequent use in cooking. Honey produced by Hyssop-fed bees is considered particularly good.

A 2-foot high evergreen shrub with dark blue flowers, Hyssop grows naturally throughout the Mediterranean region, and is cultivated elsewhere. The plant's medicinal value lies in its above-ground parts, as well as its essential oil.

Avoid If . . .

No known medical conditions preclude the use of Hyssop.

Special Cautions

Sustained use of Hyssop oil poses a slight risk of seizures. The problem has surfaced in adults after daily intake of 10 to 30 drops, and in children after administration of as little as 2 to 3 drops daily.

Possible Drug Interactions

No interactions have been reported.

Special Information If You Are Pregnant or Breastfeeding

No harmful effects are known.

How to Prepare

Although Hyssop can be taken as a crushed herb, no specific recommendations are available.

Typical Dosage

There are no guidelines on record.

Overdosage

No information is available.

Iceland Moss

Latin name: Cetraria islandica
Other name: Eryngo-leaved
Liverwort

A Remedy For

- Appetite loss
- Bronchitis
- Colds
- Cough
- Fever
- Indigestion
- Sore throat
- Tendency to infection

In folk medicine, Iceland Moss has also been used for lung disease, kidney and bladder disorders, and poorly healing wounds. Its effectiveness for these problems has not, however, been verified.

What It Is; Why It Works

Despite the name, Iceland Moss is actually a lichen. Olive, brown-green, or brown in color, it clings to the ground in northern, mountainous, and arctic regions of the northern hemisphere and in some regions of the southern hemisphere. It tastes bitter and, when wet, smells like seaweed. The organic acids in the moss work to ward off infection, soothe irritated or inflamed tissue, and—to a minor extent—kill bacteria.

Avoid If . . .

No known medical conditions preclude the use of Iceland Moss.

Special Cautions

In rare cases, external use of Iceland Moss can trigger sensitivity reactions.

Possible Drug Interactions

No interactions have been reported.

Special Information If You Are Pregnant or Breastfeeding

No harmful effects are known.

How to Prepare

To prepare a tea, pour boiling water over 1.5 to 2.5 grams (1 to 2 teaspoonfuls) of chopped Iceland Moss, steep for 10 minutes, and strain. The tea may be sweetened if desired.

Typical Dosage

The customary dosage is 4 to 6 grams (about 3 to 5 teaspoonfuls of the moss) per day.

Overdosage

No information on overdosage is available.

Immortelle

Latin name: Helichrysum arenarium
Other names: Eternal Flower, Everlasting, Yellow Chaste Weed

A Remedy For

• Appetite loss
• Liver and gallbladder problems

Immortelle is a treatment for the discomfort of gallbladder conditions, such as cramps. It is also used as a remedy for indigestion and water retention, although its effectiveness for these problems remains unconfirmed.

What It Is; Why It Works

Immortelle stimulates the production of bile and tends to ease painful spasms. It also contains antibacterial compounds. Both the dried flower and the entire plant are used medicinally.

Immortelle grows in Europe and the United States. The plant is a protected species.

Avoid If . . .

Because Immortelle promotes production of bile, you should avoid it if you have a blocked bile duct. If you have gallstones, use of the herb can cause cramps.

Special Cautions

At customary dosage levels, Immortelle poses no known risks.

Possible Drug Interactions

No interactions have been reported.

Special Information If You Are Pregnant or Breastfeeding

No harmful effects are known.

How to Prepare

To make a tea, pour boiling water over 3 to 4 grams (about 2 teaspoonfuls) of crushed Immortelle, steep for 10 minutes, then strain. Drink immediately.

Some commercial drugs for stimulating bile include Immortelle. It also is an inactive ingredient in many specialty teas.

Typical Dosage

Crushed herb: 3 grams (about 2 teaspoonfuls) daily.
Tea: Freshly brewed tea may be taken throughout the day.

Store away from light and moisture.

Overdosage

No information on overdosage is available.

Iris

Latin name: Iris species
Other name: Orris Root

A Remedy For

The root of the Iris plant is sometimes recommended for cough and bronchitis, although its value remains unproven. In homeopathic medicine, it is used for conditions of the pancreas and thyroid, digestive problems, and headaches. Asian uses include treatment of dysentery, jaundice, sore throat, and spitting up blood.

What It Is; Why It Works

With its flamboyant blossoms and wide range of colors, the Iris has been popular since the time of the Egyptian pharaohs. Its name means "rainbow" in Greek; the Romans dedicated it to Juno, the queen of heaven. The three petals of the flowers are said to signify faith, wisdom, and valor.

Although the medicinal value of Iris is debatable, there's no question that the juice of the fresh plant has a severely irritating effect on the skin and mucous membranes. Only the root and underground stem, which help loosen phlegm, should be used as a remedy.

Avoid If . . .

No known medical conditions preclude the use of Iris root.

Special Cautions

Do not experiment with fresh juice from the plant. If taken internally, it can cause vomiting, stomach pain, and bloody diarrhea, as well as severe inflammation of the mucous membranes.

Possible Drug Interactions

No interactions have been reported.

Special Information If You Are Pregnant or Breastfeeding

No harmful effects are known.

How to Prepare

Iris is an ingredient in various tea mixtures.

Typical Dosage

No recommendations are on record.

Overdosage

No information is available.

Jambolan

Latin name: Syzygium cumini
Other names: Jambul, Jamum, Java Plum, Rose Apple

A Remedy For
- Diarrhea
- Skin inflammation
- Sore throat

Only the bark of the Jambolan has proven medicinal value, although the seeds are often used as well. Taken internally, the bark relieves diarrhea. Used as a gargle, it soothes mild inflammation of the mouth and throat. Applied to the skin, it clears up mild, superficial inflammation. In folk medicine, the bark is used—without scientific validation—for congestion, asthma, and skin ulcers. Asian herbalists employ it for diarrhea, skin problems, stomach disorders, and vaginal discharge. Homeopathic practitioners recommend it for diabetes.

Jambolan seed is sometimes taken for upset stomach, although evidence of its effectiveness is lacking. It also is used in the treatment of diabetes, indigestion, gas, spasms, water retention, and failing sexual desire. In Asian medicine, it's used for diabetes, diarrhea, sore throat, and diseases of the spleen.

What It Is; Why It Works

A close relative of the clove tree *Syzygium aromaticum,* Jambolan is native to east India and the Malay Peninsula, but has spread as far as China and Australia and is grown in the Caribbean. The bark has drying effect on the tissues and has been shown to reduce blood-sugar levels in animal experiments. Similar effects have not been demonstrated for the seeds, although they do appear to have anti-inflammatory properties.

Avoid If . . .

No known medical conditions preclude the use of Jambolan.

Special Cautions

When used at customary dosage levels, Jambolan poses no risks.

Possible Drug Interactions

No interactions have been reported.

Special Information If You Are Pregnant or Breastfeeding

No harmful effects are known.

How to Prepare

You can make Jambolan bark into a tea. Mix 1 to 2 teaspoonfuls of crushed bark with about two-thirds of a cup of cold water, bring to a boil, simmer for 5 to 10 minutes, and strain. You can drink the tea, gargle with it, or use it to make compresses.

Typical Dosage

Jambolan bark can be taken internally or applied externally. The usual daily dosage is 3 to 6 grams (about 1 teaspoonful).

Overdosage

No information on overdosage is available.

Japanese Mint

Latin name: Mentha arvensis var. piperascens

A Remedy For

- Bronchitis
- Colds
- Cough
- Fever
- Liver and gallbladder problems
- Pain
- Sore throat
- Tendency to infection

Japanese Mint is taken primarily to treat respiratory inflammation and relieve gas. As a skin rub, it's used for muscle and nerve pain. In folk medicine, it has also been used for breathing difficulties and heart problems, although its effectiveness for these purposes has not been scientifically confirmed. Asian uses of unverified effectiveness include joint pain, headache, and skin diseases.

What It Is; Why It Works

Japanese Mint grows throughout northern Asia and Europe. Along with other members of the mint family, it's the source of menthol, a common ingredient in over-the-counter cough remedies, including Cepacol Sore Throat Lozenges, Hall's Cough Drops, and Vicks Cough Drops, and ointments such as ArthriCare, Eucalyptamint, and Vicks VapoRub. It exhibits antibacterial and decongestant action, relieves gas, stimulates production of bile, and has a cooling effect.

Avoid If . . .

Avoid taking Japanese Mint internally if you have blocked bile ducts, gallbladder inflammation, or severe liver damage.

Special Cautions

Do not apply Japanese Mint oil to the faces of infants or small children, especially in the nasal area. It can cause severe spasms, asthma-like attacks, and even respiratory failure, when applied to a child's face.

In adults, the oil can aggravate bronchial asthma and, when taken internally, can cause stomach discomfort.

Possible Drug Interactions

No drug interactions have been reported.

Special Information If You Are Pregnant or Breastfeeding

No harmful effects are known.

How to Prepare

Japanese Mint oil is available in oily and semi-solid preparations.

Typical Dosage

Internal use: 2 drops of oil in a glass of water, tea, or juice, 1 or 2 times daily. Take no more than 6 drops per day.

Inhalation: 3 or 4 drops in hot water.

External use: Rub a few drops on the affected area.

Overdosage

Doses of as little as 2 grams of menthol can be fatal. If you suspect an overdose, seek medical attention immediately.

Java Tea

Latin name: Orthosiphon spicatus

A Remedy For

- Kidney and bladder stones
- Liver and gallbladder problems
- Urinary tract infections

Java Tea is also taken for rheumatism and gout, although its effectiveness for these problems has not been verified.

What It Is; Why It Works

Found throughout Southeast Asia and tropical Australia, the Java Tea plant grows to a height of no more than 3 feet, producing blue to light violet flowers. Although it looks similar to peppermint, the plant has a dry, salty, bitter taste. The leaves and stem tips are used medicinally.

Java Tea has a mild diuretic action, useful for flushing the kidneys and urinary tract. It also relieves spasms of the smooth muscle in the walls of the internal organs, making it valuable for gallbladder problems. Researchers have found it to be mildly antiseptic as well.

Avoid If . . .

Do not flush out the urinary system with Java Tea or any other medication if you are retaining water due to poor heart or kidney function.

Special Cautions

At customary dosage levels, Java Tea poses no risks. However, you should be sure to compensate for its diuretic effect by drinking at least 2 quarts of liquid per day.

Possible Drug Interactions

No drug interactions have been reported.

Special Information If You Are Pregnant or Breastfeeding

No harmful effects are known.

How to Prepare

To make tea, pour 150 milliliters (a bit over half a cup) of hot water over the crushed herb, steep for 10 minutes, then strain.

Typical Dosage

Java Tea is taken internally. The usual daily dosage is 6 to 12 grams.

Overdosage

No information on overdosage is available.

Javanese Turmeric

Latin name: Curcuma xanthorrhizia

A Remedy For

- Appetite loss
- Liver and gallbladder problems

Javanese Turmeric is typically used for indigestion, particularly feelings of fullness after meals and gas. In Indian folk medicine, it has long been used for liver and gallbladder complaints.

What It Is; Why It Works

Javanese Turmeric is a leafy perennial that grows to nearly 6 feet in height. It is native to the forests of Indonesia and the nearby Malaysian peninsula.

Medicinally, Javanese Turmeric is similar to the standard variety used worldwide as a kitchen spice. It increases the flow of bile and may discourage the growth of tumors. Its fleshy underground root provides its medicinal value.

Avoid If . . .

Because of the herb's bile-stimulating properties, do not use Javanese Turmeric if you have a bile duct blockage.

Special Cautions

If you have gallstones, Javanese Turmeric could give you cramps.

Stomach problems are also a possibility after long-term use.

Possible Drug Interactions
No interactions have been reported.

Special Information If You Are Pregnant or Breastfeeding
No harmful effects are known.

How to Prepare
To make a tea, pour 1 cup of boiling water over one-half teaspoonful of Javanese Turmeric, steep for 10 minutes, and strain.

Typical Dosage
The average daily dose of the ground herb is 2 grams. The tea may be taken 2 to 3 times daily between meals.

Store protected from light.

Overdosage
The primary sign of an overdose is a stomach problem. Seek medical attention if it becomes severe.

Jimsonweed

Latin name: Datura stramonium
Other names: Apple of Peru,
  Devil's Apple, Devil's
  Trumpet, Jamestown Weed,
  Mad-apple, Nightshade,
  Stinkweed, Thornapple

A Remedy For
Jimsonweed is taken for cough and bronchitis, and has been smoked in many parts of the world as a remedy for asthma. It is also prescribed for diseases of the nerves that regulate the internal organs, and for Parkinson's disease. The plant is, however, quite poisonous, and medicinal use is therefore not recommended.

What It Is; Why It Works
Although originally found in Central America, Jimsonweed now grows in most temperate and subtropical parts of the world. Typically reaching a height of nearly 4 feet, the plant sprouts a single white flower at the tip of each branch. Its foliage has an unpleasant smell, but the flowers are fragrant. The plant's dried leaves and ripe seeds are used medicinally.

Jimsonweed has been considered a healing herb for centuries. One early commentator recommends its juice for curing burns from "fire, water, boiling lead, gunpowder, [and] that which comes by lightning." It contains atropine, a potent chemical that combats spasms and generally diminishes muscular activity in the digestive system, lungs, and other internal organs.

Atropine is among the active ingredients in the prescription drugs Donnatal, Lomotil, and Urised. In large doses, it can easily prove lethal.

Avoid If . . .
Do not take Jimsonweed if you have glaucoma or any reason to suspect it. Also avoid this herb if you have an obstruction in the outlet from the stomach, intestinal failure or blockage, an enlarged prostate, an irregular heartbeat, swelling in the lungs,

difficulty passing urine, or hardening of the arteries.

Special Cautions
Jimsonweed has a pronounced drying effect, leading to diminished urination, extreme constipation, and heat build-up due to a decline in perspiration. Other side effects (often early warning signs of poisoning) include skin reddening, dry mouth, enlarged pupils, and a fast, irregular heartbeat. Vision problems, such as difficulty focusing, are also a possibility.

Possible Drug Interactions
No interactions have been reported.

Special Information If You Are Pregnant or Breastfeeding
No information is available.

How to Prepare
Use is not recommended.

Typical Dosage
Use is not recommended.

Overdosage
Doses delivering 100 milligrams or more of atropine can be fatal. This amounts to 15 to 100 grams of Jimsonweed leaf, or 15 to 25 grams (1 to 1½ tablespoonfuls) of the seeds. Much smaller quantities will poison a child. Death occurs when the drug paralyzes the respiratory system.

Signs of overdose include restlessness, compulsive speech, hallucinations, delirium, and manic episodes, followed by exhaustion and sleep. If you suspect an overdose, seek emergency treatment immediately.

Juniper Berry

Latin name: Juniperus communis

A Remedy For
- Appetite loss
- Kidney and bladder stones
- Urinary tract infections

Juniper Berry is also used for indigestion and digestive disorders such as belching, heartburn, and bloating, as well as menstrual problems and diabetes. Its effectiveness for these conditions has not, however, been verified.

What It Is; Why It Works
This familiar household seasoning has a significant diuretic effect, flushing excess water from the body. It's this ability to increase the flow of urine that makes Juniper a useful aid in the treatment of urinary infections and kidney stones. The berries' diuretic action also tends to lower blood pressure—although not sufficiently to warrant therapeutic use.

Numerous varieties of Juniper are found throughout most of the northern hemisphere, growing from 6 to 30 feet in height. The ripe blue berries have a tangy aroma and a tangy-sweet, then bitter taste. Oil extracted from Juniper berries is the main flavoring agent in gin; in Sweden it is used in beer.

Avoid If . . .
Do not take Juniper Berry if you have a kidney inflammation.

Special Cautions
Protracted use of Juniper Berry can irritate and damage the kidneys.

Possible Drug Interactions
No interactions have been reported.

Special Information If You Are Pregnant or Breastfeeding
Do not take Juniper Berry during pregnancy.

How to Prepare
Whole, crushed, and powdered Juniper Berry can be used in teas, alcohol extracts, and wine. The essential oil is also used in remedies.

To prepare a tea, pour one teacup of boiling water over 0.5 gram of crushed Juniper Berry. Take 3 times daily.

Juniper is sometimes combined with other herbs for bladder and kidney teas. It is also used in bath salts as a treatment for rheumatism.

Typical Dosage
The usual dosage is 2 to 10 grams of crushed Juniper Berry daily. Limit use to no more than 6 weeks.

Overdosage
An overdose can damage the kidneys. If you suspect an overdose, check with your doctor immediately.

Kava

Latin name: Piper methysticum
Other name: Kava Kava

A Remedy For
- Insomnia
- Nervousness

Kava is also used to relieve anxiety, although its effectiveness as a tranquilizer has not been scientifically confirmed.

What It Is; Why It Works
One of the "new" herbs that have recently gained considerable media attention, Kava has actually been around for centuries in the South Seas, where it's used as a ceremonial beverage. The plant's fleshy underground stem is mildly intoxicating when chewed. Prepared as a nonalcoholic drink, it is said to foster a sense of contentment and well-being, while sharpening the mind, memory, and senses.

Research shows that the active ingredients in Kava (kava lactones) do in fact have a calming, sedative effect. They also appear to relax the muscles, relieve spasms, and prevent convulsions.

Avoid If . . .
Do not use Kava if you are pregnant or nursing. Also avoid it if you have a depressive disorder; Kava can deepen a depressed mood.

Special Cautions
When first taking Kava, you may notice a slightly tired feeling in the mornings.

In rare cases, Kava can cause an allergic reaction, a slight yellowing of the skin, gastrointestinal complaints, pupil dilation, difficulty focusing, or loss of balance. Because of the possibility of visual disturbances, drive with caution while using this herb.

Do not take Kava for longer than 3 months without consulting a physician.

Possible Drug Interactions

Do not take Kava when using other substances that act on the brain, such as alcohol, barbiturates, or other mood-altering drugs. Kava may increase their effect.

Special Information If You Are Pregnant or Breastfeeding

Remember, Kava should be avoided during pregnancy and nursing.

How to Prepare

Commercial extracts are the predominant form of Kava. The crushed root can also be used.

Typical Dosage

Daily doses delivering between 60 and 120 milligrams of the active ingredients are the customary recommendation. Because the potency of commercial preparations may vary, follow the manufacturer's directions whenever available.

Overdosage

An overdose is usually signaled by a lack of coordination, followed by tiredness and a tendency to sleep. If you suspect an overdose, seek medical attention immediately.

Khella

Latin name: Ammi visnaga

A Remedy For
- Bronchitis
- Cough
- High blood pressure
- Liver and gallbladder problems
- Weak heart

Khella is also used for chest pain (angina), irregular heartbeat, asthma, whooping cough, and abdominal cramps. In the treatment of kidney stones, it helps relax the ducts to the bladder, allowing the stones to pass. Externally, it's used on wounds, inflammation, and poisonous bites. For none of these problems, however, has its effectiveness ever been definitively proven.

What It Is; Why It Works

Khella combats spasms in the smooth muscles that line the walls of blood vessels, bronchial airways, and other tubes and ducts. It improves circulation in the heart muscle and gives a mild boost to the heart's pumping action.

Khella is native to the Mediterranean, and is cultivated in the United States, Mexico, Chile, and Argentina. The plant is about 5 feet tall, with flowers and small fruit. Its medicinal value lies in the dried, ripe fruit.

Avoid If . . .
There are no known medical conditions that preclude the use of Khella.

Special Cautions
Limit your exposure to sunlight and use a sunscreen when taking Khella; it can make you sensitive to sunlight.

In a few people, this herb causes jaundice (yellowing of the skin and eyes). Long-term use can bring on queasiness, dizziness, loss of appetite, headache, and sleep disorders.

Possible Drug Interactions
No drug interactions have been reported.

Special Information If You Are Pregnant or Breastfeeding
No harmful effects are known.

How to Prepare
Available in extract form.

Typical Dosage
Potency of commercial preparations may vary. Follow the manufacturer's directions.

Overdosage
Very high dosages of Khella (more than 100 milligrams of the active ingredient) can cause the same symptoms brought on by long-term use, and can also lead to liver problems.

Knotweed

Latin name: Polygonum aviculare
Other names: Allseed Nine-joints, Armstrong, Beggarweed, Bird's Tongue, Birdweed, Centinode, Cow Grass, Crawlgrass, Doorweed, Hogweed, Knotgrass, Pigweed, Red Robin, Sparrow Tongue, Swine's Grass

A Remedy For
• Bronchitis
• Cough
• Sore throat

Although its effectiveness for other purposes has not been verified, Knotweed has also been used as supportive treatment for pulmonary disorders, to inhibit perspiration in cases of tuberculosis, to promote urination, to stop bleeding in cases of hemorrhage, and to treat various skin disorders. In Asia, it is taken for gonorrhea, jaundice, itching, and dysentery.

What It Is; Why It Works
Knotweed is a sturdy annual plant found in most temperate regions of the world. The Latin name "aviculare" comes from "aviculus," the diminutive form of the Latin word for "bird"—chosen, no doubt, because of the countless birds attracted by its seeds. The plant's tiny red flowers led to the name "Red Robin." The "Swine's Grass" appellation dates from a time when farmers fed the herb to their ailing pigs.

The above-ground parts of the flowering plant, fresh or dried, are considered medicinal. The dried root is used as well. The herb exhibits an astringent, tightening action.

Avoid If . . .
There are no medical conditions known to preclude the use of Knotweed.

Special Cautions
None.

Possible Drug Interactions
No interactions have been reported.

Special Information If You Are Pregnant or Breastfeeding
No harmful effects are known.

How to Prepare
Ground Knotweed can be taken internally and applied to the skin. Knotweed extract is found in many cough syrups and diuretics (medicines used to flush excess fluid from the body).

To prepare Knotweed tea, combine 1.5 grams (about one teaspoonful) of finely cut Knotweed with cold water, bring to a simmer, steep for 5 to 10 minutes, and strain.

Typical Dosage
Knotweed tea may be taken 3 to 5 times daily. The total daily dosage of the herb should be 4 to 6 grams (about 2³⁄₄ to 4¹⁄₄ teaspoonfuls).

Overdosage
No information on overdosage is available.

Kudzu

Latin name: Pueraria lobata
Other name: Ge-gen

A Remedy For
- Hardening of the arteries
- High blood pressure

Kudzu contains ingredients known to lower blood pressure and improve circulation in the muscles of the heart. It shows promise as a treatment for alcoholism, as well.

In Chinese medicine, Kudzu is also used for allergies, migraine headache, measles, and diarrhea, but its effectiveness for these disorders has not been clinically verified.

What It Is; Why It Works
Native to the thickets and forests of China, Kudzu is a high-climbing perennial vein with an immense root (sometimes reaching the size of the human body). It is this root that's considered medicinal. It has been used in traditional Chinese medicine since at least the 1st century AD.

Certain glycosides in Kudzu are responsible for its effect on the heart and circulatory system. Two of these substances—daidzin and daidzein—have also been shown, in an animal study, to inhibit the desire for alcohol. Kudzu has, in fact, long been considered a remedy for drunkenness in traditional Chinese medicine, but human trials to verify its anti-alcohol action have not yet been conducted.

Avoid If . . .
No known medical conditions preclude the use of Kudzu.

Special Cautions
At customary dosage levels, Kudzu seems to pose no problems.

Possible Drug Interactions
No interactions have been reported.

Special Information If You Are Pregnant or Breastfeeding
No harmful effects are known.

How to Prepare
Kudzu can be taken in crushed-root or concentrated tablet form. In present-day China, tablets equivalent to 1.5 grams of crushed root are taken for the chest pain (angina) caused by hardening of the arteries.

Typical Dosage
Crushed root: 9 to 15 grams per day
Concentrated tablets: 30 to 120 milligrams 2 to 3 times per day

Overdosage
No information on overdosage is available.

Lady's Mantle

Latin name: Alchemilla vulgaris
Other names: Bear's Foot, Lion's Foot, Nine Hooks, Stellaria

A Remedy For
- Diarrhea
- Stomach and intestinal disorders

In folk medicine, Lady's Mantle has also been taken for menopausal complaints, painful menstrual periods, mouth and throat infections, eczema, and skin rashes. As a bath additive, it's used for lower-abdominal ailments. Effectiveness of these folk uses remains unproven.

What It Is; Why It Works
Found throughout the northern hemisphere, Lady's Mantle is a small shrub with clusters of small, yellow-green flowers. Its medicinal properties reside in the fresh or dried above-ground parts of the plant gathered at flowering time.

Lady's Mantle has an astringent action and slows the production of pancreatic enzymes. It has also been shown to inhibit tumors in mice.

The scientific name "alchemilla" comes from the word "alchemy," suggesting that the plant was once considered very valuable for its magical powers. It has been in use as a remedy since the Middle Ages.

Avoid If . . .
There are no known reasons to avoid Lady's Mantle.

Special Cautions
Lady's Mantle presents no health hazards or side effects when used at usual dosage levels.

Possible Drug Interactions
No interactions have been reported.

Special Information If You Are Pregnant or Breastfeeding
No harmful effects are known.

How to Prepare
Lady's Mantle can be made into a tea, using 2 to 4 grams (about one-half to three-quarters tea-spoonful) per cup. The tea can be taken up to 3 times a day between meals.

Typical Dosage
Lady's Mantle is taken orally. The usual daily dosage is approximately 5 to 10 grams (1 to 2 teaspoonfuls).

Overdosage
No information on overdosage is available.

Laminaria

Latin name: Laminaria hyperborea

A Remedy For
Laminaria is sometimes used for thyroid problems, although there has been little research on its effectiveness.

What It Is; Why It Works
Laminaria is a variety of kelp, or seaweed, found on the North Atlantic coast. Dried kelp is a source of iodine, and has been used medicinally since the beginning of the 19th century.

Avoid If . . .
No known medical conditions preclude the use of Laminaria.

Special Cautions
Be careful about the amount you take. Doses of iodine in excess of 150 micrograms a day can induce or worsen an overactive thyroid gland. Severe allergic reactions, although rare, are a possibility.

Possible Drug Interactions
No interactions have been reported.

Special Information If You Are Pregnant or Breastfeeding
No harmful effects are known.

How to Prepare
No recommendations are available.

Typical Dosage
Follow the manufacturer's directions whenever available.

Overdosage
Warning signs of excessive thyroid stimulation include thyroid enlargement, rapid heartbeat, palpitations, nervousness, agitation, increased sweating, fatigue, weakness, insomnia, increased appetite, and weight loss.

Larch

Latin name: Larix decidua

A Remedy For
- Blood pressure problems
- Bronchitis
- Colds
- Cough
- Fever
- Rheumatism

- Sore throat
- Tendency to infection

What It Is; Why It Works

Larch is a very fast-growing type of tree (six times faster than oak) native to central Europe and cultivated in North America. The medicinal part is the outer bark.

Avoid If . . .

No medical conditions are known to preclude the use of Larch.

Special Cautions

Do not inhale Larch. It can cause acute inflammation of the breathing passages. The oil can be absorbed through the skin; excessive external use can result in damage to the kidneys or the central nervous system.

Possible Drug Interactions

No interactions have been reported.

Special Information If You Are Pregnant or Breastfeeding

No harmful effects are known.

How to Prepare

Larch is used to make liquid and semi-solid preparations for external use including ointments, gels, and emulsions containing 10 to 20% essential larch oil.

Typical Dosage

For external use only.

Overdosage

No information on overdose is available.

Lavender

Latin name: Lavandula angustifolia

A Remedy For

- Appetite loss
- Insomnia
- Nervousness

Lavender has also been used internally to treat other mood disturbances and abdominal complaints, and has been used externally for circulatory disorders, but its effectiveness for these problems remains unconfirmed.

What It Is; Why It Works

Because of its wonderful fragrance, from Roman times onward Lavender has always been a popular bath additive. In fact, its name derives from the Latin "lavare" meaning "to wash." Over the centuries, it has been used in a variety of forms, including oil, distilled water, and alcohol solution (tincture). One species, Spike Lavender, is even an effective insect repellent.

Lavender's medicinal value lies in the essential oil, customarily extracted from the flowers. Taken internally, Lavender has been found to stimulate the production and flow of bile. It also has a mildly sedating effect, and gets rid of gas. Used externally, it improves circulation and brings color to the skin.

Avoid If . . .

No known medical conditions preclude the use of Lavender.

Special Cautions

Taken at customary dosage levels, Lavender presents no problems, although a few people do develop a sensitivity to the oil.

Possible Drug Interactions

No interactions have been reported.

Special Information If You Are Pregnant or Breastfeeding

No harmful effects are known.

How to Prepare

Extracts, bath additives, and crushed Lavender flowers are all available.

To prepare your own bath additive, boil 100 grams (about one-half cup) of Lavender in 2 quarts of water, then add to the tub.

Typical Dosage

The usual daily dose of Lavender for internal use is:

Crushed flowers: 3 to 5 grams
Essential oil: 1 to 4 drops

Overdosage

No information on overdosage is available.

Lemon Balm

Latin name: Melissa officinalis
Other names: Balm Mint, Bee Balm, Blue Balm, Cure-all, Garden Balm, Honey Plant, Sweet Balm, Sweet Mary

A Remedy For
• Insomnia
• Nervousness

Although officially recognized only for its ability to calm the nerves, Lemon Balm has also been used as a remedy for bloating and gas, mood disorders, bronchial inflammation, high blood pressure, palpitations, vomiting, toothache, earache, and headache.

What It Is; Why It Works

Lemon Balm's medicinal properties have been held in high regard for nearly two millennia. The Roman scholar Pliny believed Lemon Balm could prevent infection in open wounds (an action that has been clinically proven for balsamic oils in general). The noted 16th century physician Paracelsus believed Lemon Balm could heal even patients close to death.

Modern research on Lemon Balm has revealed a mild sedative effect, antibacterial and antiviral properties, and an ability to relieve cramps and gas. Only the plant's leaves are medicinal.

A perennial herb, Lemon Balm grows up to 3 feet in height. It is native to the east Mediterranean region and west Asia, but is cultivated throughout central Europe. Before flowering, it has a lemon-like taste and smell; and the fresh leaves, in addition to their medicinal applications, are commonly used in cooking.

Avoid If . . .

No known medical conditions preclude the use of Lemon Balm.

Special Cautions
When taken at customary dosage levels, Lemon Balm poses no hazards.

Possible Drug Interactions
There are no known interactions.

Special Information If You Are Pregnant or Breastfeeding
No harmful effects are known.

How to Prepare
Lemon Balm can be found in the form of dried herb, herb powder, and liquid or dry extracts, as well as various liquid and solid commercial preparations.

To make a tea, pour a cup of hot water over 1.5 to 4.5 grams (about one-quarter to 1 teaspoonful) of crushed Lemon Balm, steep for 10 minutes, and strain.

Typical Dosage
The usual daily dose of Lemon Balm is 8 to 10 grams (about 2 teaspoonfuls).

Because the strength of commercial preparations may vary, follow the manufacturer's instructions whenever available.

Lemon Balm can be stored in a well-sealed, nonplastic container protected from light and moisture for up to 1 year.

Overdosage
No information on overdosage is available.

Licorice

Latin name: Glycyrrhiza glabra

A Remedy For
- Bronchitis
- Cough
- Stomach inflammation

Both Licorice Root and Licorice Juice are used medicinally. Licorice speeds healing of stomach ulcers. The juice is also used for viral liver inflammations, and, in Asian medicine, the root is used for boils, diarrhea, headache, excessive thirst, sore throat, and swellings from infections. Their effectiveness for these disorders has not, however, been scientifically verified.

What It Is; Why It Works
Licorice contains glycyrrhizic acid, which helps heal stomach ulcers and soothes inflammation. It also loosens and thins mucus in the lungs and acts as a decongestant. There is some evidence that Licorice may help the body fight viruses by encouraging the production of interferon.

There are several varieties of Licorice growing from southeastern Europe to southwestern Asia and Iraq. The plant was introduced to the ancient Greeks by Scythians from the east. It has been used in Europe since the Middle Ages.

Avoid If . . .
Do not take Licorice if you have chronic hepatitis, cirrhosis of the liver, or any disease that impedes the flow of bile from the liver.

Avoid it also if you have abnormal muscle tension, poor kidney function, or low potassium levels in your blood. Also see "Special Information If You Are Pregnant or Breastfeeding."

Special Cautions

At recommended dosage levels, Licorice is unlikely to produce any side effects. However, when taken in high dosages (above 2 ounces per day) for an extended period of time, it will lead to excessive loss of salt from the blood, water retention, high blood pressure, and heart irregularities. Because of the possibility of these side effects, limit use of Licorice preparations to 6 weeks. The side effects disappear after the drug is discontinued.

Possible Drug Interactions

Licorice can increase the potassium loss caused by the other drugs, such as diuretics that flush excess water from the body (Diuril, Zaroxolyn, others). This potassium loss can, in turn, increase your sensitivity to drugs containing digitalis, such as the heart medication Lanoxin.

Licorice may also increase the effects—and unwanted side effects—of steroid medications such as prednisone (Deltasone).

Special Information If You Are Pregnant or Breastfeeding

Do not take Licorice preparations during pregnancy.

How to Prepare

Licorice is widely available in various commercial preparations.

To make a tea from Licorice Root, mix 1 to 1.5 grams (about one-half teaspoonful) of crushed root in cold water and bring to a boil (or pour the boiling water over the Licorice). Steep for 10 to 15 minutes and strain.

For a tea from Licorice Juice, pour 1 cup of boiling water over 1 teaspoon of juice. Steep for 5 minutes. Drink 1 cup after each meal.

Typical Dosage

Licorice is taken orally. The average daily dosage is:

Crushed Licorice Root: 5 to 15 grams (about 1½ to 5 teaspoonfuls)

Licorice Juice: 0.5 to 1 gram for sinus and throat inflammations; 1.5 to 3 grams for ulcers

Because the potency of commercial preparations can vary, follow the manufacturer's directions whenever available.

Overdosage

No information on overdosage is available.

Lily of the Valley

Latin name: Convallaria majalis
Other names: Jacob's Ladder,
  May Bells, May Lily

A Remedy For

- Circulatory disorders
- Heart palpitations
- Irregular heartbeat
- Kidney and bladder stones

- Urinary tract infections
- Weak heart

In the past, Lily of the Valley was used in folk medicine to improve labor contractions and to treat epilepsy, swelling, strokes and paralysis following strokes, conjunctivitis ("pinkeye"), and leprosy. Its effectiveness for these purposes remains unproven, and because of the herb's potential toxicity, only commercial preparations are now considered acceptable.

What It Is; Why It Works

Lily of the Valley improves the heart's efficiency, which in turn may lower blood pressure. According to Greek mythology, the plant was first discovered by the sun god Apollo, who gave it to Aesculapius, the god of medicine. In the 15th and 16th centuries, scholars believed it capable of improving the memory.

Avoid If . . .

There are no medical conditions that preclude using Lily of the Valley.

Special Cautions

Be careful to take no more than the recommended dose. Larger amounts can cause side effects such as nausea, vomiting, headache, stupor, disorders of color perception, and irregular heartbeat.

Possible Drug Interactions

The following drugs boost the effects—and side effects—of Lily of the Valley:

Calcium
Laxatives
Quinidine (Quinaglute, Quinidex)
Steroid drugs such as hydrocortisone and prednisone
Water pills such as Lasix and HydroDIURIL

Special Information If You Are Pregnant or Breastfeeding

No harmful effects are known.

How to Prepare

Commercial preparations of Lily of the Valley, typically found abroad, include alcohol solutions (tinctures), liquid extracts, and dried extracts.

Typical Dosage

Take no more than 2 grams of tincture or 200 milligrams of liquid extract in any single dose. The usual daily dosages are:

Tincture: 6 grams
Liquid extract: 600 milligrams
Dried extract: 150 milligrams

Store in an airtight container. Protect from light.

Overdosage

A massive overdose is likely to cause life-threatening disruptions of the heartbeat. If you suspect an overdose, seek emergency medical assistance immediately.

Linden

Latin name: Tilia species
Other names: Common Lime,
    European Lime

A Remedy For
- Bronchitis
- Cough

Only the flowers of the Linden tree have any proven medicinal value. In folk medicine, they have also been used to relieve stomach problems and cramps, flush excess water from the body, and calm the nerves. However, their effectiveness for these purposes has not been verified.

What It Is; Why It Works
Common in northern temperate regions, the Linden tree is prized primarily for its wood, which is used in the sounding boards of pianos. Lindens often reach a height of 80 feet. Though they are also known as Common Lime, they bear no relation to the familiar citrus fruit.

Linden flowers have several medicinal properties. They loosen phlegm, soothe irritation, and promote sweating.

Avoid If . . .
No known medical conditions preclude the use of Linden.

Special Cautions
At customary dosage levels, Linden presents no problems.

Possible Drug Interactions
No drug interactions have been reported.

Special Information If You Are Pregnant or Breastfeeding
No harmful effects are known.

How to Prepare
To make a Linden Flower tea, pour boiling water over 2 grams (about 1 heaping teaspoonful) of crushed flowers, or add them to cold water and bring to a boil. Steep for 5 to 10 minutes, then strain.

Typical Dosage
The usual daily dose is 2 to 4 grams of the crushed flowers.

Overdosage
No information on overdosage is available.

Linseed

Latin name: Linum
    usitatissimum
Other name: Flax

A Remedy For
- Constipation

Linseed is also used to soothe an irritated stomach, intestines, or bladder, and is applied externally for skin inflammation. In homeopathic medicine, it's used for throat and lung problems. Asian medicine enlists it as a remedy for chest congestion, diarrhea, gonorrhea, and irritation of the urinary tube. Aside from its use as a laxative, however, its effectiveness remains unproven.

What It Is; Why It Works

Linseed stimulates bowel movements by acting as a swelling agent within the intestines. Researchers have found that it also tends to reduce fat and sugar levels and may have preventive value against cancer.

Derived from the same plant that supplies linen, Linseed has been with us for thousands of years. Archeologists found Linseed and linen cloth in the pyramids. Homer's *Odyssey* mentions flax as the material for sails, and the Bible refers to it frequently.

Linseed is cultivated in temperate and tropical regions around the world. Its sky blue flowers open only in the morning. Only the dried seeds and their oil are routinely used for medicinal purposes.

Avoid If . . .

Do not use Linseed if you have a bowel obstruction or any narrowing of the digestive tract. Also avoid it if you have a severe inflammation of the gullet, stomach entrance, or intestine.

Special Cautions

When used in customary doses, Linseed is unlikely to cause any side effects or pose any hazards.

Possible Drug Interactions

No interactions have been reported.

Special Information If You Are Pregnant or Breastfeeding

No harmful effects are known.

How to Prepare

To treat skin inflammations, apply Linseed externally. Use 30 to 50 grams (about 2 to 3 table-spoonfuls) of Linseed meal in a hot, moist compress. Linseed oil, mixed with limewater, relieves burns and scalds.

Linseed can also be used to remove a foreign body from the eye. Moisten a single linseed and place it under the eyelid. The foreign object should stick to the mucous secretion of the seed.

Typical Dosage

For internal use, the usual dosages are:

Whole or cracked Linseed: 1 tablespoonful taken with 150 milliliters (one-half cup) of water 2 to 3 times daily

Linseed meal: 2 to 4 tablespoonfuls daily, prepared as a hot cereal

Overdosage

Large quantities of Linseed taken with too little fluid can cause a bowel obstruction.

Lobelia

Latin name: Lobelia inflata
Other names: Asthma Weed,
    Bladderpod, Gagroot, Indian
    Tobacco, Pukeweed, Vomitroot

A Remedy For

Lobelia was once taken as an asthma remedy and a way to induce vomiting, but due to a high risk of poisoning, it's no longer in use today. In Asian medicine, it is considered a remedy for cancer, snakebite, and compromised urinary function. Homeopathic practitioners, under the "like cures like" theory, prescribe it to *relieve* vomiting and nausea, and recommend it as a quit-smoking aid.

What It Is; Why It Works

Discovered by the Penobscot Indians and used widely throughout New England in the early 1800s, Lobelia enjoyed a brief period of popularity abroad at the turn of the 20th century. It's a relatively small plant—1 to 2 feet high—sporting pale violet-blue flowers lightly tinged with yellow and leaves that taste similar to tobacco. Lobelia can be found in the dry regions of the northern U.S., Canada, and eastern Siberia. The dried leaves and seeds were used medicinally.

Avoid If . . .

This herb is no longer used medicinally due to the high risk of poisoning.

Special Cautions

In very small doses, Lobelia is relatively safe. However, even a slight error could lead to overdose and poisoning. See "Overdosage" below.

Possible Drug Interactions

No interactions have been reported.

Special Information If You Are Pregnant or Breastfeeding

Use is not recommended.

How to Prepare

Use is not recommended.

Typical Dosage

Use is not recommended.

Overdosage

As little as 0.6 to 1 gram of Lobelia leaves can cause symptoms of overdose; a dose of 4 grams is fatal. Warning signs of overdose include dryness of the mouth, nausea, vomiting, diarrhea, stomach pain, burning in the urinary passages, feelings of anxiety, dizziness, headache, shivering, breathing difficulties, sweating, a feeling of burning or prickling in the extremities, irregular heartbeats, sleepiness, and muscle twitches.

If not treated, significant overdosage will end in convulsions and death. If you suspect an overdose, seek emergency treatment immediately.

Lovage

Latin name: Levisticum officinale
Other name: Sea Parsley

A Remedy For

- Kidney and bladder stones
- Urinary tract infections

In folk medicine, Lovage is also used as a remedy for indigestion, heartburn, gas, menstrual problems, and respiratory inflammation. Its value for such purposes has not, however, been confirmed.

What It Is; Why It Works

Lovage is a sturdy perennial with a fragrant fruit and leaves that give off an aromatic scent when rubbed. The plant is native to the Mediterranean region and grows wild in the Balkans and northern Greece. It is said to be named for Liguria, an Italian region where the species thrives.

The dried root is used medicinally. It has a diuretic effect that flushes out the kidneys and urinary tract. It also displays sedative and antiseptic properties, and appears to combat spasms in the smooth muscles that line the internal organs. The herb's bitter taste stimulates production of saliva and digestive juices.

Thanks to the availability of prescription remedies and other, stronger herbs, Lovage is rarely used today.

Avoid If . . .

Flushing out the urinary tract with Lovage or any other medication is not advisable if you are retaining water due to a weak heart or kidneys. Also avoid Lovage if you have an inflammation in the urinary system.

Special Cautions

To replace the water flushed out of the body by Lovage, be sure to drink plenty of liquids while taking this herb.

Be careful about your exposure to sunlight, especially if you're light-skinned. Lovage may increase your sensitivity to ultraviolet light.

Possible Drug Interactions

No drug interactions have been reported.

Special Information If You Are Pregnant or Breastfeeding

No harmful effects are known.

How to Prepare

You may find Lovage root in whole or powdered form.

Typical Dosage

Lovage is taken internally. The usual daily dosage is 4 to 8 grams.

Store in a well-sealed container protected from light.

Overdosage

No information on overdosage is available.

Luffa

Latin name: Luffa aegyptica

A Remedy For

Although sometimes proposed as a remedy for colds, nasal and sinus inflammation, and general lack of resistance, Luffa's value for these purposes has never been verified.

What It Is; Why It Works

Known primarily as a bath sponge (loofah) in the West, Luffa is also used in baskets, shoe soles, and oil filters, and has value as a sound-deadening construction material. A Luffa sponge is the *Luffa aegyptica*'s dried fruit, which contains a dense network of vascular bundles. The sponge is also the medicinal part of the plant.

Luffa probably originated in India, traveling via the Arabic world to Egypt in the Middle Ages. ("Lufa" is an Arabic word.) The plant is a climber, reaching a height of 10 to 20 feet. Nowadays it is cultivated in all tropical regions of the world.

Avoid If . . .
No known medical conditions preclude the use of Luffa.

Special Cautions
No side effects have been documented.

Possible Drug Interactions
No interactions have been reported.

Special Information If You Are Pregnant or Breastfeeding
No harmful effects are known.

How to Prepare
Usually sold as a bath sponge.

Typical Dosage
No guidelines are on record.

Overdosage
No information is available.

Lungwort

Latin name: Pulmonaria officinalis
Other name: Dage of Jerusalem

A Remedy For
• Bronchitis
• Cough

Although definitive proof is lacking, Lungwort is thought to be effective for mild upper respiratory problems. (It is no longer used for serious lung diseases such as tuberculosis.) In folk medicine, its ability to stimulate production of urine has prompted its use for kidney and urinary disorders. Applied externally, it has been used as an astringent to firm up the skin and treat wounds.

What It Is; Why It Works
As indicated by both its Latin and English names, this plant has a long-standing reputation for relieving lung problems. Indeed, it's even claimed that the plant's white-spotted leaves resemble a lung. Whether or not you'd agree with that, it's a fact that the leaves and other above-ground parts of the plant are considered the medicinal elements.

Avoid If . . .
No known medical conditions preclude the use of Lungwort.

Special Cautions
At customary dosage levels, Lungwort poses no risks.

Possible Drug Interactions
No drug interactions have been reported.

Special Information If You Are Pregnant or Breastfeeding
No harmful effects are known.

How to Prepare
To make a tea, pour boiling water over 1.5 grams (about 2 teaspoonfuls) of finely cut Lungwort,

or mix the herb with cold water and bring rapidly to a boil. Steep for 5 to 10 minutes, then strain. Used as a bronchial tea, this folk remedy may be taken with honey.

Typical Dosage
The tea may be taken repeatedly throughout the day.

Overdosage
No information on overdosage is available.

Lycium

Latin name: Lycium barbarum, Lycium chinense
Other name: Chinese Wolfberry

A Remedy For
Chinese herbalists recommend Lycium berries to improve the circulation, protect the liver and kidneys, and remedy such symptoms as dizziness, ringing in the ears, blurred eyesight, and other vision problems. Lycium root is used to reduce fever, control high blood pressure, and relieve cough and wheezing.

What It Is; Why It Works
Lycium has played a major role in Chinese medicine since at least the 1st century AD, when it was extolled in the *Divine Husbandman's Classic*. According to legend, use of Lycium (and other tonic herbs) allowed one Chinese herbalist to attain an age of 252 years!

Sporting bright red berries, and often reaching a height of 12 feet, the Lycium plant can be found throughout much of China and Tibet. The berries appear to exert a beneficial effect on the liver, protecting it from damaging toxins. The root stimulates the involuntary nervous system that governs the internal organs. The root also relaxes the walls of the arteries, allowing them to expand and thus lowering blood pressure.

Avoid If . . .
Do not take the berries if you have an inflammatory condition, poor digestion, or a tendency to become bloated.

Special Cautions
At customary dosage levels, neither the berries nor the root appears to pose risks.

Possible Drug Interactions
No interactions have been reported.

Special Information If You Are Pregnant or Breastfeeding
No harmful effects are known.

How to Prepare
Lycium berries can be eaten raw or made into teas and soups. The root can be made into tea or taken in an alcohol solution (tincture).

Typical Dosage
Lycium berry tea: For poor eyesight, take 100 milliliters (less than half a cup) daily.
Lycium root tea: For fever, take 100 milliliters daily.

Lycium root tincture: For cough and wheezing, take 3 milliliters (about one-half teaspoonful), diluted in water, 3 times a day.

Overdosage

No information on overdosage is available.

Magnolia Flower

Latin name: Magnolia liliflora
Other name: Xin yi hua

A Remedy For

Chinese herbalists use Magnolia Flower as a remedy for clogged sinus and nasal passages. In conjunction with other herbs, such as angelica, mint, and chrysanthemum, it is often recommended for upper respiratory tract infections and sinus headaches, although its effectiveness for these problems has not been scientifically confirmed.

What It Is; Why It Works

It's actually the buds—not the fully developed Magnolia blooms—that are used medicinally. In laboratory studies, the buds seem to retard certain fungal growths, but their decongestant effect remains unexplained.

A related species, *Magnolia officinalis*, has also earned a place in the traditional Chinese pharmacopoeia through the medicinal action of its bark. Called "Hou Po," this Chinese herb is used as a remedy for cramps, gas, bloating, indigestion, vomiting, and diarrhea.

Avoid If . . .

No known medical conditions preclude the use of Magnolia Flower.

Special Cautions

Magnolia buds have a hairy texture that can irritate the throat. Be sure to rub the herb with a cotton cloth or place it in cheesecloth before mixing it into a solution.

Possible Drug Interactions

No interactions have been reported.

Special Information If You Are Pregnant or Breastfeeding

No harmful effects are known.

How to Prepare

Magnolia buds can be found in some Asian markets and western-style health food stores. Choose dry, green buds free of stems or branches.

Typical Dosage

There is no standard dosage on record.

Overdosage

Signs of an overdose include dizziness and red eyes. If you suspect an overdose, seek medical attention immediately.

Maidenhair

Latin name: Adiantum capillus-veneris
Other names: Five-finger Fern, Hair of Venus, Maiden Fern, Rock Fern

A Remedy For

Maidenhair is sometimes used as a remedy for cough, bronchitis, and painful or excessive menstruation, although evidence of its effectiveness is lacking.

What It Is; Why It Works

Maidenhair has been used medicinally since the days of the Roman Empire, when it was extolled by the scholars Dioscorides and Pliny. In the Middle Ages, it was taken as a tea for various diseases of the respiratory tract, as a syrup for coughs, and as a rinse to treat thinning hair and promote healthy skin tone. The tea is still used today in parts of Europe, particularly Spain and Belgium.

A small, hardy fern with an aromatic, lily-like fragrance, Maidenhair can be found throughout southern Europe and the Atlantic coast as far north as Ireland. The dried fronds, sometimes with roots attached, are the medicinal part of the plant.

Avoid If . . .

No known medical conditions preclude the use of Maidenhair.

Special Cautions

At customary dosage levels, Maidenhair poses no problems.

Possible Drug Interactions

No interactions have been reported.

Special Information If You Are Pregnant or Breastfeeding

No harmful effects are known.

How to Prepare

To make a tea, use 1.5 grams of ground Maidenhair per cup of water.

Typical Dosage

There are no standard guidelines on record. Follow the manufacturer's instructions whenever available.

Overdosage

No information on overdosage is available.

Maitake

Latin name: Grifola frondosa
Other name: Dancing Mushroom

A Remedy For

Although ongoing research remains inconclusive, Maitake is thought to have potential value in the treatment of high blood pressure, high cholesterol, high triglycerides, and diabetes. It is also under study as an AIDS treatment and anticancer agent, and has been used as supportive treatment during cancer chemotherapy.

What It Is; Why It Works

This plate-sized mushroom grows deep in the mountains of Japan, and has long resisted cultivation. Nevertheless, organically grown Maitakes are now available in the U.S.

Mushrooms in general contain immunity-boosting compounds called polysaccharides, and those found in Maitakes are among the most potent ever discovered. The

Maitake's primary polysaccharide, beta-D-glucan, is the one considered most promising for use against cancer and the human immunodeficiency virus (HIV).

Avoid If . . .

No known medical conditions preclude the use of Maitake.

Special Cautions

At customary dosage levels, Maitake poses no risks.

Possible Drug Interactions

No interactions have been reported.

Special Information If You Are Pregnant or Breastfeeding

No harmful effects are known.

How to Prepare

Maitake can be eaten as a food or prepared as a tea. It is also available in tablets and capsules.

Typical Dosage

The usual dosage is 3 to 7 grams of Maitake supplements per day.

Strengths of commercial preparations may vary. Follow the manufacturer's labeling whenever available.

Overdosage

No information is available.

Male Fern

Latin name: Dryopteris filix-mas
Other names: Aspidium, Bear's
Paw Root, Knotty Brake,
Sweet Brake

A Remedy For

Taken internally, Male Fern root is a potent remedy for bandworms and liver flukes. However, the root is so poisonous that officials do not recommend its use, advising other, less toxic treatments instead.

Preparations of Male Fern fronds, which are one-tenth as potent as the root, are applied externally for muscle and nerve pain, earache, toothache, teething, sleeplessness, rheumatism, and sciatica. Their effectiveness has not, however, been verified.

In homeopathic medicine, Male Fern is used for worms and problems with the lymph system.

What It Is; Why It Works

For centuries, until better alternatives were discovered, Male Fern was an accepted treatment for worms. Smoke from the fern was said to drive away serpents, gnats, and "other noisome creatures." Modern research has revealed antiviral properties. The plant is found in temperate zones worldwide.

Avoid If . . .

Not for children under 4, pregnant women, the elderly, and those with anemia, diabetes, a heart condition, kidney problems, or liver disease.

Special Cautions

Even at recommended doses, Male Fern is quite toxic, producing side effects such as diarrhea, nausea, queasiness, severe headache, and vomiting.

Possible Drug Interactions
There are no known drug interactions.

Special Information If You Are Pregnant or Breastfeeding
Do not use during pregnancy.

How to Prepare
Check with your doctor. Numerous alternatives are now available.

Typical Dosage
Remember, therapeutic dosages often prove toxic.

Male Fern extract: For adults, the dose is 6 to 8 grams once daily; for children, give 4 to 6 grams. Wait several weeks before re-treatment.
Dried extract: The maximum dose is 3 grams once daily.

Strengths of commercial preparations may vary. Follow the manufacturer's labeling whenever available.

Overdosage
Overdosage can lead to heart, kidney, and liver damage, mental disorders, spasms, paralysis, and vision damage, including blindness. Fatalities have occurred, particularly among children. If you suspect an overdose, seek emergency medical attention immediately.

Manna

Latin name: Fraxinus ornus
Other name: Flowering Ash

A Remedy For
• Constipation

The ability to soften stool and ease its passage makes Manna especially helpful for people with hemorrhoids or cracks in the surface of the anus (anal fissures), as well as those who have undergone rectal surgery.

What It Is; Why It Works
Cultivated in western Sicily, the Manna tree exudes a sugary sap that has long been used as a gentle laxative (although it now serves more often as a disguise for other medicines). For medicinal use, the sap is collected from the slit bark of trees that have attained at least 8 years of growth, and is then dried and crushed.

Avoid If . . .
Do not use Manna if you have an intestinal obstruction.

Special Cautions
Do not use this or any other laxative for more than 2 weeks without your doctor's approval. Although Manna has few side effects, in some people it causes nausea and gas.

Possible Drug Interactions
No drug interactions have been reported.

Special Information If You Are Pregnant or Breastfeeding
No harmful effects are known.

How to Prepare
Manna is available in crushed form.

Typical Dosage
Manna is taken orally. The usual daily dosage is:

Adults: 20 to 30 grams (4 to 6 teaspoonfuls)
Children: 2 to 16 grams (about one-half to 3 teaspoonfuls)

Overdosage
No information on overdosage is available.

Marigold

Latin name: Calendula officinalis

A Remedy For
• Sore throat
• Wounds and burns

Marigold has enjoyed a wide variety of applications in folk medicine. It has been taken internally for inflammation, stomach ulcers, menstrual cramps, fever, convulsions, liver disease, toothache, tired limbs, eye inflammations, extreme and persistent constipation, and worm infestation, and has been used as a stimulant for the heart. Applied externally, it has been used to clean wounds and to treat enlarged and inflamed lymph glands, chronic skin inflammation, varicose veins, inflamed veins, blood clots in the veins, boils, inflammation of the rectum and anus, dry skin, eczema, and acne. While it definitely promotes wound healing, its other folk uses remain unproven.

Marigold is an ingredient in many types of skin preparations, cosmetics, and preparations for bee stings and frostbite. It is also used to flush excess fluid from the body.

What It Is; Why It Works
The familiar orange/yellow Marigold plant grows to between 12 and 20 inches tall, and has a strong, unpleasant odor. For medicinal purposes, the plant is harvested in July and dried in the shade.

Dried Marigold has been used in Europe for many years to treat a variety of skin problems. Although the active ingredient remains unknown, the flowers exhibit definite antimicrobial, antifungal, and antiviral effects, and have been shown to promote wound healing. Marigold also reduces fever and inflammation, stimulates the immune system and the production of bile, retards tumor growth, and calms the central nervous system.

Avoid If . . .
There are no known reasons to avoid Marigold at recommended dosage levels.

Special Cautions
With frequent skin contact, there is a slight risk of increased sensitivity.

Possible Drug Interactions
No interactions have been reported.

Special Information If You Are Pregnant or Breastfeeding
No harmful effects are known.

How to Prepare

A tea can be made from dried, crushed Marigold leaves using 1 cup of boiling water over 1 to 2 grams (approximately one-quarter to one-half teaspoonful) of herb and steeping for 10 minutes. Used as a gargle or mouthwash for sores in the mouth, the tea can also be poured over an absorbent cloth and applied to the skin.

Typical Dosage

The usual dosage for internal use is several cups of tea per day.

Marigold is available in alcohol solutions, liquid extracts, and ointments. Strengths may vary. Follow the manufacturer's directions whenever available.

Store away from light and moisture. Do not keep for more than 3 years.

Overdosage

No information on overdosage is available.

Marjoram

Latin name: Origanum majorana

A Remedy For

Marjoram is sometimes used as a remedy for stomach pain and the common cold, although its effectiveness for these problems has never been fully verified. Other unsubstantiated uses include treatment of headache, dizziness, and severe cough. Homeopathic practitioners recommend it for nervous conditions.

What It Is; Why It Works

This common household herb exhibits germicidal activity in lab tests, and was formerly used as a mild antiseptic. The dried leaves and flowers are considered medicinal, as is Marjoram oil.

The Latin name "origanum" is derived from the Greek words "oros" meaning mountain and "ganos" meaning joy, presumably a reference to the bright appearance that the plants lend to hillsides. A bushy little herb less than a foot high, Marjoram originated in the southeastern Mediterranean region and is now produced in Egypt, France, and central Europe.

Avoid If . . .

Do not use Marjoram salve on infants or small children.

Special Cautions

When used at customary dosage levels for limited periods of time, Marjoram poses no problems. However, you should avoid extended use.

Possible Drug Interactions

No interactions have been reported.

Special Information If You Are Pregnant or Breastfeeding

No harmful effects are known.

How to Prepare

Marjoram is taken internally as a tea, and is used externally in mouthwashes and compresses. To prepare the tea, pour 1 cup of boiling water over 1 to 2 teaspoonfuls of Marjoram, steep for 5 minutes, and strain.

Typical Dosage
Sip 1 to 2 cups of Marjoram tea throughout the day.

Dried Marjoram may be stored for up to 2 years in air-tight containers.

Overdosage
No information on overdosage is available.

Marshmallow

Latin name: Althaea officinalis
Other names: Cheeses,
*   Mallards, Mortification Root,*
*   Schloss Tea, Sweet Weed,*
*   Wymote*

A Remedy For
- Bronchitis
- Cough

In folk medicine, Marshmallow is used as a treatment for inflammations of the mouth, throat, digestive system, urinary tract, and skin, and as a remedy for ulcers, infected wounds, burns, constipation, and diarrhea. Its effectiveness for these problems has not, however, been verified.

What It Is; Why It Works
Marshmallow stimulates the immune system and the production of white blood cells. It also soothes inflammation, slows production of mucus, and reduces sugar levels in the body.

The Marshmallow plant origi-nated in central Asia, spreading westward to Europe and eastward to China. It has been known since at least the time of the Romans, who cooked it as a vegetable delicacy. In the 1st century AD, the Roman scholar Pliny wrote: "Whosoever shall take a spoonful of the Mallows shall that day be free from all diseases that may come to him." He recommended a paste made from Marshmallow leaves to reduce infection after drawing out thorns. The plant's anti-infective qualities have earned it the English name "Mortification Root," for its therapeutic effect on gangrene (mortification). The root, leaves, and flowers are all considered medicinal.

Avoid If . . .
There are no known medical conditions that preclude the use of Marshmallow.

Special Cautions
When taken at customary dosage levels, Marshmallow poses no risks. However, diabetics should be mindful of the sugar concentration of Marshmallow syrup.

Possible Drug Interactions
Marshmallow may delay the action of other drugs taken at the same time.

Special Information If You Are Pregnant or Breastfeeding
No harmful effects are known.

How to Prepare
To make a Marshmallow tea, mix 10 to 15 grams (about 2 to 3 teaspoonfuls) of crushed

Marshmallow with 150 milliliters (about one-half cup) of cold water. Allow the mixture to soak for 1½ hours, then warm it before drinking.

Typical Dosage

When taken orally, the usual dosage of Marshmallow is:

Crushed Marshmallow root: 6 grams (about 1 heaping teaspoonful) daily.

Crushed Marshmallow leaf: 5 grams (about 1 teaspoonful) daily.

Marshmallow syrup: 10 grams (about 2 teaspoonfuls) per dose. The syrup should be used only to treat dry coughs.

Marshmallow tea: Several times daily.

The potency of commercial preparation may vary. Follow the manufacturer's directions whenever available. Store away from light.

Overdosage

No information on overdosage is available.

Maté

Latin name: Ilex paraguariensis
Other names: Jesuit's Tea, Paraguay Tea, Yerba Maté

A Remedy For

- Fatigue
- Heart palpitations
- Irregular heartbeat
- Kidney and bladder stones
- Urinary tract infections
- Weak heart

Maté is also used as a treatment for mental and physical fatigue and as a diuretic for flushing water from the body.

What It Is; Why It Works

Tea made from this herb is very popular in South America, the only source of the plant. Maté is an evergreen with white flowers and red fruit. Its medicinal parts are the dried or roasted leaves, which have proven to be a rich source of caffeine. Like coffee, Maté stimulates the central nervous system and has a diuretic effect. It also increases the force of heart contractions, affects heart rhythm, and breaks down sugars and fats in the body.

Avoid If . . .

You should avoid Maté if you are sensitive to caffeine or have a health condition that is aggravated by caffeine.

Special Cautions

Maté poses no problems when taken at normal dosage levels. However, high doses of caffeine taken regularly can lead to restlessness, irritability, insomnia, palpitations, dizziness, vomiting, diarrhea, loss of appetite, and headache.

Possible Drug Interactions

No interactions have been reported.

Special Information If You Are Pregnant or Breastfeeding

Many doctors recommend limiting caffeine intake during pregnancy to the equivalent of 1 cup of coffee a day. Drinking the equivalent of 4 cups or more per day could slow the baby's development.

How to Prepare

Maté can be made into a tea by pouring boiling water over one-half teaspoonful (2 grams) of crushed Maté. Steep for 5 to 10 minutes then strain. You will find that the tea tastes better and is more stimulating if it is steeped only a short time.

Maté is available alone and in various tea combinations. It's also an ingredient in some commercial drinks.

Typical Dosage

Maté is taken orally. The usual daily dosage is 3 grams (about three-quarters of a teaspoonful).

Overdosage

Massive doses of caffeine can cause stiffness, muscle spasms, and heart irregularities, but are unlikely to be life-threatening. (The lethal dosage is the equivalent of 75 cups of coffee at one sitting.) Nevertheless, if you suspect an overdose—especially in a child—seek medical attention immediately.

Mayapple

Latin name: Podophyllum peltatum

Other names: Duck's Foot, Ground Lemon, Hog Apple, Mandrake, Raccoon Berry

A Remedy For

• Warts

Although homeopathic practitioners use Mayapple to treat various conditions of the digestive tract and liver, its effectiveness for anything other than warts has not been verified.

What It Is; Why It Works

The medicinal resin from the underground stem of the Mayapple plant serves as the active ingredient in a pair of prescription medications for external genital warts, Condylox and Podocon-25. The drug is extremely poisonous, and must never be taken internally.

Mayapple is a small perennial native to northeastern North America. The plant bears solitary white flowers between two leaves, and has an unpleasant odor. Its Latin name—from the Greek words "podos" for foot, and "phyllon" for leaf—alludes to the leaves, which resemble webbed feet.

Avoid If . . .

Pregnant women should not use this drug.

Special Cautions

Use only externally, and limit the treatment area to no more than 4 square inches (25 square centimeters). Be sure to protect the adjacent skin. Application over large areas can result in poisoning by absorption through the skin.

Mayapple is extremely irritating to the skin and mucous membranes. Common reactions to Mayapple-based prescription drugs include inflammation, burning, erosion, pain, itching, and bleeding at the site of treatment.

Possible Drug Interactions
No drug interactions have been reported.

Special Information If You Are Pregnant or Breastfeeding
There is a possibility that this drug could harm a developing baby. Do not use it during pregnancy.

It's not known whether the drug appears in breast milk, but it would cause severe reactions if it did. To avoid any possibility of harm, do not use the drug while nursing.

How to Prepare
Mayapple is available as a liquid extract or alcohol solution (tincture).

Typical Dosage
Liquid extract: Apply 1.5 to 3.0 grams (about one-half teaspoonful) daily.
Tincture: Apply 2.5 to 7.5 grams (one-half to 1¹/₂ teaspoonfuls) daily.

Overdosage
Taken internally, doses of only 200 milligrams can cause severe abdominal pain, bloody diarrhea, vomiting, dizziness, headache, disrupted coordination, and spasms, sometimes ending in coma, respiratory failure, and death. If you suspect an overdose, seek emergency medical treatment immediately.

Meadowsweet

Latin name: Filipendula ulmaria
Other names: Bridewort, Meadow-wort, Queen of the Meadow, Spireaea ulmaria

A Remedy For
• Bronchitis
• Cough

Although Meadowsweet's effectiveness for other problems remains unverified, it has been used in folk medicine to promote urination, relieve rheumatism, and alleviate gout.

What It Is; Why It Works
Once held sacred by the Druids, Meadowsweet is found throughout Europe, North America, and northern Asia. It is a perennial plant that grows from 2 to 6 feet high. Medicinal parts include the dried yellowish-white flowers, other dried above-ground parts of the flowering plant, and the entire fresh flowering plant. The herb combats inflammation and tightens the tissues.

Avoid If . . .
Do not take Meadowsweet if you are sensitive to aspirin (salicylate).

Special Cautions
At customary dosage levels, Meadowsweet shouldn't cause any problems.

Possible Drug Interactions

No interactions have been reported.

Special Information If You Are Pregnant or Breastfeeding

No harmful effects are known.

How to Prepare

Meadowsweet comes in dried, powder form for use in tea. In Europe, it's also found in many mixed teas for treatment of flu, rheumatism, and kidney and bladder inflammation.

To prepare Meadowsweet tea, pour boiling water over 3 to 6 grams (about 2 to 4 teaspoonfuls) of Meadowsweet, steep for 10 minutes, and strain.

Typical Dosage

Total daily dosages are:

Meadowsweet flower: 2.5 to 3.5 grams (about 2 teaspoonfuls)
Meadowsweet leaf: 4 to 5 grams (about 3 teaspoonfuls)
Meadowsweet tea: Several cups

Overdosage

Excessive doses of Meadowsweet can lead to queasiness and stomach problems.

Melatonin

A Remedy For

• Insomnia

Given its ability to regulate body rhythms and promote normal sleep, Melatonin has proven useful not only for insomnia, but for jet lag and seasonal affective disorder (SAD) as well.

Other roles for this natural hormone are considerably more controversial. Some advocates claim it can hold back the spread of cancer. Others say it can delay the onset of aging, improve the symptoms of Alzheimer's disease, lower cholesterol levels, and reduce high blood pressure. However, most doctors feel that its effectiveness for these purposes remains to be proven.

What It Is; Why It Works

Melatonin is a product of the pineal gland, where it is synthesized from the amino acid tryptophan. Under normal conditions, Melatonin levels foreshadow the sleep cycle, usually increasing rapidly from the late evening until midnight, then decreasing as morning approaches. In this way, Melatonin helps regulate circadian rhythm, the body's 24-hour "dark-light clock" that governs the timing of hormone production, sleep, body temperature, and more.

Not surprisingly, people with high levels of Melatonin usually sleep longer and more soundly than those with a deficiency. For example, the elderly, who produce less Melatonin than the young and middle-aged, are typically more susceptible to insomnia. Similarly, events that throw Melatonin levels out of synch—such as a jet trip between time zones—seem to interfere with production of the hormone and thus disrupt sleep. Consumption of alcohol, tobacco, and narcotics has a similar effect.

Some researchers speculate that chronically low Melatonin levels may also be linked with cancer, especially in the breast, skin, or prostate gland. They note that many cancer patients have poorly functioning pineal glands and show low levels of Melatonin. Boosting these levels, they theorize, might strengthen the immune system and stimulate it to kill malignant cells, or at least prevent the cells from dividing rapidly. Until further proof is available, however, Melatonin can at best be considered an adjunct to conventional treatment—and certainly not a substitute for it.

Avoid If . . .

Unless your doctor approves, do not take Melatonin if you have an autoimmune disease such as rheumatoid arthritis, any condition that affects your lymphatic system, AIDS, osteoarthritis, depression or any other emotional disorder, diabetes, epilepsy, heart disease, leukemia, multiple sclerosis, or serious allergies.

Couples who are trying to conceive a baby should avoid this hormone. It is also not for use in children or teenagers.

Special Cautions

Take Melatonin only at bedtime. Do not drive or operate machinery after taking a dose.

If you develop a headache, rash, or upset stomach, or find that your normal sleeping patterns are disrupted, stop taking Melatonin and check with your doctor.

Possible Drug Interactions

Check with your doctor before combining Melatonin with the following:

Beta blockers such as Inderal, Lopressor, and Tenormin
Large amounts of ibuprofen (Motrin, Advil)
Mood-altering drugs such as diazepam (Valium)
Steroid medications such as prednisone

Special Information If You Are Pregnant or Breastfeeding

Do not take Melatonin supplements during pregnancy or while breastfeeding.

How to Prepare

Melatonin is available without prescription in tablet and capsule form.

Typical Dosage

Most experts recommend taking from 1 to 3 milligrams of Melatonin approximately 20 minutes before bedtime. Controlled release formulations should be taken 2 hours before going to bed.

To determine the exact dosage best for you, ask your doctor to monitor your blood levels and adjust the dosage accordingly. Do not attempt to medicate yourself.

Overdosage

Several physicians and researchers say that dosages as high as 200 milligrams of Melatonin per day appear to do no harm.

Milk Thistle

Latin name: Silybum marianum
Other name: Our Lady's Thistle

A Remedy For
- Appetite loss
- Liver and gallbladder problems

Milk Thistle seed has demonstrated significant value in the treatment of hepatitis, cirrhosis, inflammatory liver disease, and liver damage from toxic substances. It's also an antidote for death-cap mushroom poisoning.

The rest of the above-ground portion of the plant has occasionally been used for disorders of the liver, gallbladder, and spleen, and has been taken as a stimulant and tonic, but there is little evidence that it has any effect.

What It Is; Why It Works
A compound in Milk Thistle seed dubbed silymarin has been shown to protect the liver from a variety of toxic substances. It prevents toxins from penetrating the interior of liver cells, while promoting the growth of healthy new cells to repair liver damage. It also has antioxidant properties, mopping up damaging free radicals.

Native to Europe, the Milk Thistle plant generally reaches a height of 2 to 5 feet. The Latin name "marianum" and English name "Our Lady's Thistle" stem from the color of the leaf veins, which, legend has it, were turned white by drops of the Virgin Mary's milk. Thanks to this legend, Milk Thistle was once used as a tonic for nursing mothers.

Avoid If . . .
No known medical conditions preclude the use of Milk Thistle.

Special Cautions
There are no side effects on record.

Possible Drug Interactions
No interactions have been reported.

Special Information If You Are Pregnant or Breastfeeding
No harmful effects are known.

How to Prepare
Capsules containing 140 milligrams of the active ingredient silymarin are the preferred mode of administration. Silymarin dissolves poorly in water, so tea made with Milk Thistle seed is not very effective.

If you nevertheless prefer to take tea, you should mix 3 grams (a heaping half-teaspoonful) of crushed seeds with cold water, bring to a boil, simmer 10 to 20 minutes, then strain.

Typical Dosage
The usual daily dosage is the equivalent of 200 to 400 milligrams of silymarin, or 12 to 15 grams (about 1 tablespoonful) of crushed Milk Thistle seed. Since potency of commercial preparations may vary, follow the manufacturer's instructions whenever available.

Overdosage
No information on overdosage is available.

Mistletoe

Latin name: Viscum album
Other names: All-heal, Birdlime, Devil's fuge, Mystyldene

A Remedy For:
• Rheumatism
• Tumor symptoms

Mistletoe is also believed to lower blood pressure, improve circulation, and relax tight muscles, although these effects have not yet been scientifically validated. Other unverified uses included treatment of internal bleeding, convulsions, gout, hysteria, whooping cough, asthma, dizziness, loss of menstrual cycle, diarrhea, chorea (rapid, jerky movements), and rapid heartbeat. Because of its calming effect, Mistletoe is used as a tranquilizer for various nervous conditions and for the treatment of mental and physical exhaustion. It is also used as long-term therapy to prevent hardening of the arteries.

What It Is; Why It Works
A parasitic plant, Mistletoe lives on fruit trees and poplars by tapping nutrients from the host. According to ancient folklore, the wood of the cross carried by Christ was made from Mistletoe, and the plant was therefore "punished" by being banished from the earth and forced to depend on other plants to survive. The custom of kissing under the Mistletoe is thought to be connected with the plant's legendary (and unproven) power to increase fertility. The leaves, twigs, and berries are all medicinal.

Mistletoe is used to relieve the symptoms of malignant tumors, though it will not produce a cure. Mistletoe injections are thought to relieve rheumatoid arthritis by stimulating inflamed nerve endings.

Avoid If . . .
If you have a chronic infection such as tuberculosis, a tendency to allergies, or a high fever, Mistletoe injections are not recommended.

Special Cautions
Local skin reactions such as swelling and dead skin may occur after Mistletoe injection. Other reactions may include chills, fever, headache, chest pain (angina), low blood pressure, and allergic reactions.

Possible Drug Interactions
No interactions have been reported.

Special Information If You Are Pregnant or Breastfeeding
No harmful effects are known.

How to Prepare
Mistletoe is collected in the spring and air dried or put in a drier at a maximum temperature of 106 degrees Fahrenheit. A powdered form of the herb is used to prepare solutions for injection. A medicinal tea can be

made by steeping 2.5 grams (one-half teaspoonful) of finely cut Mistletoe in 1 cup of cold water for 12 hours at room temperature. Strain the tea before use. For Mistletoe wine, mix 40 grams (8 teaspoonfuls) of the herb with 1 liter of wine. Wait 3 days before using the wine.

Typical Dosage

The maximum daily oral dosage is 10 grams (2 teaspoonfuls) of Mistletoe.

In folk medicine, the usual daily dosage is:

- 1 to 2 cups of medicinal tea
- 2 to 6 grams (one-half to 1 teaspoonful) of Mistletoe powder
- 3 to 4 glasses of Mistletoe wine

Mistletoe must be stored away from light over an appropriate drying agent.

Overdosage

No information on overdosage is available.

Motherwort

Latin name: Leonurus cardiaca
Other names: Lion's Ear, Lion's Tail, Throw-wort

A Remedy For
- Irregular heartbeat
- Weak heart

Motherwort is also used as a remedy for hyperthyroid conditions and gas, although its effec-

tiveness for such problems remains unverified.

What It Is; Why It Works

Motherwort is an unusual plant, In addition to a distinctive stem—quadrangular, grooved, hollow, often red-violet, and usually hairy—it boasts dark green leaves, small red flowers, triangular brown fruit crowned with a tuft of hair, and an unpleasant smell. Originating in central Europe, Scandinavia, Russia, and central Asia, it is now established in North America.

The plant has a mildly relaxing effect on the heart, and acts as a sedative.

Avoid If . . .

No known medical conditions preclude the use of Motherwort.

Special Cautions

At typical dosage levels, Motherwort poses no special risks.

Possible Drug Interactions

No drug interactions have been reported.

Special Information If You Are Pregnant or Breastfeeding

No harmful effects are known.

How to Prepare

Motherwort can be crushed and prepared as tablets or pellets. You also may find fluid extracts of Motherwort and solutions of Motherwort in alcohol (tinctures).

Typical Dosage

Motherwort is taken orally. Commercial preparations may vary in strength, so follow manufacturer's directions whenever available. Representative doses are:

Crushed herb: 4.5 grams (about 1 teaspoonful)
Extract or tincture: 5 drops
Tablets: 1
Pellets: 10

For acute problems, doses may be taken every 30 to 60 minutes. For chronic problems, take 2 to 3 doses a day.

Overdosage
No information on overdosage is available.

Mountain Ash Berry

Latin name: Sorbus aucuparia
Other names: Rowan Tree, Sorb Apple, Witchen

A Remedy For
There is no evidence that Mountain Ash Berry has any medicinal effect. Nevertheless, it has been used in the treatment of kidney disease, diabetes, rheumatism, gout, and constipation. It is also a folk remedy for sinus and throat inflammations, lung infections, internal inflammations, menstrual complaints, excess acid in the blood, poor metabolism, diarrhea, and vitamin C deficiency.

What It Is; Why It Works
Mountain Ash grows throughout Europe, western Siberia, parts of Asia, and North America. Only the tree's scarlet berries are thought to be medicinal. They are also a popular ingredient in marmalades, jams, jellies, fruit sauces, liqueur, and vinegar, particularly in eastern Europe and the former Soviet Union.

Avoid If . . .
No known medical conditions preclude the use of Mountain Ash.

Special Cautions
The fresh berries contain an acid that, when taken in large amounts, can cause stomach pain, queasiness, vomiting, diarrhea, kidney damage, and skin rashes. Drying the berries eliminates much of this acid, and cooking them destroys it entirely. As long as you avoid the fresh berries, you are therefore unlikely to encounter side effects.

Possible Drug Interactions
No interactions have been reported.

Special Information If You Are Pregnant or Breastfeeding
No harmful effects are known.

How to Prepare
The dried berries are found in various tea mixtures.

Typical Dosage
There are no guidelines on record.

Overdosage
No information on overdosage is available.

Mountain Flax

Latin name: Linum catharticum
Other names: Dwarf Flax, Fairy Flax, Mill Mountain, Purging Flax

A Remedy For
• Constipation

Although it has not received official recognition, Mountain Flax is an effective laxative, and can also be given to induce vomiting. In addition, it is used—without evidence of effectiveness—as a treatment for internal inflammations, rheumatic disorders, swelling due to water retention, and intestinal worms. In homeopathic medicine, it is considered a remedy for cough, hemorrhoids, and diarrhea.

What It Is; Why It Works
The purgative action of Mountain Flax has been known for centuries, a fact reflected in the Latin name "catharticum," which means "purifying" or "cleansing."

An inconspicuous little herb of less than a foot in height, Mountain Flax is found only in the wild. It grows throughout central and southern Europe, Iran, and northern Africa. The entire above-ground part of the plant is used medicinally.

Avoid If . . .
No known medical conditions preclude the use of Mountain Flax.

Special Cautions
High doses can cause vomiting, inflammation of the digestive system, and diarrhea.

Possible Drug Interactions
No interactions have been reported.

Special Information If You Are Pregnant or Breastfeeding
No harmful effects are known.

How to Prepare
Mountain Flax is taken either as a ground herb or as an extract. You can make a Mountain Flax tea by adding 2.5 grams (about one-half teaspoonful) of the ground herb to 1 cup of hot water.

Typical Dosage
Mountain Flax is taken as a single dose to remedy constipation. Follow the manufacturer's directions whenever available.

Overdosage
An overdose can be fatal. If you suspect one, seek medical attention immediately.

Mugwort

Latin name: Artemisia vulgaris
Other names: Common Wormwood, Felon Herb, St. John's Plant

A Remedy For
Mugwort has been used to treat indigestion, stomachaches, worm infections, convulsions, vomiting, poor circulation, and restlessness. The root has been taken for emo-

tional problems, including depression, anxiety, and insomnia. For none of these problems, however, has its effectiveness been verified.

What It Is; Why It Works

Found throughout most of Europe, Asia, and North America, Mugwort is the herb used in the Chinese treatment called moxibustion. In this variation of acupuncture, small cones of smoldering Mugwort are placed on the trigger points said to govern the flow of life force throughout the body. It is by redirecting and balancing this flow that moxibustion is thought to promote healing.

In medieval Europe, Mugwort was believed to be the plant used as a belt by John the Baptist during his sojourn in the desert. As such, it was thought to confer protection from evil spirits, sunstroke, fatigue, and wild beasts. In modern laboratory tests, extracts of Mugwort do in fact exhibit a protective effect—but only against microbes.

Avoid If . . .

No known medical conditions preclude the use of Mugwort.

Special Cautions

There is a remote possibility of an allergic skin reaction from contact with Mugwort.

Possible Drug Interactions

There are no known drug interactions with Mugwort.

Special Information If You Are Pregnant or Breastfeeding

No information is available.

How to Prepare

Mugwort is sometimes used as a seasoning for game. Its medicinal use is not recommended.

Typical Dosage

There are no dosage recommendations on record.

Overdosage

No information is available.

Muira-Puama

Latin name: Ptychopetalum olacoides

A Remedy For

Although this herb is sometimes recommended as a remedy for impotence, its effectiveness is debatable.

What It Is; Why It Works

Nicknamed "potency wood," by the Amazon natives who discovered it, Muira-Puama is believed to have an aphrodisiac effect. However, the makers of Viagra need not worry. None of the compounds in Muira-Puama have any physical effect.

Avoid If . . .

No known medical conditions preclude the use of Muira-Puama.

Special Cautions

No side effects or hazards have been reported.

Possible Drug Interactions
No interactions have been reported.

Special Information If You Are Pregnant or Breastfeeding
No harmful effects are known.

How to Prepare
Wood from the tree's roots and trunk is considered "medicinal."

Typical Dosage
No guidelines are available.

Overdosage
No information is available.

Mullein

Latin name: Verbascum densiflorum
Other names: Aaron's Rod, Adam's Flannel, Beggar's Blanket, Feltwort, Golden Rod, Jacob's Staff, Shepherd's Club, Torchweed, Velvet Plant

A Remedy For
• Bronchitis
• Cough

Although Mullein has also been used to treat convulsions, cramps, gout, piles, rheumatism, water retention, and wounds, only its soothing respiratory effects have been clinically verified.

What It Is; Why It Works
Mullein has been known since the time of Ulysses, who is said to have used it as protection from evil spirits. Its rigid 6-foot stem, when soaked in oil, lends itself to use as a torch (hence the name "Torchweed"). Mullein's large, yellow flowers have a honey-like fragrance and an almond-like taste. The leaves are slimy and bitter.

Mullein's medicinal value lies in its ability to soothe irritated throats and help bring up phlegm.

Avoid If . . .
No known medical conditions preclude the use of this herb.

Special Cautions
When used at usual dosage levels, Mullein poses no risks.

Possible Drug Interactions
No drug interactions have been reported.

Special Information If You Are Pregnant or Breastfeeding
No harmful effects are known.

How to Prepare
Mullein may be taken as a crushed herb or in a tea. To prepare the tea, pour boiling water over 1.5 to 2 grams (about 3 to 4 teaspoonfuls) of finely cut Mullein. Let the tea steep for 10 to 15 minutes.

Typical Dosage
The total daily oral dosage is 3 to 4 grams (about 6 to 8 teaspoonfuls) of crushed Mullein.

Store in a dark place and protect from moisture.

Overdosage
No information is available on overdosage.

Mustard

Latin name: Sinapis alba
Other name: White mustard

A Remedy For
- Bronchitis
- Colds
- Cough
- Fever
- Rheumatism
- Sore throat
- Tendency to infection

In the form of compresses and baths, mustard has also been used for flushed skin and symptoms of paralysis. Mixed with honey, it has been used to clear and brighten the voice. Its effectiveness for these purposes has not, however, been confirmed.

What It Is; Why It Works
A familiar seasoning in kitchens worldwide, Mustard is cultivated in Europe and the northern U.S. The small brown to white seeds are the medicinal element; they retard bacterial growth. Don't confuse this form of Mustard with Black Mustard, a larger plant.

Avoid If . . .
Do not use Mustard if you have stomach ulcers or inflammatory kidney disease. Not for children under 6.

Special Cautions
Because Mustard oil can irritate internal membranes, large doses may cause stomach disorders. Long-term intake of Mustard could cause nerve damage, and long-term external application could cause skin injury.

Possible Drug Interactions
No drug interactions have been reported.

Special Information If You Are Pregnant or Breastfeeding
No harmful effects are known.

How to Prepare
For internal use, Mustard can be ground into a flour and mixed with honey to form balls. Take 1 or 2 balls on an empty stomach.

For external use, Mustard can be mixed with water and applied as a warm compress. Mix 50 to 70 grams of powdered seeds with warm water just prior to use, dampen an absorbent cloth with the mixture, and apply for 10 to 15 minutes (5 to 10 minutes for children). Shorten the duration for those with sensitive skin. Limit treatment to no more than 2 weeks.

A footbath can be prepared by mixing 20 to 30 grams (approximately 1 to 2 tablespoonfuls) of mustard flour in 1 liter of water. For a mustard bath, put 150 grams (a bit more than half a cup) of mustard in a pouch and soak in the bath.

Typical Dosage
For internal use, the usual daily dosage is 60 to 240 grams (one-quarter to 1 cup)

Store in a dark, dry place.

Overdosage
No information on overdosage is available.

Myrrh

Latin name: Commiphora molmol

A Remedy For
• Sore throat

Although proven effective only for mild oral inflammations, Myrrh is occasionally used to loosen phlegm and relieve gas. In Asian medicine, it's also used for stomach pain, missed menstrual periods, indigestion, skin diseases, poor circulation, and wounds.

What It Is; Why It Works
One of the wise men's gifts to the infant Jesus, Myrrh has been used since prebiblical times in incense and perfumes. It is an ingredient in the holy oil of Jewish ceremonies, and was employed by the ancient Egyptians for embalming.

Myrrh is a resin exuded by the cut bark of *Commiphora molmol*, a shrub native to the eastern Mediterranean area and Somalia. The plant, which grows up to 9 feet high, has a thick trunk and numerous irregular knotted branches. The pale yellow resin that oozes from a wound in the bark dries to a reddish-brown mass about the size of a walnut. It has disinfectant properties, and acts as an astringent, tightening and drying the tissues.

Avoid If . . .
No known medical conditions preclude the use of Myrrh.

Special Cautions
When used at customary dosage levels, Myrrh poses no hazards.

Possible Drug Interactions
No interactions have been reported.

Special Information If You Are Pregnant or Breastfeeding
No harmful effects are known.

How to Prepare
Myrrh is available as a powder or alcohol solution (tincture) for use as a rinse or to be taken internally.

To prepare a rinse or gargle, mix 5 to 10 drops with a glass of water.

Typical Dosage
You may take the undiluted tincture 2 to 3 times daily. The strength of commercial preparations may vary, so follow the manufacturer's directions whenever available.

Store Myrrh with a drying agent in sealed containers protected from light and moisture.

Overdosage
No information on overdosage is available.

Nasturtium

Latin name: Tropaeolum majus
Other name: Indian Cress

A Remedy For
• Bronchitis
• Cough
• Urinary tract infections

What It Is; Why It Works

This vine-like plant creeps and climbs for up to 15 feet, putting forth distinctive orange flowers with flame-red stripes. The flowers are fragrant, and the leafy parts of the plant smell and taste like cress. Nasturtium is native to the warmer regions of South America, but now grows in the Mediterranean region as well. One variety has been used medicinally since 1684.

In laboratory tests, Nasturtium stops the growth of germs and fungi. Applied to the skin, it improves circulation.

Avoid If . . .

Do not give Nasturtium to infants or young children, and do not take it if you have stomach ulcers or kidney disease.

Special Cautions

High doses of the fresh plant or its oil can irritate the lining of the digestive tract. Prolonged, intensive contact with the fresh plant can also irritate the skin.

Possible Drug Interactions

No interactions have been reported.

Special Information If You Are Pregnant or Breastfeeding

No harmful effects are known.

How to Prepare

You may find preparations of the plant's seeds or leaves.

Typical Dosage

No guidelines have been published. Follow the supplier's instructions when available.

Overdosage

See "Special Cautions" above.

Niauli

Latin name: Melaleucea viridiflora

A Remedy For

- Bronchitis
- Cough

What It Is; Why It Works

Niauli kills bacteria and improves circulation.

The Niauli plant is found in tropical parts of Southeast Asia and Australia. Only oil extracted from the leaves of young plants is considered medicinal. Traces of copper in the oil lend it a slightly greenish hue. It has a fragrance similar to camphor.

Avoid If . . .

Do not take Niauli internally if you have severe liver disease or an inflammation of the stomach, intestines, or gallbladder.

Do not apply preparations containing Niauli oil to the faces of infants or small children. It can cause throat spasms, asthma-like attacks, and even asphyxiation.

Special Cautions

In rare cases, when Niauli oil is taken internally it causes nausea, vomiting, and diarrhea.

Possible Drug Interactions

Niauli oil increases the liver's ability to process drugs, leaving them less time to do their work in the body. As a result, the effect of many drugs may be diminished or shortened if they are taken with Niauli. If you are taking a prescription medication, check with your doctor before using Niauli.

Special Information If You Are Pregnant or Breastfeeding

No harmful effects are known.

How to Prepare

To make nose drops, prepare a mixture of 2 to 5% Niauli oil in vegetable oil. Preparations for external application generally contain 10 to 30% Niauli oil.

Typical Dosage

Niauli oil can be taken orally, used as a nose drop, or applied externally. For oral administration, the usual dosage is 200 milligrams up to 10 times a day.

Because the potency of commercial preparations can vary, follow the manufacturer's directions whenever available.

Overdosage

Doses larger than 10 grams (2 teaspoonfuls) can be life-threatening. Symptoms of overdose include a drop in blood pressure, circulation problems, collapse, and, finally, failure to breathe.

If you suspect an overdose, seek emergency medical assistance immediately.

Nightshade

Latin name: Solanum dulcamara
Other names: Bittersweet,
  Felonwood, Fever Twig,
  Staff Vine

A Remedy For

• Eczema, boils, acne
• Warts

Only the stems of the Nightshade plant are used medicinally. The berries are quite poisonous.

What It Is; Why It Works

Nightshade is a member of the *Solanaceae* family, which includes some of the most nutritious plants—potato, eggplant, tomato—and some of the most poisonous. Despite its toxic properties, Nightshade has been recommended for virtually every medical problem at some point in history. Its only proven value, however, lies in its ability to relieve various skin conditions.

Nightshade works at a number of levels. It tightens and dries the skin and combats the growth of germs. Some varieties of the plant also have an anti-inflammatory effect. And one of the alkaloids in Nightshade inhibits nerve impulses governing the internal organs.

Avoid If . . .

No known medical conditions preclude the use of Nightshade.

Special Cautions

Although the stem of the plant contains toxic alkaloids, the level is fairly low and no side effects are likely at customary dosage levels.

Possible Drug Interactions

No interactions have been reported.

Special Information If You Are Pregnant or Breastfeeding

No harmful effects are known.

How to Prepare

To prepare a solution for external application, use 1 to 2 grams of the chopped drug per cup of water.

Typical Dosage

When taken orally, limit daily intake to 1 to 3 grams.

Overdosage

Poisonings have occurred among children who have eaten the unripe berries. More than 10 berries will cause nausea, vomiting, enlarged pupils, and diarrhea. A dosage of about 200 berries is deadly. If you suspect a poisoning, seek medical attention immediately.

Notoginseng Root

Latin name: Panax notoginseng
Other names: San Qi,
*   Pseudoginseng Root*

A Remedy For

In Chinese medicine, Notoginseng Root is a favorite remedy for both internal and external bleeding. It is taken internally to quell nosebleeds and blood in the stools, urine, or lungs. Applied externally, it's used to relieve pain and swelling from fractures, sprains, bruises, cuts, and wounds. It's also occasionally used as a treatment for acute attacks of Crohn's disease, an inflammatory bowel condition.

Recently, Notoginseng has also shown promise as a treatment for angina (chest pain due to poor circulation in the heart muscle) and high blood pressure.

What It Is; Why It Works

By Chinese standards, Notoginseng is a relative newcomer, first appearing in the *Compendium of Materia Medica* published by Li Shizen in 1578. He pronounced the root "more valuable than gold." Modern clinical trials conducted in China appear to confirm that Notoginseng does indeed speed the clotting process. It also seems to combat the effects of hardening of the arteries, improving circulation to the heart and relieving high blood pressure.

Native to China, Notoginseng is grown commercially in the southern and central regions of the country. The portion of the plant used in remedies is the root, dug up before the plant flowers or after the fruit has ripened.

Avoid If . . .

See "Special Information If You Are Pregnant or Breastfeeding."

Special Cautions

At customary dosage levels, Notoginseng Root poses no known risks.

Possible Drug Interactions

No drug interactions are known.

Special Information If You Are Pregnant or Breastfeeding

Notoginseng Root has caused miscarriage. Avoid it during pregnancy.

How to Prepare

Notoginseng Root is sold in bulk as loose, dried roots and in tablet form. It can be made into a liniment for swelling and pain, and can be used in compresses to help heal wounds and bruises.

Typical Dosage

There are no standard guidelines on record.

Overdosage

No information on overdosage is available.

Nutmeg

Latin name: Myristica fragrans
Other name: Mace

A Remedy For

Although Nutmeg is sometimes recommended for indigestion, it is not considered a truly useful remedy. In Asian medicine, Nutmeg is also used as a treatment for inflammation, abdominal pain, impotence, diarrhea, liver disease, and vomiting—but again without clinical validation.

What It Is; Why It Works

This familiar kitchen spice comes from a 50-foot evergreen tree cultivated in Indonesia, New Guinea, and the West Indies. The dried nuts ("Nutmegs") and their oil are both used medicinally. The fleshy skin of the nuts is ground to produce the household spice called mace. A nutmeg "butter" can be made by chopping the nuts and steaming them until they form a paste.

Avoid If . . .

No known medical conditions preclude the use of Nutmeg.

Special Cautions

Contact with the nuts occasionally triggers an allergic skin reaction.

Possible Drug Interactions

No drug interactions have been reported.

Special Information If You Are Pregnant or Breastfeeding

No harmful effects are known.

How to Prepare

Not recommended for medicinal use.

Typical Dosage

Not recommended for medicinal use.

Overdosage

An overdose (1 to 3 nuts) is signaled by thirst, nausea, reddening and swelling of the face, and feelings of urgency. Altered consciousness, ranging from mild disturbances to intense hallucinations, will follow, and can last from 2 to 3 days. Seizures and shock are possible. If you suspect an overdose, seek medical attention immediately.

Oats

Latin name: Avena sativa
Other names: Groats, Oatmeal

A Remedy For
• Skin inflammation
• Warts

Oat preparations are taken internally for a wide variety of ailments, including digestive problems, gallbladder complaints, kidney disorders, rheumatism, heart disease, chest and throat complaints, fatigue, diabetes, constipation, depression, diarrhea, anxiety, stress, nerve disorders, bladder problems, sleeplessness, gout, connective tissue disorders, the symptoms of old age, and narcotic and tobacco withdrawal. However, their value for these problems remains unconfirmed; and only external use for skin conditions is considered clearly effective. Oatmeal baths are frequently given to relieve itching from local skin irritations.

The straw from oats is also used as a remedy, for inflammatory skin diseases accompanied by itch, as well as for impetigo (a contagious skin eruption), frostbite, eye problems, bladder and rheumatic disorders, gout, and disorders of the metabolism. In footbaths, it's employed as a remedy for chronically cold or tired feet, and as a tea it's taken for flu and coughs. Effectiveness of the straw has not, however, been studied.

What It Is; Why It Works
Cultivated worldwide, Oat is an annual, light green grass with a bushy root that grows from 24 to 40 inches high. Oats are used as an additive in natural cosmetics, and are found in a variety of household foodstuffs and animal feeds. Oat straw is the dried, threshed leaf and stem of the plant.

Oats have been shown to lower cholesterol and combat the production of prostaglandins (hormones that act on the blood vessels and other organs in the body).

Avoid If . . .
There are no known medical conditions that preclude the use of Oats.

Special Cautions
No health hazards have been reported.

Possible Drug Interactions
No interactions are known.

Special Information If You Are Pregnant or Breastfeeding
No harmful effects are known.

How to Prepare
Rolled oats, such as oatmeal, are the plant's dried seeds, treated with steam, then crushed.

You can make an Oat tea by mixing 3 grams (a heaping half-teaspoonful) with a cup of boiling water. Allow to cool, then strain.

To prepare a bath additive from Oat straw, add 3½ ounces of the chopped straw to 3 quarts of water, boil for 20 minutes, then add to the bathwater.

Typical Dosage

As a tea, Oats can be taken repeatedly throughout the day and shortly before bedtime.

Store away from light and moisture.

Overdosage

No information on overdosage is available.

Oleander

Latin name: Nerium odoratum
Other name: Rose Laurel

A Remedy For

Oleander is considered a remedy for heart failure. However, it is so toxic that medicinal use is not recommended.

In Asian medicine, Oleander is used to treat hemorrhoids and scabies, and homeopathic practitioners prescribe it for skin, heart, and nervous conditions. Its effectiveness for these purposes has not, however, been verified.

What It Is; Why It Works

Oleander has been used medicinally since Roman times, and was considered an important remedy in Arabic medicine. The leaves contain compounds that boost the force of the heartbeat while slowing its rate.

An evergreen shrub of up to 12 feet in height, Oleander is found throughout the Mediterranean region, and in warmer climates around the world.

Avoid If . . .

There are numerous reports of fatalities following excessive doses of Oleander. It's best to avoid this herb entirely.

Special Cautions

Side effects, which increase with the size of the dose, include nausea, vomiting, diarrhea, headache, stupor, and irregular heartbeat.

Possible Drug Interactions

Oleander boosts the action—and side effects—of a variety of drugs, including:

Calcium salts
Digitalis-type medications such as Lanoxin
Laxatives
Quinidine (Quinaglute, Quinidex)
Certain water pills (diuretics)

Special Information If You Are Pregnant or Breastfeeding

Use in pregnancy has not been studied, and is definitely not recommended.

How to Prepare

Not recommended.

Typical Dosage

Not recommended.

Overdosage

A massive overdose causes life-threatening heartbeat irregularities, with either an excessively rapid or dangerously slow heart rate. If you suspect an overdose, on the liver are thought to be due to certain compounds contained in the berries. Laboratory tests suggest that the herb may also possess a ginseng-like effect, boosting energy and fighting fatigue.

Avoid If . . .

Schisandra is not recommended for use in the early stages of coughs or rashes.

Special Cautions

Although rare, potential side effects of Schisandra include heartburn, stomach upset, decreased appetite, and skin rash.

Possible Drug Interactions

No interactions have been reported.

Special Information If You Are Pregnant or Breastfeeding

No harmful effects are known.

How to Prepare

Dried Schisandra berries are available in Asian markets and some Western health food stores. You may also find them in tablet form or as an alcohol solution (tincture).

Typical Dosage

Dried berries: 1 to 6 grams per day
Tincture: 2 to 4 milliliters per day

The strength of commercial preparations may vary, so follow the manufacturer's instructions whenever available.

Overdosage

Symptoms of overdose include restlessness, insomnia, and difficulty breathing. If you suspect an overdose, call your doctor immediately.

Scopola

Latin name: Scopolia carniolica
Other names: Belladonna
Scopola, Japanese Belladonna

A Remedy For
• Liver and gallbladder problems

Scopola is used to relieve spasms in the digestive system, the bile ducts (which carry bile from the liver to the intestine), and the urinary tract.

What It Is; Why It Works

Similar to Belladonna and Henbane in its action, Scopola blocks nerve impulses in the muscular walls of the digestive and urinary tracts, thus relaxing them and ending any spasms. It also relieves muscular tremors and rigidity, improves conduction of electrical impulses in the heart, and speeds up the heart rate. Its main active ingredient, hyoscyamine, is found in such prescription drugs as Cytospaz, Donnatal, Levsin, and Urised.

A perennial plant from 1 to 2 feet in height, Scopola's color ranges from yellowish-brown to dark brownish-gray. It is native to southeast Europe and southwest Russia. The medicinal part is the underground stem.

seek emergency medical attention immediately.

Olive Leaf

Latin name: Olea europaea

A Remedy For
Olive Leaf is sometimes used to treat high blood pressure. There is, however, no firm evidence of its effectiveness.

What It Is; Why It Works
Use olive oil as a drug? It seems improbable, but this common salad and cooking oil was indeed once prescribed for liver and gallbladder problems—until it was discovered that the "remedy" was triggering cramps in gallstone patients.

Today, only Olive Leaf is thought to have any medicinal potential. In animal tests, it has lowered blood pressure, steadied the heartbeat, and relieved spasms. Unfortunately, its value as a remedy in humans remains to be proven.

Despite its lackluster performance as a drug, the olive has been held in high esteem since ancient times. According to the Bible, Moses exempted young men from fighting in the army if they worked at cultivating olives. In many classical writings, olive oil is a symbol of goodness and purity, and it was burned in sacred temple lamps. In the ancient Olympics, it was the olive leaf that formed the victors' crowns.

Avoid If . . .
Olive Leaf can be used under any medical conditions. Avoid the oil, however, if you have gallstones.

Special Cautions
At customary dosage levels, Olive Leaf presents no risks.

Possible Drug Interactions
No interactions have been reported.

Special Information If You Are Pregnant or Breastfeeding
No harmful effects are known.

How to Prepare
To prepare an Olive tea, pour 5 ounces of hot water over 7 to 8 grams (about 2 teaspoonfuls) of crushed Olive Leaf and steep for 30 minutes.

Typical Dosage
Drink 3 to 4 cups of Olive tea daily.

Overdosage
No information on overdosage is available.

Onion

Latin name: Allium cepa

A Remedy For
• Appetite loss
• Bronchitis
• Colds
• Cough
• Fever
• Hardening of the arteries
• High blood pressure
• Indigestion

- Sore throat
- Tendency to infection

In folk medicine, Onion has also been used for whooping cough, chest pain (angina), gallbladder complaints, dehydration, menstrual problems, parasitic infections, and diabetes. It is applied externally for insect bites, wounds, mild burns, warts, boils, and bruises. These folk uses all remain unproven.

What It Is; Why It Works

It's the same ingredient that brings tears to your eyes that lends Onions their ability to fight disease. This sulfur compound thins the blood and helps prevent dangerous clots while lowering blood pressure and possibly reducing cholesterol levels. Onions also possess the ability to kill a wide variety of germs. And, for asthma victims, Onion extract may even relieve allergy-induced bronchial constriction.

Avoid If . . .

There are no known medical conditions that preclude the use of Onion.

Special Cautions

Taking large quantities can cause stomach problems. Frequent hand contact may cause eczema (a weeping, itching rash).

Possible Drug Interactions

No interactions have been reported.

Special Information If You Are Pregnant or Breastfeeding

No harmful effects are known.

How to Prepare

You can make a medicinal oil by crushing an Onion and stirring in an equal amount of fatty oil. Let the mixture stand for 48 hours, then filter the oil.

A popular form of Onion extract is made with pressed Onion juice and syrup, using 500 grams (1 pound, 1 ounce) of Onions, 500 milliliters (1 pint) of water, 100 grams (3 ounces) of honey, and 350 grams (12 ounces) of sugar.

You can prepare an Onion tincture by soaking 100 grams (3 ounces) of minced Onions in 300 milliliters (10 ounces) of alcohol for 10 days.

Typical Dosage

The usual oral dosage is:

Onion tincture: 4 to 5 teaspoonfuls daily
Onion syrup: 4 to 5 tablespoons daily
Fresh Onion: 50 grams (1²/₃ ounces) daily
Dried Onion: 20 grams (two-thirds ounce) daily

For external use, apply slices directly to the skin, cover the affected area with a juice-soaked cloth, or spread juice across the area.

When using a commercial preparation, follow the manufacturer's labeling. Strengths may vary.

Overdosage

No information on overdosage is available.

Oregano

Latin name: Origanum vulgare
Other names: Mountain Mint,
Wild Marjoram, Winter
Marjoram, Wintersweet

A Remedy For

Oregano is considered a remedy for respiratory problems such as coughs and bronchitis, although there is no conclusive proof of its effectiveness. Unverified uses in folk medicine include treatment of bloating, gas, urinary tract problems, painful menstruation, rheumatoid arthritis, swollen glands, and lack of perspiration.

What It Is; Why It Works

It's difficult to think of a common kitchen herb like Oregano as a medical remedy, but it has in fact been used as a drug since the time of the ancient Greeks and Chinese. In China, doctors prescribed it to relieve fever, vomiting, diarrhea, jaundice, and itchy skin, while the Greeks made compresses from the leaves to treat sores and aching muscles.

The primary ingredients in Oregano are thymol and carvacrol, which are also found in thyme. These compounds, researchers have found, help loosen phlegm in the lungs and relieve spasms in the bronchial passages. Many commercial cough remedies, including cough drops and skin rubs such as Vicks Vapo-Rub, contain thymol.

Harvested during the flowering season and dried on the field or under a roof, Oregano has bright purple flowers and an aromatic scent. Its medicinal value lies in the oil found in its leaves.

Avoid If . . .

No known medical conditions preclude the use of Oregano.

Special Cautions

At customary dosage levels, Oregano poses no problems.

Possible Drug Interactions

No interactions have been reported.

Special Information If You Are Pregnant or Breastfeeding

No harmful effects are known.

How to Prepare

You can make an Oregano tea by pouring 1 cup of boiling water over 1 heaping teaspoon of the dried herb, steeping for 10 minutes, then straining. The tea may be sweetened with honey.

To make an additive for the bath, pour 1 quart of water over 100 grams (3 1/3 ounces) of Oregano, steep for 10 minutes, strain, and add to a full bathtub.

Typical Dosage

Sweetened Oregano tea may be taken internally as needed. The unsweetened tea may be used as a gargle or mouthwash.

Overdosage

No information on overdosage is available.

Papaya

Latin name: Carica papaya
Other names: Melon
Tree, Papaw

A Remedy For

Although juice from Papaya leaves and fruit has been used as a treatment for digestive disorders and intestinal worms, its effectiveness for these problems has not been conclusively proven.

In Asian medicine, Papaya has also been used for constipation and leprosy.

What It Is; Why It Works

The Papaya tree, which reaches a height of 12 to 25 feet, originated in Central America, but is now cultivated in the tropics worldwide. It is prized for its large, yellow, melon-flavored fruits.

Papain, an enzyme in Papaya, is one of the active ingredients in ointments (Accuzyme, Panafil) prescribed for treatment of severe wounds and skin ulcers. Papain has the unique ability to dissolve dead tissue without damaging living cells. (It is also used as a meat tenderizer.)

Avoid If . . .

Do not take Papaya preparations during pregnancy.

Special Cautions

If you have a bleeding disorder, Papaya extracts could aggravate it. Allergic reactions are also a possibility.

Possible Drug Interactions

No interactions have been reported.

Special Information If You Are Pregnant or Breastfeeding

Remember, Papaya extracts should be avoided during pregnancy.

How to Prepare

Papain ointments for wound treatment are available only by prescription.

Typical Dosage

Follow the manufacturer's directions whenever available.

Overdosage

There is no information available.

Parsley

Latin name: Petroselinum
crispum

A Remedy For

- Kidney and bladder stones
- Urinary tract infections

Parsley seed, leaf, and root are all used medicinally, but only the leaf and root have been thoroughly tested and found effective for urinary problems.

In folk medicine, Parsley has also been used to treat stomach and intestinal disorders, jaundice, water retention, and failure to menstruate. Its effectiveness for these ailments has not, however, been scientifically proven. Juice pressed from fresh Parsley is a folk remedy for insect bites.

What It Is; Why It Works

Now grown worldwide, Parsley originated somewhere in the Mediterranean region. The ancient Greeks employed it in their funeral rites, fashioning it into wreaths for their tombs. Ironically, this most widely used of kitchen herbs was never used for cooking in ancient Greece. Instead, it was held sacred and reserved for the realms of the dead.

From Greece, Parsley spread across the Roman Empire and eventually throughout Europe. The curled-leafed variety, "crispum" was mentioned by the Roman historian Pliny. Other varieties have been known since at least the 18th century.

Although common Parsley seems an unlikely candidate for medicinal use, the oil extracted from the plant is surprisingly potent—and, in large doses, even dangerous. Parsley leaf and root help flush excess water from the body. In animal tests, they have also been found to trigger and strengthen contractions of the uterus.

Avoid If . . .

Parsley is not recommended for water retention due to a heart or kidney condition; and should not be used if you have a kidney inflammation. You should also avoid Parsley if you have ever suffered an allergic reaction to it or its active ingredient, apiole. Do not take Parsley while pregnant (see "Special Information If You Are Pregnant or Breastfeeding").

Special Cautions

When using Parsley to flush out the urinary system, be sure to drink large amounts of fluid.

There is a slight possibility that Parsley will cause a skin reaction. Contact with freshly harvested plants can increase sensitivity of light-skinned individuals to the sun.

Refined Parsley oil is considered too toxic for medicinal use (see "Overdosage").

Possible Drug Interactions

No interactions have been reported.

Special Information If You Are Pregnant or Breastfeeding

Because of Parsley's potentially abortive effects, it should not be used during pregnancy.

How to Prepare

Parsley seed can be made into a tea. Pour boiling water over 1 gram (about one-quarter teaspoonful) of freshly pressed Parsley, steep for 10 minutes, and strain. The tea should be taken 2 to 3 times a day. Crushed Parsley leaf and root may also be taken as tea.

Dry extracts are available in tablet form.

Typical Dosage

Parsley is taken orally. The usual daily dosage is:

Parsley seed: 2 to 3 grams (about one-half teaspoonful)
Parsley leaf or root: 6 grams (about 1 heaping teaspoonful)

Because the potency of commercial preparations may vary, follow the manufacturer's directions whenever available.

Store Parsley seed away from light and moisture.

Overdosage

High doses of Parsley oil—or preparations rich in the oil—can be poisonous. Symptoms of poisoning include increased contractions of the bladder, intestines, and uterus. Other side effects include excessive weight loss, bloody stools, nosebleeds, and, possibly, kidney shutdown.

If you suspect an overdose, check with your doctor immediately.

Passion Flower

Latin name: Passiflora incarnata
Other names: Granadilla,
Maypop, Passion Vine

A Remedy For
• Insomnia
• Nervousness

Although proven effective only for edginess and insomnia, Passion Flower has also been used as a remedy for depression and nervous stomach. Homeopathic practitioners prescribe it for asthma and whooping cough. Applied externally, it has been used for hemorrhoids.

What It Is; Why It Works

This perennial vine, which reaches 30 feet in length, grows naturally from the southeastern U.S. to Brazil and Argentina, and is cultivated in Europe as a garden plant. The blossoms are considered symbolic of Christ's Passion (their central corona, for instance, represents the Crown of Thorns), accounting for their name.

The above-ground parts of the plant hold its medicinal value. In animal tests, researchers found that the plant slows the passage of food through the digestive tract.

Avoid If . . .

No known medical conditions preclude the use of Passion Flower.

Special Cautions

At customary dosage levels, Passion Flower poses no risks.

Possible Drug Interactions

No interactions have been reported.

Special Information If You Are Pregnant or Breastfeeding

No harmful effects are known.

How to Prepare

Passion Flower is available as an herb for tea. It is also an ingredient in certain sedative bath additives.

To make tea, pour 150 milliliters (about two-thirds of a cup) of hot water over 1 teaspoonful of Passion Flower, steep for 10 minutes, then strain.

To prepare an external rinse, particularly for hemorrhoids, put 20 grams of Passion Flower into 200 grams (about 1 cup) of simmering water, allow to cool, then strain.

Typical Dosage

Take 2 to 3 cups of tea during the day and one-half hour before bedtime. The amount of herb used per day should total 4 to 8 grams.

Overdosage

No information on overdosage is available.

Pau d'Arco

Latin name: Tabebuia impestiginosa
Other names: Lapacho, Taheebo, Trumpet Tree

A Remedy For
• Fungal infections

In Latin America, where Pau d'Arco is grown, people use this herb to treat cancer, lupus, infectious diseases, wounds, and a variety of other ailments. In the Caribbean, it is considered a remedy for backache, toothache, sexually transmitted diseases, and low sexual drive. However, only its anti-infective properties have been verified.

What It Is; Why It Works

An inhabitant of the tropical rain forest, Pau d'Arco is a majestic tree that often reaches 125 feet in height. It owes its medicinal value to certain compounds in the bark. Called naphthaquinones, these substances show potent antifungal properties in laboratory tests. Indeed, they appear to out-perform the common prescription antifungal drug ketoconazole (Nizoral).

Although these same compounds also exhibit cancer-fighting properties, they must be taken in toxic doses to have any anticancer effect, leaving Pau d'Arco a poor choice for cancer treatment. Other compounds in the bark do, however, appear to combat bacterial, viral, and parasitic infections, and may have anti-inflammatory properties as well.

Avoid If . . .

No known medical disorders preclude the use of Pau d'Arco.

Special Cautions

The unrefined bark is much safer than extracts of the active ingredients; the whole bark has no known serious side effects.

Do not give Pau d'Arco to children for more than 7 to 10 days without your doctor's approval.

Possible Drug Interactions

If Pau d'Arco is taken in conjunction with other herbs, a reduction in dosage may be necessary.

Special Information If You Are Pregnant or Breastfeeding

Avoid Pau d'Arco while pregnant or breastfeeding.

How to Prepare

Pau d'Arco is available as capsules, tablets, alcohol solutions (tinctures), and dried bark. Because the active ingredients in Pau d'Arco are not water-soluble, a tea from the bark is ineffective.

Typical Dosage
Capsules and tablets: Three 300-milligram capsules or tablets 3 times per day.

Because the strength of commercial preparations may vary, follow the manufacturer's directions whenever available.

Overdosage
High doses of one of the naphthaquinones in Pau d'Arco can cause uncontrolled bleeding, nausea, and vomiting. If you suspect an overdose, seek medical attention immediately.

Pennyroyal

Latin name: Mentha pulegium
Other names: Lurk-in-the-Ditch,
   Mosquito Plant, Piliolerial,
   Pudding Grass, Run-by-the-
   Ground, Squaw Balm,
   Squawmint Tickweed

A Remedy For
Pennyroyal is often considered a remedy for indigestion, liver and gallbladder complaints, and skin inflammations, although there is no scientific proof of its effectiveness. It has also been used, again without validation, for gout, colds, and excessive urination. Homeopathic practitioners prescribe it for cramps and respiratory problems.

What It Is; Why It Works
This herb was evidently a favorite of royalty in early England; its name is a corruption of "puliollroyall" from the Latin "pulegium regium" or "pulegium of the king." The plant is very aromatic, and its fragrance, like that of roses, was credited with medicinal properties by the Roman scholar Pliny.

The reasons for Pennyroyal's therapeutic effects—if any—are unknown, but there's no question that it contains highly potent compounds. An overdose of oil extracted from the plant can be fatal.

Pennyroyal thrives in southern Europe, western Asia, the Middle East, and Ethiopia. A similar plant, American Pennyroyal, is found in the eastern half of the United States. Both the oil and the dried above-ground parts of the European Pennyroyal plant have been used medicinally.

Avoid If . . .
Pennyroyal has toxic effects on the liver, and is no longer recommended for use in any form.

Special Cautions
Although not recommended, the dried herb can be taken internally. The oil, however, is for external use only.

Possible Drug Interactions
No interactions have been reported.

Special Information If You Are Pregnant or Breastfeeding
Pennyroyal oil has been used to induce abortions. It's best to

avoid the herb in any form while pregnant or breastfeeding.

How to Prepare

Pennyroyal is available in powdered form, as an extract, and as an oil for external use. You can make Pennyroyal tea using 1 to 4 grams of the dried herb per cup of water.

Typical Dosage

People who insist on using this herb despite its effect on the liver are generally told to drink 1 cup of tea 3 times a day.

Overdosage

Acute poisoning from the dried herb is unlikely, but as little as 5 grams (about 1 teaspoonful) of Pennyroyal oil can cause vomiting, high blood pressure, and paralysis. Following larger doses of the oil, death from respiratory failure is a distinct possibility. If you suspect an overdose, seek medical attention immediately.

Peony

Latin name: Paeonia officinalis

A Remedy For

Peony is prescribed as a remedy for hemorrhoids and rheumatism, but its effectiveness remains unproven. Other unverified uses include treatment of diseases of the skin and mucous membranes, gout, and respiratory ailments. Peony root has also been used, without substantiation, for chronic weakness and fatigue, nerve pain, migraine, allergies, excitability, epilepsy, and whooping cough; and the flower has been used to induce vomiting and abortion. In Asian medicine, Peony is considered a remedy for menstrual disorders, discolorations on the skin, bloody vomiting, and seizures. Homeopathic practitioners use it for ulcers and hemorrhoids.

What It Is; Why It Works

The Peony has inspired more than its share of superstition. Some claimed it was of divine origin, others that it came from the moon, or that it averted evil spirits and tempests. The ancient Greek philosopher Theophrastus advised gathering Peony only at night, for if a woodpecker spies a man gathering it, "he is in danger [of losing] his eyes."

The Peony's medicinal uses seem equally overblown. The only effect that research has been able to identify is a tendency to boost muscular tension in animal tests. No painkilling action has been documented.

Avoid If . . .

No known medical conditions preclude the use of Peony.

Special Cautions

Side effects become more likely as the dosage is increased. They include such stomach complaints as vomiting, cramps, and diarrhea.

Possible Drug Interactions

No interactions have been reported.

Special Information If You Are Pregnant or Breastfeeding

Given the plant's history as an abortive agent, it would seem wise to avoid it during pregnancy.

How to Prepare

Peony root is produced as an alcohol solution (tincture). The dried flowers can be prepared as a tea, using 1 gram per cup.

Typical Dosage

The average daily dose of Peony flower is 1 gram (1 cup of tea).

Overdosage

Symptoms such as vomiting, cramps, and diarrhea could well be a sign of overdose. If you suspect an overdose, seek medical attention immediately.

Peppermint

Latin name: Mentha piperita
Other names: Brandy Mint,
  Lamb Mint

A Remedy For

Peppermint oil can be used for the following ailments:

- Appetite loss
- Bronchitis
- Colds
- Cough
- Fever
- Liver and gallbladder problems
- Sore throat
- Tendency to infection

Peppermint in leaf form is of more limited value, but still may be taken for liver and gallbladder complaints and loss of appetite.

Peppermint is also used internally for digestive cramps and irritable colon. In addition, it has been used for a number of conditions for which its effectiveness remains unproven, including nausea, vomiting, morning sickness, and painful menstruation. In homeopathic medicine, it is used for intestinal pain and skin problems.

What It Is; Why It Works

This familiar perennial is found throughout Europe and the U.S. The fresh or dried leaves and the dried branch tips can be used medicinally, but the oil extracted from the above-ground parts of the plant is more common.

Peppermint calms digestive spasms, relieves gas, boosts the flow of bile, fights bacteria, and acts as a decongestant. It has a cooling effect on the skin. The active ingredient, menthol, is found in a variety of popular over-the-counter cough remedies, including Vicks Cough Drops, Halls Cough Suppressant Drops, and Cepacol Sore Throat Lozenges, and in such common external medications as Vicks VapoRub and Mentholatum Cream.

Avoid If . . .

Do not take Peppermint internally if you have a blockage in the bile ducts, gallbladder inflammation, or liver damage. Also avoid it if you are prone to acid reflux.

Special Cautions

Peppermint can cause digestive problems, particularly in people with gallstones. The oil sometimes provokes a mild allergic reaction. Do not apply preparations containing Peppermint oil to the faces—particularly the nasal area—of infants or small children; it could cause asthma-like symptoms or even respiratory failure.

Possible Drug Interactions

No interactions have been reported.

Special Information If You Are Pregnant or Breastfeeding

No harmful effects are known.

How to Prepare

To prepare Peppermint tea, pour 150 milliliters (about one-half cup) of hot water over 1 teaspoonful of the leaves, steep for 10 minutes, and strain.

For inhalation, pour 3 to 4 drops of Peppermint oil into hot water.

Typical Dosage

The customary daily dosages are:

Oil: 6 to 12 drops
Coated capsules: 0.6 milliliter
Dried leaves: 3 to 6 grams

For external application, use an oil- or water-based cream or ointment, or rub a few drops of Peppermint oil into the affected area.

Since commercial preparations vary in potency, follow the manufacturer's directions whenever available. Store Peppermint in a cool, dry place, away from light. Do not use a plastic container.

Overdosage

Although there are no cases of Peppermint overdose on record, pure menthol can be fatal in doses of as little as 2 grams, although individuals have survived dosages as high as 8 to 9 grams (about 2 teaspoonfuls). If you suspect an overdose, seek medical attention immediately.

Periwinkle

Latin name: Vinca minor
Other name: Myrtle

A Remedy For

Periwinkle is sometimes recommended for circulatory problems—particularly in the brain—but there is no evidence of its effectiveness. In homeopathic medicine, it's used, again without evidence of effect, for hemorrhages and skin conditions.

What It Is; Why It Works

While a close relative, *Vinca rosea*, is the source of the important cancer drugs vinblastine and vincristine, *Vinca minor* has never played a major role in medicine. Used in past centuries to dry and tighten the tissues and serve as a general tonic, the herb is no longer recommended for medicinal purposes.

Originating in northern Spain, western France, and central and southern Europe, this familiar ground-hugging evergreen shrub can now be found throughout the world. Its purplish-blue flowers won it the name "Sorcerer's Violet" in the Middle Ages. It was placed on the coffins of dead children in years gone by. In German, it's therefore called the "Flower of Immortality" and in Italian the "Flower of Death."

Avoid If . . .
Large doses can be poisonous. Since the herb has no proven medicinal effect, it's best to avoid its use.

Special Cautions
Potential side effects include stomach problems and reddened skin.

Possible Drug Interactions
No drug interactions have been reported.

Special Information If You Are Pregnant or Breastfeeding
No harmful effects are known.

How to Prepare
Not recommended.

Typical Dosage
Not recommended.

Overdosage
An overdose of Periwinkle can cause a severe drop in blood pressure. If you suspect an overdose, seek medical attention immediately.

Petasite

Latin name: Petasites hybridus
Other names: Blatterdock, Bog Rhubarb, Butterbur, Flapperdock, Langwort, Umbrella Leaves

A Remedy For
• Kidney and bladder stones

The leaves and roots of the Petasite plant are both considered medicinal, but the root alone has been judged unquestionably effective. It is recommended only for the treatment of urinary stones; but it is also taken for breathing problems—such as coughs, whooping cough, and asthma—as an appetite stimulant, as a remedy for stomach and intestinal cramps, and as a cure for migraine and tension headaches.

Petasite leaf, though unproven, is used in folk medicine for treating breathing problems and diseases of the liver, gallbladder, and pancreas. It is also used as a calming drug to prevent restlessness and promote sleep. Petasite leaf compresses are sometimes applied as an external remedy for wounds and malignant ulcers.

What It Is; Why It Works
Petasite works by stopping spasms in internal organs. However, the unprocessed plant also contains cancer-causing compounds that preclude its use. As a result, you should take only purified commercial preparations (see "Avoid If . . .").

Petasite's huge leaves—the largest of any wild plant—earned

it its name. They reminded the ancient Greeks of a "petasos," the type of hat worn by Greek shepherds and the Greek god Hermes. The plant grows throughout northern Asia, Europe, and some areas of North America.

Avoid If . . .

Natural Petasite contains toxic compounds called pyrrolizidine alkaloids that cause liver damage, genetic damage, cancer, and birth defects. Even very small traces of the alkaloids are dangerous, so unprocessed Petasite should be carefully avoided.

Alkaloid-free varieties of Petasite, cultivated under laboratory conditions, permit preparation of commercial Petasite extracts that contain virtually no pyrrolizidine. Nevertheless, always check the label for pyrrolizidine content before using a Petasite product.

Special Cautions

Use only products with minimal pyrrolizidine content.

Possible Drug Interactions

No interactions have been reported.

Special Information If You Are Pregnant or Breastfeeding

Because of the danger of birth defects and harm to newborns, avoid all Petasite preparations during pregnancy and while nursing.

How to Prepare

Take only purified commercial preparations.

Typical Dosage

Follow the manufacturer's directions. The daily dose should not contain more than 1 milligram of pyrrolizidine alkaloids.

Overdosage

No information on overdosage is available.

Phyllanthus

Latin name: Phyllanthus niruri
Other name: Bahupatra

A Remedy For

• Hepatitis B

In traditional Indian medicine, Phyllanthus has been used for diabetes, gonorrhea, frequent menstruation, skin ailments, and liver disorders—generally without scientifically verified effect. For one type of liver disease, however, Phyllanthus shows genuine promise. It appears to combat the virus that causes hepatitis B.

What It Is; Why It Works

Phyllanthus niruri is the most effective of a group of closely related species that grow in India, China, and tropical locations ranging from the Philippines to Cuba. Scientists have not identified the ingredient responsible for its medicinal effect, but the herb has been shown to block an enzyme that plays a crucial role in reproduction of the hepatitis B virus. As a result, a majority of patients show an improvement in blood tests after a month of treatment.

Avoid If . . .
No known medical conditions preclude the use of Phyllanthus.

Special Cautions
To be effective, the herb must be taken regularly for a month or longer. At customary dosage levels, no side effects have been reported.

Possible Drug Interactions
No interactions have been reported.

Special Information If You Are Pregnant or Breastfeeding
No harmful effects are known.

How to Prepare
Phyllanthus is usually taken in powdered form.

Typical Dosage
In clinical trials, doses have ranged from 900 to 2,700 milligrams per day.

Overdosage
No information on overdosage is available.

Pilewort

Latin name: Ranunculus ficaria
*Other names: Figwort, Lesser
  Celandine, Smallwort*

A Remedy For
Pilewort is sometimes used as a remedy for wounds and burns, but has not gained official recognition. It is also used as a treatment for vitamin C deficiency (scurvy), bleeding gums, and swollen joints.

What It Is; Why It Works
Once considered a remedy for hemorrhoids (hence the name "Pilewort"), this herb is now used primarily as a bath additive to treat wounds, warts, and scratches. Although rich in vitamin C, the plant can be toxic when taken internally and is therefore not a particularly good choice for vitamin C supplementation.

Avoid If . . .
No known medical conditions preclude the use of Pilewort.

Special Cautions
The dried herb poses no major risks when taken in reasonable amounts. The fresh plant is a different matter. Extended skin contact with newly harvested Pilewort can lead to stubborn blisters and burns. And when the fresh herb is taken internally, it can severely irritate the stomach, intestines, and urinary tract and cause abdominal pain and diarrhea.

Possible Drug Interactions
No interactions have been reported.

Special Information If You Are Pregnant or Breastfeeding
No harmful effects are known.

How to Prepare
Pilewort is used in ground and extract forms.

Typical Dosage

Add Pilewort extract to bathwater to treat wounds and scratches. Follow the manufacturer's directions whenever available.

Overdosage

Freshly picked Pilewort contains compounds that can cause asphyxiation when taken in large amounts. However, these compounds are destroyed when the herb is dried, making the ground herb and its extracts relatively safe even in larger doses.

Pimpinella

Latin name: Pimpinella major
Other names: Burnet Saxifrage,
*   Lesser Burnet, Pimpernell*

A Remedy For
- Bronchitis
- Cough

Only the root of this plant possesses established effectiveness—and only for relief of upper respiratory irritation. In folk medicine, it is also used for a variety of urinary problems and, in bathwater, as a treatment for poorly healing wounds. The above-ground part of the plant, known as Burnet Saxifrage, has been used as a digestive stimulant, a remedy for lung ailments, and—applied externally—for varicose veins, but its effectiveness remains unproven.

What It Is; Why It Works

Fresh Pimpinella root is fairly obnoxious, with rancid odor and a taste that is tangy at first, then burning hot. Only the dried, crushed root is used medicinally. It has a decongestant effect, reducing production of bronchial secretions.

The plant is found in almost all of Europe and has been introduced to North America. It reaches a height of 2 to 3 feet and produces white flowers.

Avoid If . . .

No known medical conditions preclude the use of Pimpinella.

Special Cautions

The root can make light-skinned people more sensitive to sunlight.

Possible Drug Interactions

No drug interactions have been reported.

Special Information If You Are Pregnant or Breastfeeding

No harmful effects are known.

How to Prepare

Pimpinella root is available in crushed form for teas and as an alcohol solution (tincture).

Typical Dosage

The usual daily dosage of the root is:

Crushed Pimpinella: 6 to 12 grams
    (about 1 to 2 teaspoonfuls)
Pimpinella tincture: 6 to 15 grams

Overdosage

No information on overdosage is available.

Pine Oil

Latin name: Pinus species
Other names: Dwarf Pine,
Scotch Pine, Stockholm Tar,
Swiss Mountain Pine

A Remedy For
- Bronchitis
- Colds
- Cough
- Fever
- Nerve pain
- Rheumatism
- Sore throat
- Tendency to infection

In homeopathy, Pine Oil is considered a treatment for bronchial conditions and rheumatism.

What It Is; Why It Works
Pine Oil is extracted from several species of pine in Europe and the Near East, particularly *Pinus sylvestris*. Young Pine shoots are also used occasionally, chopped up and steeped as a tea. Oil made from turpentine from *Pinus* species can be used as a skin rub or dropped into hot water to create vapors for inhalation.

Pine Oil tends to reduce bronchial secretions and stimulate local circulation. It is mildly antiseptic.

Avoid If . . .
Do not use Pine Oil if you have bronchial asthma, whooping cough, or severe inflammation of the breathing passages. Do not use it as a bath additive if you have a large skin injury, acute skin disease, an infectious disease, heart problems, or abnormally tense muscles.

Special Cautions
Pine Oil can irritate the skin and mucous membranes, and has been known to cause breathing problems. Excessive use on large areas of the body can lead to poisoning, with damage to the kidneys or brain. Kidney damage is also a possibility when the oil is taken internally.

Possible Drug Interactions
No interactions have been reported.

Special Information If You Are Pregnant or Breastfeeding
No harmful effects are known.

How to Prepare
Pine Oil is extracted by steam distillation from fresh pine needles, branch tips, and shoots. It is used in ointments and bath salts. Oil extracted from turpentine is also available. Make sure you use only the refined medicinal oil—not raw turpentine.

Typical Dosage
PINE OIL

The oral dosage is 5 grams (about 1 teaspoonful) daily. For inhalation, add several drops to hot water and inhale the vapor. As a bath additive, use 0.025 gram per liter of water. For external use, rub several drops onto the affected area.

PINE SHOOTS

The oral dose is 9 grams daily in tea, syrup, or an alcohol solution. As a bath additive, use about half a cup of alcoholic extract (tincture).

MEDICINAL TURPENTINE OIL

For inhalation, add several drops to hot water and inhale the vapor. For external use, rub several drops onto the affected area.

Store in tightly sealed containers away from light.

Overdosage

A dose of 50 grams (less than a quarter of a cup) can be fatal in adults. Symptoms of overdose include nausea, vomiting, reddening of the face, salivation, sore throat, thirst, diarrhea, intestinal spasms, shortness of breath, dizziness, staggering, twitching, urination difficulties, and rash.

Excessive skin contact or inhalation can result in overdose, and deaths have been reported, particularly among children. If you suspect an overdose, seek medical attention immediately.

Poplar

Latin name: Populus species
Other names: European Aspen,
  Quaking Aspen

A Remedy For
• Hemorrhoids
• Wounds and burns

Although the bark, leaves, and buds of Poplar all contain the active ingredient salicylic acid, only the buds are considered unquestionably effective. They are used for frostbite and sunburn, in addition to wounds and burns.

The bark and leaves are used to treat pain, prostate problems, bladder complaints, and rheumatism. In homeopathic medicine, Poplar is prescribed for colds and disorders of the urinary system.

What It Is; Why It Works

The salicylic acid in Poplar is closely related to the familiar painkiller aspirin, and can be found in such over-the-counter skin medications as Stri-Dex, DuoFilm, and Wart-Off. Salicylic acid has anti-inflammatory and antibacterial properties. It relieves pain and eases spasms.

Poplar also contains zinc, which some researchers feel may account for its beneficial effects on the urinary system.

Avoid If . . .

Do not use Poplar if you are allergic to aspirin or the herbal product Balsam of Peru.

Special Cautions

External Poplar preparations can cause allergic skin reactions.

Possible Drug Interactions

There are no known drug interactions associated with the use of Poplar.

Special Information If You Are Pregnant or Breastfeeding

No information is available.

How to Prepare

Poplar leaves are taken internally. The buds are found primarily in preparations for external use.

Typical Dosage

Leaves: 10 grams (2 teaspoonfuls) daily
Buds: 5 grams (1 teaspoonful) daily

Strengths of commercial preparations may vary. Follow the manufacturer's labeling whenever available.

Overdosage

No information is available.

Potentilla

Latin name: Potentilla anserina
Other names: Cinquefoil, Crampweed, Goose Tansy, Goosegrass, Moor Grass, Silverweed, Trailing Tansy, Wild Agrimony

A Remedy For

- Diarrhea
- Premenstrual syndrome (PMS)
- Sore throat

In the past, Potentilla was considered a treatment for lockjaw, jaundice (liver disease), and menstrual cramps, and was used to remove freckles and prevent scarring from smallpox. Today, it is included in various tea mixtures for treating sexual disorders, nervous agitation, and nausea. Its effectiveness for such uses remains unproven.

What It Is; Why It Works

Potentilla's name is derived from the Latin word "potens," meaning powerful. Found in temperate and colder regions of the northern hemisphere, Potentilla has an almond-like fragrance and a dry taste. It has a tightening, astringent effect.

Avoid If . . .

There are no known medical conditions that preclude the use of Potentilla.

Special Cautions

Use Potentilla cautiously if you have stomach problems; it could make them worse.

Possible Drug Interactions

No interactions have been recorded.

Special Information If You Are Pregnant or Breastfeeding

No harmful effects are known.

How to Prepare

Finely cut Potentilla can be made into a tea by steeping 2 grams (about 3 teaspoonfuls) in boiling water for 10 minutes, then straining.

Typical Dosage

Potentilla is taken orally. The usual daily dosage is 4 to 6 grams (about 6 to 9 teaspoonfuls) of the herb.

Potentilla is available in crushed, powdered, and liquid herbal preparations. Strengths of commercial products may vary. Follow the manufacturer's labeling whenever available.

Overdosage

No information on overdosage is available.

Primrose

Latin name: Primula elatior
Other names: Arthritica, Butter
Rose, Cowslip, Crewel, Fairy
Caps, Key Flower, Mayflower,
Palsywort

A Remedy For

• Bronchitis
• Cough

Both the flower and root of Primrose are used medicinally, and have a variety of unproven uses in folk medicine. The flower serves as a remedy for headache, nerve pain, and tremors, and is used as a "heart tonic" for sensations of dizziness and cardiac insufficiency. Primrose root is taken for whooping cough, asthma, gout, and nerve pain. In homeopathic medicine, Primrose is prescribed for skin conditions.

What It Is; Why It Works

Referred to as "Cowslip," Primrose has earned a place in the work of many English writers, from Shakespeare's *A Midsummer Night's Dream*, to Alexander Pope ("I'll drown all high thoughts in the Lethe of Cowslip Wine"). Through the ages, it has been used to whiten and smooth the skin, and to relieve such ailments as headaches and insomnia.

The only therapeutic effects that researchers have been able to

document for Primrose are its decongestant action and its ability to thin and loosen phlegm, making it easier to expel from the lungs. The plant is native to central Europe.

Avoid If . . .

Do not take Primrose if it causes an allergic reaction.

Special Cautions

At customary dosage levels, Primrose poses little danger. However, there is a possibility of developing a sensitivity to the plant, particularly the leaves and flowers.

Possible Drug Interactions

No interactions have been reported.

Special Information If You Are Pregnant or Breastfeeding

No harmful effects are known.

How to Prepare

Primrose can be found in dried, crushed form, and in alcohol solutions (tinctures).

To make a tea from Primrose flower, pour boiling water over 2 to 4 grams (about 1 1/2 to 3 teaspoonfuls) of the crushed drug. Steep for 10 minutes, then strain. The tea may be sweetened with honey and taken repeatedly during the day.

To prepare a tea from Primrose root, place 0.2 to 0.5 gram of finely cut drug in cold water. Bring the mixture to a simmer, steep for 5 minutes, then strain. Sweeten with honey. Take every 2 to 3 hours during the day.

Typical Dosage

Primrose is taken orally. The usual daily dosage is:

Crushed Primrose flower: 2 to 4 grams (about 1½ to 3 teaspoonfuls)

Primrose flower tincture: 1.5 to 3 grams (about one-quarter to one-half teaspoonful)

Primrose root: 0.5 to 1.5 grams

Primrose root tincture: Up to 7.5 grams (about 1½ teaspoonfuls)

Because the potency of commercial preparations may vary, follow the manufacturer's directions whenever available.

Overdosage

An overdose of Primrose can lead to stomach problems, nausea, and diarrhea.

Psyllium

Latin name: Plantago isphagula
Other names: Indian Plantago, Sand Plantain, Spogel

A Remedy For
• Constipation
• Diarrhea
• High cholesterol

Psyllium is also used for irritable bowel syndrome (a stress-related disorder with alternating bouts of diarrhea and constipation). Because it will produce easy bowel movements with a loose stool, Psyllium is used by patients with anal fissures (cracks in the skin near the anus) and hemorrhoids, and is often recommended following anal or rectal surgery, during pregnancy, and as a secondary treatment in certain types of diarrhea.

What It Is; Why It Works

The medicinal part of the Psyllium plant is the ripe seed, the husk of which is a plentiful source of natural fiber. Psyllium fiber is the active ingredient in such common over-the-counter laxatives as Metamucil and Perdiem.

For diarrhea, Psyllium soaks up many times its weight in water, thereby making the stool firmer and slower to pass. For constipation, Psyllium speeds passage by adding more water, softening the hard stool, and producing more bulk. Soluble fibers such as Psyllium help lower harmful cholesterol levels in the blood. Fiber can also moderate the surge in blood sugar that follows a meal.

Avoid If . . .

Do not use Psyllium if you have a bowel obstruction or a disease that causes narrowing of any part of the digestive tract. Diabetics should avoid Psyllium if they are having problems keeping blood sugar levels under control.

Special Cautions

Taken without adequate fluid, Psyllium may swell up and block the esophagus or intestine, particularly in older adults. Take at least 5 ounces of fluid with each teaspoon of Psyllium.

Although rare, allergic reactions do occasionally occur. They include runny nose, conjunctivitis (pinkeye), asthma, and hives.

Possible Drug Interactions

If you are taking other medications, wait at least one-half to 1 hour before taking Psyllium. Otherwise, it will delay absorption of the other medications into the bloodstream.

If you must take insulin for diabetes, you may need to reduce the dosage while taking Psyllium.

Special Information If You Are Pregnant or Breastfeeding

No harmful effects are known.

How to Prepare

Soak 1 to 3 teaspoons of Psyllium in a little water and take in the morning and evenings with 1 to 2 glasses of water.

Typical Dosage

Psyllium is taken orally. Doses range from 1 teaspoonful to 1 tablespoonful, 2 or 3 times daily, depending on the preparation. Follow the manufacturer's labeling whenever available. Be sure to take 1 to 2 glasses of liquid with each dose.

Overdosage

No information on overdosage is available.

Pumpkin Seed

Latin name: Cucurbita pepo

A Remedy For

• Prostate enlargement

Pumpkin Seed relieves the urinary difficulties that develop when an enlarged prostate or prostate cancer obstructs the exit from the bladder. Although Pumpkin Seed promotes normal urination, it does not correct the underlying problem, so it's important to pursue other treatments for the condition.

Pumpkin Seed has been used for a variety of problems for which its effectiveness is unconfirmed, including kidney inflammation, intestinal parasites—especially tapeworm—and wounds. In Asian medicine it is used to treat worms, diabetes, and water retention. Homeopathic practitioners prescribe it for nausea and seasickness.

What It Is; Why It Works

Researchers do not know *why* Pumpkin Seed eases urinary problems, but clinical studies leave no doubt that it does. The seeds also exhibit antioxidant activity and anti-inflammatory properties.

Pumpkin originated in America, but is now grown worldwide. It shares its family tree with melons and cucumbers. Seeds of this group used to be ground into a paste and prescribed for fevers, bowel disorders, and urinary complaints.

Avoid If . . .

No known medical conditions preclude the use of Pumpkin Seed.

Special Cautions

At customary dosage levels, Pumpkin Seed poses no risks.

Possible Drug Interactions

No interactions have been reported.

Special Information If You Are Pregnant or Breastfeeding

No harmful effects are known.

How to Prepare

Coarsely ground Pumpkin Seed is the usual preparation. Whole seeds may also be used.

Typical Dosage

Pumpkin Seed is taken orally. The usual daily dosage is 1 to 2 heaping teaspoonfuls of ground Pumpkin Seed with liquid in the morning and evening. Your total daily intake should average 10 grams.

Store away from light and moisture.

Overdosage

No information is available.

Pygeum

Latin name: Pygeum africanum

A Remedy For

• Prostate enlargement

What It Is; Why It Works

Pygeum is an evergreen tree found in the mountains of central and southern Africa. Its bark, once used as a tea for relief of urinary disorders, has been found to contain not one, but three types of compounds that relieve the symptoms of prostate enlargement (benign prostatic hyperplasia).

Beta-sitosterol, the most important of the three, interferes with the formation of prostaglandins that cause inflammation and swelling in the prostate. *Pentacyclic terpenes* also reduce swelling. And *ferulic esters* combat enlargement by reducing levels of prolactin, a hormone which promotes uptake of growth-promoting testosterone in the prostate.

Avoid If . . .

No known medical conditions preclude the use of Pygeum.

Special Cautions

Side effects from Pygeum extract are rare, but a few men experience mild stomach irritation.

Improvement is gradual; allow 6 to 9 months for the herb to work. Remember, too, that the symptoms of enlargement can also be a sign of cancer. Check with your doctor to make sure that the problem is benign.

Possible Drug Interactions

No interactions have been reported.

Special Information If You Are Pregnant or Breastfeeding
Not for use by women.

How to Prepare
Look for a standardized extract containing 13% beta-sitosterol.

Typical Dosage
Extract: 50 to 100 milligrams 2 times per day

Overdosage
No information on overdosage is available.

Radish

Latin name: Raphanus sativus

A Remedy For
• Appetite loss
• Bronchitis
• Colds
• Cough
• Fever
• Sore throat
• Tendency to infection

The juice of this common vegetable is used primarily for digestive disorders and upper respiratory inflammation. In Asian medicine, it's also taken for headache, liver disease, and pain, but its effectiveness for these problems has not been scientifically confirmed.

What It Is; Why It Works
The thick, tangy root is the medicinal part of the plant. It promotes digestive secretions, stimulates the bowels, and helps kill germs.

Unknown in the wild, the Radish was probably domesticated in the Far East. It was already under cultivation when the pharaohs reigned in Egypt.

Avoid If . . .
Do not take large doses of Radish if you have gallstones; it could cause painful spasms in the biliary tract.

Special Cautions
High doses of radish can irritate the digestive tract.

Possible Drug Interactions
No drug interactions have been reported.

Special Information If You Are Pregnant or Breastfeeding
No harmful effects are known.

How to Prepare
Radish can be grated or pressed to produce juice. For whooping cough, grated radish can be combined with honey. Grate one radish, mix with honey, and allow the mixture to stand for 10 hours.

Typical Dosage
Radish is taken orally.

Radish juice: One-half tablespoonful of pressed juice several times a day, up to a maximum of 4 to 6 tablespoonfuls daily.
Radish/honey mixture: For whooping cough, take spoonfuls throughout the day.

Overdosage
No information on overdosage is available.

Raspberry

Latin name: Rubus idaeus

A Remedy For

Raspberry is sometimes recommended for indigestion, although there is little evidence of its effectiveness. It has also been used as a treatment for problems with the stomach, lungs, heart, mouth, and throat—again without scientific validation.

What It Is; Why It Works

Raspberry leaf tea was a traditional folk remedy for many kinds of ailments, including mouth sores, stomachache, and complications of pregnancy. The main active ingredients are tannins and vitamin C.

Avoid If . . .

No known medical conditions preclude the use of Raspberry.

Special Cautions

When taken at customary dosage levels, Raspberry poses no risks.

Possible Drug Interactions

No interactions have been reported.

Special Information If You Are Pregnant or Breastfeeding

No harmful effects are known.

How to Prepare

To make Raspberry leaf tea, pour boiling water over 1.5 grams (about 2 teaspoonfuls) of finely cut leaves, steep 5 minutes, then strain.

Raspberry is found in various laxative and "blood purifying" teas, and in fruit tea mixtures. It's also an ingredient of dietary drinks.

Typical Dosage

There are no guidelines on record.

Overdosage

No information on overdosage is available.

Rauwolfia

Latin name: Rauwolfia serpentina

A Remedy For

- Insomnia
- Nervousness

Rauwolfia is also used as a remedy for anxiety, abnormal muscle tension, and twitching. In folk medicine, it has been used for fever, diarrhea, general weakness, constipation, intestinal diseases, liver problems, rheumatism, water retention, and mental disorders. However, its effectiveness for such conditions remains unverified.

Asian medicine uses it for giddiness, high blood pressure, slow and painful urination, and wounds. In India, extracts of the plant are used as antidotes for poisonous snakebites.

What It Is; Why It Works

Reserpine, an extract of Rauwolfia, combats high blood pressure, and is found in such prescription blood pressure medications as Diupres and Hydropres. Reserpine also combats irregular heartbeat and has a sedative effect.

Rauwolfia, a small shrub sporting white to pink flowers, is native to India, Indochina, Borneo, Sri Lanka, and Sumatra. Its medicinal properties lie in the dried root. The fresh root has a very bitter and unpleasant taste.

Avoid If . . .

Rauwolfia can trigger severe depression. Do not take it when depressed.

The drug also tends to stimulate the lining of the digestive tract, so you should avoid it if you have an ulcer or ulcerative colitis.

Avoid Rauwolfia, too, if you are pregnant or nursing, or are taking a drug classified as a monoamine oxidase inhibitor, such as the antidepressants Nardil and Parnate.

Special Cautions

Side effects can include nasal congestion, depression, fatigue, impotence, and slowed reaction time. Use caution when handling machinery or driving.

Possible Drug Interactions

Never combine Rauwolfia with a monoamine oxidase (MAO) inhibitor such as Nardil or Parnate.

Rauwolfia enhances the sedative effect of alcohol and barbiturates; avoid the combination.

Taken with digitalis-based drugs such as Lanoxin, or quinidine products such as Quinaglute and Quinidex, Rauwolfia can slow the heart and cause irregular beats.

The drug is also likely to interact with levodopa (Sinemet), causing twitching and other involuntary movements. Combining it with many common flu remedies and appetite suppressants can lead to a sharp rise in blood pressure.

Special Information If You Are Pregnant or Breastfeeding

Rauwolfia may cause birth defects when taken during pregnancy; and it appears in breast milk. Avoid this drug while pregnant or breastfeeding.

How to Prepare

Rauwolfia is available in ground form and as a powder for internal use.

Typical Dosage

The usual daily dose of Rauwolfia is 600 milligrams. (Recommended dosage of the active ingredient reserpine is far smaller; 0.25 milligram is the daily maximum.)

Overdosage

Symptoms of overdosage include mental depression, heavy sedation, and a severe drop in blood pressure. If you suspect an overdose, seek medical attention immediately.

Red Clover

Latin name: Trifolium pratense
Other names: Purple Clover, Trefoil, Wild Clover

A Remedy For

- Bronchitis
- Cough
- Eczema, boils, acne

Taken internally, Red Clover is used for respiratory problems, particularly whooping cough. Externally, it's considered a treatment for chronic skin conditions such as eczema and psoriasis.

What It Is; Why It Works

Red Clover contains isoflavone compounds that theoretically could help prevent certain types of cancer, including breast and prostate cancer. However, an actual protective action in humans remains to bedemonstrated.

In the meantime, Red Clover is valued for its ability to loosen phlegm and calm bronchial spasms. A small perennial herb with fleshy red or white flowers, it is native to Europe, central Asia, and northern Africa, and is naturalized in many other parts of the world. For medicinal purposes, only the flowers are used.

Avoid If . . .

No known medical conditions preclude the use of dried, unfermented Red Clover. However, fermented preparations should be strictly avoided.

Special Cautions

At customary dosage levels, Red Clover appears to present no problems.

Possible Drug Interactions

No interactions have been reported.

Special Information If You Are Pregnant or Breastfeeding

No harmful effects are known.

How to Prepare

Red Clover is available as a dried herb, and in tablets, capsules, and alcohol solutions (tinctures).

To make a tea, pour 1 cup of boiling water over 2 to 3 teaspoonfuls of dried Red Clover flowers, cover, and steep 10 to 15 minutes.

Typical Dosage

Tea: 3 cups per day

Capsules and tablets: 2 to 4 grams 3 times per day

Tincture: 2 to 4 milliliters 3 times per day

Overdosage

No information on overdosage is available.

Red Sandalwood

Latin name: Pterocarpus santalinus

Other names: Rubywood, Sappan

A Remedy For

Red Sandalwood is sometimes recommended for indigestion, although there is no evidence of its effectiveness. It is also used—again without scientific validation—to flush excess water from the body, dry and tighten the skin, purify the blood, and relieve coughs. In Asian medicine, it's prescribed for headache, toothache, skin diseases, and vomiting, and in India is sometimes taken for diabetes.

What It Is; Why It Works
A product of southern India, Sri Lanka, and the Philippines, Red Sandalwood is valued mainly as a source of red dye. At one time, it was used to dye wool. Today, it's a brightening agent in tea mixtures and a coloring agent in toothpaste. Little is known about its effects in the body.

Avoid If . . .
No known medical conditions preclude the use of Red Sandalwood.

Special Cautions
There are no hazards on record.

Possible Drug Interactions
No interactions have been reported.

Special Information If You Are Pregnant or Breastfeeding
No harmful effects are known.

How to Prepare
Found mainly in herbal tea mixtures.

Typical Dosage
No dosage guidelines are available.

Overdosage
No information on overdosage is available.

Reishi

Latin name: Ganoderma lucidum
Other names: Ling Chih, Ling Zhi

A Remedy For
Reishi has been used in traditional Chinese medicine for more than 4,000 years to treat asthma, cough, fatigue, insomnia, and weakness. Today it's regarded as a remedy for high blood pressure and high triglycerides, and is used as a supportive treatment during cancer chemotherapy. Unconfirmed studies suggest that it may also be effective against altitude sickness and chronic hepatitis B.

What It Is; Why It Works
A wild mushroom that favors decaying logs in coastal China, Reishi is now cultivated throughout China, Japan, Korea, and North America. Although it appears in 6 different colors, the red variety is the one most commonly used.

The mushroom's active ingredients, called ganoderic acids, appear to combat high blood pressure and reduce LDL ("bad") cholesterol and triglyceride levels. They may also discourage blood platelets from clumping together, thus reducing the risk of dangerous clots.

Avoid If . . .
Because Reishi may itself delay clotting, you should not use it while taking other anticoagulant medications such as Coumadin.

Special Cautions

Continuous use of Reishi for more than 3 to 6 months can lead to dizziness, dry mouth, nosebleeds, and upset stomach.

Possible Drug Interactions

Combining Reishi with blood-thinning drugs such as Coumadin can further prolong bleeding time.

Special Information If You Are Pregnant or Breastfeeding

Check with your doctor before taking Reishi while pregnant or nursing.

How to Prepare

Reishi can be taken in dried mushroom form, or as a powder, alcohol solution (tincture), or tea.

Typical Dosage

Dried mushroom: 1.5 to 9 grams per day
Powder: 1 to 1.5 grams per day
Tincture: 1 milliliter per day

Strengths of commercial preparations may vary. Follow the manufacturer's labeling whenever available.

Overdosage

No information is available.

Restharrow

Latin name: Ononis spinosa
Other names: Cammock, Ground Furze, Stayplough, Stinking Tommy, Wild Licorice

A Remedy For

• Kidney and bladder stones
• Urinary tract infections

Restharrow is also taken for rheumatism and gout, but its effectiveness for these problems lacks verification.

What It Is; Why It Works

Restharrow is an annoying weed with a tendency to become tangled in farmers' harrows. Typically reaching a height of 1 to 2 feet, it puts out tenacious roots, bears prickly thorns, and emits a foul odor. Its only value lies in the medicinal properties of the root, which acts as a diuretic, flushing water through the kidneys and urinary tract.

Avoid If . . .

Do not flush out the urinary system with Restharrow or any other medication if you are retaining water due to poor heart or kidney function.

Special Cautions

At customary dosage levels, Restharrow poses no risks. Be sure, however, to replace lost fluids by drinking at least 2 quarts of liquid per day.

Possible Drug Interactions

No drug interactions have been reported.

Special Information If You Are Pregnant or Breastfeeding

No harmful effects are known.

How to Prepare

To make a tea, pour boiling water over 2 to 2.5 grams (about three-quarters of a teaspoonful) of finely cut or coarsely powdered

Restharrow, steep 20 to 30 minutes, and strain.

Typical Dosage
Restharrow is taken internally. The usual daily dosage is 6 to 12 grams (2 to 4 teaspoonfuls).

Overdosage
No information on overdosage is available.

Rhatany

Latin name: Krameria triandra
Other names: Krameria Root,
  Mapato

A Remedy For
• Sore throat

Applied externally, Rhatany is also used for frostbite and leg ulcers. It is sometimes taken internally for diarrhea. In homeopathic medicine, it's recommended for hemorrhoids and rectal pain. Its effectiveness for such problems has not, however, been confirmed.

What It Is; Why It Works
Rhatany is a small shrub found mostly in the mountains of Peru. Its name refers, in native Peruvian, to the creeping nature of the plant. Only the root is medicinal.

Rhatany is usually used as a gargle or mouthwash to relieve mild inflammation of the mouth, throat, and gums. It has an astringent effect, drying and tightening the tissues.

Avoid If . . .
No known medical conditions preclude the use of Rhatany.

Special Cautions
When taken internally, Rhatany can cause digestive problems. In rare cases, it has triggered allergic reactions in the mucous membranes.

Possible Drug Interactions
No drug interactions have been reported.

Special Information If You Are Pregnant or Breastfeeding
No harmful effects are known.

How to Prepare
Rhatany is available in crushed and powdered forms, and as an alcohol solution (tincture).

To make a mouthwash, mix 1.5 to 2.0 grams (about one-half teaspoonful) of powdered Rhatany with boiling water, steep for 10 to 15 minutes, then strain.

Alternatively, you can mix 1 gram of crushed Rhatany with 1 cup of water, or 5 to 10 drops of Rhatany tincture with 1 glass of water.

Typical Dosage
Use the mouthwash 2 to 3 times daily. You can also apply Rhatany tincture directly to the sore area up to 3 times daily.

Overdosage
No information on overdosage is available.

Rhubarb

Latin name: Rheum palmatum
Other names: China Rhubarb,
  Indian Rhubarb, Russian
  Rhubarb, Turkey Rhubarb

A Remedy For
• Constipation

Because it will produce easy bowel movements with a soft or loose stool, Rhubarb is used by people with anal fissures (cracks in the skin near the anus) or hemorrhoids, and is recommended following anal or rectal surgery. It can also be used to cleanse the intestines before undergoing a bowel examination or similar diagnostic tests.

What It Is; Why It Works
Not to be confused with ordinary table rhubarb, which is relatively inactive, the *Rheum palmatum* variety was discovered in the 18th century by a Dutch physician. Its medicinal value lies in the dried, underground parts of the plant, including the smaller roots and root bark.

A powerful laxative, Rhubarb stimulates secretion of fluid into the bowel, causes strong muscular contractions of the bowel wall, and hastens bowel movements.

Avoid If . . .
Do not use Rhubarb if you have an intestinal obstruction, appendicitis, abdominal pain, or an inflammatory intestinal condition such as colitis or Crohn's disease. Not for children under 12.

Special Cautions
Rhubarb may cause cramping and nausea. Long-term use can alter the body's normal balance of fluids and minerals—including those responsible for muscle contractions—ultimately triggering irregular heart rhythms. If used too often or for too long, Rhubarb may cause kidney problems and fluid retention, promote bone deterioration, and produce a laxative dependence that makes it impossible to have a bowel movement without medications such as Rhubarb. It's wise to limit use of any stimulating laxative to a period of no more than 2 weeks.

Possible Drug Interactions
Laxatives such as Rhubarb can deplete the body's potassium. This, in turn, can boost the action of certain heart medications, including digitalis and digoxin (Lanoxin).

Special Information If You Are Pregnant or Breastfeeding
Consult your doctor before using this medication.

How to Prepare
Rhubarb may be made into a laxative tea by steeping 1 to 2 grams (approximately one-quarter to one-half teaspoonful) of coarse powdered drug in a little boiling water for 5 minutes, then straining the preparation. If desired, flavor the tea with cinnamon, ginger, or peppermint oil.

Typical Dosage
Rhubarb is taken orally. The usual laxative dose is 1 to 2

grams (approximately one-quarter to one-half teaspoonful). Do not take a total of more than 1 teaspoonful per day.

Rhubarb is available as crushed, powdered, or dry extracts for teas, and as a liquid extract.

Strengths of commercial preparations may vary. Follow the manufacturer's labeling whenever available.

Overdosage

No information on overdosage is available.

Roman Chamomile

Latin name: Chamaemelum nobile
Other names: Ground Apple, Whig Plant

A Remedy For

An official review found no evidence that Roman Chamomile has any medicinal value. Specific problems for which it was rated ineffective include the common cold, upset stomach, sore throat, eczema, boils, acne, wounds, and burns.

Other uses—all unsubstantiated—include treatment of menstrual complaints, nervousness, and general weakness, and external application for sore throat, runny nose, toothache, earache, headache, and influenza.

What It Is; Why It Works

In contrast to true chamomile, the Roman variety has received little investigation. Researchers have found that its essential oil fights

bacterial and fungal infections. However, the herb also appears to cause congestion in the circulatory system.

Of the two chamomiles, the Roman is preferred in England and France, where it's a popular, if unproven, remedy for feelings of fullness, bloating, mild stomach and intestinal spasms, and sluggish bowels.

Roman Chamomile is a small plant—generally no more than a foot in height—grown throughout Europe, North America, and Argentina. In Spain, where it's called "Manzanilla," it lends its name to Manzanilla sherry, a dry wine in which it's used as a flavoring agent. The dried flowers are used medicinally.

Avoid If . . .

No known medical conditions preclude the use of Roman Chamomile.

Special Cautions

At customary dosage levels, Roman Chamomile poses no risks. There is little danger of developing a sensitivity to it.

Possible Drug Interactions

No interactions have been reported.

Special Information If You Are Pregnant or Breastfeeding

No harmful effects are known.

How to Prepare

To make tea, use 3 grams (about one-half teaspoonful) of Roman

Chamomile for each 100 milliliters (half cup) of water.

As a bath additive, use 50 grams (3 heaping tablespoonfuls) for each 2½ gallons of water.

Roman Chamomile is also supplied as a powder and in various liquid forms.

Typical Dosage

Crushed herb: 1.5 grams at main meals

Tea: 50 to 200 milliliters (about 2 to 7 ounces) per day

Store in a well-sealed glass or metal container protected from moisture.

Overdosage

No information on overdosage is available.

Rose Flower

Latin name: Rosa centifolia
Other names: Cabbage Rose, Damask Rose, French Rose

A Remedy For
• Sore throat

Although proven effective only for oral inflammations, in Asian medicine, Rose Flower is also used to treat cough, wounds, and excessive sweating.

What It Is; Why It Works

There are 10,000 known variations of the Rose, which is cultivated around the world. The medicinal value of Rose water has been recognized since the time of the 10th-century Arab physician Avicenna. The flower has astringent properties, drying and tightening the tissues.

Avoid If . . .

No known medical conditions preclude the use of Rose Flower.

Special Cautions

At customary dosage levels, Rose Flower presents no risks.

Possible Drug Interactions

There are no known drug interactions with Rose Flower.

Special Information If You Are Pregnant or Breastfeeding

There is no information available.

How to Prepare

The finely chopped flower is used for teas and mouth-rinse preparations.

Typical Dosage

Use 1 to 2 grams of crushed Rose Flower per 200 milliliters (about three-quarters cup) of water.

Strengths of commercial preparations may vary. Follow the manufacturer's labeling whenever available.

Overdosage

There is no information available.

Rose Hip

Latin name: Rosa canina
Other names: Briar Rose, Dog Rose, Eglantine Gall, Sweet Briar, Wild Brier, Witches' Brier

A Remedy For

This well-known source of vitamin C is often recommended for boosting resistance and fighting infections, although scientific proof of its effectiveness is still considered lacking.

In addition, Rose Hip *seed* is recommended for urinary tract infections, although here, too, effectiveness awaits further confirmation. Other unverified uses of the seed include treatment of rheumatism, gout, kidney disease, water retention, and sciatica (nerve pain in the lower back and thigh).

What It Is; Why It Works

Named "Dog Rose" for its purported (and discredited) effect against rabies, this prickly climber grows up to 10 feet in length, producing large white or pink flowers. The plant's seed receptacle contains its vitamin C, while the seeds themselves harbor compounds that flush excess water from the body and exert a laxative effect.

According to the Roman historian Pliny, the healing powers of this plant came to the first herbalists in a dream.

Avoid If . . .

No known medical conditions preclude the use of Rose Hip.

Special Cautions

At customary dosage levels, Rose Hip poses no problems.

Possible Drug Interactions

No interactions have been reported.

Special Information If You Are Pregnant or Breastfeeding

No harmful effects are known.

How to Prepare

Rose Hip is available in numerous vitamin preparations.

Rose Hip *seed* comes in powdered form, and is found in various diuretic products. To make a tea from the seed, pour boiling water over 1 to 2 grams (about one-half teaspoonful) of powdered Rose Hip seed, steep for 10 to 15 minutes, and strain.

Typical Dosage

Tea from the seed may be taken repeatedly throughout the day. Rose Hip itself is usually taken as a vitamin supplement. Follow the manufacturer's directions whenever available.

Overdosage

No information on overdosage is available.

Rosemary

Latin name: Rosmarinus officinalis
Other names: Compass-weed, Polar Plant

A Remedy For

- Appetite loss
- Blood pressure problems
- Liver and gallbladder problems
- Rheumatism

In folk medicine, Rosemary was used to make salves for poorly healing wounds and eczema. In homeopathic medicine, the herb is used for female sexual disorders. Its effectiveness for these purposes remains unproven.

What It Is; Why It Works

It is the essential oil of Rosemary that provides medicinal benefit. Animal tests have demonstrated its ability to control spasms in the gallbladder and upper intestine, improve the flow of blood to the heart, and strengthen the action of the heart muscle. Oil of Rosemary improves circulation when applied externally.

Among the Greeks, Rosemary had a reputation for improving memory, which led to its adoption as a sign of lovers' fidelity and its being worn at wedding ceremonies. In Italy and Spain, it was believed to ward off evil.

Avoid If . . .

No known medical conditions preclude use of this herb.

Special Cautions

Very large quantities of Rosemary leaves or oil can cause severe reactions (see "Overdosage" below). Skin reactions from contact with the herb have been observed on occasion.

Possible Drug Interactions

No interactions have been reported.

Special Information If You Are Pregnant or Breastfeeding

Do not use Rosemary if you are pregnant. It has a potentially abortive effect.

How to Prepare

Rosemary is available in ground and powdered forms, and as an extract for infusions. A medicinal wine can be prepared by combining 20 grams (about 4 teaspoonfuls) with 1 liter of wine; let stand for 5 days, shaking occasionally.

Typical Dosage

The usual daily oral dosage is 4 to 6 grams (about 1 teaspoonful).

For a bath additive, combine 50 grams (about 3 tablespoonfuls) with 1 liter of hot water.

Preparations of 6 to 10% essential oil in a semi-solid or liquid base can be applied externally.

Overdosage

Although no cases of overdose are on record, an extremely large amount (taken, for instance, to cause an abortion) could theoretically cause coma, spasm, vomiting, inflammation of the digestive tract, uterine bleeding, kidney irritation, swelling in the lungs, and possibly death. If you suspect an overdose, seek medical attention immediately.

Rue

Latin name: Ruta graveolens
Other name: Herb-of-Grace

A Remedy For

Authorities advise against Rue, which can have severe and even fatal effects when taken in excess. It is used primarily as a remedy for menstrual disorders such as

PMS, and as a means of inducing abortion.

Folk medicine employs Rue for a variety of additional ailments, including cramps, diarrhea, earache, fever, indigestion, intestinal worms, hepatitis, sore throat, skin inflammation, and toothache. It is also used as a contraceptive; and homeopathic practitioners prescribe it for strains and sprains.

What It Is; Why It Works

Although poisonous itself in large quantities, Rue was considered an *antidote* to poison from the era of the ancient Greeks until the dawn of modern times. It was also considered a defense against magic and witchcraft.

A flowering shrub 1 to 2½ feet in height, Rue is common throughout southern Europe. Its tangy aroma and hot taste make it useful as a household seasoning. For medicinal purposes, the entire above-ground part of the plant is dried and chopped.

Avoid If . . .

No known medical conditions preclude the use of Rue.

Special Cautions

Oral intake—or even contact with the skin—can cause sensitivity to light.

Possible Drug Interactions

No drug interactions are known.

Special Information If You Are Pregnant or Breastfeeding

Rue can be used to induce abortion. Avoid it during pregnancy.

How to Prepare

To prepare a tea, use approximately 3 grams (1 heaping teaspoonful) of Rue per 8 ounces (1 cup) of water.

For toothache, fresh Rue leaf may be packed into the cavity. For earache, juice from the leaf may be used as an eardrop.

Typical Dosage

Crushed Rue: The usual dose is 0.5 gram. Take no more than 1 gram a day.

Strengths of commercial preparations may vary. Follow the manufacturer's labeling whenever available.

Overdosage

Overdosage can cause liver and kidney damage, and sometimes proves fatal. Warning signs of an overdose include delirium, depression, dizziness, fainting, sleep disorders, spasm, tremor, stomach pain, and vomiting.

If you suspect an overdose, seek medical attention immediately.

Rupturewort

Latin name: Herniaria glabra
Other names: Flax Weed,
  Herniary

A Remedy For

Used in the past for hernias and kidney stones, today Rupturewort is taken primarily for urinary tract infections. It has also been used for respiratory disorders, nerve inflammation, gout, and rheumatism. For none of these problems, however, does it show any proven effectiveness.

What It Is; Why It Works

Belief in Rupturewort's efficacy is centuries old. A treatise written in 1597 recommends the herb for hernias and observes that "the powder thereof, taken with wine . . . wasteth away the stones in the kidney and expelleth them." The herb is still thought to increase urination and relieve spasms, but scientists have yet to verify these effects.

A tiny shrub—only 6 inches high—Rupturewort is found in the temperate and southern regions of Europe and Russia. It produces small yellow-white flowers that grow in clusters of 7 to 10. Only the above-ground parts of the plant are considered medicinal.

Avoid If . . .

No known medical conditions preclude the use of Rupturewort.

Special Cautions

At customary dosage levels, Rupturewort poses no risks.

Possible Drug Interactions

No interactions have been reported.

Special Information If You Are Pregnant or Breastfeeding

No harmful effects are known.

How to Prepare

Produced in crushed and extract form, Rupturewort is usually taken as tea. To prepare the tea, combine 1.5 grams (about 1 teaspoonful) of crushed Rupturewort with cold water, bring briefly to a boil, steep for 5 minutes, and strain.

Typical Dosage

As a flushing-out therapy for urinary infections, take 1 cup of tea 2 to 3 times daily.

Overdosage

No information on overdosage is available.

Saffron

Latin name: Crocus sativus

A Remedy For

Although once considered a remedy for digestive problems, Saffron is no longer used medicinally in the West. In Asian medicine, it is used to treat menstrual disorders, difficult labor, inflammation, depression, vomiting, and throat diseases.

Homeopathic practitioners recommend it to control bleeding.

What It Is; Why It Works

Produced from the tiny, dried stigma of the lily-like *Crocus sativus* blossom, genuine Saffron is worth its weight in gold. It takes as many as 4,300 flowers to yield a mere 25 grams. The spice is so expensive, in fact, that it's usually adulterated with common safflower.

Saffron has been prized for centuries as a coloring agent for food, liqueurs, cosmetics, and pharmaceuticals. Its rich golden color was extolled in Greek mythology, and in the Far East, Buddhist monks are famous for their saffron robes. The plant is native to India, the Balkans, and the eastern Mediterranean region, but is also cultivated throughout Europe and the Middle East.

In small doses, Saffron promotes production of gastric juices. Large doses cause contractions in the smooth muscle of the uterus and may induce abortion.

Avoid If . . .
No known medical conditions preclude the use of Saffron.

Special Cautions
Poisoning is a significant danger when this herb is used to induce abortion. A dose of 10 grams is needed to terminate a pregnancy, while a dose of 12 to 20 grams—not all that much more—is generally considered lethal.

Possible Drug Interactions
No interactions have been reported.

Special Information If You Are Pregnant or Breastfeeding
No harmful effects have been reported when Saffron is used as a spice or digestive stimulant.

How to Prepare
Saffron is available for household use in filament and powder form.

Typical Dosage
Medicinal use is not recommended. Store in an airtight, non-synthetic container, protected from light.

Overdosage
Warning signs of overdose include yellowing of the skin, development of red or purple blotches, dizziness, vomiting, stupor, intestinal cramping, bloody diarrhea, blood in the urine, uterine bleeding, and bleeding from the nose, lips, and eyelids.

Paralysis and death may follow. If you suspect an overdose, seek emergency medical treatment immediately.

Sage

Latin name: Salvia officinalis

A Remedy For
- Appetite loss
- Excessive perspiration
- Sore throat

In folk medicine, Sage is also taken for bloating, diarrhea, and intestinal inflammation. As a rinse and gargle, it's used for bleeding gums. Applied externally, it treats mild injuries and skin inflammation. In Asia, it's considered a remedy for hemorrhoids, blood in the urine, bloody phlegm, and fluid in the abdomen; and homeopathic practitioners prescribe it for excessive flow of breast milk. However, its effectiveness for all of these problems remains unverified.

Researchers have also been investigating the value of Sage as a treatment for Type II, non-insulin-dependent diabetes. While one study has shown positive results, further confirmation is needed.

What It Is; Why It Works

Valued in the U.S. primarily as a seasoning, Sage has a long history of medicinal use abroad. It has been taken for conditions ranging from sexually transmitted disease to insect bites, and is still used in Europe as a gargle for sore throats. It exhibits antibacterial qualities, inhibits viral and fungal growth, reduces perspiration and other secretions, and acts as an astringent, tightening and drying the tissues.

The plant's medicinal value resides in its crushed, dried leaves and the oil extracted from its flowers, leaves, and stems. Native to the Mediterranean region, Sage is now grown in all of Europe and North America.

Avoid If . . .

There are no known medical conditions that preclude the use of Sage.

Special Cautions

Although there is little danger of side effects under ordinary circumstances, extended use of Sage can produce the same symptoms as an overdose. (See "Overdosage," below.)

Possible Drug Interactions

No interactions have been reported.

Special Information If You Are Pregnant or Breastfeeding

Do not take this medication during pregnancy.

How to Prepare

Powdered Sage can be made into a remedy for bronchitis by mixing 1²/₃ ounces of the powdered drug with 2²/₃ ounces of honey.

Gargles and rinses may be prepared by mixing 2.5 grams of Sage (or 2 to 3 drops of Sage oil) with 3 ounces of water. Alternatively, use 5 grams (1 teaspoonful) of alcoholic extract in 1 glass of water. Undiluted alcoholic extract may also be applied directly to inflamed mucous membranes.

Typical Dosage

The usual daily dosage is:

Dried Sage: 4 to 6 grams (about 1 teaspoonful)

Essential oil of Sage: 2 to 6 drops

Sage tincture (alcoholic extract): 2.5 to 7.5 grams (one-half to 1¹/₂ teaspoonfuls)

Sage liquid extract: 1.5 to 3 grams (about one-quarter to one-half teaspoonful)

Sage honey: 1 teaspoonful in the morning and before bedtime

Powdered Sage: 1 capsule before each meal for excessive perspiration

Strengths of commercial preparations may vary. Follow the manufacturer's labeling whenever available.

Store away from light and humidity.

Overdosage

The danger of overdose is greater if you are taking an alcoholic extract or the essential oil. To overdose on Sage leaves, you must consume at least 15 grams.

Symptoms of overdose include a feeling of warmth, rapid heartbeat, dizziness, and convulsions. If you suspect an overdose, seek medical attention immediately.

Sandalwood

Latin name: Santalum album
Other names: Sanderswood,
* White Saunders*

A Remedy For

- Bronchitis
- Colds
- Cough
- Fever
- Liver and gallbladder problems
- Sore throat
- Tendency to infection
- Urinary tract infections

When Sandalwood is used for urinary problems, it is usually given in combination with other drugs that flush out or disinfect the urinary system.

In Asian medicine Sandalwood is also used for abdominal pain, burning sensation, difficulty in swallowing, stomach pain, headache, abnormal thirst, and vomiting. Folk uses include treatment of heat and sunstroke, gonorrhea, and excessive sex drive. Its effectiveness for these problems has not, however, been verified.

What It Is; Why It Works

Although Sandalwood is best known for its exotic fragrance,
the essential oil has several medicinal effects. It stimulates the production of urine, loosens bronchial phlegm, and exhibits a drying and disinfectant action.

The Sandalwood tree thrives in India, where it is cultivated under a government monopoly. The production process includes a waiting period of several months after the felling of a tree, allowing time for its unusable sapwood to be consumed by white ants. The essential oil is extracted only from the heartwood and the bark.

Avoid If . . .

Do not use Sandalwood if you have kidney disease.

Special Cautions

Do not take Sandalwood in high doses, or use it for an extended period of time; kidney damage could result. Side effects are uncommon, but can include itchy skin, queasiness, intestinal problems, and bloody urine.

Possible Drug Interactions

No interactions have been reported.

Special Information If You Are Pregnant or Breastfeeding

No harmful effects are known.

How to Prepare

Crushed Sandalwood can be made into a tea. The essential oil should be taken only in coated-pill form.

Typical Dosage

Sandalwood is taken orally. The usual daily dosage is:

Crushed Sandalwood: 10 grams (about 2 teaspoonfuls)
Essential oil of Sandalwood: 1 to 1¹/₂ grams

Overdosage
No information on overdosage is available.

Sanicle

Latin name: Sanicula europaea
Other name: Poolroot

A Remedy For
• Bronchitis
• Cough

Sanicle is also a homeopathic remedy for nervous problems; but its effectiveness for such conditions has not been verified.

What It Is; Why It Works
Sanicle's name comes from the Latin word "sano," meaning "I heal." Found across Europe, Asia, and Africa, the plant averages a foot in height and produces round fruit covered in barbed thorns. It has a slightly salty, bitter taste.

Sanicle loosens phlegm, making it easier to cough up. It also has a mildly astringent effect, tightening and drying the tissues. Only the leaves and flowers are medicinal.

Avoid If . . .
No known medical conditions preclude the use of Sanicle.

Special Cautions
At customary doses, Sanicle poses no risks.

Possible Drug Interactions
No drug interactions have been reported.

Special Information If You Are Pregnant or Breastfeeding
No harmful effects are known.

How to Prepare
Sanicle is prepared as a crushed herb.

Typical Dosage
Sanicle is taken orally. The usual daily dosage is 4 to 6 grams (about 1 teaspoonful).

Store the herb in a sealed container away from light.

Overdosage
No information on overdosage is available.

Sarsaparilla

Latin name: Smilax species

A Remedy For
Sarsaparilla has been used to treat urinary tract infections, psoriasis, and rheumatism, but there is no evidence that it relieves any of these problems. Unverified uses in Asian medicine include epilepsy, malignant ulcers, psoriasis, syphilis, and tuberculosis.

What It Is; Why It Works
In the 19th century, Sarsaparilla enjoyed an undeserved reputation as a cure for syphilis. Later it became a popular flavoring agent in root beer. Most recently, it has been hyped as a natural (and

legal) source of anabolic steroids for body-builders.

Actually, Sarsaparilla *does* contain steroid compounds, but they're not anabolic and don't mimic the real thing. Claims that Sarsaparilla contains testosterone (or boosts testosterone levels) are also false. The herb has revealed no ability to enhance performance or endurance.

Sarsaparilla takes its name from the Spanish words for "bramble" *(sarza)* and "vine" *(parilla)*. It is native to tropical and subtropical regions of America, eastern Asia, and India. A climbing shrub, it puts forth roots that often reach several yards in length. It's the dried roots and tubers that have been put to medicinal use.

Avoid If . . .
No known medical conditions preclude the use of Sarsaparilla.

Special Cautions
In rare cases, Sarsaparilla can cause stomach complaints and queasiness. It may also irritate the kidneys.

Possible Drug Interactions
Sarsaparilla can increase the effects of bismuth and the heart medication digitalis. Avoid these combinations.

Special Information If You Are Pregnant or Breastfeeding
No information is available.

How to Prepare
Sarsaparilla may be found in capsule and tablet form, and as an alcohol solution (tincture).

Typical Dosage
Dried root: 9 grams daily
Tincture: 3 milliliters (about one-half teaspoonful) 3 times daily

Strengths of commercial preparations may vary. Follow the manufacturer's labeling whenever available.

Overdosage
Signs of overdose include diarrhea and fluid loss leading to shock. If you suspect an overdose, seek medical attention immediately.

Savin Tops

Latin name: Juniperus sabina

A Remedy For
• Warts

Although not officially recognized as effective, this herb appears to be a valid treatment for warts.

What It Is; Why It Works
The young shoots and leaves of *Juniperus sabina* contain oils that attack the viruses responsible for warts. The oils are extremely toxic and, used carelessly, can prove highly irritating to surrounding skin.

Taken internally, the herb causes an abnormal surge of blood in the lower abdominal organs, an effect which is sometimes employed to stimulate abortion. However, the drug is so poisonous that the mother's life is often in as much jeopardy as the baby's, and numerous fatalities have occurred.

Juniperus sabina is a 14-foot evergreen shrub with blue-green needle-like leaves. It is found in southern and central Europe, southern Russia, and the northern United States.

Avoid If . . .
For external use only. Internal administration can lead to fatal poisoning.

Special Cautions
Be careful to limit application to the wart alone. Contact with the surrounding skin can cause tissue death and blistering. If the drug is absorbed through the skin, it can lead to internal poisoning.

Be aware that this herb becomes more dangerous with age. The longer the drug is stored, the more poisonous it becomes.

Possible Drug Interactions
No interactions have been reported.

Special Information If You Are Pregnant or Breastfeeding
Given the herb's use in abortion, it's wise to avoid even external application during pregnancy.

How to Prepare
The herb is applied in powder form.

Typical Dosage
Apply twice daily.

Overdosage
A mere 6 drops of the oils from this herb are enough to prove life-threatening. Early symptoms of poisoning include queasiness, irregular heartbeat, spasms, kidney damage, and bloody urine. These symptoms are followed by paralysis, coma, and, ultimately, death. If you suspect poisoning, seek emergency treatment immediately.

Saw Palmetto

Latin name: Serenoa repens
Other name: Sabal

A Remedy For
• Prostate enlargement

Saw Palmetto eases the urinary difficulties that develop when an enlarged prostate obstructs the exit from the bladder. Although this medication promotes normal urination, it will not shrink the prostate, so it's advisable to see your doctor about other forms of treatment.

What It Is; Why It Works
Benign prostate enlargement appears to be triggered by abnormally high levels of the male hormones testosterone and dihydrotestosterone (DHT) in prostate tissue. Saw Palmetto reduces absorption of these hormones within the prostate gland, while reducing inflammation and swelling. All three actions serve to relieve bladder obstruction and improve urinary flow.

Saw Palmetto's popularity has

been on an extraordinary roller coaster ride throughout the 20th century. Widely used under the name "Serenoa" until World War II, it was then completely forgotten until its rediscovery in the 1990s. The plant, a low, scrubby palm, is native to the coastal regions of the southern U.S., from South Carolina to Florida and in southern California. Its medicinal value lies in the oily compounds found in its berries.

Avoid If . . .

No known medical conditions preclude the use of Saw Palmetto.

Special Cautions

At recommended dosage levels, side effects are rare. A few stomach complaints have been reported.

Possible Drug Interactions

No interactions have been reported.

Special Information If You Are Pregnant or Breastfeeding

No harmful effects are known.

How to Prepare

The most effective preparation is an extract of the berry's oils. The crushed berry may also be taken. The berry should *not* be taken as a tea; the medicinal oils will not dissolve in water.

Typical Dosage

The usual daily dosage is 1 to 2 grams of crushed Saw Palmetto berry or 320 milligrams of Saw Palmetto extract.

Potency of commercial preparations may vary. Follow the manufacturer's instructions whenever available.

Overdosage

No information on overdosage is available.

Schisandra

Latin name: Schisandra chinensis
Other name: Wu-wei-zi

A Remedy For

• Liver disorders

Although Schisandra has not been officially declared effective, it is known to improve lab test results in cases of infectious hepatitis and other liver disorders. In traditional Chinese medicine, Schisandra is highly regarded as a remedy for wheezing, cough, insomnia, fatigue, night sweats, and allergic skin reactions. Western herbalists often use it as a tonic to counter the effects of stress.

What It Is; Why It Works

Schisandra, a member of the magnolia family, is a woody vine with numerous clusters of tiny, shiny, oily, bright red berries. The medicinal part is the fully ripe, sun-dried fruit, which is reported to have a sweet, sour, salty, hot, bitter taste. This unusual assortment of flavors is reflected in Schisandra's Chinese name "Wu-wei-zi," which means "five taste fruit."

Schisandra's beneficial effects

Avoid If . . .

Do not take Scopola if you suffer from rapid heartbeat, any narrowing or constriction in the digestive tract, or an enlarged colon. Check with your doctor before using this herb if you have glaucoma (high pressure in the eye) or a prostate tumor; in certain cases it must be avoided. Not for children under 6.

Special Cautions

Take only at the recommended dosages. High doses will cause unpleasant side effects (see "Overdosage" below).

Possible Drug Interactions

Scopola heightens the effect of certain medications. Check with your doctor before combining it with the following:

Amantadine (Symmetrel)
Quinidine (Quinaglute, Quinidex)
Tricyclic antidepressant medications such as Elavil, Pamelor, and Tofranil

Special Information If You Are Pregnant or Breastfeeding

No harmful effects are known.

How to Prepare

Scopola is available as crushed root, powder, and other preparations.

Typical Dosage

The usual daily dosage is 0.25 milligram of total active ingredient. Take no more than 1 milligram at a time. The maximum daily dosage is 3 milligrams.

Strengths of commercial preparations may vary. Follow the manufacturer's labeling whenever available.

Overdosage

The four early warning signs of an overdose are skin reddening, dry mouth, rapid heartbeat, and dilated pupils. Other problems that may develop include difficulty focusing, decreased perspiration and increased body heat, urination problems, and severe constipation.

Very high doses can cause restlessness, compulsive speech, hallucinations, delirium, and manic episodes followed by exhaustion and sleep. Doses above 100 milligrams of active ingredient for adults and 20 to 50 milligrams for children can cause asphyxiation.

If you suspect an overdose, seek medical attention immediately.

Scullcap

Latin name: Scutellaria lateriflora
Other names: Blue Pimpernel, Helmet Flower, Hoodwort, Mad-dog Weed, Madweed, Quaker Bonnet

A Remedy For

Although its efficacy has not been formally recognized, Scullcap has a mild sedative effect and is used in the treatment of anxiety and insomnia. In the past, it was also used for fever, nerve pain, muscular spasms, and epilepsy.

What It Is; Why It Works

There are several varieties of Scullcap. The type discussed here, *Scutellaria lateriflora,* is native to North America. In addition to its sedative action, this variety has the ability to calm spasms and reduce inflammation. A closely related European variety, *Scutellaria galericulata*, has similar properties. On the other hand, Chinese Scullcap (*Scutellaria baicalensis*) contains additional substances with entirely different properties. It exerts a protective effect on the liver, inhibits the growth of bacteria and viruses, and appears to relieve allergies.

The Scullcap family takes its name from its broad, disk-like flower. ("Scutella" is the Latin diminutive for "dish.") The names "Mad-dog Weed" and "Madweed" reflect a belief that the plant could cure rabies. North American Scullcap is a 2-foot-high perennial with pink to blue flowers. The entire above-ground part of the plant is pulverized for medicinal purposes.

Avoid If . . .

No known medical conditions preclude the use of Scullcap.

Special Cautions

At customary dosage levels, Scullcap presents no problems.

Possible Drug Interactions

No interactions have been reported.

Special Information If You Are Pregnant or Breastfeeding

No harmful effects are known.

How to Prepare

Scullcap is available as a dried herb and in an alcohol solution (tincture).

You can make a Scullcap tea by pouring 1 cup of boiling water over 1 to 2 teaspoonfuls of the dried herb and steeping for 10 to 15 minutes.

Typical Dosage

Dried herb: 1 to 2 grams 3 times per day
Tea: 1 cup 3 times per day
Tincture: 2 to 4 milliliters 3 times per day

Overdosage

No information on overdosage is available.

Selenicereus Grandiflorus

Latin name: Selenicereus grandiflorus
Other names: Night-blooming Cereus, Sweet-scented Cactus

A Remedy For

This herb is sometimes recommended for urinary tract infections and heart conditions such as the crushing pain of angina. Although it exhibits proven effects on the heart, its value as a remedy has not been officially recognized.

In folk medicine, Selenicereus Grandiflorus has also been used to treat the spitting up of bloody sputum, heavy or painful menstrual periods, and hemorrhages. The juice of the plant has been used for bladder infections, shortness of breath, and water retention. Applied externally, it has been used for rheumatism. And in homeopathic medicine, it's recommended for spasmodic pain and hemorrhage.

What It Is; Why It Works

Selenicereus Grandiflorus has digitalis-like effects; it boosts the heart and opens the blood vessels. It also stimulates the movement-governing nerves in the spinal cord, and may have an anti-inflammatory effect on the skin.

The plant has a snake-like, creeping or climbing stem that can reach over 30 feet in length. Its huge, sweet-smelling flowers—up to 10 inches in diameter—bloom for only 6 hours before dying. Indigenous to Central America, it is cultivated primarily in Mexico. The flowers and other above-ground parts of the plant are considered medicinal.

Avoid If . . .

No known medical conditions preclude the use of Selenicereus Grandiflorus.

Special Cautions

At customary dosage levels, extracts of Selenicereus Grandiflorus pose no problems. However, the fresh juice of the plant is said to cause itching and pustules on the skin, and, when taken internally, burning of the mouth, queasiness, vomiting, and diarrhea.

Possible Drug Interactions

No interactions have been reported.

Special Information If You Are Pregnant or Breastfeeding

No harmful effects are known.

How to Prepare

Selenicereus Grandiflorus is available as a liquid extract and an alcohol solution (tincture).

Typical Dosage

Liquid extract: Up to 0.6 milliliter 1 to 10 times daily
Tincture: 0.12 to 2 milliliters 2 to 3 times daily

Overdosage

No information on overdosage is available.

Seneca Snakeroot

Latin name: Polygala senega
*Other names: Milkwort,
    Mountain Flax, Rattlesnake
    Root*

A Remedy For

- Bronchitis
- Cough

What It Is; Why It Works

The medicinal properties of this herb were discovered around 1735, when Seneca Indians in Pennsylvania, meeting the Scottish physician John Tennant, introduced it as a snakebite remedy. A 16-inch-high perennial, the plant contains a milky liquid, hence the names Milkwort and Polygala, which means "much milk."

The medicinal part is the dried root. It acts as a decongestant and helps loosen phlegm.

Avoid If . . .
No known health conditions preclude the use of this herb.

Special Cautions
Prolonged use of Seneca Snakeroot can irritate the digestive tract.

Possible Drug Interactions
No interactions have been reported.

Special Information If You Are Pregnant or Breastfeeding
No harmful effects are known.

How to Prepare
To prepare a Seneca Snakeroot tea, mix 0.5 grams (about one-quarter teaspoonful) of the chopped root with cold water, heat to a simmer for 10 minutes, and strain.

Typical Dosage
Root: 1.5 to 3 grams (about one-half to 1 1/4 teaspoonfuls) daily

Liquid extract: 1.5 to 3 grams (about one-quarter to one-half teaspoonful) daily

Alcohol solution (tincture): 2.5 to 7.5 grams (one-half to 1 1/2 teaspoonfuls) daily

Tea: 1 cup 2 to 3 times daily, or up to every 2 hours if no side effects appear

Because potency of commercial preparations may vary, follow the manufacturer's directions whenever available.

Overdosage
Overdosage leads to nausea, diarrhea, queasiness, and other stomach complaints.

Senna

Latin name: Cassia species

A Remedy For
• Constipation

Because of its stool-softening action, Senna is especially useful for people with hemorrhoids or anal fissures. It's also recommended following rectal surgery, and can be used to cleanse the bowel prior to diagnostic procedures.

In Asia, Senna is also used for bronchitis, dysentery, seizures, fever, indigestion, and skin diseases; but its effectiveness for these disorders has never been verified.

What It Is; Why It Works
First prescribed by ancient Arabian physicians, today Senna is one of the more widely used laxatives. It's the active ingredient in such products as Senokot, Fletcher's Castoria, and Ex-Lax Gentle Nature.

Senna grows in most tropical regions of the world. Both its leaves and its seeds are medicinal. It relieves constipation by stimulating the colon, thus hastening passage of the contents. Because there's less time for fluid to be absorbed from the stool, it tends to remain soft.

Avoid If . . .

Do not use Senna if you have an intestinal blockage, appendicitis, or an inflammatory intestinal disorder such as ulcerative colitis or Crohn's disease. Not for children under 12.

Special Cautions

Senna occasionally causes abdominal cramps. Do not use it for more than 1 to 2 weeks without your doctor's approval. Long-term use can deplete the body's potassium levels, leading to such problems as muscle weakness, bone loss, kidney disorders, water retention, and blood in the urine.

Possible Drug Interactions

Loss of potassium from overuse of Senna may increase the effect of heart medications such as digitalis and digoxin (Lanoxin), and may interfere with drugs that steady the heartbeat, possibly leading to heartbeat irregularities.

Special Information If You Are Pregnant or Breastfeeding

Do not use Senna if you are pregnant or breastfeeding.

How to Prepare

Senna is available as a crushed herb, and in liquid and powdered extracts.

There are two ways you can prepare a Senna tea. Either pour hot—but not boiling—water over 0.5 to 2 grams (about one-quarter teaspoonful) of crushed herb,

steep for 10 minutes, and strain, or steep the herb in cold water for 10 to 12 hours, then strain. The slower, cold-water method is thought to leave less resin in the tea, and it's the resin that's responsible for abdominal cramps.

Allow 10 to 12 hours for the herb to take effect.

Typical Dosage

Senna is taken orally. The usual daily dosage delivers 20 to 60 milligrams of its active ingredient. The strength of commercial preparations may vary, so follow the manufacturer's directions whenever available.

Overdosage

Abdominal cramps could be a sign of overdose. If you suspect an overdose, seek medical attention immediately.

Shepherd's Purse

Latin name: Capsella bursa pastoris
Other names: Blindweed, Caseweed, Cocowort, Lady's Purse, Mother's Heart, Pepper-and-Salt, Pick-pocket

A Remedy For

- Blood pressure problems
- Irregular heartbeat
- Nosebleeds
- Premenstrual syndrome (PMS)
- Weak heart
- Wounds and burns

Shepherd's Purse is also used as a remedy for irregular or excessive menstrual bleeding, superficial bleeding from skin injuries, and headache. Additionally, in Asian medicine, it's used for swelling and urinary tract infections.

However, its effectiveness for all these conditions remains unconfirmed.

What It Is; Why It Works

Shepherd's Purse was introduced to America by the Pilgrims, who found that it would grow well in even the poorest soil. It is now found worldwide, except in tropical areas.

The plant gets its name from the appearance of its flat seed pouch, which resembles a leather purse. It blooms almost year-round with small, white flowers on a simple, upright, 16-inch stem.

Shepherd's Purse has been shown to both lower and elevate blood pressure, and to boost the force and speed of the heartbeat. It also increases uterine contractions.

Avoid If . . .

No known medical conditions preclude the use of Shepherd's Purse.

Special Cautions

At typical dosage levels, this herb presents no hazards.

Possible Drug Interactions

No drug interactions have been reported.

Special Information If You Are Pregnant or Breastfeeding

No harmful effects are known.

How to Prepare

Shepherd's Purse can be taken in crushed form, as a liquid extract, or as a tea.

Typical Dosage

Shepherd's Purse is taken orally. The usual daily dosage is :

Crushed herb: 10 to 15 grams (2 to 3 teaspoonfuls)
Liquid extract: 5 to 8 grams (1 to 1 1/2 teaspoonfuls)
Tea: Drink throughout the day

Overdosage

No information on overdosage is available.

Shiitake

Latin name: Lentinan edodes

A Remedy For

Clinical research suggests that a compound in the Shiitake mushroom effectively combats hepatitis B and certain types of cancer, particularly recurrent stomach cancer. Shiitake may also be an effective treatment for human immunodeficiency virus (HIV) infection, although clinical trials have yet to confirm this.

What It Is; Why It Works

In its native China and Japan, the Shiitake mushroom has enjoyed a long-standing reputation as a remedy for exhaustion, colds, worms, poor circulation, and liver problems. And modern research reveals that one of the mushroom's ingredients—a compound called lentinan—does in fact have unique medicinal properties. It stimulates the body's T-lymphocytes, specialized white blood cells that play a key role in the immune system's constant battle against invading germs and encroaching cancer cells.

Although the immunity-boosting action of lentinan appears to be responsible for most of Shiitake's beneficial effects, the mushroom does contain other medicinal compounds as well, including cortinelin, an antibacterial agent that kills a variety of disease-causing germs. Still other ingredients appear to have cholesterol-lowering properties.

Prized as a gourmet delicacy, Shiitakes are now cultivated worldwide. The entire dried cap is used medicinally.

Avoid If . . .
No known medical conditions preclude the use of Shiitake.

Special Cautions
At high dosages, Shiitake sometimes causes diarrhea and bloating.

Possible Drug Interactions
When combining Shiitake with other herbs, you may need to lower the dosages.

Special Information If You Are Pregnant or Breastfeeding
Safety during pregnancy has not been established.

How to Prepare
Typically, the whole, dried mushroom is used. You may also find an alcohol solution (tincture), and a concentrated lentinan extract.

To make a tea, cover a handful of the dried mushrooms with boiling water, steep for 10 to 30 minutes, and strain. The leftover mushrooms may be used in cooking.

Typical Dosage
Dried Shiitake: 6 to 16 grams per day in soup or as a tea

Lentinan extract: 1 to 3 grams 2 to 3 times per day

Tincture: 2 to 4 milliliters (about one-half to 1 teaspoonful) per day

When using a commercial preparation, remember that strengths may vary. Follow the manufacturer's instructions whenever available.

Overdosage
No information on overdosage is available.

Siberian Ginseng

Latin name: Eleutherococcus senticosus

A Remedy For
• Tendency to infection

What It Is; Why It Works
Siberian Ginseng is a relatively new addition to Western natural medicine, but has quickly gained a reputation similar to that of the better known and more expensive Chinese Ginseng. Though the chemical make-up of the two herbs differs, their effects seem

to be similar. Like its Chinese counterpart, Siberian Ginseng is taken to increase energy and concentration, relieve fatigue, and fight off infections. In tests of healthy volunteers, those who took liquid extract of Siberian Ginseng had higher levels of infection-fighting blood cells.

Found in Siberia, northern China, Korea, and Japan, the Siberian Ginseng plant grows 3 to 10 feet high with branches thickly covered in pale, thorny bristles. The root of the plant is the medicinal part.

Avoid If . . .

Don't take Siberian Ginseng if you have high blood pressure.

Special Cautions

At customary dosage levels, Siberian Ginseng poses no problems.

Possible Drug Interactions

No drug interactions have been reported.

Special Information If You Are Pregnant or Breastfeeding

No harmful effects are known.

How to Prepare

Siberian Ginseng root is available in chopped and powdered form for use in tea, and as a liquid extract.

Typical Dosage

Siberian Ginseng is taken internally. The usual daily dosage of the root is 2 to 3 grams (about one-half teaspoonful).

Overdosage

No information on overdosage is available.

Slippery Elm

Latin name: Ulmus fulva
Other names: American Elm, Indian Elm, Moose Elm, Red Elm, Rock Elm, Sweet Elm, Winged Elm

A Remedy For

- Sore throat
- Stomach inflammation
- Wounds and burns

Slippery Elm is taken orally for stomach inflammation, ulcers, and sore throat. Applied to the skin, it can be used as a treatment for wounds, burns, and skin conditions.

What It Is; Why It Works

For much of the 20th century, Slippery Elm was a popular over-the-counter remedy for sore throat and upset stomach. It was listed in *The United States Pharmacopeia* until 1960, and was declared safe and effective by the Food and Drug Administration. It disappeared from drugstore shelves only after Dutch elm disease destroyed almost all the elms in the country.

It is the powdered inner bark of the tree that provides relief. It forms a slippery, viscous coating that soothes irritation in the throat and the lining of the stomach. Its water-retaining properties also make it an ideal ingredient for a soothing compress.

Avoid If . . .

No known medical conditions preclude the use of Slippery Elm.

Special Cautions

At customary dosage levels, this herb poses no risks.

Possible Drug Interactions

No interactions have been reported.

Special Information If You Are Pregnant or Breastfeeding

No harmful effects are known.

How to Prepare

Commercial lozenges containing Slippery Elm are best for throat conditions. For stomach problems, you can make a tea by pouring 1 cup of boiling water over 1 teaspoonful of Slippery Elm powder. To apply to a wound or a burn, mix the powder with water to form a paste.

Typical Dosage

There are no formal guidelines on record. Follow the manufacturer's directions whenever available.

Overdosage

No information on overdosage is available.

Soapwort

Latin name: Saponaria officinalis
Other names: Bouncing Bet, Bruisewort, Crow Soap, Dog Cloves, Fuller's Herb, Latherwort, Old Maids' Pink,
Soap Root, Sweet Betty, Wild Sweet William

A Remedy For

- Bronchitis
- Cough

Although both the root and the leaf of this plant have been used medicinally, only the root has a verified clinical effect. In folk medicine the root is used not only for upper respiratory inflammation, but for eczema and other persistent skin problems as well. Homeopathic practitioners regard it as a remedy for colds.

What It Is; Why It Works

Soapwort gained its name from the crushed root's ability to produce suds when rubbed in water. It can actually be used as a mild detergent for fine fabrics, and was once added to beer to create a frothy head.

Researchers have found that Soapwort has both antibacterial and expectorant action: it kills bacteria and loosens phlegm, making it easier to cough up. The plant grows in the temperate regions of North America, Asia, and Europe.

Avoid If . . .

No known medical conditions preclude the use of Soapwort.

Special Cautions

Although Soapwort poses no major risks when taken at customary dosage levels, it sometimes irritates the stomach. The leaf of the plant can prove irritating to the skin and mucous membranes.

Possible Drug Interactions
No interactions have been reported.

Special Information If You Are Pregnant or Breastfeeding
No harmful effects are known.

How to Prepare
Two varieties of the root can be used, *Gypsophila* and *Rubra*. To make a Soapwort tea, use 0.4 gram (about one-eighth teaspoonful) of the *Rubra* variety.

Typical Dosage
Soapwort is taken orally. The usual daily dosages are:

Gypsophila: 1.5 grams
Rubra: 30 to 150 milligrams

Overdosage
Because of Soapwort's irritating effect on the stomach, excessive doses can cause vomiting.

Soy Lecithin

Latin name: Lecithinum ex soja

A Remedy For
• High cholesterol

In addition to lowering moderately elevated blood cholesterol levels, Soy Lecithin is used to relieve symptoms of liver disease such as loss of appetite and a feeling of pressure in the area of the liver.

In Asian medicine, the product is considered a remedy for chest fullness, fevers, fidgeting, and headache. Its effectiveness for these problems has not, however, been verified.

What It Is; Why It Works
Soy Lecithin binds chemically with cholesterol, thus reducing the amount of pure cholesterol in the bloodstream. The product is extracted from soybeans, the same crop used to produce soy sauce and tofu (soybean curd).

Soybeans have tremendous medicinal potential. They contain estrogen-like compounds that, by taking the place of human estrogen, may ease symptoms of menopause and reduce the risk of estrogen-dependent tumors such as breast cancer. Researchers have also discovered a soy ingredient called genistein that—at least in the laboratory—appears to curb the growth of tumors. Unfortunately, we still don't know the amount needed to provide a protective effect, or which soy-based foods are the richest sources.

In the meantime, at least the cholesterol-fighting role of Soy Lecithin is clear.

Avoid If . . .
No known medical conditions preclude the use of Soy Lecithin.

Special Cautions
Soy Lecithin occasionally causes mild digestive upsets, such as stomach pain, loose stools, and diarrhea.

Possible Drug Interactions
No interactions have been reported.

Special Information If You Are Pregnant or Breastfeeding
No harmful effects are known.

How to Prepare
Soy Lecithin is available as a commercial extract.

Typical Dosage
Follow the manufacturer's instructions. The product is usually taken in a single daily dose.

Overdosage
No information on overdosage is available.

Spearmint

Latin name: Mentha spicata
Other names: Curled Mint, Fish Mint, Garden Mint, Green Mint, Lamb Mint, Mackerel Mint, Our Lady's Mint, Sage of Bethlehem, Spire Mint

A Remedy For
Spearmint is considered a remedy for indigestion and gas, although its effectiveness has not been officially recognized.

What It Is; Why It Works
This member of the mint family has been held in high regard since Roman times. The ancients believed that it kept milk from souring, and used it as a bath additive, gargle, washing agent, and remedy for bee and wasp stings. The herb is named for Menthe, a nymph who, according to legend, was turned into a plant by the goddess Persephone when she learned of Pluto's love for the girl.

The medicinal oil of Spearmint is extracted from the aboveground parts of the plant by steam distillation. Today, it is used primarily as a flavoring agent in toothpaste, chewing gum, and certain food preparations. Unprocessed Spearmint leaves are used as a remedy for gas.

Avoid If . . .
No known medical conditions preclude the use of Spearmint.

Special Cautions
There is a slight possibility of developing an allergy to Spearmint oil. Aside from that, the herb appears to be safe.

Possible Drug Interactions
No interactions have been reported.

Special Information If You Are Pregnant or Breastfeeding
No harmful effects are known.

How to Prepare
Spearmint is available as an oil or concentrate.

Typical Dosage
There are no standard guidelines on record. Follow the manufacturer's directions whenever available.

Overdosage
No information on overdosage is available.

Spinach

Latin name: Spinacia oleracea

A Remedy For

Spinach is sometimes used as a remedy for indigestion and loss of appetite, but there's no evidence that it's particularly useful for these problems. It is also taken to combat anemia, stimulate growth in children, relieve fatigue, and speed recovery from illnesses.

What It Is; Why It Works

Spinach is rich in vitamins and minerals—especially iron and vitamin C—which probably accounts for its purported energizing effects. Both the fresh and dried leaves are used medicinally.

Cultivated worldwide today, Spinach was unknown in the West until the 15th century. It is believed to have originated in Iran.

Avoid If . . .

No known medical conditions preclude the use of Spinach by adults. Do not, however, give it to infants under 5 months of age. It could interfere with their ability to absorb oxygen.

Special Cautions

Spinach is relatively high in nitrates, chemical compounds which have been shown to increase the risk of cancer. This is not a reason to avoid Spinach completely. After all, we take in low levels of nitrates every day, in everything from tap water to bacon and beer. However, you might want to reserve this vegetable for times when you feel run-down.

Possible Drug Interactions

No interactions have been reported.

Special Information If You Are Pregnant or Breastfeeding

No harmful effects are known.

How to Prepare

Spinach is taken as part of the regular diet.

Typical Dosage

No guidelines are on record.

Overdosage

No information on overdosage is available.

Squill

Latin name: Drimia maritima

A Remedy For

- Irregular heartbeat
- Vein problems
- Weak heart

Squill is also used for poor kidneys and, in homeopathic medicine, for pneumonia and rheumatism. Its effectiveness for these purposes remains unproven.

What It Is; Why It Works

Squill has been used medicinally since the 6th century BC, when it was thought to be a remedy for cough. The active part of the plant is the bulb, collected after flowering, then sliced and dried.

(Bulbs are not sold whole because they tend to sprout.) The herb has a bitter, acrid taste.

Squill boosts the force of the heart while slowing the heartbeat, and can lower excessive blood pressure in the veins.

Avoid If . . .

Squill has a potent effect on the heart, and can cause dangerous problems when taken in excess. Combined with certain prescription drugs, it can increase the risk of irregular heartbeat. Check with your doctor before using this medication, especially if you have a heart condition.

Special Cautions

Even when used in standard doses, Squill can cause side effects such as digestive spasms, loss of appetite, vomiting, diarrhea, headache, and irregular pulse.

Contact with the juice of a fresh bulb can cause skin inflammations.

Possible Drug Interactions

Combining Squill with the following medications increases your risk of heart irregularities:

Asthma medications such as Alupent, Proventil, and theophylline (Theo-Dur)
Certain heart stimulants, such as Inocor and Primacor
Quinidine (Quinaglute, Quinidex)

Squill can also boost the action of water pills (diuretics), laxatives, and steroid drugs such as prednisone.

Special Information If You Are Pregnant or Breastfeeding

No harmful effects are known.

How to Prepare

Squill is taken as a powder.

Typical Dosage

Squill is taken orally. The usual daily dosage is 0.1 to 0.5 gram.

Overdosage

Warning signs of an overdose include serious heartbeat irregularities, stupor, vision disorders, depression, confusion, hallucinations, and psychosis. A massive overdose can lead to fatal cardiac arrest or asphyxiation.

If you suspect an overdose, seek emergency treatment immediately.

St. John's Wort

Latin name: Hypericum perforatum
Other names: Amber, Goatweed, Hardhay, Klamath Weed, Tipton Weed

A Remedy For

- Bruises
- Depression and anxiety
- Skin inflammation
- Wounds and burns

Although its effectiveness for other ailments has not been proven, St. John's Wort has also been used to treat sleep disturbances, gallbladder disorders, gastritis, bronchitis, asthma, diarrhea, bed-wetting, rheumatism, muscle pain, hemorrhoids; and gout. Researchers are currently studying its use in acquired immune deficiency syndrome (AIDS) patients.

What It Is; Why It Works

St. John's Wort is believed to combat depression by boosting the levels of certain chemical messengers in the brain. It works on two fronts. Like the prescription antidepressant Prozac, it seems to increase the amount of serotonin available to the nervous system. And like the monoamine oxidase inhibitor Nardil, it is thought to promote higher levels of dopamine and certain other chemical messengers.

St. John's Wort is a golden yellow perennial flower that secretes a red liquid when pinched. Cut at the start of the flowering season and processed in bunches, it must be dried quickly to preserve its oil and secretions.

This plant has been used medicinally for over 2,000 years. Ancient Greeks believed that its odor repelled evil spirits. Early Christians named the plant in honor of St. John the Baptist because they believed it released its blood-red oil on the 29th of August, the day the saint was beheaded.

Avoid If . . .

There are no known reasons to avoid St. John's Wort at recommended dosage levels.

Special Cautions

With heavy use, St. John's Wort increases sensitivity to sunlight. To avoid a sunburn, minimize your exposure to the sun while using this medication. This herb can also cause bloating and constipation.

Possible Drug Interactions

Do not use St. John's Wort while taking a prescription MAO inhibitor such as Nardil or Parnate. At least in theory, a dangerous interaction is possible. Avoid aged, pickled, and fermented food and beverages while taking MAO inhibitors. The combination could cause a sudden, dangerous surge in blood pressure.

Special Information If You Are Pregnant or Breastfeeding

No harmful effects are known.

How to Prepare

A tea can be made from the leaves and flowering tops of the plant using 2 heaping teaspoonfuls of the herb steeped in 5 ounces of boiling water for 10 minutes.

A medicinal oil can be prepared by soaking the crushed flowers in olive oil for several weeks in the sun. Once the oil acquires a reddish color, it can be taken internally or applied directly to the skin to relieve inflammation and promote healing.

Typical Dosage

St. John's Wort can be taken orally or applied to the skin. The usual daily dosage for internal use is:

- 2 to 4 grams (approximately one-half to 1 teaspoonful) of dried herb
- One 5-ounce cup of tea

For depression, take St. John's Wort for 4 to 6 weeks. If needed, repeat for another 4- to 6-week period. If you feel no improvement, check with your doctor. You may need a different therapy.

St. John's Wort is also available in powder, liquid, and solid preparations for internal use; liquid and semi-solid preparations for external use; and preparations made with fatty oils for external and internal use. Strengths for commercial preparations may vary. Follow the manufacturer's labeling whenever available.

Overdosage

No information on overdosage is available.

Star Anise

Latin name: Illicium verum
Other names: Aniseed Stars, Badiana, Chinese Anise

A Remedy For

- Appetite loss
- Bronchitis
- Cough

In Asian medicine, Star Anise is used for indigestion, facial paralysis, arthritis, and intestinal cramps. With the exception of cramps, however, its effectiveness for these problems remains unverified.

What It Is; Why It Works

Star Anise fights cough and bronchitis by loosening phlegm. It also has an antispasmodic effect on the intestines, thus relieving cramps.

Star Anise gets its name from the eight-pointed stars formed by its fruits. The dried fruit and the seeds are both medicinal, as is the oil extracted from the fruit harvested from a 30-foot evergreen tree cultivated in China and Vietnam, Star Anise is often chewed after meals to promote digestion and sweeten the breath.

Avoid If . . .

There are no known medical conditions that preclude the use of Star Anise.

Special Cautions

When taken in customary doses, Star Anise has no side effects, although a few people develop a sensitivity to it after repeated use.

Be sure to avoid confusing Star Anise with the similar, but smaller, Japanese Star Anise, which is poisonous.

Possible Drug Interactions

No interactions have been reported.

Special Information If You Are Pregnant or Breastfeeding

No harmful effects are known.

How to Prepare

You should grind Star Anise just before use.

Typical Dosage

Star Anise is taken orally. The usual daily dosage is:

Ground Star Anise: 3 grams
Essential oil of Star Anise: 300 milligrams

Overdosage

No information on overdosage is available.

Stinging Nettle

Latin name: Urtica dioica
Other names: Dwarf Nettle, Greater Nettle, Nettle Wort

A Remedy For

ROOT

• Prostate enlargement

A number of studies have confirmed the value of Stinging Nettle root for symptomatic relief of enlarged prostate. However, it's important to remember that the herb does not cure the enlargement itself, but merely relieves symptoms such as frequent urination and weak urinary flow. For treatment of the underlying problem, other drugs or surgical procedures are needed, so be sure to consult your doctor.

PLANT AND LEAF

• Kidney and bladder stones
• Rheumatism
• Urinary tract infections

The above-ground parts of the Stinging Nettle plant have no effect on the prostate, but do posses a diuretic action that increases the production of urine. This makes them useful when it's necessary to flush out the urinary system. They are applied externally as a remedy for oily hair and dandruff.

In folk medicine, the above-ground parts of the plant are taken to improve the blood, as well as serving as an ingredient in various "diabetic teas." However, there's no indication of its effectiveness for these purposes, and such uses are not recommended.

In homeopathic practice, all parts of the Stinging Nettle plant are considered an important remedy for itching, rheumatism, and conditions of the spleen.

What It Is; Why It Works

The Stinging Nettle plant, which reaches a height of 2 to 4 1/2 feet, is entirely covered with prickly hairs. It has been used medicinally in a variety of ways, including a bizarre treatment for rheumatism called "urtication" in which the patient is lashed with the above-ground parts of the plant. Today, an extract of the plant is still used externally as a dandruff remedy. All other uses require internal administration.

Avoid If . . .

Do not take the above-ground portion of the plant if you are retaining water due to a heart or kidney condition.

Special Cautions

On rare occasions, taking the above-ground portion of the plant may cause swelling or skin reactions. The root occasionally causes mild stomach and intestinal problems.

When taking the above-ground portion of the plant, be sure to drink at least 8 large glasses of fluid a day.

Possible Drug Interactions
No interactions have been reported.

Special Information If You Are Pregnant or Breastfeeding
No harmful effects are known.

How to Prepare
ROOT

To make a tea, mix 1.5 grams (about 1 teaspoonful) of coarsely powdered root with cold water, bring to a boil for 1 minute, cover, steep for 10 minutes, then strain.

PLANT AND LEAF

To make a tea, mix 1.5 grams (about 2 teaspoonfuls) of finely cut herb with cold water, bring briefly to a boil, steep for 10 minutes, then strain.

For external use, apply an alcohol solution (tincture).

Typical Dosage
ROOT

The usual daily dosage is 4 to 6 grams (about 3 to 4½ teaspoonfuls).

PLANT AND LEAF

Drink the tea several times daily. The total daily amount of cut herb to be used is 8 to 12 grams (10 to 15 teaspoonfuls).

Overdosage
No information on overdosage is available.

Strawberry

Latin name: Fragaria vesca

A Remedy For
The leaves of the Strawberry plant have been used as remedies for digestive problems and rheumatism, although there is no evidence that they have any effect. Other unsubstantiated uses include rash, diarrhea, liver disease, respiratory tract inflammation, gout, tension, kidney stones, and water retention.

What It Is; Why It Works
Enshrined in the name "Strawberry" is an obsolete form of the verb "to strew," referring to the haphazard, tangled growth of the vine. Strawberry was first used for the treatment of gout by the 18th century botanist Linnaeus. It is thought to have a diuretic effect, flushing excess water from the body, as well as a drying, tightening effect on the tissues.

Avoid If . . .
Allergies to Strawberry are fairly common. Do not attempt to use this herb if you are allergic to it.

Special Cautions
Other than allergic reactions, Strawberry poses no documented risks.

Possible Drug Interactions
No interactions have been reported.

Special Information If You Are Pregnant or Breastfeeding
No harmful effects are known.

How to Prepare
To prepare Strawberry tea, pour boiling water over 1 gram crushed Strawberry leaf, steep for 5 to 10 minutes, and strain.

Typical Dosage
As a remedy for diarrhea, drink several cups of tea per day.

Overdosage
No information is available.

Sundew

Latin name: Drosera rotundifolia
Other names: Dew Plant,
  Lustwort, Red Rot, Youthwort

A Remedy For
- Bronchitis
- Cough

Sundew has been advocated as a cure for old age and is sometimes used in combination with remedies for hardening of the arteries. In folk medicine, it has been used for asthma and warts. However, its effectiveness for any disorder other than those of the upper respiratory system has yet to be verified.

What It Is; Why It Works
A protected species in danger of extinction, Sundew ranges from 3 to 8 inches in height. It produces white flowers and has a sour, bitter, hot taste. The plant favors wet, spongy ground in most parts of the world. It has a decongestant effect and relieves bronchial spasms and coughs.

Avoid If . . .
No known medical conditions preclude the use of Sundew.

Special Cautions
When taken at customary dosage levels, Sundew poses no hazards.

Possible Drug Interactions
No interactions have been reported.

Special Information If You Are Pregnant or Breastfeeding
No harmful effects are known.

How to Prepare
Sundew is available in liquid and solid preparations for internal or external use. To prepare Sundew tea, pour boiling water over 1 to 2 grams (about one-quarter teaspoonful) of Sundew, steep for 10 minutes, and strain.

Typical Dosage
The customary dosage is 1 cup of Sundew tea 3 or 4 times daily.

Use a maximum of about 3 grams of prepared Sundew per day. Since the potency of commercial preparations may vary, follow the manufacturer's directions whenever available.

Overdosage
No information on overdosage is available.

Sweet Clover

Latin name: Melilotus officinalis
Other names: Hart's Tree, Hay
Flowers, King's Clover,
Melilot, Sweet Lucerne, Wild
Laburnum

A Remedy For
- Bruises
- Hemorrhoids
- Poor circulation in the veins

Taken internally, Sweet Clover is used to relieve the symptoms of chronic circulation problems in the veins, including pain, heaviness, night cramps, itching, and swelling in the legs. It is also used to support the treatment of people with vein inflammation and blood clots, hemorrhoids, and congestion of the lymph system. Applied externally, it is used to speed the healing of bruises.

In folk medicine Sweet Clover has been used as a diuretic, and homeopathic practitioners recommend it for hemorrhages and headache. Its effectiveness for these problems has not, however, been verified.

What It Is; Why It Works
Sweet Clover is found all over Europe, Australia, and North America, as well as in temperate regions of Asia. It is a perennial that grows from 2 to 4 feet high and produces small yellow flowers that smell like woodruff or hay. It is the principal flavoring ingredient in a particular greenish variety of Swiss cheese.

The flowering above-ground part of the plant is used medici-nally. It contains trace amounts of coumarin, the active ingredient in blood-thinning prescription drugs such as Coumadin. Sweet Clover reduces inflammation and swelling by increasing the amount of blood that flows through the veins back toward the heart. Its wound-healing properties have been confirmed in animal experiments.

Avoid If . . .
No known medical conditions preclude the use of Sweet Clover.

Special Cautions
When used in consistently high doses, Sweet Clover can cause headache and stupor. For a very small number of people, temporary liver damage is a possibility. The condition disappears when the drug is stopped.

Possible Drug Interactions
No drug interactions have been reported, but coumarin-containing prescription drugs are known to interact with a wide variety of medications. If you are taking any prescription drugs, your wisest course is to check with your doctor before using Sweet Clover.

Special Information If You Are Pregnant or Breastfeeding
Prescription drugs containing coumarin are never given during pregnancy; the drug can cause birth defects and bleeding in the developing baby. Although Sweet Clover contains relatively small amounts of coumarin, the safest

strategy is to avoid this herb during pregnancy.

How to Prepare

Sweet Clover is available as a crushed herb, and in ointments, liniments, and suppositories.

To make a tea, pour boiling water over 1 to 2 teaspoonfuls of crushed Sweet Clover, steep for 5 to 10 minutes, then strain.

Typical Dosage

When taken internally, the average daily dose should deliver from 3 to 30 milligrams of the active ingredient coumarin. This amounts to 2 to 3 cups of tea daily.

Store in a tightly sealed container away from light.

Overdosage

No information on overdosage is available.

Sweet Violet

Latin name: Viola odorata
Other name: Garden Violet

A Remedy For

Sweet Violet is sometimes used as a remedy for cough and bronchitis, although there is little evidence of its effectiveness. In folk medicine, it has also been used for colds, sore throat, asthma, migraine and other headaches, rheumatism, fever, stress, insomnia, and skin diseases. Unverified uses in homeopathic medicine include headache and rheumatism.

What It Is; Why It Works

Sweet Violet is a strongly scented plant that produces solitary, dark violet flowers. It is native to large areas of Europe and the Middle East. It is also found in parts of central Asia and North America. The dried flowers, leaves, and roots are all used medicinally.

An extract from the flowers has been found to have an antimicrobial effect, but claims that the flowers loosen phlegm, promote urination, and exert a calming effect have never been verified. The leaves and roots are said to reduce fever, loosen phlegm, and dry up secretions, but these effects also remain unverified, as does the root's ability to promote vomiting.

The plant has been known since classical times, when it was thought to quell anger. It is mentioned by both Homer and Virgil. Roman mythology tells us that Jupiter created the flower to feed his beloved Io, who had been transformed into a white heifer.

Avoid If . . .

No known medical conditions preclude the use of Sweet Violet.

Special Cautions

At customary dosage levels, Sweet Violet poses no risks.

Possible Drug Interactions

No drug interactions have been reported.

Special Information If You Are Pregnant or Breastfeeding

No harmful effects are known.

How to Prepare

To make tea from the dried flowers, use 1 heaping teaspoonful per cup of water. When using the dried leaves, use 2 teaspoonfuls per cup.

A syrup made from the flowers is used as a children's remedy.

Typical Dosage

Flower tea: Sip once or twice an hour, or drink 1 cup twice a day

Flower syrup: 1 to 2 tablespoons every 2 hours

Leaf tea: 1 cup 2 to 3 times daily

Root: The average single dose is 1 gram

Overdosage

No information on overdosage is available.

Tangerine Peel

Latin name: Citrus reticulata
*Other name: Mandarin
    Orange Peel*

A Remedy For

Chinese herbalists use Tangerine Peel to relieve indigestion, gas, bloating, nausea, vomiting, and loose stools. It is also considered a remedy for pain in the breast and side, and for the pain of hernia. Combined with pinellia root, it's used to loosen phlegm and relieve chest congestion.

What It Is; Why It Works

Tangerine Peel can be found at most Asian markets and many western-style health food stores. Aged red- or orange-colored peel is generally considered best, but it's the young, green peel that's used for hernias and pain in the breast or side. The red-colored peel is favored for control of vomiting and belching.

Avoid If . . .

You should not take Tangerine Peel if you have a dry cough or an excessively red tongue, or if you are spitting up blood.

Special Cautions

At customary dosage levels, Tangerine Peel appears to pose no risks.

Possible Drug Interactions

No interactions have been reported.

Special Information If You Are Pregnant or Breastfeeding

No harmful effects are known.

How to Prepare

Available in dried peel form, and in pills.

Typical Dosage

There are no standard guidelines on record.

Overdosage

No information on overdosage is available.

Tansy

Latin name: Tanacetum vulgare
*Other names: Bitter Buttons,
    Hindheal, Parsley Fern*

A Remedy For

Even in small amounts, this herb is highly poisonous, and its use is not recommended. The leaves and flowers are sometimes taken as a remedy for indigestion, rheumatism, intestinal worms, migraine, nerve pain, and loss of appetite, but their effectiveness has never been proven. Tansy oil has been used for indigestion, symptoms of menopause, premenstrual syndrome (PMS), and intestinal worms, but again without demonstrable value. In homeopathy, the oil is used for headache and infectious diarrhea.

What It Is; Why It Works

Despite Tansy's poisonous nature, Greek mythology credits it with conferring immortality on Ganymede, the cupbearer of the gods. In fact, the herb's name stems from "athanaton," the Greek word for immortal. Tansy also has a long-standing association with the Easter holiday; cakes made with Tansy leaves were traditionally eaten at the end of Lent.

Avoid If . . .

Due to the danger of poisoning, this herb should never be used in any significant amount.

Special Cautions

Repeated contact with the plant can lead to allergic skin reactions.

Possible Drug Interactions

No interactions have been documented.

Special Information If You Are Pregnant or Breastfeeding

Tansy has been used to trigger abortions and should be strictly avoided during pregnancy.

How to Prepare

Do not use this herb.

Typical Dosage

Do not use this herb.

Overdosage

A dose of 15 to 30 grams (1 to 2 tablespoonfuls) of the oil is sufficient to cause death. Symptoms of poisoning include vomiting, abdominal pain, severe reddening of the face, enlarged or fixed pupils, seizures, irregular heartbeat, and uterine bleeding.

Death can occur in as little as 1 to 3 1/2 hours. If you suspect an overdose, seek emergency treatment immediately.

Thyme

Latin name: Thymus vulgaris

A Remedy For

- Bronchitis
- Cough

Thyme is also used as a treatment for inflamed sinuses, nose, throat, and larynx, as a remedy for whooping cough, and as an antibacterial and deodorant skin rub. In folk medicine it has been used as a digestive aid, a urinary disinfectant, a diuretic (to flush excess fluid from the body), a remedy for intestinal worms, and an anti-gas medication. Its effectiveness for such problems has not, however, been clinically verified.

What It Is; Why It Works

Recognized today mostly for its culinary benefits, Thyme has played an important role in medicine from the Middle Ages onward. Thymol, its active ingredient, helps loosen phlegm, combats bronchial spasms, and discourages growth of bacteria. First noted by a German pharmacist in 1725, thymol eventually replaced carbolic acid as a safer, yet effective, antiseptic. Today it's found in such popular over-the-counter products as Listerine mouthwash and Vicks VapoRub.

Avoid If . . .

There are no known medical conditions that preclude the use of Thyme.

Special Cautions

No harmful effects are known with proper use.

Possible Drug Interactions

No interactions have been reported.

Special Information If You Are Pregnant or Breastfeeding

No harmful effects are known.

How to Prepare

To make a tea, mix 1.5 to 2 grams (approximately 1 to 1½ teaspoonfuls) of dried herb with boiling water. Steep for 10 minutes, then strain.

Typical Dosage

Thyme is available in crushed, powdered, and liquid extract form, and in combination with other herbs that have an expectorant action. Dosage of the liquid extract is 1 to 2 grams taken 1 to 3 times daily. Thyme tea may be taken several times a day, as needed. Take no more than 10 grams of Thyme daily.

Because strengths of commercial preparations may vary, follow the manufacturer's labeling whenever available.

Overdosage

No information on overdosage is available.

Tormentil

Latin name: Potentilla erecta
Other names: Bloodroot, English
  Sarsaparilla, Ewe Daisy,
  Septfoil, Shepherd's Knot

A Remedy For

• Diarrhea
• Sore throat

Tormentil is also used for inflammation of the stomach and intestines, although its effectiveness for this purpose has not been documented.

What It Is; Why It Works

The scientific name "potentilla" comes from the Latin word "potens," for powerful, a sign of the respect given the plant's medicinal powers. The common name "Tormentil" refers to the torment the plant supposedly can remedy.

Tormentil works by drying and tightening the tissues. A small (foot-high) perennial, it is found throughout Europe, from Scandinavia to Spain. Only the fleshy underground stem and root are used medicinally.

Avoid If . . .
No known medical conditions preclude the use of Tormentil.

Special Cautions
People with a weak stomach may develop digestive problems or vomiting after taking this herb. No other problems are likely at customary dosage levels.

Possible Drug Interactions
No interactions have been reported.

Special Information If You Are Pregnant or Breastfeeding
No harmful effects are known.

How to Prepare
To make a hot Tormentil tea, you can mix 2 to 3 grams (one-half to three-quarters teaspoonful) of finely cut or coarsely powdered root with cold water, bring rapidly to a boil, steep for a while, then strain. However, boiling this herb reduces its strength, so you may want to make a solution by soaking the drug in cold water.

Typical Dosage
Powder: 4 to 6 grams (about 1 to 1¹/₂ teaspoonfuls) per day
For sore throat: As a rinse, 10 to 20 drops of Tormentil tincture in 1 glass of water
For diarrhea: 3 to 4 cups of tea daily, or 2 to 4 grams (one-half to 1 teaspoonful) of powder mixed with red wine

Overdosage
No information on overdosage is available.

Tree of Heaven

Latin name: Ailanthus altissima
Other names: Ailanto, Chinese Sumac, Vernis de Japon

A Remedy For
This herb has garnered increasing interest as a potential treatment for malaria, although its effectiveness has not yet been proven. Other unverified uses include relief of asthma and treatment of worm infestation. In Chinese medicine, it is considered a remedy for vaginal discharges, diarrhea, and painful menstruation. In Africa, it is also used for cramps, fast heart rate, gonorrhea, and epilepsy.

What It Is; Why It Works
Originally found only in China, Tree of Heaven was introduced to Britain in 1751 and now grows throughout northern Europe, North America, and eastern Asia. A handsome, fast-growing tree, it often reaches a height of 100 feet. The satiny yellowish white wood of the full-grown tree can be used in carpentry. In France, the leaves are used to feed the Ailanthus Moth, a caterpillar that yields a

cheaper, more durable silk than the fine mulberry silk of China.

It is the bark that's used medicinally. It appears to have a drying effect and seems to calm spasms. It may also reduce fever.

Avoid If . . .

No known medical conditions preclude the use of this herb.

Special Cautions

Large doses of Tree of Heaven can cause nausea, dizziness, headache, diarrhea, and tingling in the arms and legs.

Possible Drug Interactions

No interactions have been reported.

Special Information If You Are Pregnant or Breastfeeding

No harmful effects are known.

How to Prepare

Tree of Heaven is still being researched as a drug; until now it has been used only in folk medicine.

Typical Dosage

The usual dosage is 6 to 9 grams (up to about 2 teaspoonfuls).

Store Tree of Heaven in a dry, well-ventilated location protected from moths.

Overdosage

Fatal poisonings have been observed in animal experiments. If you suspect an overdose, seek medical attention immediately.

True Unicorn

Latin name: Aletris farinosa
Other names: Ague Grass, Aloe-root, Bettie Grass, Black-root, Colic Root, Crow Corn, Devil's Bit, Star Root, Starwort

A Remedy For
• Indigestion

True Unicorn root is considered useful for poor digestion, nervous stomach, loss of appetite, and gas. In the U.S., it is also used to treat menstrual problems and symptoms of prolapsed uterus. Argentineans regard it as a remedy for bronchitis. Homeopathic practitioners also prescribe it for blood disorders.

What It Is; Why It Works

The True Unicorn plant is found throughout eastern North America, and Native Americans have long used it to relieve digestive problems and prevent threatened miscarriage. It works by stimulating activity in the digestive tract. Only the dried root is used. When fresh, the root tends to cause vomiting.

The leaves of this plant have a whitish look to them, as if dusted with flour. Hence the scientific name "farinosa," or floury. The roots are generally gathered in the wild, then air-dried in the shade.

Avoid If . . .

No known medical conditions preclude the use of True Unicorn.

Special Cautions
At customary dosage levels, True Unicorn poses no risks.

Possible Drug Interactions
No drug interactions have been reported.

Special Information If You Are Pregnant or Breastfeeding
No harmful effects are known.

How to Prepare
True Unicorn root can be found in powdered and fluid-extract form.

To make tea, use 1.5 grams (about one-quarter teaspoonful) of powdered root per half cup of water.

Typical Dosage
True Unicorn is taken orally. Typical doses range from 300 to 600 milligrams, taken 3 times daily.

Overdosage
No information on overdosage is available.

Turmeric

Latin name: Curcuma domestica

A Remedy For
- Appetite loss
- Liver and gallbladder problems

Turmeric has also been used internally for indigestion, gas, bloating, stomach pain, cramps, diarrhea, fever, swelling, bronchitis, colds, chest infections, worms, leprosy, kidney and bladder inflammation, headaches, and missed menstrual periods. Applied externally, it has been used as treatment for bruises, leech bites, festering eye infections, inflammation in the mouth, inflamed skin, and infected wounds. Its value for any of these conditions has not, however, been scientifically verified.

What It Is; Why It Works
Turmeric is more commonly used as a spice than as a medicine, though it does seem to have anti-inflammatory properties. Among its many mildly medicinal effects are antitumor and antibacterial activity, relief of liver damage, and stimulation of bile production. The medicinal part of the plant is its fleshy underground stem.

Turmeric comes from a leafy perennial with huge, lily-like leaves that grow nearly 4 feet in length. The plant is probably native to India, but today is cultivated throughout tropical southern Asia and Indonesia.

Avoid If . . .
No known medical conditions preclude the use of Turmeric.

Special Cautions
Extended use can lead to stomach problems.

Possible Drug Interactions
No interactions have been reported.

Special Information If You Are Pregnant or Breastfeeding
No harmful effects are known.

How to Prepare

To make a Turmeric tea, pour boiling water over 0.5 to 1 gram of powdered Turmeric, cover, steep for 5 minutes, then strain.

Typical Dosage

The usual daily dose of Turmeric is:

Powder: 1.5 to 3 grams (about one-quarter to one-half teaspoonful) taken in 2 or 3 smaller doses between meals

Tea: 2 to 3 cups taken between meals

Store Turmeric away from light.

Overdosage

An overdose is usually signaled by stomach problems. Seek medical attention if they become severe.

Usnea

Latin name: Usnea species
Other names: Beard Moss, Old Man's Beard, Tree Moss

A Remedy For
• Sore throat

In Asian medicine, Usnea is recommended for cough, headache, vaginal discharge, malaria, and eye irritation, and homeopathic practitioners prescribe it for headache and sunstroke. Its effectiveness for these problems has not, however, been scientifically verified.

What It Is; Why It Works

Usnea is a type of lichen found in cool, damp places worldwide. White, red, and black varieties flourish on an assortment of trees, and researchers are still trying to establish which forms are most potent. The dried tissue of the plant is used medicinally. It has a germ-killing effect.

Lichens have been used as drugs since the days of the Roman Empire, when they were considered remedies for coughs, respiratory infections, baldness, and problems in the uterus. In the 18th century, it was thought that simply holding a special type of lichen in the hands could stem bleeding.

Avoid If . . .

No known medical conditions preclude the use of Usnea.

Special Cautions

At customary dosage levels, Usnea poses no risks.

Possible Drug Interactions

No interactions have been reported.

Special Information If You Are Pregnant or Breastfeeding

No harmful effects are known.

How to Prepare

Usnea is sold in lozenges that contain the equivalent of 100 milligrams of the herb.

Typical Dosage

Usnea is taken orally. The usual dosage is 1 lozenge 3 to 6 times per day.

Overdosage

Researchers believe that an overdose could be poisonous. However, the precise effects have not yet been determined.

Uzara

Latin name: Xysmalobium undulatum

A Remedy For
• Diarrhea

What It Is; Why It Works

Uzara combats diarrhea by slowing the movement of the bowels. In high dosages, its active ingredient uzarone acts like digitalis, strengthening heart contractions and steadying the heartbeat.

Uzara is native to South Africa, where it is a traditional remedy for diarrhea and dysentery. The dried roots of 2- to 3-year-old plants are used medicinally.

Avoid If . . .

Do not use Uzara if you are taking digitalis-type heart medications such as digoxin (Lanoxin).

Special Cautions

At customary dosage levels, Uzara poses minimal risks.

Possible Drug Interactions

Uzara's possible effects on the heart, when added to those of other heart medications, could be harmful. Check with your doctor before combining this herb with any cardiovascular drugs.

Special Information If You Are Pregnant or Breastfeeding

No harmful effects are known.

How to Prepare

You can take Uzara as a liquid or dry extract.

Typical Dosage

Each dose should supply the equivalent of 1 gram of the herb, which will deliver approximately 75 milligrams of the active ingredient uzarone. The total recommended daily dosage of uzarone is 45 to 90 milligrams.

Overdosage

Poisoning following oral intake of Uzara is possible but unlikely, since the substances in the herb that affect the heart are absorbed only with difficulty and have a minimal effect. When taken intravenously, however, the herb can be fatal.

Valerian

*Latin name: Valeriana officinalis
Other names: All-heal, Amantilla, Capon's Tail, Heliotrope, Setwall, Vandal Root*

A Remedy For
• Insomnia
• Nervousness

Although its other uses have not been formally verified, Valerian is also taken for anxiety, mental strain, lack of concentration, excitability, hysteria, stress, headache, epilepsy, premenstrual syndrome, symptoms of pregnancy, problems of menopause, nerve pain, fainting, stomach cramps, colic, and uterine spasms.

What It Is; Why It Works

The ancient Greek physician Galen referred to Valerian as "Phu," an expression of disgust at the plant's smell. In medieval times, it was given the name "All-heal," reflecting its many healing properties. It was also used as a spice and an ingredient in perfume.

The medicinal parts are the carefully dried underground stem and the dried roots. The plant's strong smell is attractive to cats, who roll in it, defeating most attempts to grow it in gardens. It is equally attractive to rats and is used by some rat-catchers. Valerian is a powerful remedy for spasms. It relaxes muscles and has a sedative effect.

This plant, which produces bright pink to white flowers, grows 20 to 40 inches in height. It is native to Europe and the temperate regions of Asia, and is cultivated in Europe, Japan, and the U.S.

Avoid If . . .

Unless your doctor approves, do not bathe with Valerian extract or use the volatile oil if you have a large skin injury, an acute skin disorder, a severe infection, heart problems, or severe muscle tension.

Special Cautions

In rare instances, Valerian can cause digestive problems or an allergic reaction. Long-term use can lead to headache, restlessness, sleeplessness, pupil dilation, and heart problems.

Possible Drug Interactions

No interactions have been reported.

Special Information If You Are Pregnant or Breastfeeding

No harmful effects are known.

How to Prepare

To prepare Valerian tea, combine 3 to 5 grams (about 1 teaspoonful) of crushed Valerian with 150 milliliters hot water (about two-thirds cup), steep for 10 to 15 minutes, then strain.

To make a bath additive, combine 100 grams (about one-half cup) of crushed Valerian with 2 quarts of hot water for each full bath.

Typical Dosage

For internal use, the typical daily dose is:

Crushed herb: 15 grams (about 3 teaspoonfuls)

Tea: 2 to 3 cups daily, including 1 before bedtime

Alcohol solution: 1 to 3 milliliters (about one-quarter to one-half teaspoonful) 1 or more times per day

Alcohol solution (1:5): 15 to 20 drops in water several times daily

Pressed juice: 1 tablespoonful 3 times daily for adults; 1 teaspoonful 3 times daily for children

Because the potency of commercial preparations may vary, follow the manufacturer's directions whenever available.

Store Valerian away from light. Alcohol solutions (tinctures) and extracts must be stored in tightly closed containers.

Overdosage
No information on overdosage is available.

Veratrum

Latin name: Veratrum viride
Other names: American
  Hellebore, Bugbane, Devil's
  Bite, Earth Gall, Indian Poke,
  Itchweed, Tickleweed

A Remedy For
Veratrum does an excellent job of reducing high blood pressure, but is so toxic—even at standard dosage levels—that it is no longer used medicinally.

What It Is; Why It Works
If you're interested in trying Veratrum, consider this: It is said to have been a favorite ingredient for poisoning daggers and arrows in preindustrial Europe. It kills by paralyzing the heart.

Veratrum viride is native to swamps and moist ground throughout most of the eastern United States. Its close relative, *Veratrum album*, can be found across most of continental Europe. The plant is a handsome

perennial some 2 to 4 feet in height. The root contains the active ingredients.

Avoid If . . .
With over 100 drugs now available to control high blood pressure, there's no need to risk using Veratrum. Avoid it completely.

Special Cautions
Among Veratrum's *less* serious side effects are toxic skin reactions and severe stomach irritation. For the really bad reactions, see "Overdosage" below.

Keep in mind that even handling Veratrum can result in poisoning, since it can be absorbed through unbroken skin.

Possible Drug Interactions
No interactions have been reported.

Special Information If You Are Pregnant or Breastfeeding
Do not use Veratrum at these or any other times.

How to Prepare
Use is not recommended.

Typical Dosage
Use is not recommended.

Overdosage
The first signs of poisoning are sneezing, watery eyes, excess saliva, vomiting, diarrhea, a burning sensation in the mouth and throat, and inability to swallow. These symptoms are followed by a tingling sensation, dizziness, possible blindness, paralysis of the arms and legs, mild

seizures, slowed heartbeat, irregular heartbeat, and low blood pressure. Death occurs when the drug stops either the heart or the lungs. If you have any side effects, seek emergency medical attention immediately.

Verbena

Latin name: Verbena officinalis
Other names: Herb of Grace,
    Juno's Tears, Pigeon's Grass,
    Simpler's Joy, Vervain

A Remedy For

Verbena is sometimes recommended for cough, bronchitis, and sore throat. Its effectiveness for these problems has not, however, been scientifically confirmed.

Other uses, also unsubstantiated, include treatment of pain, cramps, fatigue, nervous disorders, digestive disorders, liver and gallbladder diseases, kidney and urinary tract complications, symptoms of menopause, menstrual problems, gout, rheumatism, asthma, and water retention. Applied to the skin, it's used to relieve arthritis, itching, and the pain of minor burns, dislocations, and bruises. In Asian medicine, it's prescribed for abdominal distention, malaria, irregular menstruation, and swelling.

What It Is; Why It Works

For centuries, Verbena was considered sacred. It played a role in the religious ceremonies of the pre-Christian Druids. Later it was said to have been found on Calvary, where it gave comfort to Christ. Its name is derived from the ancient Celtic words "fer" (to drive away) and "faen" (stone), reflecting a belief in its ability to expel kidney stones.

More recently, Verbena has been tested for antimicrobial and antiviral activity, and for possible use as an immunity booster and anticancer agent, but results are inconclusive. Researchers are also checking suggestions that it can clear bronchial passages, relieve cough, stimulate production of breast milk, flush excess water from the body, and reduce inflammation.

Though Verbena originated in the Mediterranean region, it is now cultivated worldwide, particularly in eastern Europe. The entire above-ground plant is used medicinally.

Avoid If . . .

No known medical conditions preclude the use of Verbena.

Special Cautions

At customary dosage levels, Verbena poses no risks.

Possible Drug Interactions

No drug interactions have been reported.

Special Information If You Are Pregnant or Breastfeeding

No harmful effects are known.

How to Prepare

Verbena is available as a crushed herb, as a liquid extract, and in an alcohol solution (tincture). When preparing tea, use 5 to 20 grams of Verbena per quart of water.

Typical Dosage

Dosage guidelines vary. A regimen of 2 to 4 grams up to 3 times per day is a typical recommendation. Follow the manufacturer's directions whenever available.

Store away from moisture.

Overdosage

No information on overdosage is available.

Veronica

Latin name: Veronica officinalis
Other name: Speedwell

A Remedy For

Veronica is sometimes recommended for indigestion, urinary tract infections, and rheumatism, but evidence of its effectiveness for these problems is lacking.

Other uses—also unsubstantiated—include treatment of cough and other respiratory ailments, liver disorders, kidney problems, nervous agitation, and "tired blood." As a gargle, it's used for sore throat. Applied to the skin, it's thought to speed wound healing and relieve itching, chronic skin conditions, and "sweating of the feet." In Asian medicine, it's prescribed for hepatitis, diarrhea, fever, and boils.

What It Is; Why It Works

Veronica is named not for a legendary beauty, but for an 18th-century botanist. A diminutive herb with bright blue or lilac flowers, the plant is found throughout Europe, parts of Asia, and North America. Veronica's above-ground parts are considered medicinal, but the only physical effect researchers have found to date is a tendency to prevent ulcers and speed their healing.

Avoid If . . .

No known medical conditions preclude the use of Veronica.

Special Cautions

At customary dosage levels, Veronica presents no problems.

Possible Drug Interactions

No drug interactions have been reported.

Special Information If You Are Pregnant or Breastfeeding

No harmful effects are known.

How to Prepare

Veronica is prepared as a tea for internal consumption and as a solution for external applications.

To make the tea, pour boiling water over 1.5 grams (about 1 1/2 teaspoonfuls) of finely cut Veronica, steep for 10 minutes, and strain.

To make a solution for a compress or gargle, boil 1 handful of the drug in 1 quart of water for 10 minutes.

Typical Dosage

For internal use, take 2 to 3 cups of tea daily.

Store away from light.

Overdosage
No information on overdosage is available.

Vitex

Latin name: Vitex agnus-castus
Other name: Chaste Tree

A Remedy For
• Premenstrual syndrome (PMS)

Vitex is also used for menstrual irregularity and breast pain, but its effectiveness for these problems remains unconfirmed.

What It Is; Why It Works
The ancient Greeks thought that Vitex encouraged chastity; leaves of the plant were strewn on couches during rituals associated with Demeter, the goddess of agriculture.

The plant is found throughout the entire Mediterranean region as far as western Asia, but is usually collected in Morocco and Albania. It grows 3 to 18 feet high in bush or tree form, with blue or pink flowers about 4 inches in diameter.

The medicinal parts are the ripe, dried fruit and the dried leaves. In laboratory tests, Vitex appears to inhibit production of the hormone prolactin, which stimulates the production of breast milk.

Avoid If . . .
Do not take Vitex while pregnant or breastfeeding.

Special Cautions
Tension and swelling of the breast, as well as menstrual disturbances, could be signs of a serious underlying disorder. See your doctor for a diagnosis. Don't rely on Vitex alone.

Skin rash is a potential side effect of Vitex.

Possible Drug Interactions
Vitex may interfere with the action of the digestive stimulant Reglan, as well as certain major tranquilizers, including Haldol, Prolixin, and Thorazine.

Special Information If You Are Pregnant or Breastfeeding
Avoid this herb during pregnancy and while breastfeeding.

How to Prepare
Vitex is taken as a liquid or dry extract.

Typical Dosage
Vitex is taken orally. The usual daily dosage is 30 to 40 milligrams.

Overdosage
No information on overdosage is available.

Walnut

Latin name: Juglans regia

A Remedy For
• Excessive perspiration
• Skin inflammation

Taken internally, Walnut is also used as a treatment for inflammation of the digestive tract, and intestinal worms, but its effectiveness for these problems remains unconfirmed.

In Asian medicine, Walnut is considered a treatment for eczema, herpes, tuberculosis, and syphilis.

What It Is; Why It Works

It is the leaves—not the nuts—of the Walnut tree that are used medicinally. They contain tannins that have a skin-tightening effect. Other compounds in leaves have been found to have an antifungal effect.

Walnut originated in the Middle East and Iran, but now grows worldwide. A favored source of wood for cabinetmaking, Walnut trees live up to 300 years. It was said that in the "golden age" men lived on acorns while the gods ate walnuts.

Avoid If . . .

No known medical conditions preclude the use of Walnut.

Special Cautions

At customary dosage levels, Walnut presents no known risks.

Possible Drug Interactions

No interactions have been reported.

Special Information If You Are Pregnant or Breastfeeding

No harmful effects are known.

How to Prepare

You can make a solution by adding 2 teaspoonfuls of Walnut leaf to 1 cup of water, boiling the mixture, then straining.

Typical Dosage

For external application, use 3 to 6 grams of crushed leaves daily.

Overdosage

No information on overdosage is available.

Watercress

Latin name: Nasturtium officinale
Other name: Indian Cress

A Remedy For

- Bronchitis
- Cough

High in vitamin C, Watercress is used as a general tonic, and its bitter taste is thought to stimulate the appetite and improve digestion. In Italy, compresses made from Watercress are used to treat arthritis. Homeopathic practitioners prescribe it for nervous conditions, constipation, and liver disorders. Only as a remedy for cough and bronchitis, however, has it been conclusively found effective.

What It Is; Why It Works

Known primarily for its use in salads and cooking, Watercress has a radish-like taste and emits a tangy fragrance when rubbed. Its scientific name comes from the Latin words "nasus tortus," or "screwed-up nose," describing the usual reaction to its stinging smell. The plant is found almost all over the world and is grown commercially in many regions.

Watercress contains mustard oil, a compound that flushes excess water from the body. Researchers have also shown that the herb kills bacteria.

Avoid If . . .
Do not take Watercress if you have a stomach or intestinal ulcer or a kidney inflammation. Not for children under 4.

Special Cautions
At routine dosage levels, Watercress poses no problems. However, eating large quantities of freshly harvested Watercress can irritate the stomach and intestines due to its mustard oil content.

Possible Drug Interactions
No interactions have been reported.

Special Information If You Are Pregnant or Breastfeeding
No harmful effects are known.

How to Prepare
Watercress can be made into a tea. Pour 5 ounces (about one-half cup) of boiling water over 2 grams (about one-half teaspoonful) of the crushed herb, cover, steep for 10 minutes, and strain. You can drink 2 to 3 cups daily before meals.

Typical Dosage
Watercress is taken orally. The usual daily dosage is:

Dried Watercress: 4 to 6 grams (about 1 teaspoonful)
Fresh Watercress: 20 to 30 grams (about 1 1/3 to 2 tablespoonfuls)
Watercress juice: 60 to 150 grams (about one-quarter to one-half cup)

Overdosage
No information on overdosage is available.

White Nettle

Latin name: Lamium album
Other names: Archangel, Bee Nettle, White Deadnettle

A Remedy For
• Bronchitis
• Cough
• Sore throat
• Skin inflammation

White Nettle is also used for urinary problems, digestive disorders, female sexual disorders, and menopausal complaints, although its effectiveness for these ailments has not been verified.

What It Is; Why It Works
White Nettle has an expectorant action, loosening bronchial phlegm, and also serves as an astringent, tightening and firming tissues. The medicinal parts of the plant are its leaves and its white flowers, which have a weak honey-like fragrance and a slimy-sweet taste.

White Nettle's Latin name comes from the Greek word

"laimos" for "throat," a reference to the shape of the flowers. In some places, the plant is known as "archangel," probably because it flowers around May 8th, the day dedicated to the Archangel Michael. It is common throughout Europe and central and northern Asia.

Avoid If . . .

There are no medical conditions known to preclude use of White Nettle.

Special Cautions

At customary dosage levels, White Nettle poses no danger of unwanted side effects.

Possible Drug Interactions

No interactions have been reported.

Special Information If You Are Pregnant or Breastfeeding

No harmful effects are known.

How to Prepare

White Nettle flowers and leaves are dried to form a powder for use in teas and other preparations for oral administration. It can also be used in moist compresses and rinses, and as a bath additive.

To make White Nettle tea, pour a cup of water over 1 gram of White Nettle (about one-quarter of a teaspoonful), steep for 5 minutes, and strain.

For use in a compress, pour boiling water on 50 grams (1¾ ounces) of White Nettle flowers, steep for 5 minutes, and strain.

Typical Dosage

The usual daily dose for internal use is 3 grams (about one-half teaspoonful). For bathing, add 5 grams of White Nettle (1 teaspoonful) to the water.

Overdosage

No information on overdosage is available.

White Willow

Latin name: Salix species
Other names: European Willow,
 Salicin Willow

A Remedy For

- Pain
- Rheumatism

In Asian medicine, White Willow is also considered a remedy for jaundice. Its effectiveness for this problem has not, however, been verified.

What It Is; Why It Works

White Willow has been in use since the time of the Romans. It is thought to be the original source of the drug we now call aspirin.

A tree some 20 to 50 feet in height, White Willow is native to central and southern Europe. Its medicinal value lies in the bark.

Avoid If . . .

Do not use White Willow if you are sensitive to aspirin or aspirin-like compounds.

Special Cautions

Stomach problems are the primary side effect.

Possible Drug Interactions

No interactions have been reported.

Special Information If You Are Pregnant or Breastfeeding

Since aspirin taken during the final three months of pregnancy can harm the baby or cause complications during delivery, you may also want to avoid aspirin-like products such as White Willow.

How to Prepare

To prepare a tea, put 2 to 3 grams (about 1 1/4 to 2 teaspoonfuls) of cut or coarsely powdered White Willow in cold water, bring to a boil, steep for 5 minutes, then strain.

Typical Dosage

The average daily dose is 60 to 120 milligrams of the active ingredient salicin, or 1 cup of tea 3 to 5 times a day.

Since the potency of commercial preparations may vary, follow the manufacturer's instructions whenever available.

Overdosage

No information on overdosage is available.

Wild Cherry

Latin name: Prunus serotina
Other names: Choke Cherry, Rum Cherry, Virginian Prune

A Remedy For

- Bronchitis
- Cough
- Indigestion

Wild Cherry is also used for nervous stomach and diarrhea.

What It Is; Why It Works

The bark of the Wild Cherry tree contains cyanogenic glycosides—compounds that combat spasms in the bronchial passageways and thus relieve coughs.

Native to North America, the tree is now cultivated in Europe. It is prized by cabinetmakers for its fine-grained wood.

Avoid If . . .

No known medical conditions preclude the use of Wild Cherry.

Special Cautions

At customary dosage levels, Wild Cherry poses no problems.

Possible Drug Interactions

No drug interactions have been reported.

Special Information If You Are Pregnant or Breastfeeding

No harmful effects are known.

How to Prepare

Wild Cherry is available in syrup and alcohol solution (tincture) form.

Typical Dosage

Syrup or tincture: 2 to 4 milliliters (about one-half to three-quarters teaspoonful) 3 to 4 times per day

Overdosage

A massive overdose of Wild Cherry could theoretically prove fatal, although no actual problems have been reported. If you suspect an overdose, seek medical attention immediately.

Wild Thyme

Latin name: Thymus serpyllum
Other names: Mother of Thyme, Shepherd's Thyme

A Remedy For
- Bronchitis
- Cough

Although proven effective only for bronchitis and cough, Wild Thyme has been used for a variety of other disorders. In folk medicine, it's taken to stimulate digestion, relieve intestinal gas, loosen phlegm, and treat kidney and bladder disorders. As a bath additive or liniment, it's used for rheumatism and sprains. Homeopathic practitioners prescribe it for asthma and whooping cough. And in Asian medicine, it serves as a remedy for diarrhea, itching, toothache, and vomiting.

What It Is; Why It Works

Wild Thyme's role in traditional folklore does not encourage its use: It was associated with death and was planted on graves, particularly in Wales. Nevertheless, in the 17th century, the botanist Culpeper recommended it for nightmares and headaches. Its use for uterine disorders is probably responsible for the name Mother of Thyme.

Scientific investigation has shown that Wild Thyme kills bacteria, stops spasms of the internal organs, and stimulates secretions. It grows throughout the temperate regions of Europe and Asia, and is cultivated in Albania, Hungary, and the former Yugoslavia.

Avoid If . . .

No known medical conditions preclude the use of Wild Thyme.

Special Cautions

When taken at customary dosage levels, Wild Thyme presents no problems.

Possible Drug Interactions

No interactions have been reported.

Special Information If You Are Pregnant or Breastfeeding

No harmful effects are known.

How to Prepare

Wild Thyme can be made into a tea. Pour boiling water over 1.5 to 2 grams (about 1 to 1 1/2 teaspoonfuls) of finely cut Wild Thyme. Steep for 10 minutes, then strain. A cup taken before meals is thought to stimulate digestion.

Abroad, Wild Thyme is an ingredient in commercially prepared cough suppressants. Some cough drops also contain Wild Thyme extract.

Typical Dosage

Wild Thyme is taken orally. The usual daily dosage is 4 to 6 grams (about 3 to 4 teaspoonfuls) of the finely cut herb.

Overdosage
No information on overdosage is available.

Wild Yam

Latin name: Dioscorea villosa
Other names: China Root, Colic
Root, Devil's Bones,
Rheumatism Root, Yuma

A Remedy For
• High cholesterol

An extract of Wild Yam has been shown to lower triglycerides and raise levels of the "good" HDL cholesterol that combats build-up of plaque in the arteries. Wild Yam is also considered a remedy for rheumatism, gallbladder problems, cramps, nerve pain, painful menstruation, upset stomach, and morning sickness, but its effectiveness for these problems remains to be confirmed.

What It Is; Why It Works
Wild Yam calms muscular spasms and seems to have anti-inflammatory properties. It also stimulates the flow of bile and promotes perspiration. It does not, as some believe, serve as a natural source of the female hormone progesterone. It is used in the production of artificial progesterone, but it will not yield the hormone in the absence of a chemical conversion process that the body can't supply.

Wild Yam is a member of the huge *Dioscorea* family, which includes the common potato. It is named for Dioscorides, the 1st century Greek physician whose botanical writings were the standard for more than a thousand years. Native to North America, the plant is now cultivated in tropical, subtropical, and temperate regions worldwide. The dried root is the medicinal part of the plant.

Avoid If . . .
No known medical conditions preclude the use of Wild Yam.

Special Cautions
Large doses have been known to cause nausea.

Possible Drug Interactions
There are no interactions on record.

Special Information If You Are Pregnant or Breastfeeding
No harmful effects are known.

How to Prepare
Wild Yam is available in an alcohol solution (tincture), and in capsules and tablets containing the dried root.

Typical Dosage
Tincture: 2 to 3 milliliters (about one-half teaspoonful) 3 to 4 times per day
Capsules and tablets: 1 to 2 pills 3 times per day

Because the strength of commercial preparations may vary, follow the manufacturer's directions whenever available.

Overdosage

Poisoning is conceivable. Take care to avoid excessive doses.

Wintergreen

Latin name: Gaultheria procumbens

Other names: Boxberry, Canada Tea, Checkerberry, Deerberry, Ground Berry, Hillberry, Mountain Tea, Partridge Berry, Spiceberry, Teaberry, Wax Cluster

A Remedy For

• Rheumatism

Although not officially recognized, Wintergreen is a useful external remedy for the pain of rheumatoid arthritis. In the past, it has also been used for muscle, joint, or nerve pain, stomach or back pain, various kinds of inflammation, and painful menstruation. In folk medicine, it is used as an antiseptic and taken for asthma.

What It Is; Why It Works

Once a popular painkiller, Wintergreen has been supplanted by a cheap synthetic version of its active ingredient, methyl salicylate. You can find this latter-day stand-in for Wintergreen in such aches-and-pains remedies as Bengay and Arthricare. It relieves pain by stimulating temperature-sensitive nerve endings, thus temporarily overriding nearby pain signals.

Wintergreen, a bushy little plant roughly 6 inches in height, is native to North America. Win-

tergreen oil is still produced in the United States for use in products ranging from Chinese tea to cosmetics, liniments, and bath additives.

Avoid If . . .

No known medical conditions preclude the use of Wintergreen.

Special Cautions

Both Wintergreen leaf and its oil can cause contact allergies.

Possible Drug Interactions

No interactions have been reported.

Special Information If You Are Pregnant or Breastfeeding

No harmful effects are known.

How to Prepare

Use a commercially prepared remedy such as Bengay or Arthricare.

Typical Dosage

Methyl salicylate preparations can usually be massaged into the painful area up to 3 or 4 times a day. Follow the manufacturer's directions.

Overdosage

Oral intake of as little as 4 to 6 grams of pure Wintergreen oil can prove fatal. Even its absorption through the skin can produce central nervous system problems, fluid build-up in the lungs, and collapse. Excessive intake of the leaves can lead to severe stomach and kidney irritation.

If you suspect an overdose, seek medical attention immediately.

Witch Hazel

Latin name: Hamamelis
  virginiana
Other names: Snapping
  Hazelnut, Spotted Alder,
  Tobacco Wood, Winterbloom

A Remedy For
- Hemorrhoids
- Skin inflammation
- Sore throat
- Vein problems
- Wounds and burns

In addition, Witch Hazel leaf is used in folk medicine for diarrhea and menstrual complaints, while the bark also serves as a remedy for colitis and vomiting or coughing up blood. Its effectiveness for these disorders has not, however, been verified.

What It Is; Why It Works
Witch Hazel possesses anti-inflammatory properties. It also tightens up tissues and stanches bleeding at the point of application. These effects make it a favored remedy for hemorrhoids, burns, insect bites, and skin inflammations, and have earned it a place in numerous face creams, aftershave lotions, and skin creams.

Witch Hazel originated in North America, where it has a long history among Native Americans as a compress for painful swellings. Its fruit, which looks much like a hazelnut, ripens with considerable flair, suddenly bursting and hurling its seeds up to 4 yards away. This dramatic moment is responsible for the alternative name, "Snapping Hazelnut."

Avoid If . . .
No known medical conditions preclude the use of Witch Hazel.

Special Cautions
If taken internally, the tannin in Witch Hazel can cause digestive problems. Extended internal use poses a slight risk of liver damage.

Possible Drug Interactions
No interactions have been reported.

Special Information If You Are Pregnant or Breastfeeding
No harmful effects are known.

How to Prepare
Various extracts and distillations are available as liquids, ointments, gels, and suppositories. Preparations of crushed leaf and bark may also be found.

To make a solution for compresses and rinses, steep 5 to 10 grams (1 to 2 teaspoonfuls) of crushed Witch Hazel in 250 milliliters (1 cup) of water.

Typical Dosage
Potency of Witch Hazel preparations varies. Follow the manufacturer's directions whenever available.

Overdosage
No information on overdosage is available.

Woodruff

Latin name: Galium odorata

A Remedy For

Woodruff has been used to treat urinary tract infections, edginess, insomnia, water retention, menstrual disorders, and irregular heartbeat. For none of these problems, however, has its effectiveness been confirmed.

What It Is; Why It Works

Woodruff is a 4- to 14-inch flowering plant that gives off a pleasant aroma, similar to the scent of freshly mown hay. Although native to northern Europe, Woodruff is no longer used as a drug in German-speaking countries. Only the above-ground parts of the plant have been used medicinally.

Woodruff contains coumarin— a potent drug found in prescription blood-thinners such as Coumadin—but in such tiny amounts that it's unlikely to have any effect. The herb tends to be mildly anti-inflammatory, and relieves swelling and spasms to a minor degree.

Avoid If . . .

No known medical conditions preclude the use of Woodruff.

Special Cautions

If you take Woodruff for an extended period of time, ask your doctor for periodic liver function tests. Liver damage can occur following long-term administration, and can be remedied by discontinuing use of the herb.

Possible Drug Interactions

No drug interactions have been reported.

Special Information If You are Pregnant or Breastfeeding

No information is available.

How to Prepare

To make a tea, use 1.8 grams (2 teaspoonfuls) of Woodruff per glass of water. Drink during the day or at bedtime.

Typical Dosage

The average single dose is 1 gram.

Strengths of commercial preparations may vary. Follow the manufacturer's labeling whenever available.

Overdosage

Signs of overdose include headache and disorientation. If you suspect an overdose, seek medical attention immediately.

Wormwood

*Latin name: Artemisia
    absinthium*
*Other names: Absinthe, Green
    Ginger*

A Remedy For

- Appetite loss
- Indigestion
- Liver and gallbladder problems

In folk medicine, Wormwood has also been used for poor digestion, lack of intestinal muscle tone, inflammation of the digestive tract, stomachache, liver disorders, anemia, menstrual problems, occasional fevers, and worm infestation. Externally, it has been used to aid wound healing and as a remedy for insect bites and skin ulcers and blotches. The effectiveness of these folk uses has not been scientifically verified.

What It Is; Why It Works

The medicinal parts of the Wormwood plant consist of the upper shoots and leaves. Wormwood promotes the production of cholesterol and bilirubin (a component of bile). By stimulating the bitter receptors in the taste buds of the tongue, it triggers an increase in digestive enzymes and stomach acid. The oil in the drug is thought to be antimicrobial, slowing or stopping the growth of certain bacteria.

Wormwood is used in the production of absinthe, a green liqueur with a bitter licorice or anise flavor and a high alcohol content. Production of this liqueur is prohibited in many countries because of possible health problems connected with its use.

Avoid If . . .

There are no known reasons to avoid Wormwood when taken in typical dosages.

Special Cautions

Do not use continuously.

Possible Drug Interactions

No interactions have been reported.

Special Information If You Are Pregnant or Breastfeeding

No harmful effects are known.

How to Prepare

Crushed Wormwood can be made into tea by steeping 1 gram (about one-quarter teaspoonful) of the herb in 1 cup of boiling water. You may also find fluid extracts of Wormwood, solutions of Wormwood in alcohol (tinctures), and powders and solid forms of Wormwood.

Typical Dosage

The usual oral dosage is:

Tea: 1 cup, freshly prepared, 30 minutes before each meal
Tincture: 10 to 30 drops, in water, 3 times daily
Liquid extract: 1 to 2 milliliters (about one-quarter teaspoonful) 3 times daily

Strengths of commercial preparations may vary. Follow the manufacturer's labeling whenever available.

Overdosage

Large doses of Wormwood can cause vomiting, stomach and intestinal cramps, headache, dizziness, and problems with the nervous system. If you suspect an overdose, seek medical attention immediately.

Yarrow

Latin name: Achillea millefolium
Other names: Bloodwort, Devil's
Nettle, Milfoil, Sanguinary,
Staunchweed

A Remedy For

- Appetite loss
- Gallbladder disorders
- Indigestion
- Liver disorders

Although Yarrow's effectiveness has been thoroughly documented for only the four problems listed above, it has long been used externally to stanch bleeding and relieve skin inflammation, bruises, and burns. It has also been employed as a remedy for menstrual problems and pelvic cramps.·

What It Is; Why It Works

Named in Latin for the Greek hero Achilles, who is supposed to have discovered it, Yarrow has a long history in medicine and folklore. In medieval times, it was thought to be a headache cure (through its ability to cause nosebleeds, which were considered therapeutic). People also fancied that sleeping with Yarrow under the pillow would bring visions of their future spouse.

Today, researchers have narrowed its properties down to a few key medicinal actions. It soothes the digestive system by relieving muscle spasms in the intestines, promotes the flow of digestive bile, fights bacterial invasion, and firms and tightens tissues. It is a hardy plant, about 5 feet high, with delicate, finely divided leaves and white, pink, or purple flowers. It thrives in eastern, southeastern, and central Europe, and along the southern edge of the Alps from Switzerland to the Balkans.

Avoid If . . .

Yarrow can trigger an allergic reaction in some people. Avoid it if you have this response.

Special Cautions

Aside from its allergic potential, Yarrow poses no hazards when taken at customary dosage levels.

Possible Drug Interactions

No drug interactions have been reported.

Special Information If You Are Pregnant or Breastfeeding

No harmful effects are known.

How to Prepare

To make a tea, steep 2 grams of finely cut Yarrow in boiling water for 10 to 15 minutes, covered, then strain.

For baths, use 20 grams (about 4 teaspoonfuls) of Yarrow per gallon of water.

Typical Dosage

The usual daily dosage for internal use is:

Yarrow leaf: 4.5 grams
Yarrow flower: 3 grams

Pressed juice and essential oil preparations are also available. Since potency may vary, follow manufacturer's directions whenever available. Store away from light and moisture.

Overdosage
No information on overdosage is available.

Yellow Dock

Latin name: Rumex crispus
Other name: Curled Dock

A Remedy For
- Constipation
- Liver and gallbladder problems
- Skin inflammation
- Tendency to infection

Although not officially recognized, the effectiveness of Yellow Dock has been documented for the above four conditions. In homeopathic medicine, it is used for cough, itching, pain, and respiratory tract disorders.

What It Is; Why It Works
Traditionally used as a "blood cleanser," the medicinal part of *Rumex crispus* is the root.

Avoid If . . .
No known medical conditions preclude the use of Yellow Dock.

Special Cautions
At customary dosage levels, Yellow Dock preparations pose no problems. However, the fresh root can cause vomiting.

Possible Drug Interactions
There are no known drug interactions.

Special Information If You Are Pregnant or Breastfeeding
No information is available.

How to Prepare
Yellow Dock is taken in the form of ground root or extract.

Typical Dosage
General guidelines are unavailable. Follow the manufacturer's labeling.

Overdosage
Although root preparations generally present no threat, fresh Yellow Dock leaves can be poisonous. At least one death has been reported following consumption of a soup made from Yellow Dock leaves.

Yohimbe

Latin name: Pausinystalia yohimbe

A Remedy For
Yohimbe is used primarily as a remedy for impotence. Due to its numerous side effects, it is not, however, recommended for this purpose.

What It Is; Why It Works
Yohimbine, the active ingredient in Yohimbe, is thought to increase the flow of blood to the penis, while inhibiting its outflow. The drug is available by prescription under the brand name Yocon. But with the more effective and less trouble-prone drug Viagra now on the market, de-

mand for yohimbine seems likely to wither.

Avoid If . . .

Do not use Yohimbe if you have heart disease, kidney or liver problems, or a history of ulcers.

Special Cautions

Potential side effects include agitation, anxiety, sleeplessness, tremors, dizziness, headache, queasiness, vomiting, elevated blood pressure, and fast heartbeat.

Possible Drug Interactions

Do not combine Yohimbe with mood-altering drugs such as antidepressants.

Special Information If You Are Pregnant or Breastfeeding

Yohimbe is not for use by women, and should not be used during pregnancy.

How to Prepare

The active ingredient Yohimbine is available in tablet form.

Typical Dosage

The usual recommendation is one 5.4 milligram tablet 3 times daily. If side effects appear, the doses can be temporarily reduced to one-half tablet.

Strengths of commercial preparations may vary. Follow the manufacturer's labeling whenever available.

Overdosage

An overdose can be fatal. Symptoms include salivation, dilated pupils, emptying of the bowels, low blood pressure, and irregular heartbeat ending in heart failure. If you suspect an overdose, seek emergency medical attention immediately.

Yucca

*Latin name: Yucca schidigera
(and other species)*

A Remedy For

Yucca is currently being used as a treatment for arthritis, although its effectiveness has not been officially recognized. In the past, Native Americans have used Yucca for sprains, sores, bleeding, and all sorts of inflammation. As a shampoo, it has even been used to fight dandruff and hair loss.

What It Is; Why It Works

Yucca, a desert plant related to the Joshua tree, grows primarily in the southwestern United States. The medicinal parts are the stalk and root.

Yucca can be regarded as fairly safe; it's an FDA-approved food additive, used as a foaming agent in beverages such as root beer. Researchers testing Yucca for its effect against arthritis speculate that it works by blocking intestinal release of toxins that inhibit normal formation of cartilage. In test-tube studies, an extract of one species of Yucca has been found to fight deadly melanoma cancer cells.

Avoid If . . .

Yucca poses a theoretical danger to red blood cells. In test-tube studies, ingredients in Yucca have caused the cells to burst (a process known as hemolysis). However, this problem has never been reported in humans, and the herb is considered otherwise safe under all medical conditions.

Special Cautions

Large doses may cause loose stools.

Possible Drug Interactions

No interactions have been reported.

Special Information If You Are Pregnant or Breastfeeding

No harmful effects are known.

How to Prepare

Yucca is available in root form, and in tablets and capsules containing the active ingredients (Yucca saponins).

To make Yucca tea, combine one-quarter ounce of the root with a pint of water and boil for 15 minutes.

Typical Dosage

Yucca saponins: 2 to 4 capsules or tablets per day, depending on the severity of the arthritis

Tea: 3 to 5 cups per day

Overdosage

No information on overdosage is available.

Zedoary

Latin name: Curcuma zedoaria

A Remedy For

• Indigestion

Although its effectiveness awaits conclusive proof, Zedoary appears to be a helpful remedy for digestive problems such as heartburn, bloating, nausea, gas, cramps, and stomach pain. In folk medicine it's also used for nervous diseases, and in Asia it's considered a remedy for heavy menstrual flow.

What It Is; Why It Works

The medicinal part of the plant is the fleshy underground stem. It stimulates production of digestive juices, improves the flow of bile into the digestive tract, and combats digestive spasms. Zedoary extracts are contained in many herbal combinations used to treat gastrointestinal problems and stimulate the flow of bile.

Although Zedoary comes from the same plant family as turmeric, the popular Indian spice, it has a bitter taste and plays no role in cuisine.

Avoid If . . .

No known medical conditions preclude the use of Zedoary.

Special Cautions

At customary dosage levels, Zedoary poses no problems.

Possible Drug Interactions

No interactions have been reported.

Special Information If You Are Pregnant or Breastfeeding

No harmful effects are known.

How to Prepare

You can make a tea using 1 to 1.5 grams (about one-half teaspoonful) of crushed or powdered Zedoary. Pour boiling water over the herb or mix it with cold water. Strain after 3 to 5 minutes.

Typical Dosage

Zedoary is taken orally. The usual dosage is 1 cup of tea at mealtimes.

Strengths of commercial preparations may vary. Follow the manufacturer's labeling whenever available.

Overdosage

No information on overdosage is available.

PART FOUR

Guide to Nutritional Therapy

Alpha-Tocopherol

See Vitamin E

Arginine

See Nonessential Amino Acids

Ascorbic Acid

See Vitamin C

Aspartic Acid

See Nonessential Amino Acids

Beta-Carotene

See Vitamin A

Beta-Tocopherol

See Vitamin E

Biotin

What It Is

Biotin, sometimes called vitamin H, is produced naturally within the body by normal intestinal bacteria. This supply is all that a normal, healthy adult needs. Biotin is one of the water-soluble vitamins. There is no synthetic form available.

What It Does

Biotin helps the body form fatty acids and process amino acids, starches, and sugars.

Why You Need It

Biotin helps maintain the health of the body's sweat glands, nerve tissue, blood cells, bone marrow, skin, hair, and male sex glands.

Can You Take Too Much?

Scientists currently consider natural biotin supplements to be nontoxic. Doses of 50 to 100 times the recommended intake have caused no ill effects.

Recommended Daily Allowances

The government has not yet established an official recommended dietary allowance (RDA) for biotin.

ADULTS

The estimated adequate intake for everyone 11 years of age and older is 100 to 200 micrograms per day.

CHILDREN

The following daily amounts are estimated to be adequate for children.

Infants up to 6 months:	35 micrograms
Ages 6 to 12 months:	50 micrograms
Ages 1 to 3 years:	65 micrograms
Ages 4 to 6 years:	85 micrograms
Ages 7 to 10 years:	120 micrograms

Best Dietary Sources

Biotin is found in dairy products, including butter, cheese, and milk; nuts, including cashews, peanuts, and walnuts; vegetables, including green peas, lentils, soybeans, and split peas; meats; organ meats, especially calves liver; chicken; eggs; fish, including mackerel and tuna; whole grain foods, including brown rice, bulgur, wheat, and oats; sunflower seeds; and brewer's yeast.

Branched-Chain Amino Acids

What They Are

Three essential amino acids—leucine, isoleucine, and valine—form the so-called branched chain. Amino acids are the building blocks of protein. These three are among those considered "essential" because they cannot be manufactured in the body and must be obtained through diet.

What They Do

Along with the other amino acids, the branched-chain acids are the raw material used by the body to manufacture human proteins. These proteins are a vital component of all the body's cells.

Why You Need Them

Scientific evidence shows that branched-chain amino acids may help restore muscle mass following surgery, an injury, or trauma. They also help in people who have liver disease. There currently is no evidence that extra branched-chain amino acids are beneficial for healthy individuals. However, a general deficiency of protein in the diet can cause a loss of stamina, lowered resistance to infection, slow healing of wounds, weakness, and depression.

Can You Take Too Much?

Amino acids are rarely toxic, even in large amounts.

Recommended Daily Allowances

There is no official recommended dietary allowance for the branched-chain amino acids, either separately or as a group.

The estimated adult daily requirement for leucine is nearly 9 milligrams per pound of body weight. Infants require almost 5 times that amount; children need approximately twice the adult requirement.

For isoleucine, the estimated adult daily requirement is about 6 milligrams per pound of body weight. Infants require more than 3 times that amount; the requirement for children is about twice the adult amount.

The estimated adult daily requirement for valine is also about 6 milligrams per pound of body weight. Infants require more than 4 times that amount, while children need about twice the adult requirement.

Your total daily requirement for protein in general is the number of grams equal to half your body weight. For instance, if you weigh 160 pounds, you need 80 grams of protein daily.

Best Dietary Sources

These and other amino acids are available in most meat and dairy products.

Calcifidol

See Vitamin D

Calcitriol

See Vitamin D

Calcium

What It Is

Calcium and phosphorus—the two most abundant minerals in our bodies—work together to keep our bones and teeth healthy. Calcium is found in many foods—most notably dairy products—and is also available as natural and synthetic supplements. You will need a prescription for certain forms of calcium; others can be purchased over the counter.

What It Does

Fully 99 percent of our calcium deposits are stored in the bones. In response to the body's needs, calcium moves out of the bones into the bloodstream and then back into the bones for continued storage. Most of the remaining 1 percent of our calcium supply is located in body fluids, where it helps transmit nerve impulses. Calcium also promotes blood coagulation and plays an essential role in enabling muscles, such as the heart, to relax and contract.

Why You Need It

Calcium is essential to a child's normal growth and development, and everyone needs an adequate supply to keep bones and teeth strong and healthy. Because of the part it plays in muscle activity, some people take it to prevent muscle cramps; others use it to alleviate their severe muscle spasms that accompany a disorder called tetany.

One of calcium's more recently—and widely—publicized

benefits is its ability to stave off the brittle-bone disease osteoporosis when used in combination with estrogen.

Can You Take Too Much?

Doses above 2,000 milligrams per day can lead to potentially serious problems, including development of kidney stones. A loss of appetite, constipation, drowsiness, dry mouth or a metallic taste in the mouth, headache, and a feeling of fatigue or weakness could be early warning signs that there is too much calcium in your system. Later signs may include confusion, depression, nausea, vomiting, pain in bones or muscles, high blood pressure, increased thirst or urination, increased sensitivity of the eyes or skin to light, itchy skin or rash, and a slow or irregular heartbeat. If you notice any of these symptoms and you think the amount of calcium you have been taking could be the source of the problem, stop using the supplements and call your doctor. If you think your heartbeat is either irregular or slow, seek medical attention immediately.

Recommended Daily Allowances

ADULTS

The basic allowance for everyone 18 years of age and older is 800 milligrams.

Women need an additional 400 milligrams of calcium each day during pregnancy and as long as they breastfeed. Do not take megadoses of calcium during pregnancy or while breastfeeding. Calcium does pass into the breast milk.

Many experts believe that we need more calcium than the official recommendation and suggest the following amounts: 1,000 milligrams of calcium per day for premenopausal women and, due to the risk of osteoporosis, 1,500 milligrams for postmenopausal women and for both elderly men and women past the age of 65.

CHILDREN

Infants up to 6 months:	400 milligrams
Ages 6 to 12 months:	600 milligrams
Ages 1 to 10 years:	800 milligrams
Ages 11 to 24 years:	1,200 milligrams

All calcium supplements are not created equal. The body only absorbs part of the calcium it takes in, and different forms of calcium provide varying amounts of this mineral. Calcium citrate may provide a bit more usable calcium than other forms, and is less likely to have side effects. Calcium carbonate is often recommended because it contains the highest percentage of absorbable calcium. It is also the cheapest and has the added advantage of acting as an antacid. Two 1,250- or 1,500-milligram tablets of calcium carbonate per day will provide 1,000 milligrams of what is called "available" calcium to the body.

To get the same 1,000 milligrams from other forms of calcium, you need to take up to 12 tablets a day. Divide the following amounts into more than one dose and take them after meals: two 1,600-milligram tablets of calcium phosphate, five 950-milligram tablets of calcium citrate, eleven 1,000-milligram tablets of calcium gluconate, twelve 650-milligram tablets of calcium lactate, and 12 teaspoons of calcium glubionate. Chelated calcium tablets and combinations of calcium and other vitamins and minerals such as vitamin D and magnesium offer no special advantage. Also avoid bone meal and dolomite—they may contain toxic lead, mercury, and arsenic.

Whichever supplement you choose, check the information supplied with it to determine the dosage that will supply the amount of calcium you need. Remember, too, that smoking and drinking alcohol, coffee, or tea increases the amount of calcium that your body will lose.

Best Dietary Sources

Calcium is found in dairy products, shrimp, canned salmon and sardines, green leafy vegetables, Brazil nuts and almonds, molasses, soybeans, and tofu.

One cup of yogurt contains up to 415 milligrams of calcium. There are 300 milligrams in 1 cup of skim milk, and 290 milligrams in 1 cup of whole milk. One slice of Swiss cheese provides 270 milligrams; 1 cup of cottage cheese, 230 milligrams; 1 ounce of cheddar cheese, 200

milligrams; 1 stalk of broccoli, cooked, 160 milligrams; and one 4-ounce piece of tofu, 150 milligrams.

Carotene

See Vitamin A

Chloride

What It Is

Chloride is a component of hydrochloric (stomach) acid. This mineral is also found in various salt products. Natural and synthetic supplements are available.

What It Does

Chloride helps maintain the acid balance in the body's cells and fluids.

Why You Need It

Chloride is essential to good health. Without it, the delicate chemical balance in the body will go awry.

Can You Take Too Much?

Too much—or too little—chloride in your system can lead to weakness or confusion. At the extreme, you could go into a coma.

Recommended Daily Allowances

ADULTS

The RDA for everyone 18 years of age and older is 1.75 to 5.1 grams.

CHILDREN

Infants up to 6 months:	0.275 to 0.7 grams
Ages 6 to 12 months:	0.4 to 1.2 grams
Ages 1 to 3 years:	0.5 to 1.5 grams
Ages 4 to 6 years:	0.7 to 2.1 grams
Ages 7 to 10 years:	0.925 to 2.775 grams
Ages 11 to 17 years:	1.4 to 4.2 grams

Best Dietary Sources

Most of our chloride intake comes from table salt, which contains sodium chloride; salt substitutes, which contain potassium chloride, and sea salt.

Cholecalciferol

See Vitamin D

Choline

What It Is

Choline, present to some degree in all our food, plays an important role in the nervous system. Natural and synthetic supplements are available. Choline is also a component of lecithin, another nutrient available in supplement form. It is part of the B complex of vitamins.

What It Does

The body uses choline to make acetylcholine, a substance essential for transmission of signals in many parts of the nervous system. Choline also aids in the transport of fats into the body's cells, and is vital to the health of the liver and kidneys.

Why You Need It

Although choline deficiency is rare, it can lead to internal bleeding in the kidneys, excessively high blood pressure, heart disease, and degeneration of the liver.

If you have high cholesterol and triglyceride levels and are taking nicotinic acid (a form of niacin) as a treatment, you may need choline supplements, since high levels of niacin can deplete the choline in your system.

Can You Take Too Much?

Sustained megadosing (above 6,000 milligrams) can cause dizziness, nausea, and vomiting. If you develop any of these symptoms, stop taking the choline supplement and call your physician.

Recommended Daily Allowances

The government has not yet established a recommended dietary allowance (RDA) for choline. A typical diet provides 500 to 900 milligrams daily. Taking more than 1 gram of supplementary choline per day is not generally recommended; and healthy women should not take choline supplements at all during pregnancy or while breastfeeding.

Best Dietary Sources

Foods richest in choline include cabbage, cauliflower, chickpeas, green beans, lentils, soybeans, split peas, calves' liver, eggs, rice, and soy lecithin.

Chromium

What It Is

Chromium is one of the minerals that the body needs in only trace amounts. It is found in a variety of meats, seafood, dairy products, eggs, and whole-grain foods.

What It Does

Chromium helps the body to convert blood sugar (glucose) into energy. It also makes insulin work more efficiently and effectively.

Why You Need It

Because chromium makes it easier for the body to burn glucose, chromium supplements have recently been touted as energy-boosters. In addition, chromium's alliance with insulin makes it especially important for diabetics. It can help some people who develop diabetes as older adults better tolerate glucose, thereby reducing the amount of insulin they need to control their sugar levels.

Can You Take Too Much?

The chromium in food and vitamin/mineral supplements poses no danger. Indeed, Americans are thought to not get enough. However, long-term exposure on the job has reportedly led to skin problems, perforation of the nasal septum, liver or kidney impairment, and lung cancer in some people.

Recommended Daily Allowances

The government has not yet established the recommended daily amount (RDA) of chromium. The estimated safe and adequate daily intake is as follows:

ADULTS

All adults:	50 to 200 micrograms

CHILDREN

Infants up to 6 months:	1 to 40 micrograms
Ages 6 to 12 months:	20 to 60 micrograms
Ages 1 to 3 years:	20 to 80 micrograms
Ages 4 to 6 years:	30 to 120 micrograms
Ages 7 and older:	50 to 200 micrograms

Women should avoid chromium supplements during pregnancy and while they are breastfeeding an infant.

Best Dietary Sources

You can obtain chromium from meats, including beef, chicken, and calves' liver; fish, oysters, and other seafood; cheese and other dairy products; eggs; fresh fruit; potatoes (with skin); whole grain products; brewer's yeast; and condiments such as black pepper and thyme.

Cobalamin

See Vitamin B$_{12}$

Cobalt

What It Is

Cobalt, one of the minerals we need in just trace amounts, is stored in the liver. This mineral is readily available in a well-balanced diet, and deficiencies are rare.

What It Does

Cobalt is closely related to vitamin B_{12}, and is therefore essential to the production of the red blood cells that carry oxygen throughout the body.

Why You Need It

An inadequate supply of cobalt can lead to the condition called pernicious anemia. Symptoms include digestive problems, weight loss, and a burning feeling in the tongue.

What's Too Much?

Megadoses of cobalt—in the range of 20 to 30 milligrams per day—can lead to serious problems. Cobalt toxicity can cause the thyroid gland to grow too large in infants or to become enlarged in adults. The heart may also grow too large and congestive heart failure could result. In addition, excessive cobalt exposure can lead to an abnormally high level of red blood cells.

Recommended Daily Allowances

Cobalt deficiencies are extremely rare, and the government has yet to establish a recommended dietary allowance.

Best Dietary Sources

The small amounts of cobalt in a well-balanced diet will satisfy the cobalt requirements of most people. The richest sources are meats, particularly kidney and liver; clams and oysters; milk; figs; and buckwheat. There is some cobalt available in vegetables such as cabbage, lettuce, and spinach; but strict vegetarians are at greater risk of a deficiency than others.

Copper

What It Is

Copper is one of the minerals used by the body in only trace amounts. It is an essential ingredient of proteins and enzymes.

What It Does

Copper plays a major role in the body's ability to store and use iron. This important mineral triggers the release of iron, which then forms the hemoglobin in red blood cells. The body also uses this mineral to produce various enzymes it needs to maintain its tissues.

Why You Need It

Because of its role in the production of hemoglobin, copper helps to prevent anemia. A deficiency of copper, though rare, can lead to weakness, poor respiration, and skin sores.

Can You Take Too Much?

Nausea, vomiting, stomach pain, and muscle aches may be signs that you have too much copper in your system. Excessive amounts of copper can lead to anemia in some people.

Recommended Daily Allowances

The government has not yet established a recommended dietary allowance (RDA) for copper. Estimated safe and adequate daily intake is as follows:

ADULTS

All adults:	2 to 3 milligrams

Women should not take megadoses of copper during pregnancy or while they are breastfeeding.

CHILDREN

Infants up to 6 months:	0.5 to 0.7 milligrams
Ages 6 to 12 months:	0.7 to 1 milligrams
Ages 1 to 3 years:	1 to 1.5 milligrams
Ages 4 to 6 years:	1.5 to 2 milligrams
Ages 7 to 10 years:	2 to 2.5 milligrams
Ages 11 and older:	2 to 3 milligrams

Best Dietary Sources

You can obtain copper from nuts, including Brazil nuts, cashews, hazelnuts, peanuts, and walnuts; barley and lentils; honey and black-strap molasses; mussels, oysters, and salmon; mushrooms; oats; and wheat germ.

Cyanocobalamin

See Vitamin B$_{12}$

Cysteine

See Nonessential Amino Acids

Delta-Tocopherol

See Vitamin E

DHA

See Omega-3 Fatty Acids

Dibasic Calcium Phosphate

See Calcium

Dihydrotachysterol

See Vitamin D

Docosahexaenoic Acid

See Omega-3 Fatty Acids

Eicosopentaenoic Acid

See Omega-3 Fatty Acids

EPA

See Omega-3 Fatty Acids

Ergocalciferol

See Vitamin D

Evening Primrose Oil

See Gamma-Linolenic Acid

Ferrous Fumarate

See Iron

Ferrous Gluconate

See Iron

Ferrous Sulfate

See Iron

Fiber

What It Is
Fiber is the material that gives plants their stability and structure. There are two types: soluble fiber, which dissolves within the digestive system, and insoluble fiber, which is unaffected by digestion. Both pass through the body without being absorbed.

Fiber is found to some degree in all vegetables, fruits, nuts, and grains, and is also available as a supplement.

What It Does
Fiber acts much like a sponge, and is able to absorb many times its weight in water. Soluble fiber absorbs cholesterol-containing bile from the digestive system and clears it from the body.

Why You Need It
Insoluble fiber adds bulk to bowel movements, helping to prevent constipation, hemorrhoids, diver-

ticulosis, and—over the long-term—colorectal cancer. Soluble fiber helps reduce the levels of cholesterol and triglycerides in the blood and works to moderate blood sugar levels as well.

Can You Take Too Much?
A sudden increase in fiber intake can cause bloating and gas. Tremendous amounts could cause a blockage in the large intestine, although this is a rare occurrence. A diet with 25 grams of fiber for each 1,000 calories eaten is considered high in fiber.

Recommended Daily Allowances
There is no official recommended dietary allowance (RDA) for fiber. Nutrition experts advise intake of at least 20 to 30 grams a day.

Although no problems have surfaced, women who are pregnant or breastfeeding should not use fiber supplements unless prescribed by a physician. Fiber supplements are hazardous to children younger than two years of age.

Best Dietary Sources
Good sources of fiber include: fruits and vegetables, nuts, seeds, and whole-grain products. Beans and lentils are excellent sources of soluble fiber.

Fish Oils

See Omega-3 Fatty Acids

Fluoride

What It Is
Fluoride, one of the minerals we require in only trace amounts, is best known as sodium fluoride, an ingredient in many toothpastes. Fluoride occurs naturally in some foods, and supplements are also available, with a physician's prescription.

What It Does
Fluoride helps the body retain the calcium it needs for strong bones and teeth.

Why You Need It
Fluoride supplements are prescribed to prevent dental cavities in children living where the fluoride level in the drinking water is inadequate. Children who need extra fluoride generally keep taking supplements until they are 16 years old. Physicians also use fluoride, along with calcium and vitamin D, to treat osteoporosis. It is important to note that this treatment must be supervised by a doctor.

Can You Take Too Much?
A dose of fluoride 2,500 times the standard recommendation can be fatal. Smaller overdoses can eventually lead to stomach cramps or pain, diarrhea, black stools, and vomiting, which could be bloody. A feeling of faintness, shallow breathing, increased saliva, tremors, and an unusual feeling of excitement are also potential warning signs of fluoride toxicity. Stop taking fluoride and call your doctor if you develop any of these symptoms.

Recommended Daily Allowances
The government has not yet established a recommended dietary allowance (RDA) for fluoride. The estimated safe and adequate daily intake is as follows:

ADULTS

All adults:	1.5 to 4 milligrams

The experts disagree about whether it is safe—or beneficial—to take fluoride supplements during pregnancy. At this time experts feel that breastfeeding mothers who take additional fluoride need not anticipate problems with their infants. However, it is best to discuss your specific needs with your physician and to avoid taking megadoses of fluoride while pregnant or breastfeeding.

CHILDREN

Infants up to 6 months:	0.1 to 0.5 milligrams
Ages 6 to 12 months:	0.2 to 1 milligrams
Ages 1 to 3 years:	0.5 to 1.5 milligrams
Ages 4 to 6 years:	1 to 2.5 milligrams
Ages 7 to 10 years:	1.5 to 2.5 milligrams
Ages 11 and older:	1.5 to 4 milligrams

Best Dietary Sources
Fluoride can be found in organ meats, including calves' liver and

kidneys; fish and seafood, including cod, canned salmon, and canned sardines; apples; eggs; and tea. Note, however, that the amount of fluoride in these foods can vary greatly. It is much higher in areas where the soil is rich, and the water is fluoridated.

Folacin

See Folic Acid

Folate

See Folic Acid

Folic Acid

What It Is

Folic acid is a water-soluble vitamin known by many other names—vitamin B₉, folate, folacin, and tetrahydrofolic acid. It is available in fresh leafy green vegetables and liver. Folic acid is also manufactured synthetically and is included in most multivitamin supplements. An injectable form is available by prescription.

What It Does

Folic acid is essential for the formation of the DNA that makes up our genes and the RNA that transmits their instructions. It is particularly important in the body's production of red blood cells. Folic acid deficiency results in megaloblastic anemia, an anemia similar to that caused by vitamin B_{12} deficiency. Symptoms include weight loss, digestive prob-

lems, and a burning feeling in the tongue.

Why You Need It

Folic acid helps us grow and develop normally. It also regulates nerve cell development in the embryo and the developing baby. Folic acid supplements are used to treat the anemia that may occur with alcoholism, liver disease, pregnancy, breastfeeding, or the use of oral contraceptives.

Can You Take Too Much?

Very high amounts of folic acid have been taken over long periods of time without any adverse effects. However, there is a chance that prolonged use of large amounts might lead to the formation of folacin crystals in the kidneys or cause severe neurologic problems. Symptoms such as loss of appetite, nausea, gas, and abdominal bloating may occur if you take more than 1,500 micrograms of folic acid per day.

Recommended Daily Allowances

ADULTS

For everyone 11 years and older the official recommended dietary allowance is 400 micrograms.

Women need an additional 400 micrograms of folic acid each day during pregnancy. (It is believed that folic acid supplementation during pregnancy may prevent the development of neural tube defects that can lead to mental retardation.) Breastfeeding mothers need an extra 100 micrograms of folic acid per day.

Many others may also require additional folic acid. People who do not eat a well-balanced diet, those over the age of 55, people who abuse alcohol or other drugs, and women who take oral contraceptives should discuss the need for folic acid supplementation with their physicians.

CHILDREN

Infants up to 6 months:	30 micrograms
Ages 6 to 12 months:	45 micrograms
Ages 1 to 3 years:	100 micrograms
Ages 4 to 6 years:	200 micrograms
Ages 7 to 10 years:	300 micrograms

Best Dietary Sources

Folic acid is available in green leafy vegetables such as broccoli, spinach, and romaine lettuce. It is important to note that cooking these vegetables reduces the amount of folic acid the body receives. Other natural sources of folic acid include: fruits—especially oranges and orange juice—calves' liver, brewer's yeast, wheat germ, rice, barley, beans, peas, split peas, chickpeas, lentils, soybeans, and sprouts.

One-half pound of fresh spinach contains 463 micrograms of folic acid; 1 tablespoon of brewer's yeast provides 308 micrograms. One-half cup of dry soybeans has 236 micrograms of folic acid; 1 cup of fresh orange juice provides 164 micrograms.

Gamma-Linolenic Acid

What It Is

Gamma-linolenic acid (GLA) is manufactured in the body from linolenic acid, one of the three essential fatty acids required in our diets. It is also found in oil expressed from the seeds of the evening primrose plant, and is available in a supplement called evening primrose oil.

What It Does

Gamma-linolenic acid plays a role in the production of prostaglandins, hormone-like substances that, under some conditions, may help the body fight inflammation.

Why You Need It

Some researchers believe that anti-inflammatory properties of certain prostaglandins that gamma-linolenic acid helps form may play a role in the body's ability to fight arthritis.

Can You Take Too Much?

There is currently no evidence that gamma-linolenic acid is toxic.

Recommended Daily Allowances

No recommended allowance has been established for this substance.

Best Dietary Sources

Gamma-linolenic acid is found in fish.

Gamma-Tocopherol

See Vitamin E

GLA

See Gamma-Linolenic Acid

Glutamic Acid

See Nonessential Amino Acids

Glutamine

See Nonessential Amino Acids

Glycine

See Nonessential Amino Acids

Histidine

See Nonessential Amino Acids

Inositol

What It Is

Inositol is part of the vitamin B complex. The body manufactures its own supply of this substance, which it then uses to produce lecithin, a compound that aids in the body's utilization of fats. Inositol is found in many foods and is available both as a separate supplement and as a component of lecithin supplements.

What It Does

As a component of lecithin, inositol is responsible for transferring needed fats from the liver to the body's cells.

Why You Need It

By assisting in the proper utilization of fat and cholesterol, inositol lowers blood cholesterol levels, thus protecting the arteries and heart from excessive cholesterol build-up.

Can You Take Too Much?

Inositol has not been found toxic at any dosage level.

Recommended Daily Allowances

The government has not yet established a recommended dietary allowance (RDA) for inositol, but doctors usually order no more than 500 to 1,000 milligrams daily when prescribing a supplement.

Best Dietary Sources

Inositol is found in dried beans, chickpeas, and lentils; cantaloupe and citrus fruit (other than lemons); calves' liver, pork, and veal; nuts; oats; rice; whole-grain products; lecithin granules; and wheat germ.

Iodine

What It Is

Iodine, one of the minerals that we need in only trace amounts, appears in various fish and seafood products and is also available as a natural supplement.

A physician's prescription is necessary for the larger dosage strengths.

What It Does

Iodine is an important ingredient in the thyroid hormones that regulate many bodily functions.

Why You Need It

Iodine is essential for proper functioning of the thyroid gland. Doctors use this mineral to shrink the thyroid prior to surgery and in tests to see how well the gland is working. Iodine is also useful in the treatment of goiter, an enlargement of the thyroid gland that appears as a swelling in the neck area. Iodine helps the cells function normally and keeps skin, hair, and nails healthy.

Can You Take Too Much?

Warning signs that you may have too much iodine in your system include confusion, an irregular heartbeat, and stools that are either bloody or black and tarry. If you develop any of these symptoms of potential iodine toxicity, stop taking the supplement and call your doctor.

Recommended Daily Allowances

ADULTS

All adults:	150 micrograms

Women require an additional 25 micrograms of iodine each day during pregnancy. Women who are breastfeeding an infant need an extra 50 micrograms per day.

Although pregnant women need some additional iodine, too much can have serious consequences. Excessive amounts can give the baby an enlarged thyroid or an underactive thyroid. Cretinism, a form of dwarfism accompanied by mental deficiency, is another possible birth defect related to excessive iodine intake during pregnancy.

Breastfeeding mothers should avoid taking iodine supplements and megadoses while nursing an infant. The iodine that appears in breast milk may cause a skin rash, and can keep the baby's thyroid from functioning properly.

CHILDREN

Infants up to 6 months:	40 micrograms
Ages 6 to 12 months:	50 micrograms
Ages 1 to 3 years:	70 micrograms
Ages 4 to 6 years:	90 micrograms
Ages 7 to 10 years:	120 micrograms
Ages 11 and older:	150 micrograms

Best Dietary Sources

Fish and seafood, including cod, haddock, herring, lobster, oysters, shrimp, and canned salmon are the primary sources of iodine. Other natural sources include cod-liver oil, sunflower seeds, iodized table salt, sea salt, and seaweed.

Iron

What It Is

Although we've all heard that iron is essential for good blood, it is actually one of the minerals that we need in only trace amounts. Iron is supplied in a wide range of foods and in several different supplement formulations, including ferrous fumarate, ferrous gluconate, ferrous sulfate, and, for deep muscle injections, iron dextran.

What It Does

Iron is an essential part of hemoglobin, the red part of red blood cells that carries oxygen throughout the body. Hemoglobin stores approximately 60 to 70 percent of the body's iron supply. Additional iron stored in muscle tissue helps deliver the oxygen needed to make the muscles contract.

Why You Need It

Iron deficiency leads to anemia—failure of the blood to supply sufficient oxygen to the body's cells. Signs of severe anemia include weakness, dizziness, headache, drowsiness, fatigue, and irritability.

Can You Take Too Much?

Damage from a single dose of iron is unlikely. You would need to take more than 1,000 times the RDA for the dose to be fatal. However, iron can build up to toxic levels gradually within the body, especially in older men. Early signs that you may have too much iron in your system are abdominal pain, severe nausea, diarrhea, or vomiting with blood. As iron toxicity intensifies, you may begin to feel weak or even collapse. Your skin may look pale, while your lips, hands, and fingernails begin to take on a bluish tinge. Shallow breathing and a weak, rapid heartbeat are also among the later warning signs of iron overdose. Extreme toxicity can cause convulsions and coma.

When first taking an iron supplement, you may find your stools turning black or gray. This is not a problem. However, if you notice blood in the stool, seek treatment immediately.

Emergency treatment is also essential if you have chest pain, chills, hives, shortness of breath, or a skin rash, or if you lose consciousness. If you develop these symptoms, discontinue taking the supplement and call your doctor.

Recommended Daily Allowances

ADULTS

Males 11 to 18:	18 milligrams
Males 19 and older:	10 milligrams
Females 11 to 50:	18 milligrams
Females 51 and older:	10 milligrams

Women need an extra 30 to 60 milligrams of iron each day during pregnancy and while breastfeeding. However, pregnant women should not take an iron supplement during the first trimester unless prescribed by their physician. Nursing mothers who are healthy and eat a well-balanced diet may not need an iron supplement. In any event, do not take megadoses during pregnancy or while breast-feeding, and do not give your baby an iron supplement without first checking with the doctor.

CHILDREN

Infants up to 6 months:	10 milligrams
Ages 6 months to 3 years:	15 milligrams
Ages 4 to 10 years:	10 milligrams

Best Dietary Sources

Good sources of iron include enriched bread; prune juice; nuts, including cashews, pistachios, and walnuts; caviar; cheddar cheese; egg yolks; chickpeas; lentils; pumpkin seeds; black-strap molasses; mussels; wheat germ; whole-grain products; and seaweed.

One cup of prune juice contains 10.5 milligrams of iron, a cup of cooked chickpeas nearly 7 milligrams, and a cup of cooked spinach 4.2 milligrams. Cooking in iron pots and pans greatly increases the amount of iron in your food.

Humans have trouble absorbing iron, even from foods rich in the mineral. A person with normal iron levels will probably absorb only about 10 percent of the iron available in food. A person with an iron deficiency, however, will absorb from 20 to 30 percent of the available iron. Vitamin C increases the body's ability to absorb iron.

Isoleucine

See Branched-Chain Amino Acids

L-Carnitine

What It Is

L-carnitine is a product of two of the essential amino acids that the body cannot produce on its own: lysine and methionine. It can be obtained from meat and dairy products and is also available as natural and synthetic supplements.

What It Does

Lysine, methionine, and the other essential amino acids must all be on hand before the body can manufacture the proteins needed to repair and maintain its tissues.

Why You Need It

Without the essential amino acids, including those in l-carnitine, normal growth and development is impossible. Unless you're a strict vegetarian, however, a deficiency is unlikely. Muscle weakness is the main sign that you may have a deficiency of l-carnitine in your system.

Can You Take Too Much?

Like most amino acids, l-carnitine is rarely toxic, taken in large amounts.

Recommended Daily Allowances

No allowance has been established.

Best Dietary Sources

Natural sources of l-carnitine include dairy products, avocados, and lamb, beef, and other red meats. L-carnitine is also found in the soybean product called tempeh.

Lecithin

What It Is

Lecithin is a natural compound that includes choline, inositol, phosphorus, and various fatty acids. It is found throughout the body, and is available in a variety of foods, as well as natural and synthetic supplements.

What It Does

The choline and inositol in lecithin both play important roles in the body's handling of fats. Choline is also an ingredient of acetylcholine, an essential chemical messenger in many parts of the nervous system.

Why You Need It

By promoting the normal processing of fat and cholesterol, lecithin protects against hardening of the arteries and heart disease. It also helps maintain the health of the liver and kidneys.

If you are taking nicotinic acid (a form of niacin) to lower your cholesterol, you may be advised to take lecithin as a way of boosting your choline intake. High levels of niacin tend to deplete the choline in your system.

Can You Take Too Much?

Excessive doses can cause dizziness, nausea, and vomiting. Follow manufacturers' recommendations, and if you develop any of these symptoms, stop taking the supplement and call your physician.

Recommended Daily Allowances

There is no recommended dietary allowance (RDA) for lecithin. Two tablespoons daily is the usual dosage.

Best Dietary Sources

Good sources of lecithin include cabbage, cauliflower, chickpeas, green beans, lentils, soybeans, corn, split peas, calves' liver, and eggs.

Leucine

See Branched-Chain Amino Acids

Lysine

What It Is

Lysine is one of the amino acids considered "essential" because they cannot be manufactured in the body and must be obtained through diet. Lysine is available in natural and synthetic supplement form.

What It Does

Amino acids are the raw material used by the body to manufacture human proteins. These proteins are a vital component of all the body's cells.

Why You Need It

Lysine plays an especially important role in the production of antibodies, hormones, and enzymes. It is also important for the repair of damaged tissue.

Can You Take Too Much?

Amino acids are rarely toxic, even in large amounts.

Recommended Daily Allowances

There is no official recommended dietary allowance for lysine. The estimated adult daily requirement is approximately 5.5 milligrams per pound of body weight. Infants need 8 times that amount; children, 4 times that amount.

Women who are healthy and eat a well-balanced diet do not require lysine supplementation during pregnancy or while breastfeeding. If you do use a supplement, take it in moderation.

Best Dietary Sources

Good sources of lysine include red meat, milk, cheese, eggs, fish, lima beans, potatoes, soy products, and yeast.

Magnesium

What It Is

Magnesium is one of the minerals that we require in relatively large amounts. It is particularly abundant in green vegetables, and is also available in natural supplements—some of which require a physician's prescription.

What It Does

Magnesium plays many roles in the body. It promotes absorption and use of other minerals such as calcium, helps move sodium and potassium across the cell membranes, is involved in the metabolism of proteins, and turns on essential enzymes.

Why You Need It

Magnesium helps bones grow and teeth remain strong. It enables nerve impulses to travel through the body, keeps the body's metabolism in balance, and helps the muscles—including the heart—work properly. Small amounts of magnesium work as an antacid; large amounts of magnesium work as a laxative.

Can You Take Too Much?

Although magnesium toxicity is rare, it can lead to serious problems, including severe nausea and vomiting, extreme muscle weakness, and difficulty breathing. The blood pressure can drop to an extremely low level, and the heartbeat may become irregular.

If your heartbeat seems irregular, seek emergency medical treatment immediately. Stop taking magnesium supplements and call your doctor if you notice any of the other signs of potential magnesium toxicity. You should also tell your physician if you lose your appetite, develop diarrhea, abdominal pain, mood changes, fatigue, or weakness; or if you experience discomfort when you urinate.

Recommended Daily Allowances

ADULTS

Males 11 to 14 years:	350 milligrams
Males 15 to 18 years:	400 milligrams
Males 18 and older:	350 milligrams
Females 11 and older:	300 milligrams

Women require an additional 150 milligrams of magnesium each day during pregnancy and while breastfeeding an infant. However, it is best to get the extra amount through your diet. Experts advise *against* taking magnesium supplements during pregnancy—the risk to the developing baby outweighs any benefits of supplementation.

You should also avoid taking large quantities of magnesium while you are breastfeeding. If magnesium supplements are necessary, your physician will recommend that you stop breastfeeding.

CHILDREN

Infants up to 6 months:	50 milligrams
Ages 6 to 12 months:	70 milligrams
Ages 1 to 3 years:	150 milligrams
Ages 4 to 6 years:	200 milligrams
Ages 7 to 10 years:	250 milligrams

Best Dietary Sources

Many foods are rich in magnesium. Good sources include fish and seafood, including bluefish, carp, cod, flounder, halibut, herring, mackerel, ocean perch, shrimp, and swordfish; fruits and fruit juice; leafy green vegetables; dairy products; nuts, including almonds; molasses; soybeans; sunflower seeds; wheat germ; and snails.

One-half cup of dry soybeans contains 278 milligrams of magnesium; one-half pound of spinach provides 200 milligrams. One-half of a medium avocado contains 51 milligrams; 1 cup of bottled grape juice has 30 milligrams, a cup of skim milk or buttermilk 34 milligrams, a cup of ice cream 19 milligrams.

Manganese

What It Is

Manganese is one of the minerals needed by the body in relatively small (trace) amounts. Found in many beans, nuts, and grains, it is also available by prescription in natural and synthetic supplements.

What It Does

Manganese is concentrated in the pituitary gland, liver, pancreas, kidney, and bones. It is needed for proper utilization of several of the vitamins, including vitamin C; and it plays a role in the body's production of protein, sugar, fat, and cholesterol. It helps nourish the bones and nerves.

Why You Need It

Without sufficient manganese, the body's system for processing blood sugar may falter, leading to diabetes. The nervous system may also be affected resulting in poor coordination and even seizures.

Can You Take Too Much?

Signs of manganese toxicity include depression, trouble sleeping, and impotence. Some people may develop delusions or experience hallucinations following overdoses.

When taking manganese supplements, seek emergency treatment if you have trouble breathing or suffer leg cramps. Your doctor also needs to know if you lose your appetite, have headaches, or feel unusually tired.

Recommended Daily Allowances

The government has not yet established a recommended dietary allowance (RDA) for manganese. The estimated safe and adequate daily intake is as follows:

ADULTS

All adults: 2.5 to 5 milligrams

Women who are pregnant or breastfeeding should not take supplements that contain manganese unless prescribed by their physician and should never take megadoses of this mineral.

CHILDREN

Infants up to 6
   months: 0.5 to 0.7 milligrams
Ages 6 to 12
   months: 0.7 to 1 milligrams

Ages 1 to
   3 years: 1 to 1.5 milligrams
Ages 4 to
   6 years: 1.5 to 2 milligrams
Ages 7 to
   10 years: 2 to 3 milligrams
Ages 11 and
   older: 2.5 to 5 milligrams

Best Dietary Sources

You can find manganese in vegetables, including dried beans, peas, and spinach; chestnuts, hazelnuts, peanuts, and pecans; buckwheat, bran, barley, and oatmeal; fruits, including avocados and blackberries; cloves and ginger; coffee; and seaweed.

Menadiol

See Vitamin K

Methionine

What It Is

Methionine is one of the amino acids considered "essential" because they cannot be manufactured in the body and must be obtained through diet. Worse yet for strict vegetarians, this particular amino acid is found only in meat and dairy products. However, natural and synthetic methionine supplements are available.

What It Does

Amino acids are the raw material used by the body to manufacture human proteins. These proteins are a vital component of all the body's cells.

Why You Need It

Methionine is thought to be necessary for effective use of two other amino acids, cystine and taurine.

Can You Take Too Much?

Amino acids are rarely toxic, even in large amounts.

Recommended Daily Allowances

There is no official recommended dietary allowance for methionine. The estimated adult daily requirement for methionine and cystine combined is approximately 4.5 milligrams per pound of body weight. Infants need 5 times that amount; children require twice that amount.

Women who are healthy and eat a well-balanced diet do not require methionine supplementation during pregnancy or while breastfeeding. If you do use a supplement, take it in moderation.

Best Dietary Sources

Methionine is found only in meat, fish, eggs, and milk.

Molybdenum

What It Is

Molybdenum is one of the minerals that we need in only trace amounts. It is found in certain vegetables, organ meats, and cereal grains. A molybdenum supplement is available by prescription.

What It Does

Molybdenum is part of the bones, teeth, kidney, and liver. It helps the body use its iron reserves, and plays a role in the burning of fat.

Why You Need It

Because it is an ingredient of tooth enamel, a shortage of molybdenum can contribute to tooth decay. A deficiency can also lead to anemia (oxygen starvation in the tissues), and even impotence.

Can You Take Too Much?

Regular doses of 10 to 15 milligrams of molybdenum per day—20 to 30 times the estimated safe amount—can cause the painfully swollen joints associated with gout. When people take even slightly more than the estimated safe intake of molybdenum, it can deplete the body of copper. Signs of moderate molybdenum toxicity include diarrhea and a depressed growth rate in children.

Recommended Daily Allowances

The government has not yet established a recommended dietary allowance (RDA) for molybdenum. The estimated safe and adequate daily intake is as follows:

ADULTS

All adults: 150 to 500 micrograms

CHILDREN

Infants up to 6
    months: 30 to 60 micrograms

Ages 6 to 12
 months: 40 to 80 micrograms
Ages 1 to 3
 years: 50 to 100 micrograms
Ages 4 to 6
 years: 60 to 150 micrograms
Ages 7 to 10
 years: 100 to 300 micrograms
Ages 11 and
 older: 150 to 500 micrograms

Best Dietary Sources

Molybdenum is found in dark green leafy vegetables; organ meats, including liver, kidney, and sweetbreads; beans, peas, and other legumes; and cereal grains. The actual amount of molybdenum in grains and vegetables depends on the amount in the soil when the produce was growing.

Myo-Inositol

See Inositol

Niacin

What It Is

Niacin, also known as vitamin B_3, is one of the water-soluble vitamins that need constant replenishment.

 Niacin supplements are available in two forms, nicotinic acid (the prescription drug Nicolar) and niacinamide, found in over-the-counter supplements. The nicotinic acid form of vitamin B_3 lowers the amount of cholesterol in the blood, thereby reducing the risk of heart disease. Niacinamide does not have this effect.

What It Does

Niacin helps release the energy from food and aids the body in synthesizing DNA. It works with other compounds to help the body process fat and produce sugar while aiding the tissues to rid themselves of waste products. The nicotinic acid form of the vitamin lowers the amount of cholesterol and triglycerides in the blood.

Why You Need It

Niacin helps the body's skin, nerves, and digestive system stay healthy. It is used to treat dizziness and ringing in the ears and to help prevent premenstrual headaches. Niacin supplements are also given to treat pellagra, a potentially fatal niacin deficiency disease characterized by diarrhea, mental disorders, depression, and skin problems. The nicotinic acid form of niacin is prescribed to reduce the amount of cholesterol and triglycerides in the blood.

Can You Take Too Much?

Too much nicotinic acid—more than 2,000 milligrams a day—over a long period of time may damage the liver or cause a stomach ulcer to flare up. Nausea, vomiting, abdominal cramps or pain, faintness, and a yellowish color to the skin and eyes are warning signs of excessive dosage. The niacinamide form of the vitamin does not have these effects.

Recommended Daily Allowances

ADULTS

Males 11 to 18:	18 milligrams
Males 19 to 22:	19 milligrams
Males 23 to 50:	18 milligrams
Males 50 and older:	16 milligrams
Females 11 to 14:	15 milligrams
Females 15 to 22:	14 milligrams
Females 23 and older:	13 milligrams

Women need an additional 2 milligrams of niacin each day during pregnancy. Breastfeeding mothers need an extra 4 milligrams per day.

CHILDREN

Infants up to 6 months:	6 milligrams
Ages 6 to 12 months:	8 milligrams
Ages 1 to 3 years:	9 milligrams
Ages 4 to 6 years:	11 milligrams
Ages 7 to 10 years:	16 milligrams

Best Dietary Sources

Good sources are lean meats, fish, and poultry, including beef liver, pork, veal, turkey, chicken (white meat), salmon, swordfish, tuna, and halibut. Peanuts, brewer's yeast, and sunflower seeds also provide niacin.

A 4-ounce piece of tofu contains nearly 16 milligrams of niacin. One-half cup of dry soybeans provides 11.5 milligrams. One cup of cottage cheese contains 8 milligrams—about half of the adult RDA.

Niacinamide

See Niacin

Nickel

What It Is

Nickel is one of the minerals that we require in only trace amounts. It is available in some types of food, and as a supplement.

What It Does

Nickel appears to play only a minor role in human nutrition. It is thought to be involved in the body's use of fats and the blood sugar glucose.

Why You Need It

Unlike deficiencies of most other vitamins and minerals, a lack of nickel causes few immediate symptoms. It may aggravate anemia, the condition that results when insufficient oxygen reaches the body's tissues.

Can You Take Too Much?

Although it's difficult to develop a nickel deficiency, too much can definitely be a problem. Symptoms of toxic levels include headache, vertigo, nausea, vomiting, chest pain, and coughing.

Recommended Daily Allowances

No recommendation has been established. The amount found in a normal diet can range from a few micrograms to hundreds of milligrams, depending on the nickel content of the soil in which the food is grown.

Best Dietary Sources

Foods that may contain nickel include grains, beans, vegetables, and seafood.

Nicotinamide

See Niacin

Nicotinic Acid

See Niacin

Nonessential Amino Acids

What They Are

Amino acids are the raw materials used by the body to manufacture human protein—a vital component of all the body's cells. This group of amino acids is labeled "nonessential" because, when the acids are lacking in the diet, they can be manufactured in the body.

What They Do

All the nonessential amino acids must be on hand before the body can synthesize protein; and several have additional, more specialized roles as well.

- **Arginine** turns on human growth hormone and is considered essential during childhood, when the body's production of this amino acid can't keep up with demand.
- **Cystine** is an ingredient of the body's major antioxidant, a substance called glutathione. It thereby plays an important role in neutralizing toxic pollutants and by-products within the body.
- **Glutamic acid** is another component of glutathione. It is related to glutamate, one of the nervous system's chemical messengers. Glutamate appears in our diets as the flavor enhancer MSG.
- **Glutamine** is a derivative of glutamic acid.
- **Glycine** is yet another component of the antioxidant glutathione.
- **Histidine** is needed for growth in children and is deemed essential during the childhood years, when demand outpaces the body's ability to produce this substance.
- **Taurine** helps regulate the nervous system and the muscles.
- **Tyrosine**, which is manufactured from the essential amino acid phenylalanine, plays a role in the production of three of the nervous system's messengers: dopamine, epinephrine, and norepinephrine.

Why You Need Them

Deficiencies of arginine and histidine can stunt growth in small children. Glutamine supplements are prescribed for certain digestive disorders and to treat alcoholism. Taurine is sometimes helpful in the treatment of epilepsy.

Can You Take Too Much?

Large doses of arginine may cause nausea or diarrhea; and excessive amounts of tyrosine can lead to changes in blood pressure and migraine headaches. In general, however, even large amounts of these amino acids in your system are unlikely to cause any severe problems.

Recommended Daily Allowances

There are no official recommended daily allowances for these nutrients; and it is advisable to take supplements only under a doctor's supervision. Women taking supplements while pregnant or breastfeeding should be especially careful to avoid excessive doses.

Best Dietary Sources

A complete set of all the amino acids is available in most meat and dairy products. Arginine can also be found in cereals, whole-wheat products, brown rice, chocolate, popcorn, nuts, raisins, and pumpkin and sesame seeds. Other sources of tyrosine include almonds, peanuts, bananas, avocados, lima beans, pickled herring, and pumpkin and sesame seeds.

Oil of Evening Primrose

See Gamma-Linolenic Acid

Omega-3 Fatty Acids

What They Are

This group of fatty acids, also known as fish oil, have gained popularity as a protective agent for the heart. Omega-3 supplements contain docosahexaenoic

acid (DHA) and eicosapentaenoic acid (EPA).

What They Do

The omega-3 fatty acids are believed to lower the levels of triglycerides (fats) and total cholesterol in the blood, while raising the amount of HDL (good) cholesterol. These acids also discourage unwanted clotting that can aggravate plaque buildup.

Why You Need Them

In people with a cholesterol problem, omega-3 fatty acids can help prevent the buildup of cholesterol-laden plaque that can clog the arteries and lead to heart attack and stroke.

Can You Take Too Much?

Because omega-3 fatty acids discourage clotting, excessive levels can lead to bleeding problems in case of an accident or trauma. Women who menstruate are also in greater danger of developing anemia.

Recommended Daily Allowances

There is no recommended dietary allowance (RDA) for the omega-3 fatty acids.

To increase your intake of the omega-3 fatty acids, nutritionists generally recommend eating more fish (2 to 3 times a week), rather than taking large amounts of supplements. A 7-ounce serving of certain types of fish easily provides 2 to 4 grams of omega-3 fatty acids.

Best Dietary Sources

The omega-3 fatty acids are found in cold-water fish. Best sources include cod, tuna, salmon, halibut, shark, and mackerel. Herring, bluefish, shrimp, flounder, and swordfish also provide good amounts of these acids.

A 7-ounce portion of herring contains 3.2 grams of omega-3 fatty acids. The same serving of salmon or bluefish provides 2.4 grams. Seven ounces of tuna has 1 gram.

PABA

What It Is

Also known as para-aminobenzoic acid, this water-soluble member of the vitamin B complex is closely associated with folic acid. The body receives a constant supply of PABA from friendly bacteria residing in the intestines.

What It Does

PABA plays a role in the breakdown and use of proteins, and in the formation of red blood cells. It also stimulates production of folic acid in the intestines, and helps maintain the health of the skin and hair.

Why You Need It

Unless something—such as a sulfa drug—disrupts intestinal production, there appears to be no need for PABA in the diet. If a deficiency does develop, it is signaled by fatigue, depression, nervousness, headache, and digestive disorders. In ointment form, PABA provides burn relief. It is also used as a sunscreen.

Can You Take Too Much?

Sustained megadosing can cause damage to the liver, heart, and kidneys. Symptoms of overdose include nausea and vomiting.

Recommended Daily Allowances

PABA is normally unneeded; and there is no recommended dietary allowance.

Best Dietary Sources

PABA can be obtained from liver, yeast, wheat germ, and molasses.

Pantethine

See Pantothenic Acid

Pantothenic Acid

What It Is

Pantothenic acid is a water-soluble vitamin also known as vitamin B_5 and pantethine. It is found in a variety of foods and is manufactured synthetically. Your physician can prescribe an injectable form.

What It Does

Pantothenic acid helps the body release energy from carbohydrates, protein, and fat.

Why You Need It

Pantothenic acid helps the body grow and develop normally. Some people believe that this vitamin also helps wounds heal more quickly by stimulating the cells to grow.

Can You Take Too Much?

Even at doses hundreds of times the usual amount, pantothenic acid causes no problems. However, you may develop diarrhea or retain water if you ingest megadoses of 10 grams or more.

Recommended Daily Allowances

A recommended dietary allowance (RDA) has not yet been established for pantothenic acid.

ADULTS

The estimated adequate intake for males and females 10 years of age and older is 4 to 7 milligrams per day.

Women may need additional pantothenic acid during pregnancy or while breastfeeding.

CHILDREN

The estimated adequate daily intake for children is:

Infants up to 6 months:	2 milligrams
Ages 6 months to 3 years:	3 milligrams
Ages 4 to 6 years:	3 to 4 milligrams
Ages 7 to 9 years:	4 to 5 milligrams

Best Dietary Sources

Pantothenic acid is found in all types of meats, including organ meats and especially liver. It is also available in eggs, lobster, whole-grain cereals, wheat germ, brewer's yeast, corn, peas, lentils, soybeans, peanuts, and sunflower seeds.

One-half cup of dry soybeans contains 1.8 milligrams of pantothenic acid; the same amount of lentils contains 1.3 milligrams. One tablespoon of brewer's yeast or 1 cup of fresh peas provides 1.2 milligrams.

Phenylalanine

What It Is

Phenylalanine is one of the amino acids considered "essential" because they cannot be manufactured in the body and must be obtained through diet. Natural and synthetic phenylalanine supplements are also available.

What It Does

Amino acids are the raw material used by the body to manufacture human proteins. These proteins are a vital component of all the body's cells.

Why You Need It

Phenylalanine has a special role in the production of dopamine, epinephrine, and norepinephrine, three chemical messengers that aid in transmitting signals through the nervous system. However, extra phenylalanine can be both helpful and harmful. Do not take phenylalanine supplements without consulting your physician.

Can You Take Too Much?

Potential side effects of excessive phenylalanine include high or low blood pressure and migraine headaches. If you think you may be having a reaction to phenylalanine, stop taking the supplement and call your doctor right away.

Children born without the ability to process phenylalanine can build up dangerous levels of this amino acid, resulting in mental retardation, seizures, extreme hyperactivity, and psychosis. Tests can uncover this condition, called phenylketonuria, in the newborn; and treatment is available.

Recommended Daily Allowances

There is no official recommended dietary allowance for phenylalanine. The estimated adult daily requirement for phenylalanine and the related amino acid tyrosine combined is approximately 7 milligrams per pound of body weight. Infants require almost 9 times that amount; children need 10 milligrams per pound.

Women who are healthy and eat a well-balanced diet do not require phenylalanine supplementation during pregnancy or while breastfeeding. If you do use a supplement take it in moderation.

Best Dietary Sources

Foods rich in phenylalanine include almonds and peanuts; bananas and avocados; cheese and cottage cheese; lima beans; nonfat dried milk; pumpkin and sesame seeds; and pickled herring.

Phosphorus

What It Is

Phosphorus is, after calcium, the body's second most plentiful mineral. It is a major component of the bones, and appears in every cell in the body. Supplements are available in the form of various phosphates.

What It Does

Phosphorus participates in virtually all the chemical reactions in the body. It helps the body use many of the B vitamins, and plays an important role in the utilization of fats, proteins, and carbohydrates. It stimulates muscle contraction, supports cell division and growth, and participates in transmission of nerve impulses.

Why You Need It

As one of the two major ingredients of bones and teeth, phosphorus is essential for normal growth, healing of fractures, and prevention of osteoporosis, the brittle-bone disease. It helps the body produce energy and plays an important role in the growth, maintenance, and repair of all of the tissues. A deficiency can lead to ailments ranging from weight loss and fatigue to arthritis, gum disease, and tooth decay.

Can You Take Too Much?

Phosphorus is not toxic. However potassium phosphate supplements often prescribed for kidney stones can cause side effects, including shortness of breath, an irregular heartbeat, or seizures.

When taking potassium phosphate, call your doctor immediately if you notice any of the following potential warning signs: headache; pain in the abdomen, bones, or joints; confusion; diarrhea; muscle cramps; swelling in your feet or legs; numbness or tingling in your hands and feet; unusual fatigue or thirst; or a decline in urine output.

Recommended Daily Allowances

ADULTS

All adults:	800 milligrams

Women need an extra 400 milligrams of phosphorus each day during pregnancy and while breastfeeding an infant. See your doctor before taking a supplement. Do not take megadoses of this mineral.

CHILDREN

Infants up to 6 months:	240 milligrams
Ages 6 to 12 months:	360 milligrams
Ages 1 to 10 years:	800 milligrams
Ages 11 to 17 years:	1,200 milligrams

Best Dietary Sources

Potassium phosphate occurs naturally in meats, including red meat and calves' liver; poultry; fish and seafood, including tuna, scallops, and canned sardines; milk and milk products; cheddar, pasteurized and processed cheese; eggs; almonds and peanuts; dried beans, peas, and soybeans; pumpkin and sunflower seeds; and whole-grain products.

Potassium

What It Is

Potassium is one of the key minerals required by the body to maintain its normal daily functions. Potassium supplements—often prescribed for people on blood pressure medications—are available in a variety of forms including potassium acetate, potassium bicarbonate, potassium chloride, potassium citrate, and potassium gluconate.

What It Does

Along with sodium, potassium regulates the water balance within the body and its cells. It also helps govern the body's acid balance and the electrical charge within the cells. It is essential to the healthy functioning of the brain, heart, muscles, and kidneys.

Why You Need It

Potassium keeps the heart beating normally, helps the muscles contract, and feeds the cells by controlling the transfer of nutrients from surrounding fluids. It helps the kidneys remove waste products from the body, works with phosphorus to supply oxygen to the brain, and cooperates with calcium to regulate the nerves.

Can You Take Too Much?

Too much potassium throws off the fluid and electrical balance in the cells and can lead to such serious problems as irregular or rapid heartbeat, a drop in blood pressure, and paralysis of the arms and legs. Convulsions, coma, and even cardiac arrest can follow a severe overdose. Never take more potassium than recommended or prescribed; and call your doctor if you become confused or extremely fatigued, develop nausea or diarrhea, or notice a heaviness in your legs or a numbness and tingling in your hands and feet. Seek emergency medical treatment if your stool is either bloody or black and tarry, if you are having trouble breathing, or if your heartbeat seems to be irregular.

Recommended Daily Allowances

The amount of salt you use affects your potassium requirements; and there is no standard recommended dietary allowance (RDA) for this mineral. Nutritional experts currently advise cutting back on the amount of table salt you use and increasing the amount of potassium-rich foods you eat. Many experts peg the minimum daily requirement at roughly 2,000 to 2,500 milligrams. Since a normal diet supplies from 2,000 to 6,000 milligrams daily, supplements aren't necessary unless you are taking medications that deplete the body's potassium supply.

Best Dietary Sources

Potassium is found in fruits, including avocados, bananas, citrus fruits, raisins, and dried peaches; grapefruit, tomato, and orange juice; vegetables, including fresh spinach, parsnips, and potatoes; nuts, including almonds, Brazil nuts, cashews, peanuts, pecans, and walnuts; milk; molasses; dried lentils; canned sardines; and whole-grain cereals.

One cup of cooked spinach contains 1,160 milligrams of potassium. One-half cup of raisins or one-half of a medium avocado provides 650 milligrams. One cooked potato or 1 cup of orange juice contains 500 milligrams.

Pyridoxal Phosphate

See Vitamin B$_6$

Pyridoxine

See Vitamin B$_6$

Retinol

See Vitamin A

Riboflavin

What It Is

Riboflavin, also called vitamin B$_2$, is a water-soluble vitamin commonly found in dairy products. It is also produced synthetically.

What It Does

Riboflavin plays an important role in the body's production of energy. It helps tissues breathe and get rid of waste. It also helps activate vitamin B$_6$.

Why You Need It

Riboflavin helps the body grow and develop. It keeps the mucous membranes healthy and protects the nervous system, skin, and eyes. Riboflavin is also useful in the treatment of various medical conditions, including infections, stomach and liver disorders, burns, and alcoholism. Researchers also believe that riboflavin helps the body absorb iron more efficiently. It is not uncommon for iron and riboflavin deficiencies to occur simultaneously.

Can You Take Too Much?

Riboflavin appears to be harmless no matter how high the dose. However, too much riboflavin may darken the color of your urine.

Recommended Daily Allowances

ADULTS

Males 11 to 14 years:	1.6 milligrams
Males 15 to 22 years:	1.7 milligrams
Males 23 to 50 years:	1.6 milligrams
Males 51 and older:	1.4 milligrams
Females 11 to 22 years:	1.3 milligrams
Females 23 and older:	1.2 milligrams

Women require an additional 0.3 milligram of riboflavin each day during pregnancy. Breastfeeding mothers need an extra 0.5 milligram of riboflavin per day.

People who exercise a lot—especially women—probably need extra riboflavin as well.

CHILDREN

Infants up to 6 months:	0.4 milligrams
Ages 6 to 12 months:	0.6 milligrams
Ages 1 to 3 years:	0.8 milligrams
Ages 4 to 6 years:	1.0 milligrams
Ages 7 to 10 years:	1.4 milligrams

Best Dietary Sources

The body is not able to store riboflavin, so this vitamin must constantly be replenished to prevent a deficiency.

Milk is probably the single best source of riboflavin. One quart of milk contains 1.7 milligrams of riboflavin—enough riboflavin for almost any adult or child. Other good sources of riboflavin include cheese, yogurt, chicken, organ meats, leafy green vegetables, cereal, bread, wheat germ, brewer's yeast, and almonds.

Salt

See Sodium

Selenium

What It Is

Selenium is one of the minerals required by the body in only trace amounts. It is a potent antioxidant. Supplements are available in several formulations.

What It Does
Working with vitamin E, selenium helps fend off the damage that oxidation can cause to the cells.

Why You Need It
Because selenium maintains tissue elasticity by preventing excessive cell damage, a deficiency can cause premature aging. A lack of selenium can also lead to male infertility.

Can You Take Too Much?
Sustained dosages greater than 700 to 1,100 micrograms are not recommended. Toxic levels of selenium can lead to loss of hair, teeth, and nails, a decline in energy, and even paralysis.

Recommended Daily Allowances
The government has not yet established a recommended dietary allowance (RDA) for selenium. The estimated safe and adequate daily intake is as follows:

ADULTS

All adults: 50 to 200 micrograms

Women should not take megadoses of selenium during pregnancy or while breastfeeding.

CHILDREN

Infants up to 6
    months: 10 to 40 micrograms
Ages 6 to 12
    months: 20 to 60 micrograms

Ages 1 to 3
    years: 20 to 80 micrograms
Ages 4 to 6
    years: 30 to 120 micrograms
Ages 7 and
    older: 50 to 200 micrograms

Best Dietary Sources
The amount of selenium in the following foods varies according to the amount in the soil in which they grew. Selenium is found in: vegetables, including broccoli, cabbage, celery, cucumbers, garlic, mushrooms, and onions; kidney, liver, and chicken; whole-grain products, bran, and wheat germ; egg yolks; tuna and seafood; and milk.

Sodium

What It Is
Sodium pervades our food supply. As sodium chloride it is known as salt.

What It Does
Sodium maintains the balance of water inside and outside of the body's cells. Together with potassium, it also regulates the body's acid balance and plays a role in governing the electrical charge in the nerves and muscles.

Why You Need It
Sodium prevents dehydration and is essential for proper functioning of nerves and muscles. Deficiencies are almost unheard of, but could result in digestive problems, weight loss, and arthritis.

Can You Take Too Much?

Excessive sodium levels can cause body tissue to retain water and swell. Extremely high levels of sodium can lead to dizziness, stupor, and even a coma.

For people with high blood pressure, the extra water retention caused by sodium can make the pressure worse. Blood pressure patients are therefore advised to keep their salt intake below average.

Recommended Daily Allowances

With other vitamins and minerals, the concern is a possible deficiency. With sodium, the problem is excess. The typical American diet contains as much as 12 grams of sodium per day, while we only need about 3. There is no official recommended dietary allowance (RDA) for sodium. Estimates of the minimum requirements are as follows:

ADULTS

All adults:	1.1 to 3.3 grams

According to current guidelines, healthy women need not restrict the amount of sodium in their diets during pregnancy or while breastfeeding.

CHILDREN

Infants up to 6 months:	0.11 to 0.35 gram
Ages 6 to 12 months:	0.25 to 0.75 gram
Ages 1 to 3 years:	0.32 to 1 gram
Ages 4 to 6 years:	0.45 to 1.35 grams
Ages 7 to 10 years:	0.6 to 1.8 grams
Ages 11 to 17 years:	0.9 to 2.3 grams

Best Dietary Sources

Table salt is the primary source. Other foods containing sodium include: bacon, dried and fresh beef, ham, and other meats; milk, butter, and margarine; clams and canned sardines; bread; green beans; and canned tomatoes.

Manufacturers typically add salt to improve the taste of canned vegetables and processed foods. Bouillon, soups, pickles, potato chips, and many "snack" foods are especially high in salt.

One teaspoon of salt contains 2 grams of sodium. One cup of cottage cheese provides slightly more than 0.5 gram. One cup of canned corn, 1 cup of canned tomato juice, or 1 slice of pizza (one-sixth of a 12-inch pie) each provide about 0.5 gram of sodium.

Sodium Fluoride

See Fluoride

Sulfur

What It Is

Sulfur is a component of several amino acids found naturally in protein. Our requirements are met fully through our normal diet. The only people at risk of a deficiency are strict vegetarians.

What It Does
Sulfur is one of the raw materials used by the liver to manufacture the bile required by the digestive system. It is also a component of the keratin in skin, nails, and hair.

Why You Need It
Sulfur maintains a good complexion and glossy hair.

Can You Take Too Much?
Sulfur is unlikely to cause any problems, even if your body has more than it needs.

Recommended Daily Allowances
There is no recommended dietary allowance (RDA) for sulfur and no reports of deficiency.

Best Dietary Sources
Eggs are the richest source of sulfur. It is also available in meat, fish, dried beans, cabbage, milk, and wheat germ.

Taurine

See Nonessential Amino Acids

Tetrahydrofolic Acid

See Folic Acid

Thiamin

What It Is
Thiamin, one of the water-soluble vitamins, is also called vitamin B_1. Thiamin is widely available in foods and is also produced synthetically. An injectable form is available by prescription.

A well-balanced diet should generally provide enough thiamin for healthy people. However, more adults are deficient in thiamin than in almost any other vitamin. One of the reasons this deficiency has become so common is the high rate of alcoholism. Alcohol impairs the absorption of many nutrients and is especially detrimental to the body's ability to process thiamin.

Very young children and elderly people who do not eat a well-balanced diet are also in danger of developing a serious thiamin deficiency. Although rare, an uncorrected thiamin deficiency can lead to symptoms of beriberi, a disorder that affects the nervous system and may involve the heart and circulatory systems.

What It Does
Thiamin plays an important role in converting blood sugar (glucose) into the energy needed to fuel the body. It also helps release energy from fat, and together with adenosine triphosphate, it forms a compound needed to convert carbohydrates into energy.

Why You Need It
Thiamin is important for normal growth and development. It keeps the mucous membranes healthy; and helps keep the nervous system, heart, and muscles working properly. Physicians prescribe thiamin supplements to treat beriberi. Thiamin supplements are

also important for alcoholics. The mental confusion, vision disturbances, and staggering gait typically associated with alcoholism are also symptoms of beriberi.

Can You Take Too Much?

Oral overdoses are extremely rare. People who take several hundred milligrams of thiamin daily—literally hundreds of times the recommended daily amount—may become drowsy. Large injections of thiamin occasionally cause an allergic reaction similar to anaphylactic shock.

Recommended Daily Allowances

ADULTS

Males 11 to 18:	1.4 milligrams
Males 19 to 50:	1.5 milligrams
Males 51 and older:	1.2 milligrams
Females 11 to 22:	1.1 milligrams
Females 23 and older:	1.0 milligrams

Women require an additional 0.4 milligram of thiamin each day during pregnancy. Breastfeeding mothers need an extra 0.5 milligram of thiamin per day.

CHILDREN

Infants up to 6 months:	0.3 milligrams
Ages 6 to 12 months:	0.5 milligrams
Ages 1 to 3 years:	0.7 milligrams
Ages 4 to 6 years:	0.9 milligrams
Ages 7 to 10 years:	1.2 milligrams

Best Dietary Sources

The body is not able to store thiamin very well, so it is important to constantly replenish your thiamin supply. The best sources are whole-grain cereals, rye and whole-wheat flour, wheat germ, rice bran, dried sunflower seeds, soybeans, navy and kidney beans, meat, pork, and salmon steak.

A tablespoonful of brewer's yeast provides 1.2 milligrams of thiamin; one cup of cooked kidney beans contains 0.51 milligrams; two slices of whole wheat bread have 0.15 milligrams.

Threonine

What It Is

Threonine is one of the amino acids considered "essential" because they cannot be manufactured in the body and must be obtained through diet.

What It Does

The body must have supplies of all the amino acids, including threonine, on hand in order to manufacture human proteins. These proteins are a vital component of all the body's cells and its many hormones and enzymes.

Why You Need It

The body requires a continuing supply of fresh proteins to support normal functions and maintain the tissues in good repair. Without the amino acids, production of these proteins would slow to a halt.

Can You Take Too Much?

Amino acids are rarely toxic, even in large amounts.

Recommended Daily Allowances

There is no official recommended allowance for threonine. The estimated adult daily requirement is approximately 3.5 milligrams per pound of body weight. Infants require 8 times that amount; children need about 3 times the adult requirement.

Best Dietary Sources

A complete set of all the amino acids is available in most meat and dairy products.

Tribasic Calcium Phosphate

See Calcium

Tryptophan

What It Is

Tryptophan is one of the amino acids considered "essential" because they cannot be manufactured in the body and must be obtained through diet. Natural and synthetic tryptophan supplements are also available, despite a recent incident in which contaminated supplements caused illness.

What It Does

Tryptophan is the raw material for serotonin, one of the chemicals that regulate the transmission of nerve impulses in the brain.

Why You Need It

The serotonin manufactured from tryptophan is one of the major chemicals governing mood and behavior. The well-known antidepressant drug Prozac, for instance, works by boosting serotonin levels in the brain. Serotonin also has a calming effect; and a lack of serotonin may spark a headache.

Can You Take Too Much?

When correctly manufactured, tryptophan supplements pose no danger.

Recommended Daily Allowances

There is no official recommended dietary allowance for tryptophan. The estimated adult daily requirement is less than 1.5 milligrams per pound of body weight. Infants require 7 times that amount; children need less than 2 milligrams per pound.

Best Dietary Sources

Tryptophan is particularly plentiful in bananas, dried dates, milk, cottage cheese, meat, fish, turkey, and peanuts.

Tyrosine

See Nonessential Amino Acids

Valine

See Branched-Chain Amino Acids

Vanadium

What It Is

Vanadium, one of the minerals needed in only trace amounts, can be obtained from fish, meat, whole grain, oils, and vitamin supplements.

What It Does

We do not yet know exactly how vanadium works in the body, but we do know that it's present in most body tissues.

Why You Need It

Vanadium is needed for proper development of bones, cartilage, and teeth.

Can You Take Too Much?

Megadoses can lead to anemia, eye irritation, and respiratory problems.

Recommended Daily Allowances

The government has not yet established a recommended dietary allowance (RDA) for vanadium. Adults probably need 100 to 300 micrograms of vanadium per day. Most people get more than 10 times that amount in their daily diet.

Best Dietary Sources

Vanadium is found in meat, seafood, grains, and vegetable oil.

Vitamin A

What It Is

Vitamin A, also known as retinol, is one of the fat-soluble vitamins that can be stored by the body. There are two ways of getting this vitamin from your diet: either as vitamin A itself (especially plentiful in liver) or as beta-carotene, a plant-based substance that the body can convert into vitamin A. Megadoses of vitamin A itself can be toxic. Megadoses of beta-carotene are not, since the body converts only as much as needed into vitamin A.

What It Does

Vitamin A helps regulate cell development, promotes bone growth and tooth development, and boosts the body's immune system and resistance to respiratory infections. By helping to form rhodopsin, a substance the eyes need to function in partial darkness, vitamin A enables us to see better at dusk and during the night.

Why You Need It

Vitamin A is essential for good vision, especially night vision. It helps keep the skin, hair, and mucous membranes healthy. It also promotes reproduction by helping testicles and ovaries to function properly and aiding in the development of the embryo.

Can You Take Too Much?

A large overdose of vitamin A—500,000 IU or more—can cause headache, vomiting, bone pain, weakness, blurred vision, irritability, and flaking of the skin. Long-term intake of 100,000 IU or more per day can also lead to toxicity. Symptoms include hair loss, headache, bone thickening, an enlarged liver and spleen, anemia, menstrual problems, stiffness, joint pain, weakness, and dry skin. High doses of beta-carotene, on the other hand, have no toxic effects.

Authorities recommend that pregnant women take no more than 5,000 IU of vitamin A per day. The same is true for women taking birth control pills, which tend to increase the amount of retinol in the blood. Regular doses of 25,000 to 50,000 IU or more per day may cause birth defects.

Recommended Daily Allowances

The recommended dietary allowance (RDA) for vitamin A is expressed in International Units (IU). One IU contains approximately 5 micrograms of retinol or 30 micrograms of beta-carotene.

ADULTS

Males 11 years and older:	5,000 IU
Females 11 years and older:	4,000 IU

Women need an additional 1,000 IU each day during pregnancy. Breastfeeding mothers need an extra 2,000 IU per day.

It is important to note that a daily intake of 5,000 IU may not be enough for many people. For example, people who smoke,

eat a lot of junk food, or have diabetes or an infection may need more.

CHILDREN

Infants up to 12 months:	1,875 IU
Ages 1 to 3 years:	2,000 IU
Ages 4 to 6 years:	2,500 IU
Ages 7 to 10 years:	3,300 IU

Best Dietary Sources

The average person has up to a two-year supply of vitamin A stored in the liver. However, you need to constantly replenish this supply to prevent a deficiency—and thus night blindness—from developing.

Beta-carotene, the vitamin A precursor, is available in many fruits and vegetables. Good sources include carrots, sweet potatoes, broccoli, spinach, tomatoes, lettuce, winter squash, apricots, cantaloupe, and watermelon.

One sweet potato provides almost 10,000 IU. A single carrot contains almost 5,000 IU, a cup of cooked carrots provides 15,000 IU. Liver is an excellent source of vitamin A itself. One-half pound of calves' liver provides almost 75,000 IU.

Vitamin B₁

See Thiamin

Vitamin B₂

See Riboflavin

Vitamin B₃

See Niacin

Vitamin B₅

See Pantothenic Acid

Vitamin B₆

What It Is

Vitamin B₆, also known as pyridoxine and pyridoxal phosphate is one of the water-soluble vitamins that the body can't store. You need a continued daily supply from food or supplements. A synthetic form is available.

What It Does

Vitamin B₆ helps the body process the protein, fat, and carbohydrates in our diet. It works with other vitamins and minerals to supply the energy used in our muscles, and plays a role in cell growth, including the body's production of red blood cells and cells of the immune system.

Why You Need It

Vitamin B₆ plays a crucial role in maintaining the body's immune system. It helps the brain work properly and assists in maintaining the proper chemical balance in the body's fluids. It also helps the body resist stress. Physicians prescribe this vitamin to treat certain types of anemia and to counteract poisoning from the prescription drugs cycloserine and isoniazid.

Can You Take Too Much?

There is currently little evidence that more than 50 milligrams of vitamin B₆ per day will do the body any extra good. However, a total daily intake of more than 500 milligrams can lead to serious nerve damage. Clumsiness and numbness in the hands and feet are signs that you may be getting too much vitamin B₆. To be on the safe side, experts recommend that you avoid taking supplements of more than 200 milligrams per day.

Recommended Daily Allowances

ADULTS

Males 11 years and older:	2.2 milligrams
Females 11 years and older:	2.0 milligrams

Women need an additional 0.6 milligram of vitamin B₆ each day during pregnancy. Breastfeeding mothers need an extra 0.5 milligram per day.

CHILDREN

Infants up to 6 months:	0.3 milligrams
Ages 6 to 12 months:	0.6 milligrams
Ages 1 to 3 years:	0.9 milligrams
Ages 4 to 6 years:	1.3 milligrams
Ages 7 to 10 years:	1.8 milligrams

Best Dietary Sources

Vitamin B₆ is available in meats; fish, including salmon, shrimp, and tuna; whole grains, including bran, whole-wheat flour, wheat germ, and rice; bananas; vegetables, including avocados and carrots; and brewer's yeast, hazelnuts, lentils, soybeans, and sunflower seeds.

One-half cup of soybeans provides 0.85 milligram of vitamin B$_6$; a medium banana has 0.61 milligram; one-half of a medium avocado has 0.46 milligram; and one-quarter cup of wheat germ provides 0.3 milligram.

Vitamin B$_9$

See Folic Acid

Vitamin B$_{12}$

What It Is

Vitamin B$_{12}$, a water-soluble vitamin, is also called cobalamin and cyanocobalamin. It is found in meat, fish, dairy products, and eggs—but cannot be obtained from plant-based foods. People who follow a strict vegetarian or macrobiotic diet are at serious risk of developing a vitamin B$_{12}$ deficiency. This is of particular concern for children. A synthetic form of vitamin B$_{12}$ is available, but a prescription is necessary if your physician decides you need high doses or must take it by injection.

What It Does

Vitamin B$_{12}$ helps the body process and burn fats and carbohydrates. It also helps the nervous system work properly and aids in growth and cell development—especially blood cells. It is also necessary for production of the protective sheath that covers nerve cells, and helps the body process DNA.

Why You Need It

Vitamin B$_{12}$ is essential to the body's growth and development. This vitamin is also useful in the treatment of some types of nerve damage and pernicious anemia. Supplements can help prevent a deficiency in strict vegetarians. Vitamin B$_{12}$ supplementation is particularly important to assure normal growth and development in children who follow a vegetarian diet.

Can You Take Too Much?

Very few problems have been reported with vitamin B$_{12}$—even when people take as much as 1,000 milligrams per day. However, if you take vitamin B$_{12}$ along with large amounts of vitamin C, you may develop a nosebleed, bleeding from the ears, or a dry mouth.

Recommended Daily Allowances

ADULTS

The RDA for everyone 11 years and older is 3 micrograms. Women need an extra 1 microgram of vitamin B$_{12}$ each day during pregnancy and while they are breastfeeding an infant.

CHILDREN

Infants up to
6 months: 0.5 micrograms

Ages 6 to	
12 months:	1.5 micrograms
Ages 1 to	
3 years:	2 micrograms
Ages 4 to	
6 years:	2.5 micrograms
Ages 7 to	
10 years:	3 micrograms

Best Dietary Sources

The best sources of vitamin B$_{12}$ are fish, including clams, flounder, herring, mackerel, sardines, and snapper; dairy foods, including milk and milk products, blue cheese, and swiss cheese; organ meats, especially kidney and liver; other meats, such as beef, pork, and liverwurst; and eggs.

One-half cup of cottage cheese, packed, provides 1 microgram of vitamin B$_{12}$. One cup of whole or skim milk or one large egg contains 1 microgram. One ounce of cheddar, brick, or mozzarella cheese has 0.28 microgram.

Vitamin C

What It Is

Vitamin C, one of the water-soluble vitamins, is also called ascorbic acid.

Some nutritionists have extolled vitamin C as a "cure" for the common cold. While there is no proof for this claim, some studies have indicated that vitamin C can help prevent colds from developing and also ease the symptoms if you do get one.

Researchers may not be convinced, but a great many people believe in vitamin C—it is esti-mated that more than half of all adults take vitamin C supplements. Taking large doses once a day could, however, be a waste of money, since the body tends to get rid of supplemental vitamin C very quickly. Taking smaller doses several times a day could prove to be more effective.

What It Does

Vitamin C plays an essential role in the manufacture of collagen, a substance in connective tissue that essentially holds the bones together. Vitamin C also helps repair damaged tissue and has antioxidant properties.

Why You Need It

Vitamin C may or may not cure the common cold, but it is definitely valuable in many other ways. This vitamin helps the body absorb more iron and is, therefore, useful in the treatment of iron-deficiency and other types of anemia. Vitamin C plays a role in the production of hemoglobin and red blood cells, works to keep the gums and teeth healthy, helps heal broken bones and wounds, and is one of the substances physicians choose to treat urinary tract infections.

Vitamin C continues to be used to treat the deficiency disease scurvy. Although scurvy was much more common in the 19th century, it has not disappeared. Symptoms include muscle weakness or wasting, bleeding or swollen gums, loss of teeth, rough skin, delayed wound healing, fatigue, and depression.

Can You Take Too Much?

The body rids itself of extra vitamin C very quickly. Daily doses of as much as 5,000 to 10,000 milligrams taken for several years have failed to produce any serious side effects. However, if too much vitamin C accumulates in the body, facial flushing, headaches, stomach cramps, nausea, or vomiting are possibilities. At a dose of more than 1,000 milligrams per day, you may also notice that you have to urinate more frequently or start having mild diarrhea. Dizziness and faintness may occur following a vitamin C injection.

Recommended Daily Allowances

ADULTS

The RDA for everyone 15 years of age and older is 60 milligrams.

Women need an additional 20 milligrams of vitamin C each day during pregnancy—a developing baby needs the vitamin to support the growth and formation of its bones, teeth, and connective tissue. Breastfeeding mothers need an extra 40 milligrams of vitamin C per day to pass on to their rapidly growing babies. If you are pregnant or breastfeeding, your physician will determine the exact amount of vitamin C that you need to take.

People over the age of 55 and smokers may also need a vitamin C supplement.

CHILDREN

Infants up to 12 months:	35 milligrams
Ages 1 to 10 years:	45 milligrams
Ages 11 to 14 years:	50 milligrams

Best Dietary Sources

Most people know that oranges and orange juice contain vitamin C, but the vitamin is also available in many other fruits, and even in vegetables. Sources of vitamin C include broccoli, brussels sprouts, cabbage, grapefruit, green peppers, lemons, potatoes, spinach, strawberries, sweet and hot peppers, tangerines, and tomatoes.

One cup of orange juice provides 120 milligrams of vitamin C; a medium orange contains 66 milligrams. One stalk of raw broccoli has 160 milligrams of vitamin C; a medium green pepper, raw, provides 70 milligrams.

Vitamin D

What It Is

There are two forms of vitamin D: ergocalciferol, which is found in a relatively small selection of foods; and cholecalciferol, which the body manufactures when exposed to the sun. Vitamin D is fat-soluble, can build up inside the body, and therefore is highly toxic when taken in large doses for a long time. Milk fortified with vitamin D is our major dietary source.

What It Does

Vitamin D helps to control the formation of bone tissue. It

increases the amount of calcium and phosphorus the body absorbs from the small intestine and thus helps regulate the growth, hardening, and repair of the bones.

Why You Need It

Vitamin D is essential for the normal growth and development of the teeth, bones, and cartilage in children. It's also needed to keep adult teeth and bones in good repair. Vitamin D prevents rickets, a deficiency disease characterized by malformations of bones and teeth in children and by brittle, easily broken bones in adults.

Can You Take Too Much?

For adults, doses of 50,000 IU per day can prove toxic; and doses of 25,000 IU daily are risky. For a small child, as little as 1,800 IU per day can cause harm. Longterm overdose of vitamin D can cause *irreversible* damage to the kidneys and cardiovascular system, and can retard growth in children. Excessive amounts of the vitamin may lead to high blood pressure and premature hardening of the arteries. Nausea, abdominal pain, loss of appetite, weight loss, seizures, and an irregular heartbeat may be signs that you are taking too much. If you have any concerns, stop taking the vitamin right away and consult your physician.

Vitamin D produced by sunlight is not a concern. Overexposure to the sun does not cause vitamin D toxicity among healthy people.

Recommended Daily Allowances

ADULTS

Ages 19 to 22 years:	600 IU
Ages 23 years and older:	400 IU

Women need an extra 400 IU each day during pregnancy and while they are breastfeeding an infant. The additional vitamin D is important for the baby's normal growth. Do not increase dosage beyond this point, however. Too much vitamin D during pregnancy may cause abnormalities.

People over the age of 55 may also need to take a vitamin D supplement—especially women who have completed menopause.

The increasing use of sunscreens protects against the harmful ultraviolet rays that cause skin cancer; unfortunately, this sensible practice also limits the body's production of vitamin D. If you live in an area that does not typically have a lot of sunshine, you may want to check with your doctor about the possible need for extra vitamin D. This is especially important for children, whose bones and teeth need vitamin D to grow properly.

CHILDREN

Through age 18:	800 IU

Best Dietary Sources

Sunlight is the best source of vitamin D, but you can also boost your body's supply by drinking fortified milk. Other sources include herring, mackerel, salmon, sardines, and cod- and halibut-liver oils.

Vitamin E

What It Is

Vitamin E, also known as alpha-tocopherol, is a leading antioxidant. Although it is one of the fat-soluble vitamins that can build up in the body, it has proven safe in much larger than standard doses. A synthetic form of vitamin E is available, and your doctor can also prescribe vitamin E injections.

What It Does

Vitamin E protects the fats found in cell membranes throughout the body from oxidation, or spoilage. Because of this ability to inhibit the natural cell destruction that occurs with age, vitamin E is being tested as a treatment for many of the chronic diseases of the elderly.

Why You Need It

In addition to preventing the oxidation of cells and tissue, vitamin E helps to prevent blood clots, thereby reducing the risk of heart disease. It may also discourage development of some types of cancer; and it is needed for production of normal red blood cells. It helps children grow and develop normally and is used to treat vitamin E deficiency in premature or low-birthweight babies.

Can You Take Too Much?

Even at doses of 1,500 IU per day (50 times the RDA), vitamin E

has no harmful effects. However, at doses of 2,400 IU per day, it may cause bleeding problems due to its clot-preventing ability. Too much vitamin E may also reduce your body's supply of vitamin A, alter the immune system, and impair sexual function.

Because they can impede formation of blood clots, vitamin E supplements should be avoided for 2 weeks before and after surgery. You should also forego large doses when taking anticoagulant medications.

Recommended Daily Allowances

ADULTS

Males 18 or older:	30 IU
Females 18 or older:	24 IU

Women need an additional 6 IU each day during pregnancy. Breast-feeding mothers need an extra 9 IU per day.

People over the age of 55, smokers, and people who abuse alcohol may need to take vitamin E supplements.

CHILDREN

Infants up to 12 months:	9 to 12 IU
Ages 1 to 10 years:	15 to 21 IU
Ages 11 to 18 years:	24 IU

Best Dietary Sources

Vegetable oils, including corn, cottonseed, and peanut oils, are the best source of vitamin E. Almonds, hazelnuts, safflower nuts, sunflower seeds, walnuts, wheat germ, whole-wheat flour, and margarine are also rich in vitamin E. Various fruits and vegetables—spinach, lettuce, onions, blackberries, apples, and pears—also contain this vitamin.

Vitamin H

See Biotin

Vitamin K

What It Is

There are two forms of vitamin K: phylloquinone, which is found in green leafy vegetables; and menaquinone, which is produced within the body by "friendly" bacteria that reside in the intestinal tract. A deficiency may result if antibiotics or an intestinal disease destroys these bacteria.

What It Does

Vitamin K is an essential element in the blood's normal clotting process. It promotes production of the clotting factors, such as prothrombin, that stop us from bleeding.

Why You Need It

Vitamin K helps prevent abnormal bleeding, and is given to newborns as a precaution against hemorrhagic (bleeding) disease. It is also prescribed to correct deficiencies that result in bleeding disorders.

Can You Take Too Much?

Doses as high as 500 times the usual recommendation have failed to cause any ill effect. However, allergic-type reactions have been reported; and the vita-min could interfere with the liver's ability to function, although liver problems are not very common. Infants who receive an excessive amount may suffer brain damage.

Recommended Daily Allowances

The government has not yet established the recommended dietary allowance (RDA) for vitamin K.

ADULTS

The estimated adequate daily intake for everyone 18 years of age and older is 70 to 140 micrograms.

There is currently no information on the safety and effectiveness of vitamin K supplements during pregnancy. If you are pregnant or are breastfeeding, do not take vitamin K without consulting your physician.

CHILDREN

The estimated adequate daily intake of vitamin K for children is as follows:

Infants up
   to 6 months: 12 micrograms
Ages 6 to 12
   months: 10 to 20 micrograms
Ages 1 to
   3 years: 15 to 30 micrograms
Ages 4 to
   6 years: 20 to 40 micrograms
Ages 7 to 10
   years: 30 to 60 micrograms
Ages 11 to 17
   years: 50 to 100 micrograms

Best Dietary Sources

Vitamin K is found in brussels sprouts, cabbage, cauliflower, oats, soybeans, spinach, cheddar cheese, egg yolks, and green tea.

Zinc

What It Is

Zinc is one of the minerals that we require in just trace amounts. It is found in a variety of meat and grain products. Supplements are available as well.

What It Does

Zinc is part of the molecular structure of more than 80 enzymes, and works with the red blood cells to transport waste carbon dioxide from body tissue to the lungs for exhalation. It is essential for the production of the RNA and DNA that governs the division, growth, and repair of the body's cells.

Why You Need It

Zinc is an extremely important mineral: It helps the body grow and develop, and also promotes normal fetal growth. It preserves our sense of taste and smell, helps wounds heal, and keeps the right amount of vitamin A in our blood. It is also a component of the insulin that regulates our energy supply.

Can You Take Too Much?

Doses of more than 40 times the RDA cause few, if any, problems. Nausea, vomiting, and diarrhea may follow sustained overdosage. Other consequences include drowsiness, sluggishness, light-headedness, and restlessness. Difficulty writing or walking can also be warning signs of zinc toxicity.

Recommended Daily Allowances

ADULTS

All adults:	15 milligrams

Women need an additional 5 milligrams of zinc each day during pregnancy. Women who are breastfeeding an infant should take an extra 10 milligrams per day. Since women may not get all the zinc they need from their diet, it is important that they discuss the possibility of supplementation with a physician.

CHILDREN

Infants up to 6 months:	3 milligrams
Ages 6 to 12 months:	5 milligrams
Ages 1 to 10 years:	10 milligrams
Ages 11 and older:	15 milligrams

Best Dietary Sources

Zinc can be obtained from meat, including beef, lamb, and pork; poultry; seafood, including herring and oysters; egg yolk; milk; maple syrup and black-strap molasses; sesame and sunflower seeds; soybeans; whole-grain products; wheat bran; wheat germ; and yeast.

PART FIVE

Treatment Finder

Alternative Therapies Indexed by Illness

This index presents you with the leading alternatives for a host of specific medical problems. Only treatments that have been scientifically verified—or show promise—have been included. Unsubstantiated and disproven treatments do not appear. Some entries are considered the mainstream therapy of choice. In most cases, however, the treatments are used as supplementary measures, or as second-line therapy when orthodox treatments fail to work or are deemed inappropriate.

Shoulder pain
Feldenkrais Method, 134
Hellerwork, 142
Hypnotherapy, 158
Myotherapy, 189
Sinus headache
See Headache, sinus
Skin grafts, non-healing
Oxygen Therapy, 212
Smoke inhalation
Oxygen Therapy, 212
Sneezing
Environmental Medicine,
122
Soft tissue injuries
Hydrotherapy, 148
Sprains and Strains
Magnetic Field Therapy,
177
Myotherapy, 189
Reconstructive Therapy,
225
Stiffness
Alexander Technique, 57
Feldenkrais Method, 134
Qigong, 219
Rolfing, 231

Tai Chi, 237
Yoga, 252
Stress-related disorders
Alexander Technique, 57
Aromatherapy, 65
Aston-Patterning, 70
Guided Imagery, 139
Hellerwork, 142
Massage Therapy, 181
Qigong, 219
Reflexology, 228
Rolfing, 231
Sound Therapy, 233
Yoga, 252
Stroke rehabilitation
*See Rehabilitation,
stroke*
Surgical pain
Hypnotherapy, 158
Swallowing difficulties
Biofeedback, 76
**Temporomandibular joint
disorder**
Biofeedback, 76
Energy Medicine, 116
Feldenkrais Method, 134
Myotherapy, 189

Tendency to infection
Juice Therapy, 164
Naturopathic Medicine, 192
Tension
Aromatherapy, 65
Aston-Patterning, 70
Biofeedback, 76
Guided Imagery, 139
Hypnotherapy, 158
Massage Therapy, 181
Meditation, 185
Qigong, 219
Therapeutic Touch, 242
Trager Integration, 246
Yoga, 252
Tension, muscle
See Muscle tension
Tobacco addiction
See Addiction, tobacco
Tourette syndrome
Biofeedback, 76
Ulcers
Biofeedback, 76
Weight reduction
See Excess weight
Wounds, non-healing
Oxygen Therapy, 212

Natural Medicines
Indexed by Illness

For each ailment shown below, this index lists the remedies most likely to provide significant relief. The majority have been pronounced effective by the German Health Authority's herbal "Commission E." Those which have not been reviewed by the commission are included on the strength of especially promising research. The index does not include unverified uses in folk medicine and homeopathy. For a summary of these uses, please turn to the individual profiles.

Natural Medicines Indexed by Common Name

Use this index to quickly locate the entry on any herb (or other natural medicine). All are profiled alphabetically under their common name in Part Three of this book.

Natural Medicines
Indexed by Latin Name

If you know an herb only by its scientific name, this index will steer you to the appropriate profile. For each Latin title, it supplies the corresponding common name, plus the page number of the profile.

Nutritional Supplements Index

Use this index to locate entries on the vitamins, minerals, and other nutritional elements profiled in Part Four of this book. Substances are listed by both their most common and their alternate names.

The PDR® Family Guide Encyclopedia of Medical Care™

Now the most trusted name in medical publishing—the source physicians and pharmacists turn to—puts expert guidance and information at your fingertips. With a comprehensive alphabetical listing of common and unusual ailments that afflict both children and adults—plus a unique index that matches your signs and symptoms to possible conditions—this is a reassuring home health care reference. Inside you'll find

- Detailed instructions for home care

- Possible causes of ailments

- When to call your doctor for further care

- And much more

Published by The Ballantine Publishing Group.
Available in bookstores everywhere.

The PDR® Family Guide to Over-the-Counter Drugs™

For the first time, the most trusted name in medical publishing, *Physicians' Desk Reference®*, has produced a comprehensive, authoritative, and reliable consumer guide to over-the-counter drugs. Its features include

- The uses, active ingredients, proper dosages, and side effects of each medication

- Handy comparison tables to help you select the best product for each ailment

- Symptoms of vitamin deficiency—and the signs of overdose

- Special cautions for seniors, expectant mothers, and infants

- And much more!

Published by The Ballantine Publishing Group.
Available wherever books are sold.

The PDR® Family Guide to Common Ailments™

The publishers of the *Physicians' Desk Reference®* have created this easy-to-use A-to-Z guide filled with the information you need on one hundred common ailments. *The PDR® Family Guide to Common Ailments* explains the health problems your family is likely to encounter—injuries, aches and pains, chronic disorders, infectious diseases, and the ailments of childhood and old age—and tells you what you should do next. Inside you'll find:

- A comprehensive overview of conventional treatment options

- Advice on herbal remedies, nutritional supplements, and complementary therapies

- Descriptive listings of prescription drugs

- Signs and symptoms that signal an emergency

- And much more!

Published by The Ballantine Publishing Group.
Available wherever books are sold.